TEACHING IN NURSING

TEACHING IN NURSING

A Guide for Faculty

✣

FOURTH EDITION

Diane M. Billings, EdD, RN, FAAN
Chancellor's Professor Emeritus
Indiana University School of Nursing
Indianapolis, Indiana

Judith A. Halstead, PhD, RN, ANEF, FAAN
Professor and Executive Associate Dean for Academic Affairs
Indiana University School of Nursing
Indianapolis, Indiana

ELSEVIER

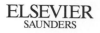

3251 Riverport Lane
St. Louis, Missouri 63043

TEACHING IN NURSING: A GUIDE FOR FACULTY   ISBN: 978-1-4557-0551-1

Notices

Knowledge and best practice in this field are constantly changing. As new research and experience broaden our understanding, changes in research methods, professional practices, or medical treatment may become necessary.

Practitioners and researchers must always rely on their own experience and knowledge in evaluating and using any information, methods, compounds, or experiments described herein. In using such information or methods they should be mindful of their own safety and the safety of others, including parties for whom they have a professional responsibility.

With respect to any drug or pharmaceutical products identified, readers are advised to check the most current information provided (i) on procedures featured or (ii) by the manufacturer of each product to be administered, to verify the recommended dose or formula, the method and duration of administration, and contraindications. It is the responsibility of practitioners, relying on their own experience and knowledge of their patients, to make diagnoses, to determine dosages and the best treatment for each individual patient, and to take all appropriate safety precautions.

To the fullest extent of the law, neither the Publisher nor the authors, contributors, or editors, assume any liability for any injury and/or damage to persons or property as a matter of products liability, negligence or otherwise, or from any use or operation of any methods, products, instructions, or ideas contained in the material herein.

Library of Congress Cataloging-in-Publication Data

Teaching in nursing : a guide for faculty / [edited by] Diane M. Billings, Judith A. Halstead.—4th ed.
   p. ; cm.
Includes bibliographical references and index.
ISBN 978-1-4557-0551-1 (pbk. : alk. paper)
I. Billings, Diane McGovern. II. Halstead, Judith A.
[DNLM: 1. Education, Nursing—methods. 2. Faculty, Nursing. 3. Teaching—methods. WY 18]
LC classification not assigned
610.73076—dc23
                              2011030662

Acquisitions Editor: Robin Carter
Developmental Editor: Angela Perdue
Publishing Services Manager: Jeff Patterson
Project Manager: Megan Isenberg
Design Direction: Karen Pauls

Printed in the United States of America

Last digit is the print number: 9   8   7   6   5   4   3

*To all nurse educators who are engaged in teaching
the future of our profession—our students.*

Contributors

Marsha Howell Adams, DSN, RN, CNE, ANEF
Assistant Dean of Undergraduate Programs
and Professor
Capstone College of Nursing
The University of Alabama
Tuscaloosa, Alabama
Chapter 29

Donna L. Boland, PhD, RN, ANEF
Associate Professor and Associate Dean
for Evaluation
School of Nursing
Indiana University
Indianapolis, Indiana
Chapters 8 and 9

Wanda Bonnel, PhD, RN, ANEF
Associate Professor
School of Nursing
University of Kansas
Kansas City, Kansas
Chapter 27

Mary P. Bourke, PhD, RN, MSN
Assistant Dean of Graduate Programs
School of Nursing
Indiana University
Kokomo, Indiana
Chapter 24

Nancy Burruss, PhD, RN, CNE
Associate Professor and BSN Program Director
School of Nursing
Bellin College
Green Bay, Wisconsin
Chapter 2

Lori Candela, EdD, RN, APRN, BC, CNE
Associate Professor and Chair
Department of Psychosocial Nursing
School of Nursing
University of Nevada, Las Vegas
Las Vegas, Nevada
Chapter 13

Kay E. Hodson-Carlton, EdD, RN, ANEF, FAAN
Professor; Associate Director, School of Nursing;
and Simulation and Information Technology
Center Director
School of Nursing
Ball State University
Muncie, Indiana
Chapter 19

John M. Clochesy, PhD, RN, FCCM, FAAN
Independence Foundation Professor of Nursing
Education
Francis Payne Bolton School of Nursing
Faculty Diversity Officer
Case Western Reserve University
Cleveland, Ohio
Chapter 20

Diann A. DeWitt, PhD, RN, CNE
Professor of Nursing and Director of BSN Program
School of Nursing
Colorado Christian University
Lakewood, Colorado
Chapter 25

Nancy Dillard, DNS, RN
Assistant Professor in Nursing and
Baccalaureate Program Director
School of Nursing
Ball State University
Muncie, Indiana
Chapter 5

Linda M. Finke, PhD, RN
Professor and Senior Director of Interprofessional
Education and Practice
College of Health and Human Services
Purdue University
Fort Wayne, Indiana
Chapters 1 and 8

Natasha Flowers, PhD
Clinical Assistant Professor of Teacher Education
School of Education
Indiana University
Indianapolis, Indiana
Chapter 17

Betsy Frank, PhD, RN, ANEF
Professor Emeritus
College of Nursing, Health, and Human Services
Indiana State University
Terre Haute, Indiana
Chapter 4

Barbara M. Friesth, PhD, RN
Director of Learning Resources and Clinical
Associate Professor
School of Nursing
Indiana University
Indianapolis, Indiana
Chapter 22

Nancy Nightingale Gillespie, PhD, RN
Dean
School of Health Sciences
University of Saint Francis
Fort Wayne, Indiana
Chapter 28

Barbara A. Ihrke, PhD, RN
Dean
School of Nursing
Indiana Wesleyan University
Marion, Indiana
Chapter 24

Pamela R. Jeffries, PhD, ANEF, FAAN
Associate Dean for Academic Affairs
School of Nursing
Johns Hopkins University
Baltimore, Maryland
Chapter 20

Elizabeth G. Johnson, DSN, RN
Assistant Professor and Coordinator of Owensboro
Campus
School of Nursing
University of Louisville
Louisville, Kentucky
Chapter 3

Jane M. Kirkpatrick, PhD, RN
Associate Dean of the College of Health and Human
Sciences and Head of the School of Nursing
Purdue University
West Lafayette, Indiana
Chapter 25

Amy Knepp, NP-C, MSN, RN
Chair and Assistant Professor
Department of Nursing
University of Saint Francis
Fort Wayne, Indiana
Chapter 28

Gail C. Kost, MSN, RN, CNE
Education Specialist
Community Health Network
Indianapolis, Indiana
Chapter 18

Susan Luparell, PhD, CNS-BC, CNE
Associate Professor
College of Nursing
Montana State University
Great Falls, Montana
Chapter 14

Alexander Muehlenkord, MBA
Instructional Technology Manager
Department of Public Health
School of Medicine
Indiana University
Indianapolis, Indiana
Chapter 21

Carla Mueller, PhD, RN
Professor
Department of Nursing
University of Saint Francis
Fort Wayne, Indiana
Chapter 12

Ann Popkess, PhD, RN, CNE
Assistant Professor
School of Nursing
Southern Illinois University Edwardsville
Edwardsville, Illinois
Chapter 2

Connie J. Rowles, DSN, RN
Visiting Clinical Associate Professor
School of Nursing
Indiana University
Indianapolis, Indiana
Chapters 15 and 16

Marcia K. Sauter, PhD, RN
Director of Institutional Effectiveness and
Accreditation
University of Saint Francis
Fort Wayne, Indiana
Chapter 28

Martha Scheckel, PhD, RN
Assistant Professor
College of Nursing and Health Sciences
Winona State University
Winona, Minnesota
Chapter 11

Linda Siktberg, PhD, RN
Director of the School of Nursing and
RN to BS Track Program Director
School of Nursing
Ball State University
Muncie, Indiana
Chapter 5

Lillian Gatlin Stokes, PhD, RN, FAAN
Associate Professor Emeritus
School of Nursing
Indiana University
Indianapolis, Indiana
Chapters 17 and 18

Prudence Twigg, MSN, RN, APRN, BC
Adjunct Lecturer
School of Nursing
Indiana University
Nurse Practitioner
Advanced Healthcare Associates
Indianapolis, Indiana
Chapter 26

Theresa M. "Terry" Valiga, EdD, RN, ANEF, FAAN
Professor and Director, Institute for Educational
Excellence
Nursing Education Specialty Lead Faculty
School of Nursing
Duke University
Durham, North Carolina
Chapter 7

Linda M. Veltri, PhD, RN
Assistant Professor
University of Portland
Portland, Oregon
Chapter 6

Joanne Warner, PhD, RN
Dean and Professor
University of Portland
Portland, Oregon
Chapter 6

Karen M. Whitney, PhD
President
Clarion University
Clarion, Pennsylvania
Chapter 14

Enid Errante Zwirn, PhD, MPH, RN
Associate Professor Emerita
School of Nursing
Indiana University
Indianapolis, Indiana
Chapter 21

Reviewers

Amanda L. Alonzo, PhD, BSN, MS, RN
Assistant Professor
School of Nursing
Oklahoma Wesleyan University
Bartlesville, Oklahoma

Mary Barrow, MSN, RN
Assistant Professor
Charity School of Nursing
Delgado Community College
New Orleans, Louisiana

Phyllis Clayton, EdD, EdS, MSHRD, BSW
Faculty
School of Education
Capella University
Minneapolis, Minnesota

Tina Covington, MN, RN, ACNS-BC, CCRN, CNE
Associate Professor
Charity School of Nursing
Delgado Community College
New Orleans, Louisiana

Michelle De Lima, MSN, RN, APRN, CNE, CNOR
Assistant Professor
Charity School of Nursing
Delgado Community College
New Orleans, Louisiana

Kristina Thomas Dreifuerst, PhD, RN, ACNS-BC, CNE
Assistant Professor
Indiana University School of Nursing
Indianapolis, Indiana

Cris Finn, PhD, RN, FNP
Assistant Professor
School of Nursing
Regis University
Denver, Colorado

Wendy Garretson, BSN, MN, RN, CCRN, CNE
Assistant Professor
Charity School of Nursing
Delgado Community College
New Orleans, Louisiana

Phyllis K. Graham-Dickerson, PhD, RN, CNS
Professor
School of Nursing
Regis University
Denver, Colorado

Joannie S. Hebert, MSN, RN, CNE
Faculty
School of Nursing
Our Lady of the Lake College
New Orleans, Louisiana

Denise G. Hirsch, MSN, RN
Director and Instructor
Nursing Resource Center
Amarillo College
Amarillo, Texas

Edna Hull, PhD, MSN, RN, CNE
Associate Professor and Program Director
School of Nursing
Our Lady of the Lake College
Baton Rouge, Louisiana

Maria E. Lauer, MSN, RN, CNE
Nursing Instructor
School of Nursing and Allied Health Professions
Thomas Edison State College
Trenton, New Jersey

Lisa McConlogue, MSN, PMHCNS-BC
Director
Mental Health Services
Capital Health Regional Medical Center
Trenton, New Jersey

Frances Donovan Monahan, PhD, RN, ANEF
Faculty
Excelsior College
Albany, New York
Adjunct Faculty
University of Arkansas at Little Rock
Little Rock, Arkansas

Diane B. Monsivais, PhD, CRRN
Assistant Professor, Nursing
University of Texas at El Paso School of Nursing
El Paso, Texas

Gina Oliver, PhD, APRN, FNP-BC, CNE
Assistant Teaching Professor
MU Sinclair School of Nursing
Columbia, Missouri

Bridget Parsh, EdD, MSN, RN, CNS
Assistant Professor
Division of Nursing
Sacramento State
Sacramento, California

Patricia S. Smart, MN, RN-BC, CNE
Professor of Nursing
Charity School of Nursing
New Orleans, Louisiana

Rachel E. Spector, PhD, RN, CTN-A, FAAN
Associate Professor, Retired
School of Nursing
Boston College
Chestnut Hill, Massachusetts

Jason T. Spratt, MA, BA
Dean of Students
Indiana University-Purdue University Indianapolis
Indianapolis, Indiana

Brent W. Thompson, PhD, MS, BSN, RN
Associate Professor
Department of Nursing
West Chester University of Pennsylvania
West Chester, Pennsylvania

Kim Uddo, MN, RN, CCRN, CNE, CDE
Professor
Charity School of Nursing
Delgado Community College
New Orleans, Louisiana

Kathleen D. Wagner, EdD, MSN, RN
Lecturer
College of Nursing
University of Kentucky
Lexington, Kentucky

Krista A. White, PhD, RN, CCRN
Instructor
School of Nursing
Lancaster General College of Nursing and Health Sciences
Lancaster, Pennsylvania

Mary E. Wombwell, EdD, RN, CNE
Associate Professor
School of Nursing
Holy Family University
Philadelphia, Pennsylvania

Preface

There has never been a more exciting or challenging time to have a career in nursing education. Health care reform demands new competencies of the graduates from our nursing programs and, in turn, demands new competencies of nurse educators. Landmark reports on nursing and health care have focused attention on the critical role of the nurse educator in preparing competent practitioners with the requisite skills to work in complex health care systems and have challenged us to reconsider what, how, and where we teach our students. These same reports have emphasized the importance of preparing qualified nurse educators who not only possess clinical expertise, but also have been educationally prepared in the art and science of teaching. We need nurse educators who fully understand the many aspects of the role and who are willing to create student-centered learning environments and engage in new and innovative ways of teaching.

We have developed this edition of *Teaching in Nursing* to prepare nurse educators to embrace the role in its entirety and respond to the needs of an increasingly diverse student body as well as recommendations from commissions, studies, and task forces about curriculum changes, and to use the increasing evidence that guides nurse educator practice. For example:

- The scope and standards of the advanced practice role of the nurse educator have been more clearly defined and supported with the development of evidence-based core competencies. Certification as a nurse educator is now a credential that is possible to achieve. The chapter on faculty role reflects this recent emphasis on evidence-based faculty competencies.
- Educators must be prepared to teach in classrooms as students of diverse ages, generations, genders, ethnic backgrounds, races, religions, languages, and learning styles are recruited to and enter nursing programs. Faculty must be able to respond to a variety of student needs, engage in inclusive teaching, choose learning strategies to appeal to a variety of groups and individuals, integrate technology into their teaching, and manage classes with larger numbers of students. To respond to these issues, we have substantively updated chapters on meeting the diverse needs of students, proactively managing the classroom learning environment, and engaging in multicultural education.
- New clinical models, such as the dedicated educational unit and residency programs, are being developed and tested with the goal of more closely aligning nursing education with the realities of the practice setting. At the same time there is a dramatic increase in the use of preceptors and adjunct and part-time faculty to support clinical teaching, all of whom must be oriented and welcomed as they transition to faculty roles. New content in this edition about clinical teaching will assist all educators working with students in clinical settings.
- As nurse educators respond to the need for new types of academic programs, most notably the proliferation of doctorate in nursing practice (DNP) degrees, chapters on curriculum development and program evaluation assume new importance. The faculty must be able to establish dynamic and fluid curriculum structures and processes that can accommodate rapid changes and respond to meet health care delivery needs. To this end we have included updated information on curriculum development and added a chapter on course design. Recognizing the importance of continuous quality improvement and meeting standards for quality established by state boards and national accrediting agencies, we also have added a new chapter on program accreditation.
- There continue to be calls for increasing the numbers of highly educated and well-prepared nurses. In response, faculty are establishing or redesigning mobility and transition programs to facilitate academic progression and must be prepared to develop seamless education systems. This edition of the book includes revised chapters on curriculum design and developing competencies for graduates at all levels of the curriculum continuum.

- The nurse of the future must be able to access, evaluate, and synthesize vast amounts of information, use clinical decision support tools, communicate effectively with patients as a member of an interdisciplinary health care team, and make clinical decisions for safe patient care. Preparing this nurse requires educators to guide students to higher-order learning, the deep and applied learning that prepares students for the complex health care settings in which they will be employed. Chapters on teaching and evaluation strategies as well as an updated chapter on using simulations to promote learning will guide faculty to use active learning approaches.

- Students and faculty are seeking educational experiences that are accessible, engaging, and interactive and educators now find themselves in high-tech campus classrooms with multimedia projection capabilities, using electronic response systems, and integrating smart phone applications into the lesson plan. Educators will find themselves equally teaching online and hybrid courses and using webinars and video conferencing to reach learners worldwide. We have extensively updated the chapters on teaching in the learning resource center, using media and digital media, and teaching at a distance and online to prepare educators to effectively use the now pervasive information technologies and learning resources that create and support these needs.

This edition of *Teaching in Nursing* has been written for nurses who are preparing to teach, for nurses who have recently become faculty members or staff educators and who are searching for answers to the daily challenges presented in their role as educators, as well as for experienced faculty members who are transforming teaching practices for the future. This book is also written for nurses who are combining clinical practice and teaching as preceptors or part-time or adjunct faculty and for graduate students or teaching assistants who aspire to assume a full-time teaching role. Given the current shortage of nurse educators, it is crucial that we continue to prepare and mentor future nursing faculty now. It is our hope that this book can help influence that preparation by providing guidance on the competencies essential to the effective implementation of the educator role.

Since we wrote the first edition of this book, the science of nursing education has evolved and best practices for teaching and learning are beginning to emerge. This edition continues to draw on foundational work while integrating findings from recent research in nursing, education, and related fields. We have attempted to provide a balance of the practical and the theoretical, and urge readers to not only seek new evidence, but also test its application in their classrooms.

We continue to consider this book to be a guide, bringing under one cover an overview of models and approaches for assuming the faculty role; working with students; developing curricula; designing learning experiences; using learning resources; and evaluating students, faculty, courses, and programs. Although the book is organized in five units, teaching in nursing is an integrative process and we encourage readers to select chapters as appropriate for their needs and teaching practice.

We suggest that readers use the book as a guide and resource but recognize that implementation must be adapted to the values and missions of the institutional settings and the personal style and philosophy of the faculty. We intend for this book to stimulate faculty to engage in the scholarship of teaching by reflecting on their own teaching practices, implementing and evaluating new approaches to creating an interactive learning community, and conducting their own educational research in classroom and clinical settings.

We still believe this is an exciting time to teach nursing—a time that is filled with many challenges, opportunities, and rewards for those who step forward to accept the responsibility. It is our hope that this book provides those who engage in the rewarding activity of teaching the future of our profession— our students—with a resource that will lead to greater fulfillment of the teaching role.

Diane M. Billings
Judith A. Halstead
April 2011

Acknowledgments

We thank the contributors to the fourth edition of this book who shared their experience and expertise with us and the readers. We continue to value and build on the work of the original chapter authors, recognize the work of sustaining contributors, and welcome contributors who are new to the book. We also thank those who served as reviewers of the book for their insightful comments, as well as the many nurse educators who have used the book over the past few years. *Teaching in Nursing* is a public and peer-reviewed work and we appreciate the feedback from a variety of readers.

Many thanks, as well, to those who made the production process easier. We especially thank Jenny Parliament for her administrative support—her organizational skills were a tremendous assistance to us in the preparation of the manuscript—and Cindy Hollingsworth, who provided us with significant support in editing the manuscript. We also acknowledge the editorial support at Elsevier: Robin Carter, Angela Perdue, Megan Isenberg, Sandra Clark, and Deanne Dedeke.

As always, we thank our families and colleagues for their continued support and encouragement throughout this project. We also offer special thanks to our students, who continue to be our own guides to teaching in nursing.

Diane M. Billings
Judith A. Halstead

Contents

UNIT V   Evaluation

Teaching in Nursing: The Faculty Role

Linda M. Finke, PhD, RN

As the demands of society have changed, the faculty role in higher education has grown from the singular colonial unitarian mission of teaching to a multifaceted challenge of teaching, scholarship, and service. Over time, as nursing education has moved from the service sector to college and university campuses, the role of nursing faculty has evolved, becoming increasingly complex. As higher education and the science of nursing have developed, the impact on nursing education has been tremendous.

Today higher education and nursing education are poised on the brink of sweeping changes. The forces driving these changes are numerous and difficult to isolate: the increasing multiculturalism of society; decreasing financial resources in education and health care; changes in the delivery of health care through health care reform; the integration of evidence-based practice and the need for more nurses with higher degrees; expanding technology and the accompanying knowledge explosion; the need for lifelong learning; a shifting emphasis to learning, instead of teaching; and the increasing public demand for accountability of educational outcomes. These are just a few of the issues that educators must consider as they fulfill the responsibilities of their role. There has been a call by the federal government and others to build more points of student assessment into postsecondary education to provide the evidence that outcomes are being met in an effort to hold colleges and universities accountable for the learning experiences they provide (Dwyer, Millett, & Payne, 2006).

The need of nurse educators to maintain strong clinical skills while there continues to be a critical shortage of nurses that is projected to last for decades has created an additional hurdle for nurse educators. To meet projected demand for registered nurses, nursing programs must increase their graduation rates, specifically for nurses with higher degrees (U.S. Department of Health and Human Services, 2010). The recent Future of Nursing report released by the Institute of Medicine (2010) issued a call for a nursing workforce in which 80% of the nurses have a bachelor's degree in nursing by 2020 as well as double the number of nurses prepared with a doctorate. At the same time, the Tri-Council for Nursing (2010)—made up of the American Association of Colleges of Nursing, American Nurses Association, American Organization of Nurse Executives, and National League for Nursing—reports a scarcity of prepared nursing faculty. The demand for more nurses with advanced degrees for health care delivery and a scarcity of prepared nursing faculty have placed a tremendous burden on nursing education and the faculty trying to meet the growing needs. Nursing education is entering a crisis with no end in sight, overloaded by the demand to teach more students with fewer faculty members.

As faculty in higher education face these challenges, they need to find new ways to teach and implement their role. Benner, Sutphen, Leonard, and Day (2010) call for "radical transformation" of nursing education. They made 26 recommendations to transform nursing education, calling for a major paradigm shift in nursing education. Nursing faculty of the future need to embrace innovation and be advocates for change and forward movement. This chapter provides a brief historical perspective of the faculty role, identifies faculty rights and responsibilities, and describes the process of faculty appointment, promotion, and tenure within the current context. In addition, faculty development of the competencies related to teaching as a scholarly endeavor is discussed, and implications for change in the faculty role needed to meet current and future expectations and demands are addressed.

Historical Perspective of Faculty Role in Higher Education

The role of the faculty member in academia has developed through time as the role of higher education in America has changed. If one reviews the history of American higher education, three phases of overlapping development can be identified (Boyer, 1990).

The first phase of development occurred during colonial times. Heavily influenced by British tradition, the role of faculty in the colonial college was a singular one: that of teaching. The educational system "was expected to educate and morally uplift the coming generation" (Boyer, 1990, p. 4). Teaching was considered an honored vocation with the intended purpose of developing student character and preparing students for leadership in civic and religious roles. This focus on teaching as the central mission of the university continued well into the nineteenth century.

Gradually, however, the focus of education began to shift from the development of the individual to the development of a nation, signaling the beginning of the second phase of development within higher education. Legislation such as the Morrill Act of 1862 and the Hatch Act of 1887 helped create public expectations that added the responsibility of service to the traditional faculty role of teaching. This legislation provided each state with land and funding to support the education of leaders for agriculture and industry. Universities and colleges took on the mission to educate for the common good (Boyer, 1990). Educational systems were expected to provide service to the states, businesses, and industries. It was in the 1870s that the first formal schools of nursing began to appear in the United States. Nursing programs were established in hospitals to help meet the service needs of the hospitals. Nursing faculty were expected to provide service to the institution and to teach new nurses along the way. Nursing students were expected to learn while they helped staff the hospitals.

In the mid-nineteenth century, a commitment to the development of science began in many universities on the East Coast (Boyer, 1990), thus beginning the third phase of development in higher education. Scholarship through research was added as an expectation to the role of faculty. This emphasis on research was greatly enhanced in later years by federal support for academic research that began during World War II and continued after the war.

Gradually, as expectations for faculty to conduct research spread throughout institutions across the nation, teaching and service began to be viewed with less importance as a measurement tool for academic prestige and productivity within institutions. Faculty found it increasingly difficult to achieve tenure without a record of research and publication, despite accomplishments in teaching and service. As nursing education entered the university setting, nursing faculty began to be held to the same standards of research productivity as faculty in other more traditionally academia-based disciplines. Because of the prominence of practice in nursing, the integration of scholarship into the role of nursing faculty grew slowly initially. The emphasis on research in higher education as evidence of faculty productivity has continued to this day.

Currently a rapidly changing political environment and health care reform are having a dramatic effect on the role of nursing faculty. Universities are facing a "new and sometimes hostile world" (Association of Governing Boards of Universities and Colleges, 1996, p. 2). Diminishing resources and increasing public scrutiny and expectations place a heavy burden on faculty in higher education. Changes in health care will demand that nursing faculty critically evaluate the design of curricula and the competencies of graduates. There is increasing emphasis on the teaching role of faculty with an accompanying expectation that outcomes of the educational process will be regularly assessed at the institutional and program levels. The balance among teaching, research, and service is being reexamined in many institutions for its congruence with the institution's mission.

Further changes in higher education include a revolution in teaching strategies. Sole reliance on the use of lecture is no longer an accepted teaching method. Instead faculty are integrating the use of technology into their teaching and promoting the active involvement of students in the learning process. Computer-mediated courses and the use of simulation are the future of higher education and the norm in nursing as movement is made away from the structured classroom to the much larger learning environments of the home, community, and clinical setting. Distance education strategies play an increasingly important role in the education of learners.

Furthermore, nursing care delivery is changing to a community-based, consumer-driven system. The shift from acute care to the important role of primary care has had an impact on the curricula of undergraduate and graduate nursing education. There also is a continuing gap in the representation of minorities in nursing education programs, with the percentage holding at 10% for decades. There is a need to expand the number of graduates from baccalaureate nursing programs and to increase the numbers of graduates from underrepresented populations. As the minority population continues to grow, all nurses must increase their skills to meet the needs of this underserved population. Application of cultural competency content requires major revision of some nursing curricula (Amen & Pacquiao, 2004; Campinha-Bacote, 2005).

The American Association of Colleges of Nursing (2010) reports that there is a growing need for increased numbers of nurses prepared at the doctoral level, not only to teach but also to collect and analyze data necessary to evaluate the effectiveness of health care and to identify trends of future development. The clinical movement toward advance practice nurses holding the Doctor of Nursing Practice degree creates an overwhelming need for nurses prepared with a doctorate. The majority of nursing programs (61.4%) reported not being able to accept more students because of the need for qualified faculty, with the programs predicting a growing need. All of these issues place nursing faculty at the heart of the nursing shortage.

Faculty Rights and Responsibilities in Academia

In the academic environment, faculty have traditionally enjoyed a number of rights, including the right to self-governance within the university setting. Governance may include participation on department and university committees and "using . . . professional expertise to solve community problems" (Gaff & Lambert, 1996, p. 40). Self-governance includes developing policies for faculty behavior, student affairs, and curriculum; performing administrative activities; and providing advice to administrators or student groups. Serving on committees or task forces at the department, school, or university level is also an expectation of faculty (Tucker, 1992). Faculty, in cooperation with administrators, share in addressing the issues that face the university and the community it serves.

As constituents place more and more expectations on faculty for productivity, faculty governance is not as highly valued by those outside of academia (Plater, 1995). However, the new environment for higher education demands new forms of governance, including representative forms. Methods must be instituted to maintain the participation of faculty in governance while allowing for less of a time commitment. The change that must permeate all other aspects of the role of twenty-first-century faculty must also permeate governance.

The core responsibility of faculty is the teaching and learning that takes place in the institution. Boards and administrators delegate decisions about most aspects of the teaching–learning process to faculty. This responsibility includes not only the delivery of content but also curriculum development and evaluation, development of student evaluation methods, and graduation requirements (Association of Governing Boards of Universities and Colleges, 1996). Faculty also have the responsibility to create the standards for promotion and tenure of faculty. Tenured faculty have the right and responsibility to mentor more junior colleagues and to approve standards or criteria for appointment and promotion of faculty in non-tenure tracks.

Intellectual property, copyright, and fair use laws govern faculty and student use of works developed by faculty, students, and others. The easy online access of course content has added to this complicated issue. Most academic settings have policies that guide the development of "works for hire," which may include course content, written works, and products. Many institutions of higher learning now lay claim to works developed by faculty because the faculty member was hired to develop the content. A wise faculty member is well informed about these institutional policies so that there is no misunderstanding about ownership of course materials and other works developed by the faculty member.

Evaluation is a major responsibility of faculty. Faculty engage in the evaluation of students and of colleagues. Peer evaluation is a vital aspect of faculty development and is part of the documentation data considered in the decision-making process for promotion and tenure. Faculty are involved in the development of fair and equitable evaluation criteria on which to base these judgments. Effective teaching is the gold standard that all faculty must meet. Excellence in research and service is the added value.

Another responsibility of faculty is mentoring. Nursing faculty mentor not only nursing students but also other faculty members in their development as teachers and scholars. The mentoring of students may include not only formal academic advisement but also the coaching, supporting, and guiding of protégés through the academic system and into their professional careers. The mentoring of faculty members also involves coaching, supporting, and guiding as they develop in their role as faculty. When starting at a new institution, even an experienced faculty member has some culture shock and requires mentoring (Lieb, 1995). Lieb (1995) defines mentoring as helping another to reach his or her potential.

The mentoring of new faculty members is an especially important responsibility because nurses are not usually prepared in graduate nursing programs for a role in academia. Faculty are dropped into an environment with unspoken rules and expectations that can be markedly different from those of their previous practice environment. Faculty know the role of the student from experience but see the faculty role from a distance. Mentoring is needed to assist new faculty members as they learn to balance all aspects of their complex role.

The responsibilities of nursing faculty include teaching and scholarship, as well as service to the school, university, community, and the profession of nursing. Nursing faculty have the responsibility to expand their service beyond the university and local community to active participation in professional nursing organizations at local, regional, and national levels. Nursing faculty often provide the leadership for these organizations and set national public policy agendas. As a faculty member climbs the promotion and tenure ladder, service responsibilities increase and leadership at the national level is required.

True success as a faculty member is measured by the person's ability to juggle all aspects of the faculty role. Although some educational settings emphasize teaching, many require that faculty meet established criteria in all aspects of the role—teaching, research, and service. With careful planning and selection of activities, nursing faculty can integrate clinical interests into scholarship, service, and teaching, thus meeting the expectations of the role. On initial appointment to a faculty position, the faculty member will be well served by the development of a 5- to 6-year career plan designed to ensure that he or she will meet the criteria for all aspects of the role.

Some faculty do work in a unionized environment. The American Association of University Professors (AAUP) is probably the best known faculty union. Faculty can also be members of AAUP without belonging to a union. In a setting that has a union, faculty rights and responsibilities can be affected by the negotiated contract.

Faculty Appointment, Promotion, and Tenure

Faculty are appointed by the governing body of the college or university and are responsible, in cooperation with the administration of the institution, for teaching, scholarship, and service (Association of Governing Boards of Universities and Colleges, 1996). Faculty are appointed to fulfill various responsibilities to meet the mission and goals of the college or university and the school of nursing and, according to their degrees and experience, are promoted and tenured on the basis of achievement of specified criteria. Faculty may hold appointments in more than one unit of the institution, including other academic units or service units. Criteria for promotion and tenure are based on the institution's overall mission and thus vary among institutions.

Appointment

Faculty may be appointed to a variety of full-time and part-time positions. Faculty positions are described as *tenured* or *tenure-probationary appointments* or as *non-tenured, nonprobationary instructional appointments* such as adjunct, distinguished, emeritus, and other part-time, temporary, or otherwise designated positions. Appointment in the tenure tracks may lead to tenure and a permanent position at the school of nursing; other positions require reappointment at specific intervals (e.g., yearly or every 3 to 5 years). Reappointment and continued service in tenured positions are based on evaluation of teaching and other faculty activities, such as scholarship and service.

Ranks

Appointment ranks, or tracks, have been developed to specify the responsibilities of the faculty member in relation to teaching, scholarship, and service. The ranks may include tenure, clinical, or research scientist. Each rank has its own criteria for teaching, scholarship, and service and for promotion within the rank.

The *tenure* track is established for faculty whose primary responsibilities are teaching and research. There is expectation of a promise of excellence and the ability to be promoted to senior ranks. A doctoral degree is generally required for appointment to the tenure track at most schools of nursing. Faculty appointed to this rank are considered *tenure probationary* until they have obtained tenure.

The *clinical* track has been developed at some institutions for those faculty members whose primary responsibility is clinical supervision of students and/or clinical practice. The increased use of clinical faculty is a growing trend as the shortage of nurses prepared with a doctorate deepens. The focus of the clinical track is on health care delivery, and it is used to integrate faculty practice into the traditional university faculty structure (Paskiewicz, 2003; Riley, Beal, Levi, & McCausland, 2002). This track may also be developed as an educator track, clinical educator track, or educator/practitioner track, depending on the primary focus of the responsibilities of the faculty appointed into this track. Appointment to this track is based on teaching and clinical skills. A doctoral degree may not be required for appointment to a clinical track. The clinical track usually does not include the protection of tenure, but does facilitate promotion through the ranks of assistant, associate, and professor based on leveled criteria.

The *research scientist* track is for faculty whose primary responsibilities are generating new knowledge and disseminating the findings. Although research scientists may have responsibilities for working with students, serving on dissertation committees, teaching in the area of their expertise, or providing service to the school, campus, or profession, their time is protected for research. Appointment is based on evidence of or promise of a program of research. A doctoral degree and at least beginning research experience are prerequisites for appointment to this track.

Within these ranks, faculty are appointed at the levels of instructor (rarely used), assistant professor, associate professor, and professor. Each school of nursing defines the criteria for appointment and promotion to these levels. These criteria specify the responsibilities associated with teaching, scholarship and service, or other frameworks used to define the faculty role.

Schools of nursing may also develop temporary and other positions to which faculty can be appointed. *Visiting* positions may be held at any rank and designate someone who has a limited appointment (1 or 2 years), who is on leave from another institution, who is employed on a temporary basis, or who may be under consideration for a permanent position within the school. The *lecturer* position is used for faculty who lack necessary credentials (usually degrees) for appointment to a tenure track position. *Adjunct* faculty are courtesy appointments for individuals whose primary employment is outside the school of nursing but who have responsibility for teaching students or working with students on research projects.

Emeritus is a title that may be conferred on faculty who are retired. Faculty with emeritus status may be granted specific privileges, such as use of the library, use of computing services, and an office and secretarial support.

Students may also be employed in teaching positions. These appointments, such as *teaching assistant* and *associate instructor*, are temporary and usually part-time. These students are responsible only for teaching or assisting faculty with teaching. They do not have the same level of responsibility as full-time faculty. Teaching assistants must be assigned to work with a faculty member who will assume responsibility for the quality of their work.

The Appointment Process

The appointment process in universities and schools of nursing is somewhat different from that for positions in nursing service, and nurses who are applying for teaching positions in schools of nursing should be cognizant of this. The interview is conducted by a search and screen committee appointed by the dean or other university administrator. Interested applicants submit an application and curriculum vitae that are screened by this committee. Potential candidates are invited for an interview with the search committee, faculty and administrators at the school of nursing, and others at the college or university as appropriate. Depending on the requirements of the position for which they are applying, applicants may be asked to make a presentation of their research or to demonstrate teaching skills. At the time of appointment to rank, the applicant's records are reviewed by the appointment, promotion, and tenure committee, or other appropriate committee, for recommendation to the dean about appointment.

Tenure and Promotion

Tenure

Tenure to the university is a reciprocal responsibility on the part of the university and faculty. The expectation is that the faculty member will remain competent and productive and maintain high standards of teaching, research, service, and professional conduct. Tenure also assumes that the faculty member is promotable, and typically promotion to the next level and tenure occur at the same time. Tenure, then, provides the faculty member protection of academic freedom. Academic freedom is the "freedom . . . to explore new ideas and theories unimpeded" (Whicker Kronenfield, & Strickland, 1993, p. 14). Academic freedom guarantees the protection of faculty against efforts by government, university administration, students, and even public opinion to influence their expression of opinions in class. On the other hand, academic freedom does not give faculty unbounded rights; for example, a faculty member does not have the right to alter the curriculum, sequence, or content of established courses or to subject students to discussions that are irrelevant to the course. Tenure can be withdrawn for reasons of financial exigency on the part of the school or university and for behavior that is unprofessional. Finally tenure does not mean not having to participate in performance review, and most institutions and their schools of nursing have instituted a posttenure review process (Suess, 1995).

Tenure is granted after a review by peers and administrators using published criteria of the evidence submitted by the faculty member (a curriculum vitae and dossier). This review is typically held in the faculty member's sixth year, with tenure granted in the seventh year. At appointment, faculty with a record of exceptional achievement may be granted a specific number of years toward tenure, thus shortening the time for the tenure review.

The tenure process is specific to each school of nursing, and faculty who are appointed to a tenure track should familiarize themselves with the criteria and process before appointment. Although the tenure and promotion process may seem mysterious, there are in fact clear and specified criteria. The current attitude is to employ faculty who show high promise for attaining tenure and being promoted and to provide support and mentoring that will facilitate their developing into successful and fully capable members of the academic community. Although at one time tenure was an unquestioned right of faculty, currently both prospective faculty and the academic community are questioning its true benefit, and some institutions of higher education have abandoned the notion altogether.

Promotion

Promotion refers to advancement in rank. As with the tenure review process, faculty must submit evidence of excellence in teaching, scholarship and service, or other criteria established by the school and be judged by a committee of peers, school and university administrators, and governing bodies. Criteria and processes for promotion, like those for tenure, are established by faculty committees and are made public. In most schools of nursing, tenure-probationary faculty who are appointed as assistant professors are expected to be able to be promoted to the rank of associate professor at the time tenure is granted.

Faculty should familiarize themselves with promotion criteria and processes at the time of appointment and establish a relationship with the primary appointment, promotion, and tenure (APT) committee and the department chair, whose role it is to inform faculty about APT policies and procedures. As noted earlier, an expectation of senior faculty is to guide and mentor junior faculty through the tenure and promotion process. Some schools of nursing assign mentors at the time of appointment; if a mentor is not assigned, the newly appointed faculty member should seek one.

Teaching as a Scholarly Endeavor

Redefining the Faculty Role

The faculty role has been redefined in the twenty-first century, in response to emerging societal trends such as technology and an emphasis on outcomes; new definitions of the faculty role have been proposed to facilitate this role transformation. For example, Norris and Dolence (1996) described numerous ways that the faculty role needed to change to meet the needs of the learners in the information age. They described the faculty role as one encompassing the synthesis of knowledge and a broader range of scholarship, with faculty assuming the role of "learning mentors" who guide learners through individualized programs of study and evaluate the mastery of learners. In such a role, faculty need to develop expertise in flexible, fluid curricula design and outcome assessment. In the same vein, Barr and Tagg (1995) described a shift from a "teaching paradigm" to a "learning paradigm" to "create environments and experiences that allow students to discover and construct knowledge for themselves" (p. 15). These changes in the faculty role, first addressed in the '90s, have indeed transpired. Teaching, although always an important aspect of the faculty role, has continued to assume an even greater significance in recent years.

Boyer (1990) first proposed a new paradigm for scholarship that encompassed all aspects of the faculty role but placed a renewed emphasis on teaching as a scholarly endeavor. In *Scholarship, Reconsidered: Priorities of the Professorate*, Boyer called for the development of a balance between research and teaching when measuring the faculty member's success in academia. He described four types of scholarship in which faculty engage: the scholarship of *discovery*, the scholarship of *integration*, the scholarship of *application*, and the scholarship of *teaching*. In these four types of scholarship, the previously narrow view of scholarly productivity that rested only on the careful discovery of new knowledge through research has been greatly expanded. Boyer's model supports the practice model of nursing, which calls for more than the discovery of knowledge; it also calls for the application and integration of knowledge into clinical practice. As Boyer stated:

> We believe the time has come to move beyond the tired old "teaching versus research" debate and give the familiar and honorable term "scholarship" a broader, more capacious meaning, one that brings legitimacy to the full scope of academic work. Surely, scholarship means engaging in original research. But the work of the scholar also means stepping back from one's investigation, looking for connections, building bridges between theory and practice, and communicating one's knowledge effectively to students. Specifically, we conclude that the work of the professorate might be thought of as having four separate, yet overlapping, functions. These are: the scholarship of discovery; the scholarship of integration; the scholarship of application; and the scholarship of teaching. (p. 16)

The Scholarship of Discovery

The scholarship of discovery is the traditional definition of original research or discovery of new knowledge (Boyer, 1990). The scholarship of discovery may be considered the foundation of the other three aspects of scholarship because new knowledge is generated for application and integration into the discipline, as well as for teaching (Brown et al., 1995).

It is through the scholarship of discovery that scientific methods are used to develop a strong knowledge base for the discipline. Evidence-based practice in nursing builds on the knowledge generated by the scholarship of discovery. Most federal funding traditionally has been appropriated for the scholarship of discovery, and until recently tenure decisions in many universities have been based primarily on the faculty member's engagement in the generation of new knowledge. The scholarship of discovery remains an important aspect of the role of many faculties, including nursing faculties. At the federal level, research efforts in nursing are supported by the National Institute of Nursing Research and content-specific institutes such as the National Institutes of Health and the National Institute of Mental Health.

The Scholarship of Integration

The scholarship of integration involves the interpretation and synthesis of knowledge within and across discipline boundaries in a manner that provides a larger context for the knowledge and the development of new insights (Boyer, 1990). The scholarship of integration requires communication among colleagues from various disciplines who work together to develop a more holistic view of a common concern. The combined expertise of all who are involved leads to a more comprehensive understanding of the issue and results in more thorough recommendations for solutions to the phenomena of concern.

Nursing faculty have long integrated knowledge from various disciplines into their practice (Brown et al., 1995) and have many competencies that enable them to be productive members of interdisciplinary teams studying a variety of health problems and issues. With the emphasis in today's world on the development of collaborative, team-building, and knowledge-sharing efforts across disciplines, the scholarship of integration assumes an ever-increasing importance for faculty who must remain at the fore-front of the information age. This is especially true for health care professionals and faculty in this era of rapidly changing health care delivery systems and accompanying complex health care issues that require innovative solutions. Nursing content often builds on the knowledge students have learned from other disciplines such as the biological and social sciences. The scholarship of integration involves the designing of learning models that guide the students to apply their previously learned knowledge to clinical situations such as the use of patient care plans or care maps (Kirkpatrick et al., 2001).

The Scholarship of Application

The scholarship of application, which connects theory and practice, is an area of scholarship in which nursing faculty should also excel. In the scholarship of application, faculty must ask themselves, "How can knowledge be responsibly applied to consequential problems?" (Boyer, 1990, p. 21). Service activities that are directly connected to a faculty member's areas of expertise warrant consideration as application scholarship. It is in the performance of service activities that practice and theory interact, thus leading to the potential development of new knowledge.

For example, in nursing, clinical practice and expertise that result in the development of examples of nursing interventions and positive patient care outcomes meet the definition of scholarship of application (Paskiewicz, 2003; Riley et al., 2002). Activities that encourage students to use critical decision making and self-reflection and self-evaluation are examples of the scholarship of application in teaching. Faculty practice in nursing centers is another example. Faculty should disseminate the knowledge gathered through practice and service activities by publishing in professional journals.

The scholarship of application, which includes service to the profession of nursing at the local, regional, national, and international levels, also involves developing policies and practices for nursing and health care. Nursing faculty often provide leadership in professional organizations and on community or national panels and boards.

The Scholarship of Teaching

The heart of the faculty role can be found in the scholarship of teaching. An important attribute of any scholar is having the ability to effectively communicate the knowledge he or she possesses to students. Boyer's (1990) definition of scholarship provides a model through which the special competencies and skills that are an integral part of the scholarly endeavor of teaching are acknowledged. Developing innovative curricula, using a variety of teaching methods that actively involve students in the learning process, collaborating with students on learning projects, and exploring the most effective means of meeting the learning needs of diverse populations of students are all examples of the scholarship of teaching.

The scholarship of teaching requires evidence of effective teaching and dissemination of the knowledge that is acquired as a result of teaching. Faculty should share their teaching expertise with their colleagues through publication and presentation of their innovative teaching methods and the outcomes of their working with students.

The scholarship of teaching brings many exciting opportunities for nursing faculty in classroom and clinical settings. It is based on the scholarship of discovery, integration, and practice (Shoffner, Davis, & Bowen, 1994). At a time when health care practice arenas are rapidly changing—curriculum models are being designed to meet the needs of a global society, use of technology in education is increasing, and perspectives on teaching and learning are changing—the scholarship of teaching provides nursing faculty with the opportunity to demonstrate their innovation and creativity. It also provides a means for recognizing the effort spent preparing students to be competent health care providers for the future.

Summary

Although the role of the faculty member remains complex, Boyer's (1990) broad description of scholarship provides a model that legitimizes all aspects of the faculty role. Boyer has given credibility to aspects of the faculty role that extend beyond the creation of new knowledge through research to include teaching and service to the university, community, and profession. As a scholarly endeavor, teaching is the synthesis of all types of scholarship described by Boyer. Faculty can combine the role of researcher with the integration, application, and dissemination of knowledge. The ability to teach is an important criterion for the evaluation of faculty at most universities (Gaff & Lambert, 1996; Kirkpatrick et al., 2001; Stull & Lantz, 2005). Boyer has provided a model for nursing faculty to use to develop their expertise in teaching as a scholarly endeavor (Shoffner et al., 1994). Nursing education has moved from the notion that there is only one way to do something to a broader perspective that recognizes the creativity and uniqueness of each student. The teacher is no longer the only expert but instead is someone who joins with the student in the learning process.

Faculty Development for the Teaching Role

Teaching in nursing is a complex activity that integrates the art and science of nursing and clinical practice into the teaching–learning process. Specifically, teaching involves a set of skills, or competencies, that are essential to facilitating student learning outcomes. These competencies can be developed through educational preparation, faculty orientation programs, and faculty development opportunities. Most graduate programs in nursing, unless they are specifically preparation for the educator role, do not prepare the graduate to teach. Therefore mentoring of new faculty and strong professional development programs are essential for the preparation of nursing faculty.

Teaching Competencies

Teaching competencies are the knowledge, skills, and values that are critical to the fulfillment of the teaching component of the faculty role. Several authors have identified general competencies for teaching in nursing (Billings, 1995; Choudhry, 1992; Davis, Dearman, Schwab, & Kitchens, 1992) and Kirschling et al. (1995) have identified domains of teaching effectiveness that can be used as standards for evaluating teaching competence. Promotion and tenure criteria articulate specific expectations of teaching competence and excellence at each school of nursing. Teaching and related role competencies include the following competencies.

Competencies Related to Curriculum Development; Teaching; Using Teaching, Learning, and Information Resources; and Evaluating Student Outcomes

These competencies include being knowledgeable about the content area; setting learning objectives; designing learning activities; being well organized in the selection and presentation of learning experiences; selecting and using appropriate learning strategies; understanding and using theories of teaching and learning; teaching in the clinical setting; communicating expectations clearly; providing helpful and timely feedback; assisting students to develop critical thinking skills; using information

technologies such as databases, spreadsheets, statistical software, electronic communications (e-mail), presentation systems, test-authoring programs, and videoconferencing applications; developing appropriate evaluation measures; and evaluating fairly (Billings, 1995; Choudhry, 1992; Davis et al., 1992; Kirschling et al., 1995).

Competencies Related to Professional Practice

Competencies related to professional practice include being knowledgeable about the content area and clinical practice, having the ability to influence change in nursing and health care by selecting appropriate strategies, and facilitating relationships with clinical agencies to benefit students (Choudhry, 1992; Kirschling et al., 1995).

Competencies Related to Relationships with Students and Colleagues

Competencies in this area include being an advocate for students; advising and counseling students; accepting student diversity; showing consideration for students; having a sense of humor; conveying a sense of caring to students; serving as a mentor and role model; facilitating student development; and developing collaborative, collegial relationships with students characterized by mutual respect (Choudhry, 1992; Halstead, 1996; Kirschling et al., 1995). Competence as a colleague means serving as a mentor to junior faculty, assisting colleagues with professional duties, conducting one's professional life without prejudice toward others, and respecting the views of others (Balsmeyer, Haubrich, & Quinn, 1996).

Competencies Related to Service and Faculty Governance

Competencies related to service and faculty governance include understanding institutional structure, policies, and procedures; understanding and assuming the rights and responsibilities of a faculty member; serving on committees and performing work necessary to the operation of the department; and serving on committees or providing leadership to the school, college or university, and profession (Balsmeyer et al., 1996; Choudhry, 1992; Davis et al., 1992).

Competencies Related to Scholarship

Scholarship, a larger component of the faculty role, may or may not be a requirement of the teaching role depending on the position description. Competencies related to the scholarship of teaching include conducting research about teaching (and the area of content expertise), publishing about teaching and learning issues, presenting at national meetings, and consulting about teaching and learning issues (Choudhry, 1992; Davis et al., 1992).

The National League for Nursing (2005) has developed core competencies for nurse educators. The competencies focus on eight areas: facilitating learning, facilitating learner development and socialization, using assessment and evaluation strategies, participating in curriculum design and evaluation of program outcomes, functioning as change agents and leaders, pursuing continuous quality improvement in the nurse educator role, engaging in scholarship, and functioning within the educational environment. A statement of the competencies can be found in Box 1-1. These competencies guide the development of graduate nursing programs that focus on the preparation of nurse educators, enhance recruitment and retention of nurse educators, influence public policy efforts affecting nurse educators and nursing education, and identify scholarship and research priorities related to the nurse educator role. Further information can be found on the National League for Nurses website at www.nln.org. Faculty can also become certified as a Nurse Educator through the National League for Nursing.

Preparation to Teach

Developing competent faculty requires an investment on the part of both the individual faculty member and the school of nursing. Preparation for teaching requires participation in classroom and clinical experiences to acquire the competencies previously identified. These experiences may take place in teacher education courses or in focus areas in master's and doctoral degree programs in nursing schools or schools of education. Participating in orientation programs, teaching institutes, or continuing education offerings and working as a teaching assistant are other ways of preparing to teach. The mission of the particular college or university and its school of nursing determines the expectation of teaching experiences, competencies, and appointment, as well as how faculty prepare for these. Appointment in tenure track and clinical positions requires proven teaching competencies and a commitment to teaching as a scholarly endeavor.

Orientation Programs and Faculty Development

Orientation to the teaching role and the school of nursing for newly appointed faculty, as well as ongoing faculty development for all faculty, is assuming renewed importance as rapid changes in higher education and health care and the use of information technologies are creating new environments for teaching and changes in the faculty role. Most schools of nursing have established orientation programs and instituted mechanisms for faculty development and renewal.

Orientation Programs

Comprehensive orientation programs are necessary to assist new faculty to acquire teaching competencies, facilitate socialization to the teaching role of the faculty, and support faculty members as they develop as fully participating members of the faculty (Genrich & Pappas, 1997; Norton & Spross, 1994; Sheehe & Schoener, 1994). Orientation programs should include information about the rights and responsibilities of the faculty and institution, information about school- and department-specific policies and procedures, an overview of the curriculum with an orientation to the instructional technologies and computer-mediated instruction used at the school, and orientation to teaching assignments and clinical facilities. Orientation is particularly important for part-time faculty members, who have fewer opportunities for contact with the school and faculty colleagues.

Orientation programs are most effective when they occur over time and provide for ongoing support (Genrich & Pappas, 1997). Some schools of nursing have school-, department-, or course-developed programs. Orientation to the teaching aspect of the faculty role also can be facilitated through a mentor relationship. Many schools of nursing have formal mentor programs in which each new faculty member is assigned to a senior faculty member, who guides the new faculty member. Other mentoring relationships can occur on an informal basis.

Faculty Development

Faculty development refers to a planned course of action to develop all faculty members, not only those newly appointed for current and future teaching positions. Faculty development is assuming new importance as faculty prepare for teaching in

---

BOX 1-1 National League for Nursing Nurse Educator Competencies (2005)

COMPETENCY 1: FACILITATE LEARNING

To facilitate learning effectively, the nurse educator:
- Implements a variety of teaching strategies appropriate to learner needs, desired learner outcomes, content, and context
- Grounds teaching strategies in educational theory and evidence-based teaching practices
- Recognizes multicultural, gender, and experiential influences on teaching and learning
- Engages in self-reflection and continued learning to improve teaching practices that facilitate learning
- Uses information technologies skillfully to support the teaching–learning process
- Practices skilled oral, written, and electronic communication that reflects an awareness of self and others, along with an ability to convey ideas in a variety of contexts
- Models critical and reflective thinking
- Creates opportunities for learners to develop their critical thinking and critical reasoning skills
- Shows enthusiasm for teaching, learning, and nursing that inspires and motivates students
- Demonstrates interest in and respect for learners
- Uses personal attributes (e.g., caring, confidence, patience, integrity, and flexibility) that facilitate learning
- Develops collegial working relationships with students, faculty colleagues, and clinical agency personnel to promote positive learning environments
- Maintains the professional practice knowledge base needed to help prepare learners for contemporary nursing practice
- Serves as a role model of professional nursing

COMPETENCY 2: FACILITATE LEARNER DEVELOPMENT AND SOCIALIZATION

To facilitate learner development and socialization effectively, the nurse educator:
- Identifies individual learning styles and unique learning needs of international, adult, multicultural, educationally disadvantaged, physically challenged, at-risk, and second-degree learners
- Provides resources to diverse learners that help meet their individual learning needs
- Engages in effective advisement and counseling strategies that help learners meet their professional goals
- Creates learning environments that are focused on socialization to the role of the nurse and facilitate learners' self-reflection and personal goal setting
- Fosters the cognitive, psychomotor, and affective development of learners
- Recognizes the influence of teaching styles and interpersonal interactions on learner outcomes

- Assists learners to develop the ability to engage in thoughtful and constructive self and peer evaluation
- Models professional behaviors for learners including, but not limited to, involvement in professional organizations, engagement in lifelong learning activities, dissemination of information through publications and presentations, and advocacy

COMPETENCY 3: USE ASSESSMENT AND EVALUATION STRATEGIES

To use assessment and evaluation strategies effectively, the nurse educator:
- Uses extant literature to develop evidence-based assessment and evaluation practices
- Uses a variety of strategies to assess and evaluate learning in the cognitive, psychomotor, and affective domains
- Implements evidence-based assessment and evaluation strategies that are appropriate to the learner and to learning goals
- Uses assessment and evaluation data to enhance the teaching–learning process
- Provides timely, constructive, and thoughtful feedback to learners
- Demonstrates skill in the design and use of tools for assessing clinical practice

COMPETENCY 4: PARTICIPATE IN CURRICULUM DESIGN AND EVALUATION OF PROGRAM OUTCOMES

To participate effectively in curriculum design and evaluation of program outcomes, the nurse educator:
- Ensures the curriculum reflects institutional philosophy and mission, current nursing and health care trends, and community and societal needs, so as to prepare graduates for practice in a complex, dynamic, multicultural health care environment
- Demonstrates knowledge of curriculum development including identifying program outcomes, developing competency statements, writing learning objectives, and selecting appropriate learning activities and evaluation strategies
- Bases curriculum design and implementation decisions on sound educational principles, theory, and research
- Revises the curriculum based on assessment of program outcomes, learner needs, and societal and health care trends
- Implements curricular revisions using appropriate change theories and strategies
- Creates and maintains community and clinical partnerships that support educational goals

Continued

BOX 1-1 National League for Nursing Nurse Educator Competencies (2005)—cont'd

- Collaborates with external constituencies throughout the process of curriculum revision
- Designs and implements program assessment models that promote continuous quality improvement of all aspects of the program

COMPETENCY 5: FUNCTION AS A CHANGE AGENT AND LEADER

To function effectively as a change agent and leader, the nurse educator:
- Models cultural sensitivity when advocating for change
- Integrates a long-term, innovative, and creative perspective into the nurse educator role
- Participates in interdisciplinary efforts to address health care and educational needs regionally, nationally, or internationally
- Evaluates organizational effectiveness in nursing education
- Implements strategies for organizational change
- Provides leadership in the parent institution as well as in the nursing program to enhance the visibility of nursing and its contributions to the academic community
- Promotes innovative practices in educational environments
- Develops leadership skills to shape and implement change

COMPETENCY 6: PURSUE CONTINUOUS QUALITY IMPROVEMENT IN THE NURSE EDUCATOR ROLE

To develop the educator role effectively, the nurse educator:
- Demonstrates commitment to lifelong learning
- Recognizes that career enhancement needs and activities change as experience is gained in the role
- Participates in professional development opportunities that increase one's effectiveness in the role
- Balances the teaching, scholarship, and service demands inherent in the role of educator and member of an academic institution
- Uses feedback gained from self, peer, student, and administrative evaluation to improve role effectiveness
- Engages in activities that promote one's socialization to the role
- Uses knowledge of the legal and ethical issues relevant to higher education and nursing education as a basis for influencing, designing, and implementing policies

and procedures related to students, faculty, and the educational environment
- Mentors and supports faculty colleagues

COMPETENCY 7: ENGAGE IN SCHOLARSHIP

To engage effectively in scholarship, the nurse educator:
- Draws on extant literature to design evidence-based teaching and evaluation practices
- Exhibits a spirit of inquiry about teaching and learning, student development, evaluation methods, and other aspects of the role
- Designs and implements scholarly activities in an established area of expertise
- Disseminates nursing and teaching knowledge to a variety of audiences through various means
- Demonstrates skill in proposal writing for initiatives that include, but are not limited to, research, resource acquisition, program development, and policy development
- Demonstrates qualities of a scholar: integrity, courage, perseverance, vitality, and creativity

COMPETENCY 8: FUNCTION WITHIN THE EDUCATIONAL ENVIRONMENT

To function as a good "citizen of the academy," the nurse educator:
- Uses knowledge of history and current trends and issues in higher education as a basis for making recommendations and decisions on educational issues
- Identifies how social, economic, political, and institutional forces influence higher education in general and nursing education in particular
- Develops networks, collaborations, and partnerships to enhance nursing's influence within the academic community
- Determines own professional goals within the context of academic nursing and the mission of the parent institution and nursing program
- Integrates the values of respect, collegiality, professionalism, and caring to build an organizational climate that fosters the development of students and teachers
- Incorporates the goals of the nursing program and the mission of the parent institution when proposing a change or managing issues
- Assumes a leadership role in various levels of institutional governance
- Advocates for nursing and nursing education in the political arena

From: National League for Nursing. (2005). *The scope of practice for academic nurse educators.* New York: National League for Nursing. Included with the permission of the National League for Nursing, New York, NY.

new and reformed health care environments and community-based settings, delivering instruction in new ways and using new teaching and learning technologies (Riner & Billings, 1996).

Faculty development is a shared responsibility of the individual faculty members, the department chair and other academic officers, and the school or university. It may include the school providing formal and informal workshops and sessions, credit courses, and informal "brown bag lunches" and encouraging faculty to attend local and national conferences related to teaching, as well as providing the financial support to do so. Because effective teaching also requires clinical competence, faculty are encouraged to maintain clinical expertise through faculty practice and by keeping abreast of changes in the field through literature review and attending professional meetings related to the practice area. Sabbatical leaves provide another opportunity for faculty renewal.

Evaluation of Teaching Performance

To ensure competent teaching, the faculty members themselves, as well as administrators, peers, colleagues, and students, regularly review their teaching performance. Evaluation of teaching is a critical component of tenure (and posttenure) review. Results of this evaluation may also be used in making decisions about reappointment, merit raises, and awards that recognize and honor excellence in teaching.

Evidence for review of teaching effectiveness can be provided by a number of sources, including student evaluations of teaching, peer and colleague observations of teaching and teaching products (e.g., syllabi, case studies, publications, videotapes, computer-mediated lessons, Internet-based courses, study guides), letters from former students, success of graduates in employment, publications of students, teaching awards, administrative review, and self-evaluation (Kirschling et al., 1995; Lashley, 1993; Melland & Volden, 1996; Suess, 1995). Methods for gathering data for evaluation include promotion and tenure review, peer and colleague review, posttenure review, and the use of a teaching portfolio or dossier. These methods are explained in Chapter 24.

SUMMARY

Because of the various aspects of the faculty role, the demands of a career in academia can be challenging and require the ability to develop and change with the needs of the learner. To be successful, individuals aspiring to the role of a faculty member must be clear about the expectations of the role. This chapter described the various competencies expected of faculty members, as well as their rights and responsibilities.

Many nursing faculty have found that the rewards of the role greatly outweigh the demands and expectations. The challenges of the role provide many creative and innovative opportunities for faculty, leading to a career filled with diversity and productivity. Whether it be through teaching a new generation of nurses the art and science of nursing; providing service and consultation to constituents within a local, regional, national, or even international community; or generating new knowledge that has an impact on the delivery of quality patient care through evidence-based nursing, being a member of the academic community provides faculty with stimulation and the opportunity to debate and collaborate with colleagues from their own discipline and others. Faculty are given a "laboratory" to explore new technology and solutions to the problems found in society and health care, while meeting an important societal need. In what other role could a nurse touch the lives of patients and future generations of nurses while developing a knowledge base that will assist in the further evolution of nursing and health care? The career of a faculty member is indeed a rewarding one.

▮▮ REFLECTING ON THE EVIDENCE

1. Describe the conceptual framework that would guide your implementation of the nursing faculty role.
2. Describe nontraditional teaching strategies you would use to teach nursing content to prepare students for their future role as nurses.
3. Compare the faculty role expectations for tenure in a university that has a primary focus on research and in one that has a primary focus on teaching.
4. Develop a project that would fit into the Boyer model as the scholarship of teaching.

REFERENCES

Amen, M. M., & Pacquiao, F. (2004). Contrasting experience with child health care services by mothers and professional caregivers in transitional housing. *Journal of Transcultural Nursing, 15*(3),217–224.

American Association of Colleges of Nursing. (2010). *Final data from 2009 survey.* Washington, DC: Author.

Association of Governing Boards of Universities and Colleges. (1996). *Renewing the academic presidency.* Washington, DC: Author.

Balsmeyer, B., Haubrich, K., & Quinn, K. (1996). Defining collegiality within the academic setting. *Journal of Nursing Education, 35*(6), 264–267.

Barr, R. B., & Tagg, J. (1995). From teaching to learning: A new paradigm for undergraduate education. *Change, 27*(6),13–25.

Benner, P., Sutphen, M., Leonard, V., & Day, V. (2010). *Educating nurses: A call for radical transformation.* Princeton, NJ: The Carnegie Foundation for the Advancement of Teaching.

Billings, D. M. (1995). Preparing nursing faculty for information-age teaching and learning. *Computers in Nursing, 13*(6),264–269.

Boyer, E. (1990). *Scholarship reconsidered: Priorities of the professorate.* Princeton, NJ: The Carnegie Foundation for the Advancement of Teaching.

Brown, S. A., Cohen, S. M., Kaeser, L., Levine, C., Littleton, L. Y., Meininger, J. C., . . . Rickman, K. J. (1995). Nursing perspective of Boyer's scholarship paradigm. *Nurse Educator, 20*(5), 26–30.

Campinha-Bacote, J. (2005). A biblically based model of cultural competence in health care delivery. *Journal of Multicultural Nursing and Health, 11*(2), 16–22.

Choudhry, U. K. (1992). New nurse faculty: Core competencies for role development. *Journal of Nursing Education, 13*(6), 265–272.

Davis, D. C., Dearman, C., Schwab, C., & Kitchens, E. (1992). Competencies of novice nurse educators. *Journal of Nursing Education, 31*(4),159–164.

Dwyer, C., Millett, C., & Payne, C. (2006). *A culture of evidence: Postsecondary assessment and learning outcomes.* Princeton, NJ: ETS.

Gaff, J., & Lambert, L. (1996). Socializing future faculty to the values of undergraduate education. *Change, 28*(4),38–45.

Genrich, S. J., & Pappas, A. (1997). Retooling faculty orientation. *Journal of Professional Nursing, 13*(2),84–89.

Halstead, J. A. (1996). The significance of student-faculty interactions. In K. Stevens (Ed.), *Review of Research in Nursing Education* (Vol. 2, pp. 67–90). New York, NY: National League for Nursing.

Institute of Medicine. (2010). *The future of nursing: Leading change, advancing health.* Washington, DC: The National Academies Press.

Kirkpatrick, J., Richardson, C., Schmieser, C., Schafer, K. S., Valley, K. S., & Yehle, K. T. (2001). Building a case for promotion of clinical faculty. *Nurse Educator, 26*(4),178–181.

Kirschling, J., Fields, J., Imle, M., Mowery, M., Tanner, C., Perrin, N., & Stewart, B. (1995). Evaluating teaching effectiveness. *Journal of Nursing Education, 34*(9),401–410.

Lashley, M. E. (1993). Faculty evaluation for professional growth. *Nurse Educator, 18*(4),26–29.

Lieb, M. (1995). Mentoring: Making a difference in nursing education. In P. Bayles & J. Parks-Doyle (Eds.), *The web of inclusion: Faculty helping faculty.* New York, NY: National League for Nursing.

Melland, H. I., & Volden, C. M. (1996). Teaching portfolios for faculty evaluation. *Nurse Educator, 21*(2),35–38.

National League for Nursing Task Group on Nurse Educator Competencies. (2005). *Competencies for nurse educators.* New York, NY: Author.

Norris, D. & Dolence, M. (1996). IT leadership is key to transformation. *Cause/Effect, 19*(1), 12–20.

Norton, S. F., & Spross, J. (1994). From advanced practice to academia: Developmental tasks and strategies for role socialization. *Journal of Professional Nursing, 33*(8),373–375.

Paskiewicz, L. (2003). Clinical practice: An emphasis strategy for promotion and tenure. *Nursing Forum, 38*(4),21–26.

Plater, W. (1995). Future work: Faculty time in the 21st century. *Change, 27*(3),23–33.

Riley, J., Beal, J., Levi, P., & McCausland, M. (2002). Revisioning nursing scholarship. *Journal of Nursing Scholarship, 34*(4), 383–389.

Riner, M. E., & Billings D. M. (1996). *Faculty development for teaching in a changing health care environment: A statewide needs assessment.* (Unpublished manuscript). Indiana University School of Nursing, Indianapolis.

Sheehe, J. B., & Schoener, L. (1994). Risk and reality for nurse educators. *Holistic Nursing Practice, 8*(2),53–58.

Shoffner, D. H., Davis, M. W., & Bowen, S. M. (1994). A model for clinical teaching as a scholarly endeavor. *IMAGE: Journal of Nursing Scholarship, 26*(3),181–184.

Stull, A., & Lantz, C. (2005). An innovative model for nursing scholarship. *Journal of Nursing Education, 4*(11), 493–497.

Suess, L. R. (1995). Attitudes of nurse-faculty toward post-tenure performance evaluations. *Journal of Nursing Education, 34*(1),25–30.

Tri-Council for Nursing. (2010). *New consensus policy statement on the educational advancement of registered nurses.* New York, NY: Author.

Tucker, A. (1992). *Chairing the academic department: Leadership among peers* (3rd ed.). New York, NY: American Council on Education/Macmillan.

U.S. Department of Health and Human Services. (2010). *The registered nurse population: Initial findings from the 2008 national sample survey of registered nurses.* Washington, DC: Author.

Whicker, M., Kronenfield, J., & Strickland, R. (1993). *Getting tenure.* Newbury Park, CA: Sage Publications.

The Diverse Learning Needs of Students

2

Nancy Burruss, PhD, RN, CNE

Ann Popkess, PhD, RN

Students in today's college classrooms represent a wide array of diversity in learning needs and expectations. Nursing faculty not only are faced with the challenges of teaching students from varied backgrounds, of varied ages, and with an array of life experiences, but also are faced with the challenges of teaching students with significant technological experience and demands on their time. Faculty must continually think creatively as they develop interactive learning environments to foster students' successful integration into an ever-changing health care system. This chapter presents a brief profile of today's nursing students and describes the unique demographic characteristics of students along with strategies to improve success in nursing programs. Also, the chapter provides information about students' learning styles, thinking skills, and cognitive abilities. Specific teaching and learning strategies related to students' diverse needs are presented to enable faculty to plan effective learning experiences for all students.

Profile of Contemporary Nursing Students

The profile of nursing students in the new millennium is markedly different from that of the past. There are generational differences, more men in nursing schools, and increasing racial and ethnic diversity. Planning effective learning experiences to meet the needs of these students has implications for faculty as they contemplate the development of curricula and determine the resources necessary to support the academic performance of students.

Enrollment Demographics

The most recent National League for Nursing (NLN) (2009a) survey of nursing programs indicated that only 14% of baccalaureate students were over the age of 30. In contrast, the percentage of prelicensure students over age 30 enrolled in associate degree and diploma programs remains high at nearly 50%. More than 60% of students enrolled in graduate nursing programs are over the age of 30, and nearly 70% of those in doctoral programs are over the age of 40. This wide range of age diversity among students in nursing offers unique challenges to nurse educators when these students are mixed in classrooms.

Degree transition and graduate programs in nursing have seen an increase in enrollment. Baccalaureate completion programs, such as RN to BSN and accelerated option programs, have incurred increased popularity with steady increases in enrollment of 8.2% and nearly 10%, respectively (American Association of Colleges of Nursing [AACN], 2009). In 2008, nursing master's degree programs saw an increase of nearly 18% enrollment as well (U.S. Department of Education, 2009). The college student population is also becoming more representative of the increasing cultural diversity that exists in American society. Of all college students, 32.2% are minority students (U.S. Department of Education, 2009). In nursing, baccalaureate minority representation remains high at 26%, and master's programs have increased to 24% (AACN, 2009).

Competition for admission into baccalaureate, associate, and master's degree nursing schools remains significant, which also shifts the demographic profile of the student nurse. Of all qualified applications submitted to prelicensure nursing schools in 2007–2008, only 42.3% were accepted (AACN, 2009). The major reasons for turning away qualified applicants, as reported by nursing schools, include a shortage of faculty, insufficient clinical teaching sites, limited classroom space, lack of preceptors, and budget cuts (AACN, 2009). At the same time, faculty and administrators are challenged to continue to recruit qualified, diverse student bodies and to maintain high academic standards and outcomes despite a critical shortage of resources.

Different Generations

Students in nursing classrooms represent a variety of generations, each with unique perspectives and learning needs. The generation of the student also may be different from that of the faculty.

Millennials or Generation Y

Millennials, or *Generation Y*, are persons born between the late 1970s and mid to late 1990s. They are described as "the next great generation" and outnumber any previous generation at around 76 million strong (U.S. Census Bureau, 2007). Millennials grew up as highly valued children of the Generation X "baby busters" and are generally described as optimistic, team-oriented, high-achieving rule-followers. Aptitude test scores among this group have risen across all grade levels, and the pressure to succeed has risen likewise (Howe & Strauss, 2000). Millennials characteristically have good relationships with their parents and families and share their interests in music and travel. Parents of Millennials are involving their children in academic and sports activities at younger ages to prepare them for success. Millennials are accustomed to living highly structured lives planned by their parents and have had very little free time. By the time they reach college, they have learned how to work with others and be a member of a team. Group grades for projects and assignments are something they are used to and expect (Johnson & Romanello, 2005). Implications for nurse educators in dealing with this generation include providing immediate feedback and structure in the classroom, providing for the safety of the students on campus and in clinical sites, and providing opportunities for service and giving back to their communities.

Millennial learners are technologically savvy and comfortable with multitasking, and value doing rather than knowing. They are "digital natives," having grown up with technology (Elam, Stratton, & Gibson, 2007); however, this can sometimes be a barrier to critical thinking, as students may have difficulties refining their abilities to focus on priority issues. Millennials as a group are more diverse than previous generations: 36% are nonwhite or Hispanic (Walker et al., 2006) and 20% have an immigrant parent (Howe & Strauss, 2000). The parents of this generation expect that their children's schools and universities will reflect diversity and thus provide a richer learning experience.

Graduate and second degree students like the use of distance technologies such as web-based courses. Such teaching modalities can result in positive student perceptions, high satisfaction, and achievement of learning outcomes. These nontraditional students often find the convenience of online or hybrid formats (those offered online and face-to-face) more convenient for their lifestyles (Ali, Hodson-Carlton, & Ryan, 2004).

Generation X or "Baby Busters"

Generation Xers represent a smaller cohort (50 million) of those born between 1965 and 1976 (U.S. Census Bureau, 2009). They are more diverse in race and ethnicity than previous generations, but not as diverse as their counterpart Millennials. These are children of baby boomers and their work ethics and loyalty differ from those of their parents. Many are children of divorced parents and thus "latchkey" kids. This generation was the first to demonstrate a need for work–life balance and self-sufficiency, coining the phrase "what's in it for me?" Generation Xers are comfortable with change and technology, as their members have participated in the development of Google, YouTube, and Amazon (Johnson & Romanello, 2005; Stephey, 2008). See Table 2-1 for a comparison of demographic characteristics of Generation X and Generation Y students.

The implications of such generational demographics are significant to nursing faculty and the profession as a whole. Teaching strategies that successfully engage the Millennial learner need to be interactive, group focused, objective, and experiential (Elam et al., 2007). Older students who are returning to school with multiple role responsibilities may require support resources such as tutoring,

TABLE 2-1 Generation X and Generation Y Demographic Characteristics, 2009

Population	Generation X	Generation Y
Males	24,982,122	39,180,752
Females	24,678,179	37,189,278
Total	49,660,301	76,370,030
Non-Hispanic, White	62%	60%
Non-Hispanic, Black	12%	14%
Non-Hispanic, Asian	6%	4%
Hispanic	18%	19%
Other	2%	3%

Data from: U.S. Census Bureau, National Population Estimates and Projections.

remediation, day care, and the opportunity for part-time study (Swail, 2002). Graduate students may find that the use of online or hybrid programs meets their scheduling demands much better than traditional classroom formats (Ali et al., 2004). Incorporating a variety of teaching strategies, such as the teacher-centered lecture, as well as entertaining interactive, web-based media, that appeal to multi-generational students recognizes both groups' learning needs and preferences. Faculty can benefit from the diverse generational component in their classes. A prime example would be to have inter-generational students respond to questions as a group, which would demonstrate the varying perceptions related to life experiences (Johnson & Romanello, 2005). Faculty must prepare for an increasingly diverse student body by closely examining the changing demographics of their student body, the adequacy of support services for the adult learner in their institution, and the flexibility of nursing curricula in their program.

Men in Nursing

Currently men occupy about 6.6% of the nurse population (U.S. Department of Health and Human Services, 2010) and nearly 14% of the pre-licensure student population (NLN, 2009a). Numbers continue to grow through increased enrollment in schools of nursing due to the job flexibility and diverse career opportunities (Ellis, Meeker, & Hyde, 2006). According to the NLN (2009c), men comprise 12% of students in baccalaureate programs, 11% of master's students, and 10% of students in doctoral programs. While encouraging, there remains an imbalance in gender enrollment in nursing programs as well as evidence of male students not completing their respective educational programs (Stott, 2007). Various studies indicate the possibility of barriers in the professional schools that lead male students to feel marginalized and, in some cases, even to abandon their career choice before graduating (Bell-Scriber, 2008; Ellis et al., 2006; O'Lynn, 2004; Smith, 2006; Stott, 2007). Nursing faculty are compelled to recognize barriers perceived by men in schools of nursing and seek to rectify them.

Male nursing students present with their own perceptions and needs. In a study performed by Smith (2006), an interview of 29 male nursing students identified three major themes: (1) pressures of balancing family, work, and school, (2) perceptions of nursing, and (3) clients refusing to be cared for by a male nurse. Bell-Scriber (2008) identified that use of sexist language in the classroom and textbooks creates a less inviting classroom for male students. In another study, Ellis et al. (2006) determined that curricula in nursing programs are designed for female learners. As one respondent suggested, the curriculum was "set up by women, for women," especially in relation to testing, classroom lecture and discussion, and course structure. O'Lynn's (2004) study identified that male nursing history is not emphasized in classroom discussion and lecture. In addition, textbooks frequently underrepresent men in the nursing profession and faculty refer to nurses in a female context in the classroom. Stott (2007) used tape-recorded interviews and diaries written by the participants to determine factors influencing male nursing students' course completion. The presence of male role models in nursing education was identified as important for student support and inspiration (Stott, 2007). However, lack of these role models creates self-doubt and social isolation in male students, potentially contributing to increased drop-out rates. The use of sexist language, lack of role models, and a biased curriculum all present as barriers to the successful recruitment and retention of male students in schools of nursing and, subsequently, the profession.

Smith (2006) offered several strategies for nursing programs to develop and implement in order to respond positively to the minority of men in nursing: (1) develop peer support systems, (2) link male students with academic leadership to share experiences and concerns, (3) collect data regarding client refusal of care by male students and develop guidelines to address such issues, and (4) select texts and case studies that reflect both males and females in the nursing profession. These strategies could also be implemented for other minority students.

Racial and Ethnic Diversity

In 2004 the Sullivan Commission on Diversity in the Healthcare Workforce, in its report *Missing Persons: Minorities in the Health Professions*, described a lag in the ethnic diversity of all health professions. While nearly 25% of the population is represented by African Americans, Hispanics, and American Indians, these groups account for less than 9% of nurses and even lower percentages of physicians and dentists. Despite an emphasis on recruitment of ethnically diverse students, there continues to be an underrepresentation of minorities in schools of nursing and in the profession. According to the Health Resources and Services Administration survey of registered nurses (U.S. Dept of Health and Human Services, 2010), nearly 16.8% of practicing RNs identified themselves as belonging to a minority group. In 2008–2009 data collected on the ethnicity of baccalaureate nursing students, 26.3% of students were identified as minority students. Of that population, 14% were black, 4% were Pacific-Asian, 6% were Hispanic, and 1.5% were American Indian. The proportion of minority students in master's and doctoral programs increased to 25.6% and 23.0%, respectively (AACN Annual Report, 2009). Although there was a 3% increase in minority enrollment from 2005 to 2009 (NLN, 2009b), the profession is challenged to continue to meet the demands of a growing workforce need and recruitment of minorities and males into the profession.

Barriers that Influence the Success of Racially and Ethnically Diverse Students

Students with racially and ethnically diverse backgrounds can face a number of barriers that hamper their ability to succeed in college. Cultural differences between and within faculty and student groups, gender and generational differences as previously discussed, and a lack of rigorous academic preparation are thought to contribute to the difficulty of teaching a diverse student body (Bednarz, Schim, & Doorenbos, 2010). The most common barriers are the lack of racially and ethnically diverse faculty, lack of student finances, and lack of academic preparedness (Beacham, Askew, & Williams, 2009; Gardner, 2005a; Martin-Holland et al., 2003).

Lack of Faculty Diversity

There is a parallel need to recruit more faculty from diverse racial, ethnic, and gender minorities. According to 2009 data from AACN member schools, only 11.6% of full-time nursing faculty members come from minority backgrounds and only 5.1% are male. A lack of racial, ethnic, and gender diversity among faculty represented in nursing is a reflection of the failure to recruit and retain the same diversity in the undergraduate and graduate student population. Furthermore, the lack of ethnically diverse faculty can perpetuate a culture of insensitivity to the needs of those ethnically diverse students. In a research study analyzing perceived existing educational barriers in nursing schools, 26 faculty and 17 ethnically diverse nurses who graduated from an associate or baccalaureate nursing program within the last 2 years were interviewed (Amaro, Abriam-Yago, & Yoder, 2006). Throughout the interview process, several themes related to educational barriers emerged: (1) personal needs (lack of finances, time issues, family responsibilities and obligations, and difficulties related to language and communication); (2) academic needs (workload); (3) language needs (difficulty reading and understanding assignments, prejudice due to accents, verbal communication barriers); and (4) cultural needs (expectations related to assertiveness and cultural norm, lack of diverse role models, and difficulty with communication). Intolerance by faculty and peers were found to exist for these nurses during their educational experience. Faculty need to embrace the cultural differences of their students and use available resources to foster a successful learning environment. Collaboration with ethnic student associations on campus could assist faculty to promote learning among their culturally diverse student population. Furthermore, faculty could work to promote student success by offering access to role models, peer support and encouragement, tutoring opportunities, and communication strategies.

Lack of Financial Resources

Financial problems are a major stressor for minority students. Rising tuition costs and other fees, coupled with a reduction in government support for higher education, affect all students but may be particularly difficult for minority students. Minority students are often the first in their family to seek higher education. They often come from low-income households and therefore their families may lack the necessary financial resources to support their education. Financial aid in the form of loans or scholarships is becoming more competitive, and less money is available (Brown, Santiago, & Lopez, 2003).

Lack of Rigorous Academic Preparation

Insufficient academic preparation and lack of support can also prevent ethnically diverse students from completing their program of study. Many Latino youth are in schools with few academic and physical resources and are thus not prepared for the academic challenges of a nursing program (Brown et al., 2003). Many colleges offer special enrichment programs to help students achieve basic academic skills, as well as adjust to the college learning environment. Through academic advisement, skills assessment, and assistance with developing study skills, students can be helped to achieve a better academic record. For example, Mount Carmel's Learning Trail student success program assists Hispanic students to be successful by providing mentoring, tutoring, counseling, and follow-up. More than 80% of the students in the program graduate (Martinez & Martinez, 2003).

Stewart and Cleveland (2003) described a program to introduce middle and high school students to college and nursing. The Wisconsin Youth in Nursing program recruited minority youth with a high grade point average (GPA) and the motivation to complete the program. Twenty-three students participated in the 2-week summer residential program on a college campus. The program included general education and nursing courses, and the students were in class all day, 5 days a week. The nursing segment included classes on careers in nursing, introduction to nursing, pathophysiology, and case studies. Students also worked on computers and were taught some nursing skills, including physical assessment skills. Students evaluated the program as being very successful. Faculty will follow the participants to determine how many were successful in gaining admission to a nursing school.

Lack of Language Skills

For many students, English is an additional language (EAL), and the students may speak one language at home and English at school. Most studies of EAL have examined Hispanic, Asian, and American Indian students, but ignored other significant immigrant African students. Several studies have found that EAL students experience several barriers such as lack of self-confidence, reading/writing and learning difficulties, isolation, prejudice, and lack of family and financial support (Starr, 2009).

Strategies to Increase the Success of Racially and Ethnically Diverse Students

Role Models and Mentors

Although the recruitment and retention of racially and ethnically diverse students in the nursing profession is an important issue, little research is available on the effectiveness of various recruitment and retention efforts directed toward these students (Gardner, 2005a; Villarruel, Canales, & Torres, 2001). It is important to acknowledge that many nursing programs rely on standardized tests and GPAs as criteria for admission. These types of recruitment strategies do not take into account the educational experience of many minority students and constitute a "relentless exclusion based on academic adequacy and who will pass the NCLEX-RN exam" (McQueen & Zimmerman, 2004, p. 52). It is painfully obvious to potential applicants who are socially or economically disadvantaged, particularly when a limited number of admission slots are available, that they will be excluded when admissions are determined by GPA alone. Such a selection process also has been called a biased response to scarce resources (McQueen & Zimmerman, 2004). The outcome is that only a few diverse students are admitted, and many of those tend to be labeled "high-risk."

In a study conducted by Soroff, Rich, Rubin, Strickland, and Plotnick (2002), the absence of diverse role models for nursing students affected both recruitment and retention efforts to increase diversity within their student population. It was important for students to see faculty from their racial or ethnic group functioning successfully in a variety of leadership positions in the university setting (Soroff et al., 2002). Practicing minority nurses can be encouraged to function as role models and mentors. Many nursing students plan to practice in a hospital or community setting after graduation, and matching them with a practicing nurse is a way to instill confidence in them that they can be successful. Nursing school faculty could work with their school's alumni association and with diverse nursing groups to provide role models for students.

Faculty commitment is crucial to the success of all students, and those students who must also overcome barriers need a student–faculty relationship with a faculty member who is not responsible for assigning a grade to them. An example of successful mentoring is a program developed by the University of Southern California. At the beginning of each semester, at-risk students are identified and offered study skills workshops, peer tutors, study groups, and faculty coaches. Success was determined by the evidence that at-risk minority students were passing at similar rates to students who were not considered at risk (Peter, 2005). It is essential for all faculty members and administrators to develop sensitivity with regard to the diversity of the students on their campus and awareness of the needs of these students. Faculty commitment to student success results in more successful students.

Faculty members who represent the dominant race at the school can also assist in the recruitment and retention of minority students by modeling a commitment to developing cultural competence among the faculty (Campinha-Bacote, 2010; Pacquiao, 2007). Assessment of faculty cultural competence is an important step in gaining commitment and support of the value of working with racially and ethnically diverse students and colleagues. Campinha-Bacote (2010) developed a cultural competence assessment tool (IAPCC-M) according to her model of cultural competence to assist in developing a culturally competent mentoring program for faculty. Use of culturally conscious mentoring programs can help improve the success of minority and other diverse students in nursing programs. In the model, cultural competence is viewed as a process that involves the integration of cultural awareness to achieve competence in mentoring. Using the ASKED (Awareness, Skill, Knowledge, Encounters, and Cultural Desire) model as a basis for developing

a mentoring program could help address the critical need for increasing and retaining diverse students in nursing programs. (See also Chapter 17.)

Faculty can also advocate for policies and procedures and support services that assist students and support an institutional faculty "mix" that is diverse. Faculty members need to remember that many students feel isolated in their educational experience and therefore faculty may need to be more assertive in establishing and maintaining open lines of communication with minority students. Helping students to access campus support services will help students feel more connected to the institution.

Support Systems

Participating in special support programs can increase the chance of academic success for culturally diverse students. Many schools of nursing have identified and implemented strategies focused on securing the success of the culturally diverse student. At California State University, a Minority Retention Project (MRP) was developed to improve the retention and success of its minority students (Gardner, 2005b). The MRP was designed based on Dr. Vincent Tinto's Theory of Student Retention (1993) that those students who felt connected and committed to their educational institution were more likely to be successful in their academic pursuits and achieve graduation. Building upon that premise, California State University then identified the role that faculty played in providing a safe, warm, and nurturing learning environment, both in the didactic and clinical settings (Gardner, 2005b).

This project developed several support services that students could access. For example, the position of Retention Coordinator was developed to check in with students frequently and offer support and resources. A Minority Pre-Nursing Student Outreach Committee was developed to communicate with minority students considering the nursing profession. Also created was a Family Night to bring together students, their spouses, and significant others at a monthly potluck dinner to foster a sense of connectedness and belonging. Students experiencing language barriers could be involved in a Language Partnership, which paired students with mentors who were proficient in speaking the student's language. During the academic year 2003–2004, California State University experienced a 100% retention success for their nursing students (Gardner, 2005b).

Support for EAL students was provided at one historically black university in the form of language, academic, faculty, and social activities to enhance student ability to be successful in nursing school (Brown, 2008). Preliminary results of the program indicated increased retention of EAL students along with higher scores in standardized exit and first-time NCLEX exam scores and improved perceptions of climate (Brown, 2008).

Summary

The recruitment of an academically qualified and diverse student body has been a recent emphasis of many nursing schools. The data are beginning to show that while recruitment is effective, there is concern that minority students appear to be less successful than white students in graduating from nursing programs. It is important for nurse educators to reexamine their minority student recruitment efforts as well as the support services that are available for these students. Recruiting diverse faculty and developing them as role models and mentors is essential to the successful recruitment and retention of diverse students.

Understanding Learning Style Preferences

The NLN's Core Competencies for Nurse Educators (Competency 2) states that educators must facilitate current student development and socialization by identifying individual learning style preferences and the unique learning needs of students who are culturally diverse (including international), traditional versus nontraditional, and at risk (e.g., educationally disadvantaged, learning and/or physically challenged, experiencing social and economic issues) (Finke, 2009; Kalb, 2008; NLN, 2005). Given the significant shortage of nurse faculty and increasing class sizes, nurse educators are challenged to identify learning style preferences and develop appropriate learning experiences that will meet the complex needs of the current nursing student (Fountain & Alfred, 2009; Ironside & Valiga, 2006). Learning style preferences should be identified early in the undergraduate nursing curriculum with the intent to empower individual students to use their knowledge of learning style preferences

in order to achieve positive outcomes (Holstein, Zangrilli, & Taboas, 2006), especially in large classes where students at risk may go unnoticed. As a group, underrepresented minority students have diverse learning style preferences (Hassouneh, 2008). Since a diverse environment is central to the mission and the academic goals of many institutions, strategies that maximize the potential for success of all students need to be tailored to fit each individual's learning style preferences (Evans, 2008).

Acknowledgment of diverse students' learning style enhances the learning environment while supporting academic achievement (Choi, Lee, & Jung, 2008). Currently, obtaining knowledge of the learner and his or her characteristics is a vastly underused approach to improving teaching–learning strategies. To address this concern, faculty should understand their students' learning style preferences (Slater, Lujan, & DiCarlo, 2007). Learning style is defined as the way individuals concentrate on, absorb, and retain new information (Dunn & Griggs, 2000). It is the manner in which a learner perceives, interacts with, and responds to the learning environment. Components of learning style are the cognitive, affective, and physiological elements, all of which may be strongly influenced by a person's cultural background.

Faculty are held responsible for assuring quality learning experiences in their courses and need to consider strategies for facilitating learning even when course enrollment increases. With the Bureau of Labor Statistics projecting the need for more than 1 million new and replacement registered nurses by 2016, nursing schools around the country are exploring creative ways to increase student capacity and reach out to new student populations. The challenge inherent in these efforts is to quickly produce competent nurses while maintaining the integrity and quality of the nursing education provided (AACN, 2008). Nurse educators would be wise to determine the learning styles of the students in their nursing courses (Emerson & Records, 2008), whether in the traditional classroom or online. These data will provide evidence as to how faculty should design their courses in order to retain and maximize student success, particularly in view of large enrollments.

Learning environments must be evidence-based, respectful of students' differences, and aligned with changes in health care reform (Wellman, 2009). In programs with high numbers of adult students, there may be a larger number of students who leave the program because of family problems or job-related issues (Sauter, Johnson, & Gillespie, 2009). A further concern is that achievement gaps continue to exist for diverse students. For instance, there are lower graduation rates among institutions serving high proportions of minority, low-income, and first-generation college students. Current students are striving to reduce achievement gaps, and it is important that educators augment their efforts (Brown & Marshall, 2008). A one-size-fits-all educational accommodation is likely to stress and discomfort many students who, otherwise, might perform well if their individual uniqueness were recognized and responded to instructionally (Reese & Dunn, 2007).

Students are diverse in their experiences, cultural backgrounds, and traditional versus nontraditional and at-risk status. As a result of this diversity, it is unlikely that any single teaching style would be effective for all or most students in a class of 25 or more. Although faculty vary the approaches they use, they tend to differentiate instruction for the entire class rather than for individuals (Dunn & Griggs, 2000). In a large class, where students are likely to have every learning style represented, if faculty teach in the manner they were taught, they are very likely to turn off large numbers of students (Heppner, 2007). Students may experience a difficult transition due to the loss of individuality in large classes in which they receive a lack a personal recognition. The lack of mastery of course concepts may be an outcome of the professors' lack of awareness of how differently students in the same class actually learn.

Definitions of Learning Style

Learning style is defined as the cognitive, affective, and psychological traits that serve as relatively stable indicators of how learners perceive, interact with, and respond to the learning environment (Keefe, 1987) and individuals' preferred ways of perceiving and processing information (Kolb, 1984). Kolb defined learning style as a student's consistent way of responding to and using stimuli in the context of learning (Claxton & Murrell, 1987). Honey and Mumford (1992) adapted a variation on the Kolb (1984) definition. They defined learning style as a description of the attitudes and behavior that determine an individual's preferred way of learning.

Dunn, Dunn, and Price (1986) defined learning style as the way in which each learner begins to concentrate on, process, and retain new and difficult information, which is a biologically and developmentally imposed set of personal characteristics or traits. Their definition incorporated environmental, emotional, sociological, physical, and psychological preferences that affected how individuals learn new and difficult information and skills (Dunn & Dunn, 1999).

Grasha (1996) defined learning styles as personal qualities that influence a student's ability to acquire information, to interact with peers and the instructor, and otherwise to participate in learning experiences. Learning preference related to the "likes and dislikes" that an individual had for a particular sensory mode or condition for learning, including a preference for certain learning strategies (Sutcliffe, 1993). Learning style may be defined as an attribute or characteristic of an individual who interacts with instructional circumstances in such a way as to produce differential learning outcomes (Linares, 1999). Aragon, Johnson, and Shaik (2002) defined learning style as the combination of the learner's motivation and information processing habits while engaged in the learning process and how individuals acquire information and how it is processed or acted upon once acquired (Ames, 2003).

Learning Style Frameworks and Models

Several learning style models guide faculty in their understanding of student preferences. Curry (as cited in Claxton & Murrell, 1987) defined four areas of learning styles in an "onion" model: personality factors, social interaction preference, informational processing, and instructional preference. The Witkin's and Myers-Briggs models are described as the innermost personality factors models.

The *Witkin's model* is a bipolar measure of field-dependent/field-independent cognitive style that assesses the manner in which students perceive and process information and classifies them along a continuum of field dependence to field independence. Noble, Miller, and Heckman (2008) reported statistically significant differences in the Witkin's Groups Embedded Figures Test (GEFT) mean scores of undergraduate nursing students. Undergraduate nursing students scored higher on the GEFT than did RN to BSN or graduate nursing students. Moreover, nursing students were classified as more field dependent than students in other health-related disciplines. Due to their cognitive processing requirements, field-dependent nursing students may be at risk for academic failure. Therefore instructional strategies tailored to students' needs should be incorporated into the nursing curriculum. The *Myers-Briggs Type Indicator* (MBTI) defines 16 personality types via the use of four factors. The factors used by this model are extroversion (focus on people)/introversion (ideas), sensors (detail oriented)/intuitors (imagination oriented), thinkers/feelers, and judgers/perceivers (Felder, 1996). It is a helpful tool, as it encourages individuals to recognize their strengths and understand their areas to improve.

Information processing models such as the *Kolb Model of Experiential Learning* (1978) classifies students in two basic dimensions: concrete experience (CE) or abstract conceptualization (AC) and active experimentations (AE) or reflective observation (RO). Using this model, students are classified into one of four types based on how they perceive information (CE/AC) and how they learn information (AE/RO). This theory states that students use any of the four styles some of the time by claiming that the classification is a preferred method, not an exclusive one. Kolb's Learning Style Inventory (LSI) categorizes students according to this model (Willcoxson & Prosser, 1996). The Kolb Learning Style Inventory (LSI-IIa Survey) is a survey developed from Kolb's (1978) four-stage model of experiential learning. Kolb believed that learning required different abilities that include concrete experience, reflective observation, abstract conceptualization, and active experimentation (Hauer, Straub, & Wolf, 2005). The Kolb LSI is one of the most commonly used LSIs in nursing education, as well as in other disciplines.

Gregorc's model (1982) is similar to Kolb's, except that the two dimensions rate perception from abstract to concrete and ordering from sequential to random. The classification of the learner is one of four states, again similar to Kolb, using the Gregorc Style Delineator. Honey and Mumford (1986, 1992) developed their learning styles questionnaire as a variation on Kolb's model. The four learning styles are Activist (immediate experiences, here and now), Reflector (observer of experiences, analyzes thoroughly), Theorist (logical approach), and Pragmatist (practical approach, problem-solver).

The *Grasha-Reichmann model* (Reichmann & Grasha, 1974) focuses on the social interaction aspect of students' response toward learning, classroom procedures, and faculty/peer interaction. The three bipolar dimensions include: (1) independent–dependent, those who preferred working alone and were confident and self-directed *versus* those who preferred an authority figure to provide guidance; (2) collaborative–competitive, those who enjoyed working cooperatively with others *versus* those who competed with their peers; and (3) participant–avoidant, those who took part in learning activities and classroom interactions *versus* those who demonstrated little interaction.

Theories by Canfield (1980) and Dunn and Dunn (1978) are based on instructional preference. The *Canfield model* (1980) is based on four learner scales: conditions of learning (affiliations and orientation toward goals), content (numbers and language), mode of learning (preference for listening, reading, direct experience), and expectation (expected grade). *Dunn, Dunn, and Price's Learning Style Model* (1993, 1996) is multidimensional and takes into account environmental, emotional, sociological, perceptual, physiological, and psychological elements.

The Dunn, Dunn, and Price Productivity Environmental Preference Survey (PEPS) (Dunn et al., 1986) provides information about patterns through which learning occurs. The theory underpinning development of the PEPS is that students possess biologically based physical and environmental learning preferences that, along with well-established trait-like emotional and sociological preferences, combine to form an individual learning style profile.

An adaptation of the PEPS (Dunn et al., 1986) was created by the Assessment Technologies Institute (ATI, 2000). The Self-Assessment Inventory (SAI) assesses a student's personal characteristics and attitudes as they relate to qualities of a successful nursing candidate. The SAI is composed of a number of subscales designed to measure the individual in four areas: critical thinking, learning styles, professional characteristics, and work values. The learning styles content area has a subscale with factors such as physical (visual, auditory, tactile) and sociological (individual and group) that parallels the PEPS elements.

Fleming's model (2001) suggests four categories that reflect the experiences of the students. The acronym VARK indicates the following categories: Visual (V), Auditory (A), Read/write (R), and Kinesthetic (K). The VARK questions and results focus on the ways in which people like information to come to them and the ways in which they like to deliver their communication. Fleming's (2001) VARK tool was suggested by the NLN's Certified Nurse Educator Preparation Workshops and Examination Information as one way that nurse educators might examine learning styles (NLN, 2008).

Learning Style Characteristics

Achievement may be optimized when the student's learning style is matched with a similar teaching style (Slater et al., 2007). In a recent meta-analysis, Lovelace (2005) concluded that matched learning styles instruction usually increased the achievement and motivation of the students. Choi et al. (2008) concurred that it was important to redesign teaching methods based on learners' preferred styles so that the learning outcome would be maximized.

When instruction matches students' learning style preferences, students may achieve higher scores than when instruction and learning style are mismatched. Student examination scores and students' attitude toward learning scores were significantly higher when presentation was matched with student learning styles (Slater et al., 2007). But should students use only their matched preferred learning style and risk becoming rigid and unable to learn differently? Mismatching is suggested as an occasional teaching strategy employed to stimulate interest, and not as an alternative or replacement for matching. Akdemir and Koszalka (2008) found that matches between students' learning styles and instructional strategies did not affect the learners' perception of their learning achievement, level of effort and involvement, and level of interactions in the course.

Incorporating a variety of teaching techniques acknowledges the full spectrum of learning styles and narrows the performance differences that are brought about by reliance on one teaching methodology (Flanagan & McCausland, 2007). Engaging students with different learning styles in different types of instructional strategies that either match or mismatch their preference did not prompt any difference in perceived learning engagement (Akdemir & Koszalka, 2008; Cook, Gelula, Dupras, & Schwartz, 2007).

As Bandura (1986) explained with his theory of reciprocal determinism, the environment affects behavior, which may influence learning performance.

Environmental factors such as interaction with instructor and peers, general atmosphere of the classroom, class size, and diverse backgrounds may influence learning style. It may be possible that individual characteristics were not stable and therefore learning styles may change over time. Liu (2007) concluded that the preferred learning styles of graduate students taking an online course tended to change from the beginning of the semester to the end of the semester as opposed to face-to-face graduate students, who demonstrated that over a 2-year period learning styles tended to be relatively stable (Salter, Evans, & Forney, 2006).

A variety of teaching strategies can be used to appeal to different learning styles and thus maximize student learning. The idea of teaching students to recognize their own learning style and possibly to modify their approach to learning has critical implications for developing nursing curricula. By strategizing with students to become aware of their own cognitive style and its implications about learning, students will be better able to select optimal instructional strategies that are consistent with their own style or adapt to a given instructional environment (Noble et al., 2008). Rassool and Rawaf (2007) reported that the predominant learning style for undergraduate nursing students was the Reflector (observer of experiences; analyzes thoroughly), and 30% were noted to have a dual learning style, meaning they scored high on two different learning style categories. These findings were similar to those of Butler and Pinto-Zipp (2005), who studied nursing and non-nursing graduate students in online environments. Over one half of the subjects studied by Slater et al. (2007) preferred multimodal learning yet the modality combinations were not statistically significant, as opposed to Wehrwein, Lujan, and DiCarlo (2007), who reported that females preferred unimodal learning while males preferred multimodal learning.

Using the Results of Learning Style Inventories

Nursing faculty should implement a variety of teaching strategies appropriate to content, setting, learner needs, learning style, and desired learner outcomes (Finke, 2009; NLN, 2005). Nursing educators should tailor teaching strategies to current students and provide more options in courses that will enhance retention and graduation rates. Among the strategies for educators to consider when designing classes or learning activities are the students' characteristics, preferences, and values (Emerson & Records, 2008).

Learning style inventories should be administered prior to entering a program or early in the curriculum. Once an educator knows a student's preferred learning style, that information can be used to strategize ways to be successful. For example, if a student has difficulty studying or taking tests, the educator should counsel the student to use the study methods that would be most helpful for students with his or her preferred learning style.

Burruss (2010) reported on the variables associated with the intent to use learning style preference information by undergraduate nursing students. The findings indicated that intent was significantly greater for students in 4-year programs as opposed to accelerated programs, those with fewer overall years of education, those whose learning style results were shared with the student by an academic adviser rather than faculty, those who perceived their learning style assessment as useful, and those who had a high ability to explain their learning style preference information. Evaluation of fiscal resources required for administration of learning style inventories and perceived usefulness of the information by students was critical. Implications from this study include ensuring students' ability to understand and explain their learning style preference information, as well as providing strategies that students can use throughout their curriculum.

Faculty should assist individual students to identify their learning style preferences, help them to improve study habits, and aid them in the selection of courses or work environments that are compatible with their learning styles. Students might profit substantially from knowledge on how to accommodate their own learning style. This information should guide students toward doing their homework with strategies responsive to their individual styles (Reese & Dunn, 2007). In class, some students may benefit from increased interaction with the faculty, the scheduling of periodic meetings, and frequent feedback on submitted assignments. Faculty may recommend that a student complete an assignment independently, in a pair, or in a small group. Additionally, information about preferred learning styles should help administrators to plan more appropriately when scheduling

theory and clinical courses for current students (Reese & Dunn, 2007).

Understanding Students' Multiple Ways of Thinking

Students also vary in the way they approach thinking and problem solving. The ability to think critically and make individualized but safe clinical judgments is a significant outcome in nursing programs. Benner, Sutphen, Leonard, and Day (2010) recommend that students develop a variety of thinking skills, including critical thinking, clinical reasoning, and clinical imagination. Faculty can assess students' cognitive development as well as their dispositions and abilities to think critically and make clinical decisions in order to guide students to think like a nurse.

Critical Thinking

The NLN (2007) and the AACN (2008) consider critical thinking an outcome criterion for baccalaureate nursing education. Professional nursing practice requires critical thinking skills and problem-solving abilities. The emphasis of nursing curriculum has shifted toward guiding students to become lifelong, independent critical thinkers (Lee, 2007). The application of nursing knowledge within the nursing process is enhanced through use of the process of critical thinking (NLN, 2007). Nurse educators remain accountable for creating and implementing curricula that produce graduate nurses who are able to use critical thinking skills to formulate appropriate clinical and nursing judgments (NLN, 2007).

Critical thinking has been discussed in the nursing literature for the past several years. However, experts on critical thinking cannot agree on a definition for it, nor is there one way to measure it or the impact it has on patient care. Critical thinking is defined by all or part of the process of questioning, analysis, synthesis, interpretation, inference, inductive and deductive reasoning, intuition, application, and creativity (AACN, 1998). Critical thinking underlies independent and interdependent decision making. The critical thinker must have the attitude or desire to approach the problem and to accept that the problem needs to be solved. Next, the critical thinker must have knowledge of the problem's subject matter. The critical thinker then must have the necessary skills to use and manipulate this knowledge in the problem-solving process (Bradshaw & Lowenstein, 2011).

In the nursing literature, there is an emphasis on reflection as being both an essential component of critical thinking and promoting the development of it. Riddell (2007) identified four commonalities among the various process descriptions of critical thinking. These four commonalities include reflection; identification and appraisal of assumptions; inquiry, interpretation and analysis, and reasoning and judgment; and consideration of context. Critical thinking is not a single way of thinking but rather a complex process. Critical thinking is an attribute that enhances one's skill in problem solving and decision making (Romeo, 2010). As nursing educators seek to assess their students' knowledge and critical thinking abilities, they must clearly remain focused on evidenced-based practice and outcomes management.

Suliman (2006) explored the critical thinking disposition and the learning style of students in both a traditional and an accelerated nursing program. The majority of students in this Saudi Arabian accelerated (second degree) nursing program evidenced a different learning style than the majority of students in the traditional program. Students in the accelerated program were mostly Kolb's (1978) Convergers and relied on thinking and demonstrating, while the traditional students were Divergers and relied on watching and feeling. Students in the accelerated program were significantly better critical thinkers than the traditional students whose critical thinking appeared inadequate.

Rush et al. (2008) reported that simulation used by distance delivery cultivated critical thinking in RN to BSN students. Compared with generic BSN students, the critical thinking skills of RN to BSN students and students with an associate degree in nursing were significantly lower, regardless of the measure of critical thinking used (Shin et al., 2006).

Critical Thinking Inventories

Despite the difficulty of defining critical thinking, several critical thinking inventories have been developed. These inventories have been used in nursing and include the Watson-Glaser Critical Thinking Appraisal (WGCTA), the California Critical Thinking Skills Test (CCTST), and the California Critical Thinking Disposition Inventory (CCTDI). A brief description of each follows. The reader

should bear in mind that these inventories have been tested with predominantly white middle-class groups and therefore may not work well when used with ethnically or racially diverse populations.

Watson-Glaser Critical Thinking Appraisal

The Watson-Glaser Critical Thinking Appraisal (WGCTA) is a tool available to measure critical thinking as a composite of attitudes, knowledge, and skills. Three different forms of the instrument are available. The original version of the test (Form A and Form B) is composed of 80 items and can be completed in 60 minutes. Form A and Form B are parallel tools available for use as pretest and posttest measurements, and Form S is the latest, shortest version of the instrument reporting a Cronbach's alpha coefficient of 0.81 (Wacks, 2005). The WGCTA Form S is composed of 40 items and can be completed in 45 minutes. The WGCTA consists of a number of objective items that involve problems, statements, arguments, and interpretations. The assessment has five subsets: inference, recognition of assumptions, deduction, interpretation, and evaluation of arguments. The WGCTA scores (maximum score is 80) have been found to be significant predictors of NCLEX-RN performance. Wacks (2005) reported that the correlation of the American College Test (ACT) to WGCTA ($p < 0.001$) and WGCTA to NCLEX-RN ($p < 0.002$) were significant in associate degree nursing students. These findings suggest that WGCTA is a strong predictor of NCLEX-RN performance; however, the tool may not be appropriate as a reliable and valid measure of critical thinking abilities in all nursing students (Romeo, 2010).

California Critical Thinking Skills Test

The California Critical Thinking Skills Test (CCTST) College Level (Facione, 1990) is a 34-item multiple-choice test taken in 45 minutes that measures overall critical thinking skills, in addition to five subscales that specifically assess analysis, evaluation, inference, deductive reasoning, and inductive reasoning. The maximum score is 34 on the skills test (Brunt, 2005). Reliability has been reported as 0.68 to 0.70, using the Kuder-Richardson internal reliability coefficient (Facione, 1990). The CCTST measures critical thinking in realistic problem situations and provides an objective measure of critical thinking skills. Different questions progressively invite analysis or interpretation of information presented in order to draw accurate and warranted inferences. Students then evaluate inferences and explain why they represent strong reasoning or weak reasoning, or explain why a given evaluation of an inference is strong or weak. Critical thinking can be manifested in the successful application of one's skills to a wide range of images and graphical elements into the content of questions, thus enabling test-takers to demonstrate the range as well as the depth of their critical thinking skills (Insight Assessment, 2010).

Giddens and Gloeckner (2005) reported a positive relationship between critical thinking skills and NCLEX-RN success when this tool was used. McMullen and McMullen (2009) reported on the critical thinking skills of master's prepared nurse practitioner students. The findings indicated change in student critical thinking skills based on scores from the evaluation, inference, and analysis subscales on the CCTST. During the students' educational program, patterns of change in critical thinking skills varied for different students depending on the level of critical thinking skills upon entrance into the program. Students at higher and median skill levels at program entry exhibited modest increases in evaluation skill, stable inference skills, and a sharp decline in analytic skills as compared to students reporting lower levels of total critical thinking skills who demonstrated substantial growth in all three critical thinking skills.

California Critical Thinking Disposition Inventory

The California Critical Thinking Disposition Inventory (CCTDI) is a tool that surveys the dispositional aspects of critical thinking. The CCTDI asks respondents to indicate the extent to which they agree or disagree with 75 statements expressing beliefs, values, attitudes, and intentions that relate to the reflective formation of reasoned judgments. The CCTDI can be administered in 20 minutes (Insight Assessment, 2010). There are seven dispositions that are the elements of one's character that move one toward using critical thinking skills. For each of the seven subscales, a score below 40 indicates a general weakness in that area and a score above 50 represents a consistent strength. A total CCTDI score below 280 represents overall deficiencies in the students' critical thinking dispositions and a score above 350 shows overall strengths (Giddens & Gloeckner, 2005). The seven dispositions are noted in Table 2-2.

Construct validity of the CCTDI was established by Facione and Facione (1992). Cronbach's alpha

for the overall instrument is .91; for the individual subscales, alphas ranged from .71 to .80. Giddens and Gloeckner (2005) investigated the relationship of critical thinking to performance on the NCLEX-RN exam. Baccalaureate nursing students ($N = 218$) completed the CCTST and CCTDI. Results showed that there was a difference between those who passed and failed the NCLEX-RN on both the entry and exit CCTST; however, neither instrument was useful in the prediction of NCLEX-RN performance. There were no differences reported between pass and fail groups for age or gender.

Clinical Reasoning

Critical thinking has been defined as the process of purposeful thinking and reflective clinical reasoning through which nurses examine ideas, assumptions, principles, beliefs, and actions in the context of practice (Brunt, 2005). Nursing needs

TABLE 2-2 Critical Thinking Dispositions

Disposition Subscales	Description
Truth seeking	A person's eagerness to seek knowledge and ask questions.
Open-mindedness	Reflects a person's tolerance of opinions different from his or her own and sensitivity to his or her own bias.
Analyticity	A person's awareness of potential problems, ability to anticipate consequences, and ability to use reason to solve dilemmas.
Systematicity	Reflects how organized, orderly, and focused a person is when approaching problems or specific issues.
Self-confidence	Reflects the level of trust a person has in his or her own ability to reason.
Inquisitiveness	A person's desire for learning. It also reflects how intellectually curious a person is and how well informed he or she is on a variety of issues.
Maturity	A preference for exercising judiciousness when making decisions. The cognitively mature person approaches problems with the attitude that there may be more than one solution and the realization that some problems are ill structured.

to focus on multiple ways of thinking with a greater emphasis on clinical reasoning. Clinical reasoning is the process by which nurses and other clinicians make their judgments, and includes the deliberate process of generating alternatives, weighing them against the evidence, and choosing the most appropriate one (Tanner, 2006). These judgments are used to assimilate information, analyze the patient data, and make decisions regarding patient care (Simmons, Lanuza, Fonteyn, & Hicks, 2003). Clinical reasoning is also defined as reasoning across time about particular situations, through changes in the patient's condition or concerns and/or changes in the clinician's understanding of the patient's clinical condition or concerns (Benner et al., 2008).

Reflective clinical reasoning is essential for deconstructing situations of practice breakdown and for questioning information that is received that requires reform or innovation. Critical reflection and the use of evidence-based knowledge will assist nurses to understand patient needs and take definitive action. Nurse educators should shift their approach from an exclusive emphasis on critical thinking to an emphasis on clinical reasoning and multiple ways of thinking (Benner et al., 2008). Use of learning activities that incorporate analysis, application, and clinical reasoning is beneficial. This type of experiential learning applies a concept in a clinical context that is consistent with integrative pedagogy (Giddens, 2010).

Assessing patient needs by analyzing data to identify and frame problems within the clinical environment reflects students' clinical reasoning ability. The Outcome-Present State Test (OPT) Model of Clinical Reasoning is a nursing process model designed to assist students in developing clinical reasoning skills (Pesut & Herman, 1999). By using this model, not only did students gain clinical reasoning skills, but they also used and learned more about the North American Nursing Diagnosis Association, Nursing Interventions Classification, and Nursing Outcomes Classification languages. Bland et al. (2009) reported significant improvements in undergraduate nursing students' ability to frame the patient's story and identify the correct keystone issues in a psychiatric course. They recommend the comparison of the OPT model with a standard care plan used in the clinical component of other nursing courses, allowing further insight into students' thought processes.

Measuring nursing students' critical thinking outcomes using a tool such as the CCTDI would be a useful comparison with outcomes from the OPT model (Bartlett et al., 2008).

Nursing programs are struggling with how to incorporate educational content and practice strategies to promote safe, quality care for patients seeking health care (Miller & LaFramboise, 2009). In an effort to change how nurses are educated with regard to safe, quality patient care, the Robert Wood Johnson Foundation support a nationwide project entitled Quality and Safety Education for Nurses (QSEN), which incorporates the Institute of Medicine (IOM) competencies. The AACN has made the IOM and QSEN competencies a substantial component of *The Essentials for Baccalaureate Education for Professional Nursing Practice* (AACN, 2008). The *Essentials* has stated several assumptions regarding how baccalaureate graduates are prepared, including using clinical reasoning to address patient situations that range from simple to complex (AACN, 2008).

Clinical Judgment

Clinical judgment is the outcome of critical thinking in nursing practice. Clinical judgments begin with an end in mind. Judgments are about evidence, meaning, and outcomes achieved (Pesut, 2001). Clinical judgment also means the conclusion about a patient's needs, concerns, or health problems, and the decision to take action (or not), use or modify standard approaches, or improvise new ones as deemed appropriate by the patient's response (Tanner, 2006). Clinical judgment is case-based, contextually bound, interpretive reasoning. It is always in the context of the particular patient, a deep understanding of the patient's experience, and preferences and values, within the ethical standards of the discipline. The emergence of simulation is an example of case-based teaching, providing students with real-time experience of thinking in action. Case-based teaching holds great promise for helping learners to develop habits of thought that our profession has identified as central to our practice—evidence-based practice, critical thinking, and clinical judgment—learning to draw on these skills in the context of realistic clinical situations (Tanner, 2009).

In many communities, the number of nursing students exceeds the number of clinical placements available. Students are assigned a patient and prepare a care plan prior to direct contact with the patient. Students then provide patient care for an entire clinical day. In the current health care environment, the patient for whom students so diligently prepared may already be discharged before students arrive on the clinical unit (Nielsen, 2009). Teacher–student contact time may be consumed with checking preparations and asking key questions to ensure students are safe in the clinical environment, thus decreasing time available for more meaningful interaction that promotes deeper understanding of the clinical situation and supports development of clinical judgment (Randall, Tate, & Lougheed, 2007).

Cognitive Development

Cognitive development has been defined as "the way in which individuals reason, view knowledge, manage diversity of opinion and conflicting points of view, and relate to authorities or experts" (McGovern & Valiga, 1997, p. 29). The level of a student's cognitive development can have an impact on his or her ability to think critically and make autonomous clinical decisions.

Historically, schools of nursing have used GPAs as their only criterion for admission and subsequently student retention, academic success, and quality and diversity of the student population might be affected adversely (McNelis et al., 2010). GPA and standardized test scores, such as Scholastic Aptitude Test (SAT) and ACT scores, have often been used to determine a student's overall cognitive abilities. However, sole reliance on grades and standardized test scores is not enough. These need to be considered in conjunction with other assessments to determine a student's overall potential. A student who scores well on standardized tests or earns high grades may or may not do well with the affective or psychomotor aspects of nursing. Conversely, a student who does well with the affective and psychomotor aspects of nursing may not be able to analyze and synthesize all of the information needed to make appropriate clinical decisions.

McNelis et al. (2010) evaluated the implementation of a revised admission policy to a baccalaureate nursing program. In addition to a weighted GPA, criteria were added to include an interview, a writing sample, and a service requirement. Revised admission criteria were the student's critical, analytical, and science GPA; nursing GPA; interview; and service experience. Results suggested that the revised approach to student admission was successful in its initial implementation.

Several assessment activities can be used to determine the cognitive abilities of students before they begin a program. These activities can be used to determine students' current level of knowledge and skill development and can occur at the institutional, program, or course level. Data gathered from such activities can be used to recommend and plan a student's program of study and other more specific learning experiences. For example, at the course level, the best way to determine whether a student has a particular psychomotor skill is to have the student demonstrate the skill. Further learning activities can then be planned based on the level of psychomotor skill the student has demonstrated. A written pretest can be effective in determining a student's cognitive knowledge level about a specific concept. If there is not enough time in a course to have each student demonstrate a skill or to conduct a pretest, asking the students as a whole whether they are able to perform certain skills or can demonstrate certain levels of cognitive knowledge may suit the faculty's purposes.

A more inclusive testing process provides a more comprehensive student profile that can be used to design learning experiences. At the institutional and program levels this would include testing of prospective students before acceptance or as part of the acceptance process to the institution, the nursing major, or both. The testing could include assessment of learning style preferences, mathematical abilities, reading and writing abilities, stress and coping strategy preferences, and critical thinking abilities. A program could then be developed to maximize the fit to the student profile.

Several issues are related to the selection and use of assessment and diagnostic instruments. Initially, faculty must consider the time and expense of administering the instrument. Some instruments may require that scoring be performed by the company that sells the tools. This can create a delay in having the results returned to faculty, which could make it difficult for faculty to make programming decisions in a timely fashion. Other issues include whether all students should take the tests and, if not, which students would benefit the most from the results of the testing information. Faculty need to be diligent in sharing assessment results with students and ensuring students understand and are able to explain their results. Further, faculty should strategize with students on how to use their results to improve academic outcomes.

Fostering Development of Cognitive Abilities

McGovern and Valiga (1997) recommended a systematic approach to developing the cognitive abilities of students. If faculty view cognitive development as an ongoing process that occurs throughout the program, it is reasonable to assume that any systematic approach to the cognitive development of students will require frequent assessment of students' abilities, along with appropriate feedback to students.

Within the educational program itself, fostering the development of cognitive abilities in students requires faculty to shift the major focus of concern from content to the student. It will be imperative that faculty continually "rethink" their approach to "teaching" and use varied learning methods to meet the needs of all students. Equally important is the need to continually revisit the level of student abilities and creatively offer more challenging and clinical reasoning opportunities as students progress through their program (Green, 2006). Learning experiences that require active involvement in the learning process, such as reflective writing, simulations, and concept mapping, are more appropriate for developing cognitive abilities. Such student-centered efforts can help foster the development of self-assessment skills in students, as well as the development of lifelong learning skills.

One of the NLN's Hallmarks of Excellence in Nursing Education is for students to be excited about learning and exhibit a commitment to lifelong learning (Ironside & Valiga, 2006). Current students need to be empowered to be efficient lifelong learners who remain marketable and constantly broaden their knowledge and skills. This knowledge may involve becoming open to different methods of learning, moving from their comfort zone of being a passive learner to a more active learner. Lifelong learning is the only answer for a competitive future (NLN, 2005).

SUMMARY

This chapter describes the demographic characteristics of the current population of nursing students and the unique needs of students from varied generations, men in nursing, and students who are not in the racial or ethnic majority in their classrooms. The chapter also provides information related to understanding learning styles, multiple ways of thinking, and the cognitive abilities of students. Faculty are responsible for establishing an environment that is conducive to learning. Likewise, students are responsible for identifying environments that will best help them to learn. Understanding students' diverse needs will help faculty and students develop collaborative partnerships that will foster the acquisition of the attitudes, knowledge, and skills necessary to become a nurse.

REFLECTING ON THE EVIDENCE

1. Assess learning style preferences with instruments that fit the needs of your students. Do you share the results of the learning style preference assessment with the students? Do you ask the students if they intend to use their learning style preference information and counsel them on strategies that will help them to be successful?

2. Engage students in creative learning environments that appeal to their diverse needs and learning styles. Do you offer several options for instructional strategies? Do you provide your students a choice of delivery method?

3. Assess critical thinking in students and assist them to use this knowledge to problem-solve and make sound clinical and nursing decisions. Do you create opportunities for students to develop their critical thinking?

4. Teach students multiple ways of thinking, with greater emphasis on clinical reasoning and clinical judgment. Do you create opportunities for students to develop their clinical reasoning and clinical judgment skills?

5. Assessing cognitive development may aid in determining a student's overall potential and fit to your nursing program. Do you foster the development of students' cognitive abilities by establishing a creative environment that meets the needs of diverse students? Are you promoting student-centered learning and development of lifelong learners?

REFERENCES

Akdemir, O., & Koszalka, T. (2008). Investigating the relationships among instructional strategies and learning styles in online environments. *Computers & Education, 50*, 1451–1461.

Ali, N., Hodson-Carlson, K., & Ryan, M. (2004). Students' perceptions of online learning: Implications for teaching. *Nurse Educator, 29*(3). 111–112.

Amaro, D., Abriam-Yago, K., & Yoder, M. (2006). Perceived barriers for ethnically diverse students in nursing programs. *Journal of Nursing Education, 45*(7), 247–254.

American Association of Colleges of Nursing. (1998). *The essentials of baccalaureate education for professional nursing practice*. Washington, DC: Author.

American Association of Colleges of Nursing. (2008). *The essentials of baccalaureate education for professional nursing practice*. Washington, DC: Author.

American Association of Colleges of Nursing. (2009). *The annual report advancing higher education in nursing*. Retrieved from http://www.aacn.nche.edu/Media/Annualreport.htm

Ames, P. (2003). Gender and learning style interactions in students' computer attitudes. *Journal of Educational Computing Research, 28*(3), 231–244.

Aragon, S., Johnson, S., & Shaik, N. (2002). The influence of learning style preference on student success in online vs. face-to-face environments. *The American Journal of Distance Education, 16*, 227–44.

Assessment Technologies Institute. (2000). *Technical manual for the self assessment inventory*. Overland Park, KS: Author.

Bandura, A. (1986). *Social foundations of thought and action: A social cognitive theory*. Englewood Cliffs, NJ: Prentice Hall.

Bartlett, R., Bland, A., Rossen, E., Kautz, D., Benfield, S., & Carnevale, T. (2008). Evaluation of the outcome-present state test model as a way to teach clinical reasoning. *Journal of Nursing Education, 47*, 337–344.

Beacham, T., Askew, R. & Williams, P.R. (2009).Strategies to increase racial/ethnic student participation in the nursing profession. *The ABNF Journal, 20*(3), 69–72.

Bednarz, H., Schim, S., & Doorenbos, A. (2010). Cultural diversity in nursing education: Perils, pitfalls, and pearls. *Journal of Nursing Education, 49*(5), 253–260.

Bell-Scriber, M. (2008). Warming the nursing education climate for traditional-age learners who are male. *Nursing Education Perspectives, 29*(3), 143–150.

Benner, P., Sutphen, M., Leonard, V., & Day, L. (2010). *Educating nurses: A call for radical transformation*. San Francisco, CA: Jossey-Bass.

Benner, P., Sutphen, M., Leonard-Kahn, V., & Day, L. (2008). Formation and everyday ethical comportment. *American Journal of Critical Care, 17*(5), 473–476.

Bland, A., Rossen, E., Bartlett, R., Kautz, D., Carnevale, T., & Benfield, S. (2009). Implementation and testing for the OPT model as a teaching strategy in an undergraduate psychiatric nursing course. *Nursing Education Perspectives, 10*, 14–21.

Bradshaw, M., & Lowenstein, A. (2011). *Innovative teaching strategies in nursing and related health professions* (5th ed.). Sudbury, MA: Jones and Bartlett.

Brown, J. (2008). Developing an English-as-a-second language program for foreign-born nursing students at an historically black university in the United States. *Journal of Transcultural Nursing, 19*, 184–191. doi: 10.1177/104365960731297

Brown, J., & Marshall, B. (2008). Continuous quality improvement: An effective strategy for improvement of program outcomes in a higher education setting. *Nursing Education Perspectives, 29*, 205–211.

Brown, S., Santiago, D., & Lopez, E. (2003). Latinos in higher education. *Change, 35*(2), 40–46.

Brunt, B. (2005). Critical thinking in nursing: An integrated review. *Journal of Continuing Education in Nursing, 36*(2), 60–67.

Burruss, N. (2010). *Variables associated with intent to use learning style preference information by undergraduate nursing students*. Unpublished doctoral dissertation, Indiana University, Indianapolis.

Butler, T., & Pinto-Zipp, G. (2005). Students' learning styles and their preferences for online instructional methods. *Journal of Education Technology Systems, 34*, 199–221.

Campinha-Bacote, J. (2010). The Process of Cultural Competence in the Delivery of Healthcare Services. In M. Douglas and D. Pacquiao (Eds.) Core Curriculum in Transcultural Nursing and Health Care. *Journal of Transcultural Nursing, 21*(1), 119S–127S.

Canfield, A. (1980). *Learning styles inventory manual*. Ann Arbor, MI: Humanics Media.

Choi, I., Lee, S., & Jung, J. (2008). Designing multimedia case-based instruction accommodating students' diverse learning styles. *Journal of Educational Multimedia and Hypermedia, 17*(1), 5–25.

Claxton, C., & Murrell, P. (1987). *Learning styles: Implications for improving educational practices*. Washington, DC: George Washington University, School of Education and Human Development.

Cook, D., Gelula, M., Dupras, D., & Schwartz, A. (2007). Instructional methods and cognitive and learning styles in web-based learning: Report of two randomized trials. *Medical Education, 41*(9), 897–905.

Dunn, R., & Dunn, K. (1978). *Teaching students through their individual learning styles: A practical approach*. Upper Saddle River, NJ: Prentice Hall.

Dunn, R., & Dunn, K. (1999). *The complete guide to the learning styles in-service system*. Boston, MA: Allyn & Bacon.

Dunn, R., Dunn, K., & Price, G. (1986). *Productivity environmental preferences survey*. Lawrence, KS: Price Systems, Inc.

Dunn, R., Dunn, K., & Price, G. (1993). *Productivity environmental preference survey*. Lawrence, KS: Price Systems.

Dunn, R., Dunn, K., & Price, G. (1996). *Productivity environmental preference survey*. Lawrence, KS: Price Systems, Inc.

Dunn, R., & Griggs, S. (2000). *Practical approaches to using learning styles in higher education*. Westport, CT: Bergin & Garvey.

Elam, C., Stratton, T., & Gibson, D. D. (2007). Welcoming a new generation to college: The millennial students. *Journal of College Admission*, Spring, 21–25.

Ellis, D., Meeker, B., & Hyde, B. (2006). Exploring men's perceived educational experiences in a baccalaureate program. *Journal of Nursing Education, 45*, 523–527.

Emerson, R., & Records, K. (2008). Today's challenge, tomorrow's excellence: The practice of evidence-based education. *Journal of Nursing Education, 47*, 359–370.

Evans, B. (2008). The importance of educational and social backgrounds of diverse students to nursing program success. *Journal of Nursing Education, 47*, 305–313.

Facione, P. (1990). *The California critical thinking skills test: College level.* Millbrae, CA: California Academic Press.

Facione, P., & Facione, N. (1992). *The California critical thinking dispositions inventory.* Millbrae, CA: California Academic Press.

Felder, R. (1996). Matters of style. *American Society for Engineering Education, 6*(4), 18–23.

Finke, L. (2009). Teaching in nursing: The faculty role. In D. Billings & J. Halstead (Eds.), *Teaching in nursing: A guide for faculty* (3rd ed., pp. 3–17). St. Louis, MO: Saunders.

Flanagan, N., & McCausland, L. (2007). Teaching around the cycle: Strategies for teaching theory to undergraduate nursing students. *Nursing Education Perspectives, 28,* 310–314.

Fleming, N. (2001). *Teaching and learning styles: VARK strategies.* Christchurch, New Zealand: Neil D. Fleming.

Fountain, R., & Alfred, D. (2009). Student satisfaction with high-fidelity simulation: Does it correlate with learning styles? *Nursing Education Perspectives, 30*(2), 96–98.

Gardner, J. (2005a). Barriers influencing the success of racial and ethnic minority students in nursing programs. *Journal of Transcultural Nursing, 16,* 155–162.

Gardner, J. D. (2005b). A successful minority retention project. *Journal of Nursing Education,44 (12),* 566–568.

Giddens, J. (2010). The immunity game: Conceptual learning through learner engagement. *Journal of Nursing Education, 49,* 422–423.

Giddens, J., & Gloeckner, G. (2005). The relationship of critical thinking to performance on the NCLEX-RN. *Journal of Nursing Education, 44,* 85–89.

Grasha, A. (1996). Teaching with style. *College Teaching, 47*(4), 130–135.

Green, D. (2006). A synergy model of nursing education. *Journal of Staff Development,22 (6),* 277–283.

Gregorc, A. (1982). *Gregorc style delineator: Development, technical and administrative manual.* Maynard, MA: Gabriel Systems, Inc.

Hassouneh, D. (2008). Reframing the diversity question: Challenging eurocentric power hierarchies in nursing education. *Journal of Nursing Education, 47,* 291–292.

Hauer, P., Straub, C., & Wolf, S. (2005). Learning styles of allied health students using Kolb's LSI-IIa. *Journal of Allied Health, 34*(3), 177–182.

Heppner, F. (2007). *Teaching the large college class: A guidebook for instructors with multitudes.* San Francisco, CA: Jossey-Bass.

Holstein, B., Zangrilli, B., & Taboas, P. (2006). Standardized testing tools to support quality educational outcomes. *Quality Management in Health Care, 15,* 300–308.

Honey, P., & Mumford, A. (1986). *Using your learning styles.* Maidenhead, Berkshire, UK: Peter Honey Publications.

Honey, P., & Mumford, A. (1992). *The manual of learning styles.* Maidenhead, Berkshire, UK: Peter Honey Publications.

Howe, N., & Strauss, W. (2000). *Millennials rising: The next great generation.* New York, NY: Vintage Books.

Insight Assessment. (2010). California critical thinking disposition inventory. Retrieved from http://www.insightassessment.com/Scales%20CCTDI.html

Ironside, P., & Valiga, T. (2006). National survey on excellence in nursing education. *Nursing Education Perspectives, 27*(3), 166–169.

Johnson, S. & Romanello, M. (2005). Generational diversity, *Nurse Educator30 (5),* 212–216.

Kalb, K. (2008). Core competencies of nurse educators: Inspiring excellence in nurse educator practice. *Nursing Education Perspectives, 29*(4), 217–219.

Keefe, J. (1987). *Learning styles theory and practice.* Reston, VA: National Association of Secondary School of Principals.

Kolb, D. (1978). *Learning style inventory: Technical manual* (Rev. ed.). Boston, MA: William McBee.

Kolb, D. (1984). *Experiential learning: Experience as the source of learning and development.* Englewood Cliffs, NJ: Prentice Hall.

Lee, K. (2007). Online collaborative case study learning. *Journal of College Reading and Learning, 37*(2), 82–100.

Linares, A. (1999). Learning styles of students and faculty in selected health care professions. *Journal of Nursing Education, 38,* 407–414.

Liu, Y. (2007). A comparative study of learning styles between online and traditional students. *Journal of Educational Computing Research, 37*(1), 41–63.

Lovelace, M. (2005). Meta-analysis of experimental research based on the Dunn and Dunn model. *The Journal of Educational Research, 98*(3), 176–183.

Martin-Holland, J., Bello-Jones, T., Shuman, A., Rutledge, D. N., & Sechrist, K. R. (2003). Ensuring cultural diversity among California nurses. *Journal of Nursing Education, 42*(6), 245–248.

Martinez, T., &. Martinez, A. (2003). Nursing schools ratchet up recruitment of Hispanics. *Hispanic Outlook, 13,* 10–13.

McGovern, M., & Valiga, T. (1997). Promoting the cognitive development of freshman nursing students. *Journal of Nursing Education, 36,* 29–35.

McMullen, M., & McMullen, W. (2009). Examining patterns of change in the critical thinking skills of graduate nursing students. *Journal of Nursing Education, 48,* 310–318.

McNelis, A., Wellman, D., Krothe, J., Hrisomalos, D., Mcelveen, J., & South, R. (2010). Revision and evaluation of the Indiana University School of Nursing baccalaureate admission process. *Journal of Professional Nursing, 26*(3), 188–195.

McQueen, L., & Zimmerman, L. (2004). The role of historically black colleges and universities in the inclusion and education of Hispanic nursing students. *The ABNF Journal, 15*(3), 51–54.

Miller, C., & LaFramboise, L. (2009). Student learning outcomes after integration of quality and safety education competencies into a senior-level critical care course. *Journal of Nursing Education, 48,* 678–685.

National League for Nursing. (2005). *Core competencies of nurse educators with task statements.* Retrieved from http://www.nln.org/facultydevelopment/pdf/corecompetencies.pdf

National League for Nursing. (2007). *Critical thinking in clinical nursing practice/RN examination.* Retrieved from http://www.nln.org/testproducts/pdf/CTinfobulletin.pdf

National League for Nursing. (2008). *Certified nurse educator (CNE) candidate handbook.* New York, NY: Author.

National League for Nursing. (2009a). Percentage of basic RN students and U.S. college students over age 30 by program type. NLN DataView™. Retrieved from http://www.nln.org/research/slides/xls/AS0809_f18.ppt

National League for Nursing. (2009b). Percentage of minorities enrolled in basic RN programs by race-ethnicity. NLN DataView™. Retrieved from http://www.nln.org/research/slides/xls/AS0809_f19.ppt

National League for Nursing. (2009c). Percentage of students enrolled in nursing programs by sex and program type. NLN DataView™. Retrieved from http://www.nln.org/research/slides/xls/AS0809_f19.ppt

Nielsen, A. (2009). Concept-based learning activities using the clinical judgment model as a foundation for clinical learning. *Journal of Nursing Education, 48*, 350–354.

Noble, K., Miller, S., & Heckman, J. (2008). The cognitive style of nursing students: Educational implications for teaching and learning. *Journal of Nursing Education, 47*, 245–253.

O'Lynn, C. (2004). Gender-based barriers for male students in nursing education programs: Prevalence and perceived importance. *Journal of Nursing Education, 43*, 229–236.

Pesut, D. (2001). Clinical judgment: Foreground/background. *Journal of Professional Nursing, 17*(5), 215.

Pesut, D., & Herman, J. (1999). *Clinical reasoning: The art and science of critical and creative thinking.* New York, NY: Delmar.

Peter, C. (2005). Learning—whose responsibility is it? *Nurse Educator, 30*(4), 159–165.

Randall, C., Tate, B., & Lougheed, M. (2007). Emancipatory teaching–learning philosophy and practice education in acute care: Navigating tensions. *Journal of Nursing Education, 46*, 60–64.

Rassool, G., & Rawaf, S. (2007). Learning style preferences of undergraduate nursing students. *Nursing Standard, 21*(32), 35–41.

Reese, V., & Dunn, R. (2007). Learning style preferences of a diverse freshman population in a large, private, metropolitan university by gender and GPA. *Journal of College Student Retention, 9*(1), 95–112.

Reichmann, S., & Grasha, A. (1974). A rational approach to developing and assessing the construct validity of a student learning style scale instrument. *The Journal of Psychology, 87*, 213–223.

Riddell, T. (2007). Critical assumptions: Thinking critically about critical thinking. *Journal of Nursing Education, 46*, 121–126.

Romeo, E. (2010). Quantitative research on critical thinking and predicting nursing students' NCLEX-RN performance. *Journal of Nursing Education, 49*, 378–386.

Rush, K., Dyches, C., Waldrop, S., & Davis, A. (2008). Critical thinking among RN-to-BSN distance students participating in human patient simulation. *Journal of Nursing Education, 47*(11), 501-507.

Salter, D., Evans, N., & Forney, D. (2006). A longitudinal study of learning style preferences on the Myers-Briggs Type Indicator and Learning Style Inventory. *Journal of College Student Development, 47*, 173–184.

Sauter, M., Johnson, D., & Gillespie, N. (2009). *Educational program evaluation.* St. Louis, MO: Saunders Elsevier.

Shin, K., Jung, D., Shin, S., & Kim, M. (2006). Critical thinking dispositions and skills of senior nursing students in associate, baccalaureate, and RN-to BSN programs. *Journal of Nursing Education, 45*(6), 233-237.

Simmons, B., Lanuza, D., Fonteyn, M., & Hicks, F. (2003). Clinical reasoning in experienced nurses. *Western Journal of Nursing Research, 25*, 701–719.

Slater, J., Lujan, H., & DiCarlo, S. (2007). Does gender influence learning style preferences of first-year medical students? *Advances in Physiology Education, 31*, 336–342.

Smith, J. (2006). Exploring the challenges for nontraditional male students transitioning into a nursing program. *Journal of Nursing Education, 45*, 263–269.

Soroff, L., Rich, E., Rubin, A., Strickland, R., & Plotnick, H. (2002). A transcultural nursing educational environment: An imperative for multi-cultural students. *Nurse Educator, 27*(4), 151–154.

Starr, K. (2009). Nursing education challenges: Students with English as an additional language. *Journal of Nursing Education, 48*, 478–487.

Stephey, M. J. (2008, April 16). Gen-X: The ignored generation. *Time.* Retrieved from http://www.time.com/time/arts/article/0,8599,1731528,00.html

Stewart, S., & Cleveland, R. (2003). A pre-college program for culturally diverse high school students. *Nurse Educator, 28*(3), 107–110.

Stott, A. (2007). Exploring factors affecting attrition of male students from an undergraduate nursing course: A qualitative study. *Nursing Education Today, 27*, 325–332.

Suliman, W. (2006). Critical thinking and learning styles of students in conventional and accelerated programs. *International Nursing Review, 53*, 73–79.

Sutcliffe, L. (1993). An investigation into whether nurses change their learning style according to subject area studied. *Journal of Advanced Nursing, 18*, 647–658.

Swail, W. (2002). Higher education and the new demographics. *Change, 34*(4), 15–23.

Tanner, C. (2006). Thinking like a nurse: A research-based model of clinical judgment in nursing. *Journal of Nursing Education, 45*, 204–211.

Tanner, C. (2009). The case for cases: A pedagogy for developing habits of thought. *Journal of Nursing Education, 48*, 299–300.

Tinto, V. (1993). *Leaving college: Rethinking the causes and cures of student attrition.* Chicago: University of Chicago Press.

U. S. Census Bureau, (2007). Age Distribution of the Population by Sex and Generation. Retrieved from http://www.census.gov/population/www/socdemo/age/age_sex_2007.html

U.S. Department of Education, National Center for Education Statistics. (2009). *Digest of education statistics, 2008.* (NCES 2009-020).

U.S. Department of Health and Human Services, Health Resources and Services Administration. (2010). *The registered nurse population: Initial findings from the 2008 National Sample Survey of Registered Nurses.* Retrieved from http://www.bhpr.hrsa.gov/healthworkforce/rnsurvey/initialfindings2008.pdf

Villarruel, A., Canales, M., & Torres, S. (2001). Bridges and barriers: Educational mobility of Hispanic nurses. *Journal of Nursing Education, 40*(8), 245–251.

Wacks, G. (2005). *Relationships among pre-admission characteristics in associate degree nursing programs as predictors of NCLEX-RN success.* (Unpublished doctoral dissertation). The University of Alabama, Birmingham.

Walker, J., Martin, T., White, J., Elliott, R., Norwood, A., Mangum, C., & Haynie, L. (2006). Generational (age) differences in nursing students' preferences for teaching methods. *Journal of Nursing Education, 45*, 371–374.

Wehrwein, E., Lujan, H., & DiCarlo, S. (2007). Gender differences in learning style preferences among undergraduate physiology students. *Advances in Physiology Education, 31*, 153–157.

Wellman, D. (2009). The diverse learning needs of students. In D. Billings & J. Halstead (Eds.), *Teaching in nursing: A guide for faculty* (3rd ed., pp. 18–32). St. Louis, MO: Saunders Elsevier.

Willcoxson, L., & Prosser, M. (1996). Kolb's learning style inventory: Review and further study of validity and reliability. *British Journal of Educational Psychology, 66*, 247–257.

3 The Academic Performance of Students: Legal and Ethical Issues

Elizabeth G. Johnson, DSN, RN

Nursing faculty have many things to consider as they assist students in the learning process. Developing curriculum content, choosing teaching strategies, and developing student evaluation plans can be major areas of focus. However, in carrying out these functions, faculty must also consider the legal and ethical concepts that influence the process and product of nursing education.

Just as nurses in practice have guidelines, nurse educators are guided by legal and ethical principles and policies. Nursing faculty are responsible for understanding the broad legal and ethical principles that apply in all circumstances, as well as those specific to their own setting. Major problems can occur if faculty lack an understanding of these principles and policies and are unable to apply them appropriately.

Many potential problems can be avoided if faculty take a proactive approach to anticipate student concerns. Faculty members who treat students with respect, provide honest and frequent communication about progress toward course goals and objectives, and are fair and considerate in evaluating performance are less likely to encounter student challenges. A learning environment that supports student growth and questioning is likely to reduce the incidence of problems, especially litigation. Suggestions for avoiding such problems are discussed later in this chapter.

The goal of the educational experience remains that students develop knowledge, skills, and values that will enable them to provide safe, effective nursing care. Nursing faculty who are able to apply general legal and ethical principles are much more likely to play their part in effectively meeting that goal.

This chapter provides an overview of the legal and ethical issues related to student academic performance that nurse educators most commonly face in the classroom and clinical setting. The chapter includes a discussion of the importance of student–faculty interactions and the legal and ethical issues related to academic performance, including the provision of due process, the student appeal process, assisting the failing student, and academic dishonesty.

Student–Faculty Interactions

The student–faculty relationship that is developed during the teaching and learning process is a very important one. Students have often identified student–faculty relationships as the relationships that most often affect learning. The Sullivan Commission Report (2004) identified several factors that "significantly determine the quality of the educational experience" (p. 84) and the student–faculty relationship is among those. There is little doubt that a positive interaction between faculty and students is likely not only to decrease legal issues but also to promote student success.

The National League for Nursing (2005) has asserted that the focus of the faculty should be on establishing a learning environment that is "characterized by collaboration, understanding, mutual trust, respect, equality, and acceptance of differences" (p. 4). Such a learning environment fosters professional growth and development on the part of both students and faculty.

Faculty in the classroom and in clinical settings encounter students whose backgrounds and learning

The author acknowledges the work of Judith A. Halstead, PhD, RN, ANEF, in the previous edition(s) of the chapter.

needs are extremely diverse. Faculty who are able to address the needs of students from an educational perspective as well as establish positive interpersonal relationships with students of varied backgrounds will make positive contributions in assisting students to meet the desired outcomes. The challenge for faculty in assisting students is to identify ways to address these varied needs. To successfully assist students, faculty must understand and appreciate cultural diversity and be able to use multiple learning strategies to assist students with varying learning styles and needs. The student role in the educational process has changed and must be one of active involvement. When faculty view students as partners or colleagues in an educational experience, they promote the development of a relationship that supports student growth and development and the attainment of educational goals and objectives.

The first step in the process of developing a learning environment that encourages collaborative and positive student–faculty interactions requires faculty to carefully examine and develop an awareness of their own beliefs and values about the teaching–learning process. Working collaboratively with students will require faculty to adopt strategies that involve active student participation and do not place faculty in the role of having sole responsibility for determining learning experiences. Activities such as cooperative group work, debate and discussion, role playing, and problem-solving exercises are examples of interactive teaching strategies that shift the focus from the faculty to the student. Such a pedagogical shift in teaching may also require faculty to leave behind the "safety" and control of the classroom lecture and develop more fully the skills necessary to successfully incorporate interactive teaching strategies into the classroom. Chapter 15 provides further discussion of teaching strategies that promote active learning.

Another important step in the process of developing a positive learning environment is examining attitudes and beliefs that students bring to the learning environment. Students may lack confidence of their abilities in the academic environment, especially those who are first-generation college students and lack role models who have been successful in pursuing higher education. Empowerment of students can occur when faculty demonstrate a sense of caring and commitment to students, and use courtesy and respect in interactions. Having a role in

developing their own learning experiences can also prove to be an empowering experience for students.

How can nursing faculty successfully incorporate this concept of empowerment and equity into student–faculty relationships? Educators can design learning activities and projects that demonstrate collaborative learning and collegial interactions between faculty, students, and nurses in practice settings (Halstead, 1996). For example, the use of computer-mediated communication, such as e-mail and online discussion forums, tends to remove the elements of status and power from communication, thus allowing a freer exchange of information. Integrating content and discussion about empowerment, collaboration, collegiality, and teamwork throughout the curriculum can also help nurture positive student–faculty interactions. Faculty involvement in orientation programs, mentoring initiatives, academic advising, and student organizations can help promote positive student–faculty interactions outside the classroom (Halstead, 1996). Ongoing, open dialogue with students that results in clear communication of mutual expectations and responsibilities is an essential component of all successful student–faculty interactions, as is illustrated in the remaining sections of this chapter.

Legal Considerations of Student Performance

An established responsibility of faculty in nursing education programs is the evaluation of student performance in the classroom (didactic) and clinical setting. This responsibility carries with it accountability because the outcomes of such evaluation have a major impact on the student's progress in the course and even status in the program. In addition, faculty serve as the safeguard for society at large from practitioners who have not demonstrated the ability to practice safely. The courts have consistently affirmed faculty members' responsibility for evaluation and have for the most part practiced "judicial deference"—meaning that the court has not interfered with the faculty's expertise in evaluation of student academic performance—as long as due process has been provided and evaluation is deemed fair and just (Smith, 2005). However, the evaluation process must be based on principles that ensure that students' rights are not violated.

Student Rights

Faculty must be aware that students enter the educational experience with rights, just as faculty have rights. The concept of "student rights" is a relatively new one in the legal system, developing over the last 5 decades (Brent, 2001). However, there is increasing evidence of the judicial system's perception that student rights are important, and cases supporting and detailing this concept are increasing (for information about specific cases, see Brent [2001] and Guido [1997]). Rights of students that are addressed here are due process, fair treatment, and confidentiality and privacy.

Due Process

Student rights in the broadest sense are protected by the Fourteenth Amendment of the U.S. Constitution, which limits the restrictions that government may impose on an individual. This amendment states that no citizen may be deprived of life, liberty, or property without due process of law and requires that the federal government provide due process for all citizens.

Due process, then, involves assurances that procedures are "fair under the circumstances" (Brent, 2001, p. 428). Because the Fourteenth Amendment refers to state or government action, a public institution is always accountable for due process. Private institutions may not be held to these same standards because they are not considered a government arm. However, many private institutions have adopted policies ensuring due process for their students. Although private institutions may not always be held to the due process standards, to avoid problems and potential litigation, all institutions must ensure that faculty actions are not perceived as "arbitrary, capricious, or discriminatory" (Brent, 2001, p. 428).

Student rights have their foundation in two categories of due process: procedural due process and substantive due process. Procedural due process refers to process steps and requires that "individuals whose rights are affected be entitled to appropriate notice and a hearing" (Osinski, 2003, p. 56). These guidelines mandate that individuals be provided with notification of the concerns and provided with an opportunity to be heard—or to present their case to involved parties in the decision-making process.

Substantive due process involves the basis for the decision itself (or the substance of the decision) and is based on the principle that a decision should be fair, objective, and nondiscriminatory. Students who might challenge on this principle would seek to prove that a faculty decision was arbitrary or impulsive.

Other legal concepts that influence student rights come from contract law or theory. Students may also use these concepts in seeking action against an institution. Contract law is applied in this circumstance with the understanding that when students enter a university or college, they actually enter into a contract with the school. If students complete the degree requirements and follow the required procedures, then a degree will be awarded. The implied contract between the student and the school forms the basis for much student rights–oriented precedent law.

There is a difference between student concerns or grievances based on academic performance and those based on disciplinary circumstances. Academic concerns are based solely on grades or clinical performance, whereas disciplinary misconduct is based on violation of rules or policies within the school or department. Osinski (2003) reported that due process for academic challenges requires that students be informed of the problems and the need to improve, be given a time frame for doing so, and have an understanding of the consequences if they do not. When disciplinary action is considered, different rules apply. In this circumstance the individual must receive notice of the specific charge that is being made and the policy and code that has been violated. The student must have an opportunity to present a defense against the charges, usually at a formal hearing, but at least in writing. Because disciplinary dismissals may have more long-lasting effects on the individual, more complicated due process rules apply. Consider the due process rights of the student illustrated in the following scenario:

> Jane Short is a sophomore nursing student who has completed the first nursing course with a barely passing grade. She had difficulty in performing the basic nursing skills, stating that having someone watch her made her nervous. She did not come to college with a strong academic background and has struggled in making the adjustment to the required higher-level

thinking and need for decision making. However, she was able to complete the course requirements in the basic nursing course, although at a minimal level. As she progresses to the next course, she is having more difficulty. Her study skills need development and she has missed several classes. She is not doing well on tests and has been late for clinical on two occasions in the first three weeks of class. Her instructor has asked to meet with her to discuss these concerns. She informs Jane of the issues of concern and relates what needs to be done to address these concerns. She suggests some new study strategies and asks that Jane practice in the lab to become more comfortable with the procedures and skills. She also relates that continued absences and tardiness will negatively affect Jane's classroom performance and her clinical evaluation. She reminds Jane of the School of Nursing Policy that states that students who miss one third of the clinical experiences will be automatically dismissed from the program. The faculty member tells Jane that she needs to demonstrate improvement in these areas within the next three weeks. The faculty member asks Jane to add her comments to the documents containing all this information and gives Jane a copy of the document explaining the concerns and including the suggestions for improvement as well as the consequences if no change occurs. The faculty member schedules times to provide regular feedback to Jane about her progress.

What has the faculty done to uphold Jane's due process rights in this circumstance? The faculty member has made Jane aware of the situation and what needs to be done to improve it. She has made suggestions for improvement and provided Jane with a written copy of those suggestions and the consequences if no change occurs. Jane has been informed and duly notified and her due process rights have been addressed.

Fair Treatment

Students have the right to expect that they will be treated fairly, consistently, and objectively. Standards of expectations for the course provide the objective guide for evaluation and must be communicated to students early and often. Course requirements should be consistent for all students, including classroom and clinical assignments. Students should receive equivalent assignments, even if they are not identical, that allow them to demonstrate progress toward meeting course objectives. In addition, students must be provided with opportunity and appropriate time to demonstrate the outcomes required in the course. Students cannot be held accountable for end of course outcomes on the first day of class and the same principle applies in the clinical setting. Students must be provided with time to learn and then evaluation can take place; students must clearly understand the difference in the learning and the evaluation portion of the clinical experience.

Confidentiality and Privacy

Legislation that has been passed to protect health information and the privacy of patients should remind faculty of their obligation to protect information from and about students. The need for confidentiality in the faculty role is based in the same code of ethics that guides all nurses. Students have a right to expect that information about their progress in the program, their academic and clinical performance, and their personal concerns will be kept confidential.

In the course of the teaching role, faculty are often privy to information about students that is of a personal and private nature. Students often confide in faculty about events that may influence their performance in the classroom or may simply seek advice from persons they feel they can trust. This information, as in a nurse–patient interaction, must be guarded and held in confidence. Morgan (2001) pointed out the conflicts that nursing faculty often feel when deciding whether it is in the student's best interest to divulge information of a personal nature. She suggested that there should be a "compelling professional purpose" (p. 291), such as protection of patients or helping the student achieve the goal of successful completion of the program, for disclosing confidential personal information. Faculty must exercise good judgment in sharing information, making certain that it is in the student's best interest to do so and obtaining permission whenever possible. Faculty are often anxious to share a student's strengths and weaknesses with other faculty members who will have the student in subsequent semesters. Faculty must seriously consider the implications of such a practice as a standard approach. A student's performance or challenges in one class will not necessarily follow him or her to the next class. Informing other faculty members about an individual student's strengths or weaknesses may provide prejudicial information and could be interpreted as unjust. However, alerting faculty to information that may affect patient or student safety may warrant discussion.

In addition to confidentiality, privacy, especially of student records, is essential. The Buckley Amendment (often referred to as FERPA or the Federal Educational Rights and Privacy Act) provides the basis for protection of student records. This law was enacted to assure that students older than age 18 have access to their educational records and to ensure that they have some input about who can receive information in that record without their consent. The amendment also mandates that a procedure be in place that allows students to contest information in the record that is inaccurate or that they do not agree with. In actual practice, one of the most frequent applications of this law comes when parents seek information about student progress or grades without student permission. Parents are often dismayed to find that they have no "right" to information about student progress, unless the student provides permission. It is imperative that faculty understand the components of this legislation and follow it implicitly. For example, faculty cannot post grades in any form in public, leave graded materials for students to retrieve in a public place, or circulate a printed class list with student IDs or social security information as an attendance list. All of these constitute violations of FERPA and make faculty and their institutions subject to prosecution.

Schools of nursing must follow the guidelines of the institution regarding FERPA but they must also give particular attention to guarding student health records. These health records are usually kept in a separate file and should follow Health Insurance Portability and Accountability Act of 1996 (HIPAA) guidelines. Student records and evaluation notes maintained by faculty during the process of course evaluation must also be guarded to protect privacy.

Guidelines for Providing Due Process to Students

Due Process for Academic Issues

The potential for litigation always exists, even in the best of circumstances; therefore it is prudent to take actions and establish policies that decrease the likelihood that litigation will occur as a result of academic failure or dismissal. The following practices help keep students informed of faculty expectations and their progress in coursework and provide the basis for ensuring that students receive the information they need.

1. *Provide a copy of student and faculty rights and responsibilities in formal documents.* On admission to the program, students should be given a copy of rights, responsibilities, policies, and procedures that apply to students and faculty. Although institutions have the right to establish policies, they also have the responsibility to communicate those policies and guidelines to students and faculty. Policies and procedures that are in effect for all students in the institution, as well as those that are specific to a program, should be available and must be congruent. Policies should address progression, retention, graduation, dismissal, grading, and conduct. Students should also be informed of circumstances that will interfere with progression and those that would result in termination from the program. They should learn the process to follow in filing a grievance. These policies should be readily available and are usually published in faculty and student handbooks. Strategies that ensure that students have read and understand the information contained in these documents should be a part of the orientation process. In every course, faculty should plan to reinforce this information, including providing specific expectations for the course. Written specifics of requirements should be contained in the course syllabus and discussed with students on the first day of class.

2. *Review and update policies in the handbook and catalog periodically.* Published materials given to students and faculty should contain current information about academic policies and procedures. This serves to keep students and faculty informed about the policies and procedures they are subject to, and it is a requirement of institutional and program accreditation agencies. Regular review by faculty of policies and procedures ensures that faculty are aware of current policies and increases the likelihood that they will be consistent in following them.

3. *Course requirements and expectations should be clearly established and communicated at the beginning of the course.* The course syllabus should explain course requirements, critical learning experiences, and faculty expectations of student performance to satisfactorily complete the course. Schools commonly establish guidelines for information to be included in all syllabi developed for nursing courses, and faculty should follow these criteria. A course syllabus should include the following information, at a minimum: description of the course, course objectives, course credit hours, faculty responsible for the course, class schedule, attendance policies, teaching strategies used in the course, topical outlines, evaluation tools and methods, due dates for assignments, late work policy, and standards that must be met for students to pass the course. Many institutions also require that course syllabi include a statement about the need for students to notify faculty about desired accommodations for a disability. The syllabus for a course should be distributed on the first day of class to provide students the opportunity to understand and clarify course requirements.

4. *Retain all tests and written work in a file until the student has successfully completed at least the course requirements, and in some cases the program requirements.* Student assignments, tests, and evaluations are invaluable, especially in cases of academic deficiency that may result in a student challenge. All evidence of a student's performance in a class should be kept at least until that course is completed. Faculty must be aware of institutional policy or standards that govern maintenance of records and should follow those. There are no universal rules for how long student files should be maintained, and the policy may vary from institution to institution. Student clinical evaluations often become a part of the student's permanent file, although in some programs these are only retained until the student completes the program. The maintenance of files of student work and tests may also serve to decrease the likelihood of plagiarism of other students' work. Knowing that faculty keep a copy of assignments and tests may make students less likely to attempt to claim other students' work as their own. Files of student work may also serve as examples of assignments to share with evaluators during accreditation visits or to assist in outcome assessment efforts. Samples of student work may also be used to provide positive examples to other students. Faculty must obtain a student's permission to share his or her work with others. Some schools choose to have students sign a standard form granting such permission and to keep this on permanent file.

5. *Students should have the opportunity to view all evaluation data that are placed in the student file.* Students have the right to see all documentation that has been used to determine an evaluation of their performance. Students also have the right to disagree with the appraisal of their performance and should be provided with an opportunity to respond to the comments of the evaluation with comments of their own. Faculty should ask students to sign and date the evaluation form to indicate that the evaluation has been discussed with them, while providing an opportunity for them to register their own comments on the form.

6. *When students are not making satisfactory progress toward course objectives and the potential for course failure or dismissal exists, students must receive notification of and information about their academic deficiencies.* Students should receive regular feedback about the progress they have made toward meeting class and clinical objectives throughout the course. If deficiencies occur, students must receive details of what behavior is unsatisfactory, what needs to be done to improve the behavior, and the consequences if improvement does not occur. Faculty should hold formal conferences with students who are in academic jeopardy, identify the deficiencies in writing, and work with the student to determine a plan to address the deficiencies. Both the faculty member and the student should sign the document to indicate mutual involvement in and agreement to the plan. Subsequent follow-up conferences should be held to note progress or lack of progress made toward achieving the agreed-upon goals and note revisions or

additional strategies employed. All conferences should be documented in writing, and both parties should receive a copy of the documentation. An example of how this might occur was presented in the earlier example relating to Jane Short.

Faculty who fail to evaluate a student's unsatisfactory performance accurately, through either a reluctance to expose the student to the experience of failure or a fear of potential litigation, are guilty of misleading the student, potentially jeopardizing patient care, and placing faculty peers in a difficult situation. Nursing faculty and even the university are responsible for preparing safe and competent practitioners and can be held accountable if they relinquish their responsibility for doing so (Smith, McKoy, & Richardson, 2001). Student deficiencies will eventually be identified and dealt with by faculty. Students might legitimately ask why they were not notified earlier in the educational experience of these deficiencies and accuse the "failing" faculty of prejudicial behavior. It is much fairer to inform students of their unsatisfactory behaviors when such behaviors are first identified. Informing students of deficiencies in a caring, constructive manner allows them the opportunity to improve performance; to not inform them denies them this opportunity and right.

These procedures help ensure that students receive the due process related to academic failure that is their right by law. Maintaining open lines of communication with a student who is not progressing is a key component in resolving such situations satisfactorily and decreasing faculty liability. Students are much less likely to sue if they perceive that they have been treated in a fair and impartial manner and have been given information throughout the process.

Due Process for Disciplinary Issues

Students who are dismissed because of misconduct or disciplinary reasons should receive additional assurances that due process has been followed. A disciplinary action occurs when a student violates a regulation or law or has engaged in activity that is not allowed. Students must receive in writing a copy of the charges or concerns that are cited (Osinski, 2003). The information should include details about what policy or rule was violated, and enough information must be provided to ensure that the student can develop a defense against the charges. Osinski (2003) reports that students are usually granted the opportunity to speak on their own behalf and provided an opportunity to explain their actions. Students often are allowed to hear the evidence against them and to present oral or written testimony, and they may be allowed to call witnesses in their defense (Smith et al., 2001). If the student desires, legal counsel can be present to provide the student with advice but not to question or interview other participants in the proceedings. Legal counsel for the institution is usually available as well. No action should be taken by the faculty or university until a formal hearing has occurred. Depending on the institution, a councilor committee usually decides the outcome of the charges. Courts may be more likely to become involved in disciplinary actions since they involve less professional judgment and evaluation.

In the example presented earlier, if Jane Short's absences continue in clinical and she misses enough clinical days that she is dismissed from the program, then the provision for due process as a disciplinary event must include more faculty action. The faculty member must provide written information about the school policy that has been violated (although she has hopefully done that at the earlier conference) and provide an opportunity for Jane to respond to the accusations. The process must provide for Jane to present a "defense" for her actions or an opportunity to explain her actions to those persons who will make the final decision about the outcome of her situation. In this circumstance, since the issue is a disciplinary one, faculty must take additional steps to ensure that due process rights are protected.

Grievances and the Student Appeal Process

Even when a student has been treated in accordance with due process with a clear communication of policies and expected academic standards, it is possible that the student may wish to seek legal recourse in the face of an academic failure or dismissal. In such cases, the student may appeal to the court on the basis that faculty has acted in a capricious or arbitrary manner. Courts have traditionally not overturned academic decisions unless the student can prove that faculty did not follow "accepted academic norms so as to demonstrate the person or committee responsible did not actually exercise professional judgment" (*Regents of University of Michigan* v. *Ewing*, 474 U.S. 214 [106 S. Ct 507 1985]). In this case, a student who was dismissed from medical school brought suit against the university, citing that university faculty moved to dismiss him based on circumstances that were not rational and were capricious. The court ruled that the university faculty did have cause to dismiss the student and thus a "substantive due process claim" had not occurred.

There are other reasons that students may choose to bring suit against an institution. Breach of contract, described earlier, may be charged by students, particularly in private institutions, who may not be provided with due process protections. The court has generally followed the "well-steeled rule that relations between a student and a private university are a matter of contract" (*Dixon* v. *Alabama Board of Education*, 294 F. 2d 150 [5th Cir. 1961]). However, there is inconsistency in court cases that address grievances of contract issues depending on the substance of the case. Students may also make charges of defamation or violation of civil rights, including discrimination. Courts generally have not hesitated to analyze cases in which discrimination based on any parameter (e.g., race, gender, age, or disability) has been charged. Brent (2001) reported that the best way to avoid such litigation is to maintain policies that clearly demonstrate adherence to the institution's and program's guidelines, which must be in compliance with all federal and state laws regulating civil rights.

Goudreau and Chasens (2002) pointed out that recent cases in which nursing faculty have been charged with negligence in terms of protecting students from injury have also occurred. Student safety in the classroom, in the clinical area, and on clinical experiences must be a consideration of nursing faculty. Students must receive adequate preparation and instructions to avoid foreseeable risks and, as these authors stated, "Faculty members are obligated to be as concerned about students' personal safety as they are about patient safety" (p. 45).

The Student Appeal Process

Before seeking the assistance of the court system, students must first use all available recourse within the institution. Guido (1997) reported that the courts have generally relied on academic institutions to deal with grade disputes and have intervened only when due process questions come into consideration. Institutions of higher learning have established policies for hearing student grievances and appeals. See Box 3-1 for an example of such a procedure. The purpose of these guidelines is to establish common procedures to ensure that students are provided due process and that faculty rights are supported.

Institutional and program policies related to student appeals and grievance procedures should be made available in writing to students and faculty. Faculty are usually given this information in the faculty handbook on orientation to the institution and should refer to them periodically as changes are made.

Likewise, students should be informed that a formal grievance process policy exists and that it is their responsibility to initiate the procedure. It is recommended that programs distribute this information to students when they are first admitted to the institution and document that students have received such notification. Students may choose not to initiate the grievance procedure that is their right, but they should always be aware of the option of doing so. Information about the appeal process should be reviewed with an individual student if the situation warrants.

When a grievance occurs and the appeal process is implemented, there are two possible outcomes. It is possible that the appeals board may review the information provided and find that there are insufficient grounds for the student's charge and that the assigned grade or faculty action should stand. The other option is that a recommendation for corrective action may be made based on a review of evidence that indicates that the student's charges have merit. This may mean a change of grade or an opportunity for further evaluation. Implementation of the recommendations may vary depending on the specific charges and circumstances. If, at the conclusion of the institutional appeal process, the student is not satisfied with the outcome, the student has the right to pursue further recourse in the court system.

Faculty Role in the Appeal Process

Being involved in the appeal process can be a stressful experience for both the faculty member involved and the student. When a student indicates

BOX 3-1 Grades Appeal Policy – Indiana University School of Nursing, Indianapolis

The purpose of the Subcommittee on Appeals is to provide a grade appeal system that affords recourse to a student who has evidence or believes that evidence exists to show that an inappropriate grade has been assigned **as a result of prejudice, caprice, or other improper conditions** such as mechanical error, or assignment of a grade inconsistent with those assigned to other students. Additionally, a student may challenge the reduction of a grade for alleged scholastic dishonesty. In essence, the grade appeals system is designed to protect students from grade assignments that are inconsistent with policy followed in assigning grades to others in the course.

A grade will not be raised because a faculty member graded tests very severely, provided the faculty member applied the same rigorous standards to all students. Nor will proof that a faculty member has been antagonistic toward the student be sufficient cause to raise a grade unless evidence exists that such antagonism did in fact result in a lower grade. The grounds for appeal are limited. If you are not certain whether you have grounds for appeal, you should discuss your case with the Chair of the CCNF Undergraduate Student Affairs Committee.

GENERAL PROCEDURE:

The grade appeals procedure for IUSON requires that you resolve the dispute at the lowest possible level.

1. The student is required to talk to the faculty member within 5 business days of notification of the failing grade.
2. If the grade issue is not resolved after the first meeting, the faculty will assist the student to schedule a meeting with the next appropriate administrative representative (For example: the Department Chair, Assistant Dean, or Division Head) on each respective campus.
3. The student, faculty, and appropriate administrative representative or designee will meet within 5 business days. If the grade is still not resolved, begin the formal grade appeal process by completing the Student Form.
4. File a formal appeal with the Chair of the CCNF Undergraduate Student Affairs Committee. You must give notice that you plan to appeal not later than 10 days after the beginning of the semester following the semester in which the original grade was awarded. You then have 10 days from the time you file notice to prepare your appeal.

PROCEDURE FOR PREPARING A WRITTEN APPEAL:

The outcome of a case depends on the quality of the written appeal. The following points should be presented in the appeal.

1. First, state the basis for the appeal, i.e., whether you believe there was prejudice on the part of the faculty member, a mechanical error, or inconsistent grading practices. Be explicit. The appeals committee must know your grounds for appeal.
2. Second, state the evidence in support of your appeal. Present only the facts. Physical evidence should be included, such as your personal records, or tests, papers, comparisons of your score and grade scores of other students and their grades.

SCHOOL GRADE APPEALS PROCEDURE

Prior to the Hearing:

1. When first approached by a student, the Chair of the CCNF Student Affairs Committee shall provide a copy of "Suggestions to students who are preparing a grade appeal at the IUSON."
2. When the Chair of the CCNF Student Affairs Committee receives the student's written appeal, he/she contacts the Chair of the department where the grade was issued or his/her designated representative to determine whether the student has exhausted informal means of resolving the disagreement.
3. The Chair of the CCNF Student Affairs Committee shall provide the faculty member with a copy of the student's written statement, a copy of "Suggestions to Faculty who are party to a grade appeal" and request a statement in response. The faculty member shall furnish class records required to resolve the dispute along with his/her written response.
4. The Chair of the CCNF Student Affairs Committee shall contact the parties to the appeal and members of the grade appeal subcommittee to set a hearing date. All committee members should understand that grade appeals hearings are high-priority meetings. Any hearing held without a full committee as described in the Student Handbook may be challenged on the basis of procedural irregularity.
5. The Chair of the CCNF Student Affairs Committee shall furnish copies of the written statements to each committee member and involved parties in advance of the hearing. These materials are confidential and must be treated as such. They can be distributed only to those committee members who will hear the appeal and copies must be returned to the Chair at the conclusion of the hearing.

Schedule of Events:

a. The involved faculty member should be notified of the appeal on the date a written appeal from the student is received by the Chair of the CCNF Undergraduate Committee. The faculty member will complete the Faculty Form.
b. Written statements by the student and the faculty member should be distributed to the committee members and involved parties within a week of the receipt of the written appeal.

BOX 3-1 Grades Appeal Policy – Indiana University School of Nursing, Indianapolis—cont'd

c. The hearing would be held within two weeks of receipt of the written appeal.

d. Members for the appeal will consist of 3 undergraduate faculty and 3 undergraduate students.*

e. The procedure described in the School Grade Appeals Hearing Procedure shall be furnished to members of the committee and the involved parties in advance of the hearing.

f. Note*: Guiding principles statement:
   i. Faculty on APG Subcommittee will not be on the grade appeal subcommittee.
   ii. Corridor representation of faculty and students will be on the appeal subcommittee.
   iii. Place preference for the meeting will be based on the student's residence.

SCHOOL GRADE APPEALS HEARING PROCEDURE

(Proceeding in steps II–IV must be recorded on tape.)

I. Closed Session. Prior to the hour scheduled for the hearing, the committee shall meet in closed session to identify the issues in the case. Specific points that require clarification should be identified.

II. Statement by the Chair of the CCNF Student Affairs Committee. The involved parties shall then be admitted to the hearing, which will open with a statement by the Chair that describes the committee's understanding of the relevant issues and, where appropriate, those issues considered relevant. The Chair shall then ask the student and faculty member to identify and clarify issues that have been overlooked and/or justify consideration of issues the committee has identified as irrelevant.

III. Open Questioning. During this period the student, faculty member, and/or committee members may ask questions of either involved party and/or their witnesses.

IV. Summary Statements. After questions have ceased, or when the Chair is satisfied that additional questions will not provide further clarification of issues, the student and faculty member will be given an opportunity to make summary statements. Such statements should be brief and in no case exceed 5 minutes.

V. Closed Hearing. At this point, interested parties and witnesses shall be dismissed and committee members shall deliberate the outcome in a closed session.

VI. Balloting. After deliberations a secret ballot shall be taken, including a rational statement for the vote, and the vote recorded. In the case of a tie, Roberts Rules of Order will be followed.

VII. Reporting. The Chair prepares a written statement of the committee decision (including the vote of the committee), the basis for the decision, and the reasoning used by the committee shall be kept on file by the Chair. Copies of the report shall be sent to the student, the faculty member, and the Associate Undergraduate Dean.

AFTER THE HEARING:

1. The Chair will notify the student and faculty of the committee decision via e-mail within 2 business days.

2. The Chair shall collect all copies of the written statements from the committee.

3. The Chair shall retain the tape recording of the hearing, one copy of all written materials pertaining to the case, and the report of the committee decision for a period of at least one year.

4. The Chair shall submit a copy of the report of the committee decision to the Associate Undergraduate Dean.

5. A certified letter concerning the decision will be sent to the student including a statement of the rationale for the decision.

6. Higher appeal of the Subcommittee's recommendation may be made through the Associate Dean of Undergraduate Programs at IUSON.

Used with permission of Indiana University School of Nursing (2011).

---

dissatisfaction with an assigned grade or evaluation and is considering an appeal, the faculty member should give consideration to reevaluation. If the faculty member finds that the student's evidence is legitimate and that the student truly deserves a higher grade, then the grade should be changed. If the faculty member believes no changes are justified after reviewing the situation and finding that all procedures and standards have been applied consistently and justly, then the faculty member should maintain the assigned grade. However, a faculty member should not act in haste or out of fear in reaction to the threat of a grievance procedure. Changing a grade without justification sets a dangerous precedent and should be avoided. Clear, consistent use of standards for grading that are made known to students will help effectively support grades that are assigned. Planning before the implementation of a course assignment or activity and providing clearly established grading criteria may help decrease student misunderstanding.

Academic Performance in the Clinical and Classroom Settings

One major responsibility of nursing faculty is the evaluation of student academic performance. In many circumstances faculty are charged with evaluating students in both classroom (didactic) and clinical settings. Student evaluation is an expectation of faculty at all levels and requires careful consideration for many reasons.

The outcome of evaluation has a major impact on students, and faculty must always be aware of this. Boley and Whitney (2003) report that university faculty do take this responsibility seriously, contrary to what students may believe. The outcome of an evaluation usually means that students progress in the program; however, an unsatisfactory evaluation means that students may face having to repeat a course, a delay in their education, or removal from the program. These outcomes have financial, emotional, and other costs for students. In addition, faculty may also experience negative consequences, such as emotional distress, pressure from administration to maintain numbers, and a sense of personal failure when it is necessary to assign a failing grade. In the context of this stressful situation for all involved, faculty must be aware of the legal concepts important to the evaluation process.

Academic Failure in the Clinical Setting

Faculty who teach clinical nursing courses are responsible for guiding students in the development of professional nursing skills and values. Faculty must ensure that the learning experiences chosen provide the student with the opportunity to develop those skills that ensure that they will become safe, competent practitioners. Applying a theoretical knowledge base, developing psychomotor skills, using appropriate communication technique with patients and staff, exhibiting decision-making and organizational skills, and behaving in a professional manner are examples of the types of competencies that nursing students are expected to achieve through their clinical experiences. Faculty are also expected to make judgments and decisions about the ability of students to satisfactorily meet the objectives of the clinical experience. When students are unable to satisfactorily meet the objectives of the clinical experience, faculty have the legal and ethical responsibility to deny academic progression.

Legal and ethical grounds exist for dismissal of a student who is clinically deficient. Nurse Practice Acts exist in all states to regulate nursing practice and nursing education within a given state. Successful graduation from a nursing program should indicate that the student has achieved the minimum competencies required for safe practice.

When providing clinical care, nursing students are held to the same standards as the registered nurse (RN); that is, what would the reasonably prudent nurse with the same education and experience do (Guido, 1997)? Patients should expect that the care provided be safe, quality care at the level that is needed. In addition, students and faculty are expected to follow professional standards of practice and codes of ethics that have been developed to guide the profession, even though the students' educational experiences are not completed. Individual students are also accountable for their actions and may be held liable for their negligence (Guido, 1997). Students do not "practice on the instructor's license" and are accountable for their own actions, assuming that they have received adequate information and orientation to the clinical assignment.

When engaged in clinical learning experiences, the nursing student is under the supervision of the clinical faculty, with input from agency staff. The nursing staff in the facility have ultimate control over patient care that is delivered, so there must be constant and appropriate communication between staff, faculty, and students. The clinical agency contract that allows the school to use the facility for learning experiences may also contain a clause stipulating that the school of nursing will provide supervision of students. It is also common for the agency to retain the right to request removal of students and faculty if the level of performance does not meet the standard of care acceptable to the institution, and could result in the loss of the clinical agency as a site for future clinical experiences. Faculty must accept responsibility for ensuring that students practice with an acceptable level of competence. Failure of clinical faculty to intervene when an unsafe situation exists with a student's level of performance could conceivably place the faculty member, the clinical agency, and the educational institution in a legally liable situation (Guido, 1997).

Clinical faculty have several responsibilities related to the instruction of students. First, clinical faculty must set clear expectations for student performance and communicate these expectations to students before the onset of any learning experience. These expectations must be reasonable for students to meet and must be consistently and equitably applied to all of the faculty member's assigned students. Second, faculty must determine the amount of supervision to provide to students. When determining the appropriate level of supervision, faculty should consider the severity and stability of the assigned patient's condition, the types of treatments required by the patient, and the student's competency and ability to adapt to changing situations in the clinical setting. Another responsibility of clinical faculty is to judge the ability of the student to transfer classroom knowledge to the clinical setting.

Application of theory to nursing care is an important component of safe nursing practice, and faculty must engage in data collection to determine the level of student performance in this area. Faculty may collect data in multiple ways. For example, before providing care, students may be asked to develop written care plans and provide the rationale for their proposed nursing interventions. Faculty may also verbally ask students to explain the significance of patient assessment data they have gathered, or students may be asked to keep a weekly journal that provides insight into their clinical decision making. Chapters 18 and 25 provide further discussion of clinical teaching and evaluation. Whatever data collection methods are used by faculty to assess student performance must be consistently applied to all students. It is the clinical faculty's responsibility to remove students from the clinical setting if their performance is unsatisfactory and potentially harmful to patients (Boley & Whitney, 2003).

Fearing legal action, faculty may hesitate to fail a student who performs poorly in the clinical setting. However, federal and state courts have frequently upheld the responsibility and right of faculty to evaluate students' clinical performance and dismiss students who have failed to meet the criteria for a satisfactory performance. The courts have indicated that faculty, as experts in their profession, are best qualified to make decisions about the academic performance of students (Brent, 2001; Guido, 1997; Smith et al., 2001). When teaching a clinical course, faculty must clearly establish and communicate the course and clinical objectives; they must document student performance and effectively communicate with students on an ongoing basis about their progress in the clinical area. These measures are discussed in greater depth in Chapter 18. Key to the success of any of these measures is that there has been clear communication of expectations to students.

As part of this communication, faculty should clearly identify at the beginning of the course, along with the clinical objectives, the level of clinical competence that students will be expected to achieve. These requirements should be stated in the course syllabus, along with information about how the clinical grade will be determined for the course. It is also important to identify in writing the types of data that will be used to determine the clinical grade, such as preceptor evaluations, written care plans, patient feedback, direct observation, participation in clinical conferences, skills testing, professional behavior and appearance (Smith et al., 2001), and any other data used in the evaluation process. Chapter 27 provides more information about the process of clinical evaluation. Students must be informed about how data will be obtained and whether the clinical evaluation will be formative and/or summative. Students must receive continuing input through a formative evaluation process, periodically receiving information about progress and suggestions for improvement. Students must have time to demonstrate the course competency requirements during the clinical experiences and cannot be required to master those competencies until the end of the course. The consequences of not meeting objectives should also be clearly communicated to students.

Written records of all clinical experiences and student–faculty conferences should be kept for each student during the course. Smith et al. (2001) noted that anecdotal records make a significant contribution to the process of clinical evaluation.

Written records of a student's learning experiences provide documentation that the student has been provided with adequate opportunity to meet the clinical objectives. If opportunities to meet clinical objectives have not been provided, students cannot be evaluated or failed on unmet objectives.

Anecdotal records should be objectively written, describe both positive and negative aspects of a student's performance, and address the objectives of the course. Faculty should avoid commenting on the personality of the student but instead should reflect on what the student has or has not accomplished in relation to the course objectives. Dwelling on the negative aspects of the student's performance to the exclusion of any positive aspects could convey the impression that the faculty member is negatively biased toward the student (Smith et al., 2001). Notes of the student's daily and weekly assignments should be based on fact and should be nonjudgmental. Documenting both aspects of performance indicates that the student's total performance was taken into account when the final clinical grade was assigned.

Throughout the clinical experience, faculty should provide consistent, constructive feedback to students. Identifying positive aspects of a student's clinical performance and areas needing improvement will help that student develop self-esteem and confidence as a practitioner. Feedback is best conveyed in privacy, away from peers, staff, and patients, thus maintaining student confidentiality. Persistent clinical deficiencies should be addressed in conferences with the student, ideally away from the clinical setting. Written records of student–faculty conferences are used to document areas of faculty or student concern that have been discussed, along with the measures that are being taken to correct these deficiencies. Information about the progress the student makes toward correcting clinical deficiencies and any lack of progress should be included in follow-up notes. Both the faculty member and the student should sign these written records.

Communicating effectively with a student who is not performing satisfactorily can be difficult. When feedback is given to a student about deficiencies in performance, it is essential for the faculty member to convey to the student a sense of genuine concern about helping the student to improve his or her performance, as well as to convey the faculty member's responsibility for ensuring patient safety in the clinical setting. McGregor (2007) addressed the importance of the student–faculty relationship in which faculty are supportive when helping students cope with a clinical failure while at the same time retaining a sense of their self-worth and dignity. Students should be allowed the opportunity to clarify and respond to the feedback given by the faculty member. Sometimes an objective third party, such as a department chairperson or course coordinator, can assist by providing an objective perspective of the circumstances and serving as an impartial witness to what was said by both the faculty member and the student.

When notifying a student that course requirements are not being met and failure of the course may result, the faculty member must follow the institutional guidelines that have been established for such situations. Informing a student of unsatisfactory clinical performance can produce a stressful situation for the student. However, it also provides the due process that is the student's right in cases of academic deficiency. It enables the student to understand that his or her performance is unsatisfactory and provides the student with the opportunity to correct deficiencies. It is equally important that the faculty member communicate information about the student's performance to other faculty who are administratively responsible for the course.

Assisting the Failing Student in the Clinical Setting

How do clinical faculty determine when a student's clinical performance is unsatisfactory and warrants failure of the course? How many opportunities should the student be given to learn before being evaluated? These are questions that have been debated in nursing education for decades without resolution. Faculty are responsible for evaluating the cognitive, psychomotor, and affective behaviors of students during clinical learning experiences. Even with reliable and valid evaluation tools, it can be difficult to objectively evaluate the behavior of students, especially in the affective domain.

Scanlan, Care, and Gessler (2001) reported that nursing faculty have great difficulty defining behaviors that make a student "unsuited" to nursing. However, once having determined that a student's performance is unsatisfactory and that failure of the course is likely to occur, faculty must implement actions to protect the student's right to due process and assist the student through what will undoubtedly be a stressful experience.

Faculty may use several guidelines when working with students whose clinical performance is unsatisfactory. For example, as previously mentioned, unsatisfactory clinical behaviors should be identified and discussed with the student as early as possible. Documentation of the student's performance and all conferences with the student should be maintained. At this time, faculty should cite the positive aspects of the student's performance in addition to the unsatisfactory aspects (Smith et al., 2001).

Working in collaboration with the student, faculty should develop a plan or "learning contract" in which the needed areas of improvement are identified, along with appropriate measures to ensure improvement of performance. The student should be made aware that isolated instances of good or inadequate performance will not lead to a passing or failing grade. Instead, it is essential that the student strive to develop a consistency of behavior that portrays continuing improvement in performance and the delivery of safe patient care. The student should also understand that successful completion of any remedial work identified in the plan may not be sufficient to ensure a passing grade for the course; satisfactory completion of the course objectives will be required. After the plan has been detailed in a document, both the student and faculty should sign and date it. The student should be given a copy of the plan for his or her own records and reference.

Frequent feedback sessions are essential during this time, as the student attempts to make an improvement in performance. The number of sessions depends on the situation, but it is often helpful to agree to meet on a regular basis, for example, weekly. The faculty member should maintain objective and factual records of all sessions held with the student, including a description of strategies for intervention that were developed. Student self-appraisal should be a part of the process.

The student should also understand that during this period of evaluation, increased supervision and observation by faculty may be necessary to continue to ensure that patient safety is maintained. The student may report feeling treated unfairly or harassed and indicate that the increased faculty supervision is creating a stressful situation. It may be helpful at this time to refer the student to a counselor or other qualified individual for assistance with stress management. The clinical faculty member should refrain from assuming the role of counselor to the student because a conflict of interest could develop that would interfere with the objective and unbiased judgment of the instructor. Morgan (2001) cautioned that faculty, like counselors and therapists, have a responsibility to avoid assuming dual roles, such as counselor and faculty supervisor, when establishing relationships with students.

At times, a clinical instructor may experience a sense of concern about a student's performance but have difficulty clearly identifying the unsatisfactory behaviors. The instructor may wish to seek input from another faculty member about the student's performance. Faculty have the right, but no legal responsibility, to obtain an objective evaluation by another faculty member. If this is done, the faculty member must make the student aware of the purpose of this observation and that the results of the objective evaluation may have an impact on the grade awarded.

If the student continues to provide unsafe patient care despite the interventions to improve performance, faculty can withdraw the student from the course before the end of the semester. Students who might qualify for removal from the clinical setting are those who demonstrate a consistent lack of understanding of their limitations, those who clearly and repeatedly cannot anticipate the consequences of their actions or lack of action, and those who consistently fail to maintain appropriate communication with faculty and staff about patient care. If a student is dishonest with faculty and staff about the care provided to a patient, serious legal and ethical implications occur.

In all of these cases, patient care may be jeopardized and unsafe situations may be created for patients. Clinical faculty can refuse to allow a student to continue to provide care in the clinical setting; however, if the student's performance is safe, the student must be allowed to complete the clinical requirements of the course, even if the student is not meeting course objectives. Students are not required to achieve course objectives until the end of the course.

Following the mentioned procedures helps ensure that a student's right to due process has been upheld. Maintaining effective communication with the student throughout the experience may be difficult but is essential to achieving a satisfactory resolution to the situation for both faculty and student. When students perceive that they have been treated fairly and objectively, most will accept that they were unable to satisfactorily meet the objectives required of the course. Faculty should avoid excessive self-blame for the clinical failure of a student. Scanlan et al. (2001) stated, "Failing students can be viewed as an uncaring practice, when, indeed, it may be more caring to fail students than to allow them to continue" (p. 26).

Academic Failure in the Classroom Setting

Nursing program curricula are by necessity academically rigorous. Academic classroom failure, with a subsequent attrition from the nursing program, is not uncommon, and retention of nursing students is a familiar concern of nurse educators. However, faculty have a responsibility to uphold academic standards and must at times assign a failing grade in a course.

The reasons for academic failure in the classroom are numerous. First, students may initially underestimate the amount of time that they will need to devote to course study to be successful in the pursuit of a nursing degree. Students may be unprepared and lack the study and time management skills necessary to organize their schedules and study time appropriately. Students can quickly become overwhelmed with the academic demand of a nursing program, and the resulting stress serves to further increase anxiety and the inability to deal with course requirements.

Second, many of today's nursing students are attempting to fulfill numerous roles, simultaneously juggling the responsibilities and demands of work, family, and school. Role overload becomes excessive, and the students' grades are adversely affected. Students are often forced to make difficult decisions and may be ill-equipped to identify appropriate priorities when addressing these issues.

Third, some students have difficulty with the level of cognitive ability required in nursing courses. Although adept at memorizing facts and information, they are not able to apply the concepts and develop the appropriate decision-making abilities. This is usually demonstrated by their inability to perform well on tests that demand application, analysis, and synthesis levels of cognition. Students who have never before been required to think on these levels may become frustrated when they spend much time memorizing information but still do not perform well on tests.

Some students may have learning disabilities that affect their ability to read with comprehension, successfully take tests, memorize information, or maintain concentration. Some students have satisfactory clinical performance but are unable to perform well in the classroom setting. See Chapter 4 for further discussion of students with learning disabilities. Students for whom English is a second language may also experience these difficulties.

Faculty have an ethical responsibility to identify students who are considered to be at high risk for academic failure in the classroom. Examples of high-risk characteristics include low grade point average, low standardized test scores, decreased critical thinking skills, attendance at several universities without attaining a degree (Donovan, 1989), and difficulty achieving satisfactory grades in required science courses (Wolkowitz & Kelley, 2010). When students who have these characteristics are accepted into a nursing program, academic support services must be provided to increase their chances of success. Students who are working more than 16 hours a week and those who have English as a second language have also been documented to be at increased risk for lower academic performance (Salamonson & Andrew, 2006).

Faculty also have the responsibility for developing and providing academic support services that increase students' chances for success and thus increase student retention in the nursing program. Examples of services that can assist students academically are tutoring programs, individual course study sessions, study skills workshops (Hopkins, 2008), faculty–student mentoring programs, test taking support, and time and stress management training. Faculty should be aware of resources within other departments in the institution that can offer valuable assistance to students in need. They should also encourage activities that provide a support system for students, such as participation in student clubs and organizations. Peer mentoring can also be an effective educational strategy that benefits both the student serving as the mentor and the student being mentored (Dennison, 2010; Robinson & Niemer, 2010). Developing and providing support services for students with academic difficulties helps ensure that students receive the assistance they need at the earliest possible intervention point.

Assisting the Failing Student in the Classroom Setting

When designing intervention programs that will assist students to be academically successful in a nursing program, faculty must consider the academic experience from the perspective of the student because this may have major implications for student retention and success. Faculty should obtain feedback from students in the program about their areas of concern, both academic and nonacademic. For example, if students believe that large class size is interfering with their ability to learn, strategies that provide students with access to faculty in small groups could be implemented. Student focus groups can provide much feedback, and faculty can use this information to develop interventions.

Faculty also need input about what programs or interventions are working (e.g., tutoring services, orientation programs, peer-to-peer study assistance groups) so that these can be continued or eliminated according to their success. Faculty need to know what concerns students have that can be addressed with appropriate resources. Using this information, faculty would be able to develop a retention intervention program designed to maximize students' positive experiences and enhance academic success.

More specifically, faculty can implement several proactive strategies that support students' academic efforts in the classroom. First, faculty should remain aware of the changing student population and students' different learning styles. Nurse educators need to develop innovative, flexible programs designed to support the academic needs of the increasing numbers of nontraditional adult learners, graduate students, and culturally diverse students.

Flexible class scheduling, the use of technology to provide learning at convenient times for students, campus child care, recognition of students' life experiences, and support for students with English as a second language can all help students achieve their educational goals. The learning expectations and strategies of today's college students are likely to be different than those of students of the past. Much literature has been published that addresses the varying learning styles of the current generation, and information gained from those studies should be used to provide meaningful learning experiences for students.

Students who are successfully integrated academically and socially into the academic environment will more likely be retained in the system. Institutions must realize that students bring diverse needs to the educational process. The role of the faculty adviser is key in assisting students to successfully adjust to their academic responsibilities. Faculty need to be informed about academic policies that have an impact on student advisement so that they are able to provide accurate, timely information.

Williams (1993) also emphasized the importance of the faculty adviser in aiding student retention in nursing programs. In addition, Williams suggested that improving the cultural competence of faculty and developing orientation programs and support services for new students can assist in decreasing student anxiety and increase the likelihood of success in nursing studies. Nursing associations or organizations can be a source of encouragement for students and can serve as a vehicle for socializing students into the nursing profession.

Individually, faculty members can take several steps to assist students who are doing poorly in the classroom. When a student demonstrates evidence of a lack of understanding of content of the course, such as failing a test or not completing an assignment properly, the faculty member should meet with the student to identify the student's perspective of the problem. Students are often able to recognize the problem themselves, such as not enough time spent in preparation, lack of understanding of the material, or personal problems. Each of these reasons for poor performance requires the use of different intervention strategies, and the student should be involved in determining what actions are to be taken. Tests should be reviewed to assess the areas of difficulty and to determine whether the problem is potentially related to, for example, lack of knowledge about content, reading difficulties, anxiety associated with test taking, poor study skills, or personal difficulties. Once the potential causes have been identified, intervention strategies can be designed and implemented to help correct the situation.

Faculty must realize that it is the student's responsibility to learn as well as the student's responsibility to use the resources available to improve academic performance. Students must take responsibility for carrying out the plan of action developed in conjunction with the faculty member. Faculty cannot assume responsibility for ensuring that all students are successful in the course, but they must make certain that students are active participants in identifying concerns, developing strategies to address deficiencies, and improving performance. Faculty should always be willing to listen to student concerns and suggestions in a respectful manner, even if it is not always possible to carry out the suggestions (Paterson & Lane, 2000).

If, despite various efforts, a student cannot satisfactorily meet the course requirements, faculty have no alternative but to assign a failing grade. At this point, the student will require guidance and support as the available options are reviewed. If this is the first nursing course that the student has failed, it is commonly program policy to allow one retake of the course. If this is the second nursing course failure for the student, the student may be dismissed from the program. The student should receive appropriate academic advice as he or she plans future educational goals.

Ethical Issues Related to Academic Performance

Many ethical principles that influence student–faculty relationships and interactions are the same ones that guide interactions between nurses and patients. The relationship should be characterized by mutual respect and open communication. Faculty have a responsibility to conduct themselves in a manner that is exemplary, fair, nonjudgmental, and just, and should serve as role models for students in demonstrating honest academic conduct. It is apparent, though, that there is the potential for student–faculty conflict to develop in these interactions. Faculty should consider the ethical implications that

exist in relationships developed with students. This section addresses ethical issues that can develop in student–faculty relationships, including academic dishonesty and the nature of interactions occurring between students and faculty. Suggestions for avoiding the development of unethical situations are provided.

Academic Dishonesty

A student copies from another student during a test or uses "crib" notes; another student agrees to help an academically weaker student by providing answers to a test. Lacking the time it takes to write a term paper, a student turns in a paper written by another student, yet another student plagiarized portions of a term paper, taking the chance that the professor will not detect the omission of appropriate reference citations. During a clinical experience, a student forgets to administer a medication on time. Fearing the consequences of admitting the error, the student instead documents it as "given." These are all examples of academic dishonesty, or "cheating," representing one of the most difficult situations faculty have to deal with in their interactions with students.

Unfortunately, such incidents are not uncommon and as technology has developed and students have become more proficient, the methods of cheating have become more complicated and complex (DiBartolo & Walsh, 2010; Sifford, 2006). Harper (2006) reported that the use of highly sophisticated, high-tech methods of cheating has become almost commonplace and can involve the use of cameras, computer equipment, and even hacking into faculty computers. Numerous reports detail alarming statistics that demonstrate an increasing occurrence and acceptance of cheating in schools at every level. McCabe (2009) reported that while nursing faculty might think that nursing students are less likely to participate in academic dishonesty since they are engaged in a helping profession, that belief is not supported in research. Nursing faculty may be particularly concerned about academic dishonesty since a link between unethical classroom behavior and unethical clinical behavior exists.

McCabe (2009) pointed out that schools and faculty have a major role to play in addressing the issues of academic dishonesty. However, Groark, Oblinger, and Choa (2001) reported that although it is believed that cheating has significantly increased in the last two decades, there has not been a proportional increase in the number of infractions reported by faculty. Fontana (2009) noted that the cost to nursing faculty who discover and take action when academic dishonesty occurs is significant. She reported that faculty feel they have significant changes in student relationships, that there is a significant risk associated with confronting students, and that even collegial relationships are altered. However, most faculty acknowledged their responsibility to identify and address the issue, viewing themselves as "gatekeepers of the nursing profession" (Fontana, 2009, p. 182).

There are many factors that may influence a student's decision to cheat; however, many authorities note that an alarming number of students do not consider their behavior to be unethical or cheating but see it as acceptable and common. Arhin (2009) noted that while nursing students were more consistent about perceptions of cheating on formal examinations, there was greater variety in what behaviors were identified as unethical in terms of course assignments, paper writing, and laboratory reporting. This should be of great concern, since dishonesty in clinical settings has serious implications for patient safety.

Tippitt et al. (2009) have suggested that strategies to address academic dishonesty should begin with faculty review of their own behaviors in terms of academic dishonesty. For example, do faculty cite sources on materials presented to students in class? Are student contributions to research and publications appropriately acknowledged? Is there discussion about the importance of values and value development in students, or do these discussions occur only when a crisis situation has occurred? These authors point to the importance of a learning environment that integrates ethics into the entire curriculum and the use of learning strategies that work to develop values and behaviors in students that have lasting consequences. Maintaining civility in student–faculty interactions is another important action that faculty can take to serve as positive role models for students (DiBartolo & Walsh, 2010) and to create learning environments that engender respect for all individuals.

Faculty can take a number of actions to deter cheating in their courses. One of the most common forms of academic dishonesty is cheating on classroom tests. This may be done by copying from another student's test, with or without the cooperation of the other student, concealing and bringing into the classroom potential answers to the test, or obtaining test questions from students who were previously enrolled in the course. Developing alternate test forms that can be used in subsequent semesters can help decrease the likelihood of questions being shared between classes of students. Alternative test forms can also be used among students in the same class, thus decreasing the chance that students can cheat by looking at the test of the student sitting next to them. Requiring students to leave books and other personal items at the front of the classroom or under their desks and rearranging the seating can also make it more difficult for students to cheat. Directing students to look only at their own tests can serve to remind students that their behavior is being observed and that they are responsible for not conveying the appearance of cheating.

Another common method of cheating is plagiarism of written work, through either the use of papers written by other students or the inappropriate citation of references. Students may be unclear about what constitutes plagiarism; therefore faculty should consider clarifying this at the beginning of the course, including how and when citing is to be done and what consequences will take place if plagiarism occurs. The proactive approach has been shown to be more successful, especially when tied to the development of an environment of academic honesty, often linked to an honor code or honor system. This may reduce the number of "I did not know that was wrong" excuses from students. Requesting that copies of the references cited in written work be turned in with the assignment can facilitate faculty review of the materials and reduce the likelihood that students will deliberately plagiarize. Keeping on file copies of past student papers can also decrease the likelihood that students will be able to represent a previous student's work as their own.

Sometimes students are pressured into helping another student cheat on coursework, either through a misguided sense of feeling sorry for and wanting to "help" the student or sometimes through fear. It can be helpful to periodically review the institution's policy on academic dishonesty with students in the class, especially if the faculty member suspects there may be a problem. Many students do not realize that institutional policies commonly state explicitly that a student participating in and enabling another student to cheat is also guilty of academic dishonesty and may be disciplined as well. Also, most institutions have policies that provide guidance for students who feel that they are being verbally and otherwise harassed by another student.

Solomon and DeNatale (2000) described the use of a program-wide convocation to discuss the issue of academic dishonesty, maintaining that drawing the analogy between academic dishonesty and professional ethics is an important first step in socializing students into the nursing profession. Academic honor codes can be used as a proactive stance to discourage dishonesty and to foster the development of a professional value system within an institution. An academic honor code should define what activities constitute academic misconduct, what disciplinary action could result if the student engages in such activity, and the student grievance and appeal procedure. McCabe and Trevino (1996) reported that evidence exists to suggest that the presence of a campus academic honor code creates an environment where cheating is not a socially acceptable behavior and decreases the number of incidences of student dishonesty. They also point out that student involvement in the outcomes (i.e., student hearings, student courts) may also deter cheating.

It is also helpful if written statements on course syllabi are used to remind students of the institution's policy on academic dishonesty and the academic code of honor, if one exists. The consequences of cheating and violating the honor code should also be clearly delineated in course syllabi. If cheating has occurred, does the student get an F for the assignment or an F for the course? Or are other options a possibility? This information can be included in the evaluation section of the syllabus and lets students know that any incidents of cheating will be taken seriously by the faculty member. It is important that these outcomes be guided by school policy and procedure; all course policies must be congruent with those of the broader school guidelines.

If a faculty member has evidence that a student has engaged in some form of academic dishonesty, it becomes necessary for him or her to confront the student about the incident. Jeffreys and Stier (1995) recommended that the following steps be followed when discussing an incident of academic dishonesty.

Privacy should first be ensured for the student when initiating discussion of the incident. It is appropriate to include an impartial third party, such as the department chairperson or another faculty member, in the discussion. Faculty must clearly communicate to the student the identified dishonest behavior and the potential consequences resulting from this behavior. It is important that faculty convey this information in an objective manner, avoiding blame or anger. The student should be informed of institutional policies and the importance of adhering to professional standards of conduct. The conference should be documented by the faculty member. As mentioned previously in the section regarding disciplinary action and due process, the student's right to due process should be ensured before any action is taken.

Student–Faculty Relationships

As discussed earlier in this chapter, the nature of the relationships that students develop with faculty in the classroom and clinical setting can have a profound influence on the quality of the students' education experiences. The relationship of the student to faculty in nursing may be closer than in other disciplines because of the increased amount of individual contact that occurs between students and faculty. Novice faculty often are uncertain about how to appropriately develop relationships with students. This can have a major impact on the success of faculty in the classroom and their personal satisfaction with their role as an educator. Faculty may indeed be very knowledgeable about the content they teach, but if they cannot relate in a positive manner to students, the students may not listen to the substance of the information being conveyed. Novice faculty should be encouraged to seek guidance on how to develop an effective interpersonal style with students (Halstead, 1996).

Behaviors that help develop effective relationships with students are those that have been described throughout this chapter. Open, ongoing dialogue with students throughout the educational process is essential. Students have the right to expect from faculty respect for their ideas and opinions (although not necessarily agreement); constructive, helpful feedback on their academic performance; a willingness to answer questions and address concerns the student may have; and a respect for student confidentiality. Displaying an appropriate sense of humor and warmth with students is also important and allows students to see the human side of faculty.

Behaviors that are inappropriate and unethical in the teaching situation include using sarcasm or belittling the student, threatening the student with failure, criticizing the student in front of others, acting superior, discussing confidential student issues with other faculty, and displaying inappropriate sexual behavior. Standards and guidelines addressing sexual harassment are part of each institution's policies and procedures. Nursing faculty must be informed about such policies and must follow them explicitly. Faculty may also serve to assist students to access appropriate resources should students have issues with sexual harassment by other members of the university community and need such assistance.

Showing favoritism in the treatment or grading of students, refusing to answer students' questions, behaving rudely, and being authoritarian are other examples of unethical teaching behaviors. Student–faculty interactions that are based on the inappropriate use of power and control cannot result in caring, collegial relationships. In some institutions, policies govern the contact that is appropriate between students and faculty. Those policies must always guide decisions about appropriate student contact and interaction.

Faculty can foster the development of positive student–faculty relationships through the design of learning experiences that promote collaborative, collegial learning exchanges between faculty and students. Faculty need to examine their beliefs about the teaching–learning process and student–faculty relationships to gain an understanding of their own attitudes. The first step in the process of fostering a learning environment that is empowering for both faculty and students is conceptualizing the student–faculty relationship as a collaborative partnership instead of an authoritarian one (Halstead, 1996).

SUMMARY

This chapter provides an overview of the legal and ethical issues that are related to the academic performance of students. The development of positive student–faculty interactions and the faculty role in evaluation of student performance is discussed. The legal and ethical concepts that guide student and faculty interactions and relationships are explained. Academic failure in the classroom and clinical setting is discussed, as are methods of assisting students through this difficult experience while ensuring their rights to due process. The importance of clear, mutual communication of expectations between students and faculty is emphasized.

Nursing students in today's classroom exhibit different characteristics from those of faculty when they were nursing students. Today's diverse students bring a richness of life experiences to the learning experience. Each student is an individual possessing a variety of knowledge, skills, values, beliefs, and needs that will help form the nursing professional that the nursing student wishes to become. It is important for nurse educators to meet the needs of these students by establishing professional relationships that are positive and empowering in nature, ultimately providing students with a learning environment that supports their personal and professional goals.

REFLECTING ON THE EVIDENCE

1. Under what circumstances would it be appropriate to share personal information you have gained from a student with your direct supervisor? With colleagues? Under what circumstances, if any, should it be mandatory that you would do so?

2. What "boundaries" should guide the development of the student–faculty relationship? Are there any activities that are "off limits"?

3. What actions should be considered when a faculty member suspects a student has cheated on an assignment? Is that different than "cheating" in a clinical venue (e.g., altering data, recording data that was not assessed)? Should these situations be treated differently? Why or why not?

REFERENCES

Arhin, A. (2009). A pilot study of nursing student's perceptions of academic dishonesty: A generation Y perspective. *The ABNF Journal, 20*(1), 17–21.

Boley, B., & Whitney, K. (2003). Grade disputes: Considerations for nursing faculty. *Journal of Nursing Education, 42*(5), 198–203.

Brent, N. (2001). *Nurses and the law: A guide to principles and applications.* Philadelphia, PA: W. B. Saunders.

Dennison, S. (2010). Peer mentoring: Untapped potential. *Journal of Nursing Education, 49*(6), 340–342.

DiBartolo, M., & Walsh, C. (2010). Desperate times call for desperate measures: Where are we in addressing academic dishonesty? *Journal of Nursing Education, 49*(10), 543–544.

Dixon v. *Alabama State Board of Education*, 294 F. 2d 150 (5th Cir. 1961.).

Donovan, M. (1989). The "high-risk" student: An ethical challenge for faculty. *Journal of Professional Nursing, 5*(3), 120.

Fontana, J. (2009). Nursing faculty experiences of students' academic dishonesty. *Journal of Nursing Education, 48*(4), 181–185.

Goudreau, K. A., & Chasens, E. R. (2002). Negligence in nursing education. *Nurse Educator, 27*(1), 42–46.

Groark, M., Oblinger, D., & Choa, M. (2001). Term paper mills, anti-plagiarism tools and academic integrity. *Educause Review, 36*(5), 40–48.

Guido, G. (1997). *Legal issues in nursing.* Stamford, CT: Appleton & Lange.

Halstead, J. (1996). The significance of student-faculty interactions. In K. Stevens (Ed.), *Review of research in nursing education* (*Vol 7*, pp. 67–90). New York, NY: National League for Nursing.

Harper, M. (2006). High tech cheating. *Nurse Education Today, 26*(8), 672–679.

Hopkins, T. H. (2008). Early identification of at-risk nursing students: A student support model. *Journal of Nursing Education, 47*(6), 254–259.

Jeffreys, M. R., & Stier, L. A. (1995). Speaking against student academic dishonesty: A communication model for nurse educators. *Journal of Nursing Education, 34*(7), 297–304.

McCabe, D. (2009). Academic dishonesty in nursing schools: An empirical investigation. *Journal of Nursing Education, 48*(11), 614–623.

McCabe, D. L., & Trevino, L. K. (1996). What we know about cheating in college: Longitudinal trends and recent developments. *Change, 28*(1), 28–33.

McGregor, A. (2007). Academic success, clinical failure: Struggling practices of a failing student. *Journal of Nursing Education, 46*(11), 504–511.

Morgan, J. E. (2001). Confidential student information in nursing education. *Nurse Educator, 26*(6), 289–292.

National League for Nursing. (2005). *Transforming nursing education.* New York, NY: Author.

Osinski, K. (2003). Due process rights of nursing students in cases of misconduct. *Journal of Nursing Education, 42*(2), 55–58.

Paterson, C., & Lane, L. (2000). An analysis of legal issues concerning university based nursing education programs. *Journal of Nursing Law, 7*(2), 7–18.

Regents of University of Michigan v. Ewing, 474 U.S. 214 (106 S. Ct 507 1985.).

Robinson, E., & Niemer, L. (2010). A peer mentor tutor program for academic success in nursing. *Nursing Education Perspectives, 31*(5), 286–289.

Salamonson, Y., & Andrew, S. (2006). Academic performance in nursing students: Influence of part-time employment, age and ethnicity. *Journal of Advanced Nursing, 55*(3), 342–349. doi:10.1111/j.1365–2648.2006.03863.x

Scanlan, J., Care, W., & Gessler, S. (2001). Dealing with the unsafe students in clinical practice. *Nurse Educator, 26*(1), 23–27.

Sifford, K. (2006). Academic integrity and cheating. *Nursing Education Perspective, 27*(1), 35–36.

Smith, M. (2005). *The legal, professional, and ethical dimensions of higher education.* Philadelphia, PA: Lippincott, Williams & Watkins.

Smith, M., McKoy, M., & Richardson, J. (2001). Legal issues related to dismissing students for clinical deficiencies. *Nurse Educator, 26*(1), 33–38.

Solomon, M., & DeNatale, M. (2000). Academic dishonesty and professional practice: A convocation. *Nurse Educator, 25*(6), 270–271.

Sullivan Commission Report. (2004). *Missing persons: Minorities in the health professions.* Washington, DC: Report of the Sullivan Commission on Diversity in the Workforce.

Tippitt, M., Ard, N., Kline, J., Tilghman, J., Chamberlain, B., & Meagher, G. (2009). Creating environments that foster academic integrity. *Nursing Education Perspectives, 30*(4), 239–244.

Williams, R. P. (1993). The concerns of beginning nursing students. *Nursing and Health Care, 14*(4), 178–184.

Wolkowitz, A., & Kelley, J. (2010). Academic predictors of success in a nursing program. *Journal of Nursing Education, 49*(9), 498–503.

Teaching Students with Disabilities

Betsy Frank, PhD, RN, ANEF

4

Almost 40 years ago, Congress passed the Rehabilitation Act (1973). This act states that any program or activity that receives federal funding cannot deny access or participation to individuals with disabilities. Section 504 of this act specifically addresses higher education and prohibits public postsecondary institutions receiving federal funds from discriminating against individuals with disabilities. Furthermore, just over 20 years ago Congress enacted the Americans with Disabilities Act (ADA) (1990). This act was further updated in 2008 (Summary of key provisions, n.d.). Because of these two laws, colleges and universities have experienced an increased number of students with disabilities admitted to their programs, including nursing programs. In the 2007–2008 academic year, 10.8% of undergraduates and 7.6% of graduate and first professional degree students had some form of disability (National Center for Education Statistics, n.d.).

Nursing students with special needs present a challenge to nursing faculty in both the classroom and clinical settings. Students who have special needs include those who have a physical disability, such as a visual or hearing impairment; a chronic illness; a learning disability; or a chemical dependency problem. Many nursing programs have had some experience in meeting the needs of these students. More than 15 years have passed since Colon (1997) surveyed schools of nursing and discovered over half had admitted students with a variety of physical, cognitive, and emotional disabilities. A survey by Sowers

and Smith (2004b) suggested that even though faculty had experience with students with special needs, faculty had many concerns regarding whether students with special needs could be successful in achieving success in nursing programs. On the other hand, others, such as Maheady (2003) and Arndt (2004), have challenged nursing faculty to adopt a more open attitude in accommodating those students with disabilities. In fact, Nichols and Quaye (2009) have suggested that societal culture and norms provide the framework in which disabilities are defined, not the person who may have a disability. As more students with disabilities seek admission to nursing programs, and as those within the profession age, retaining nurses with disabilities in the workforce will be essential. Patient safety concerns notwithstanding, without an open attitude toward students with disabilities, much nursing talent may be lost.

This chapter addresses the issues related to the education of students with disabilities. It specifically focuses on common problems experienced by college students and nursing students: learning disabilities, physical disabilities, mental health problems, and chemical impairment issues. The Rehabilitation Act of 1973, the ADA as amended in 2008 (Summary of key provisions, n.d.), and the significance of these acts to nursing education are also addressed.

Legal Issues Related to Students with Disabilities

Faculty should be aware of the legal issues associated with teaching students with disabilities. The ADA protects the rights of individuals with disabilities in the arenas of education, employment,

The author acknowledges the work of Judith A. Halstead, PhD, RN, ANEF, in the previous edition(s) of the chapter.

and environmental accessibility. Higher education institutions must guarantee individuals with disabilities equal access to educational opportunities. Discrimination against individuals with physical and mental disabilities is prohibited by the ADA. However, the ADA does not guarantee that an admitted student will achieve academic success—only that the student has the *opportunity* to achieve academic success. A university or college has the obligation to maintain academic and behavioral standards for all students, disabled or not (Wolf, Brown, & Bork, 2009).

The full impact of the ADA on professional education continues to be determined as more potential students with disabilities seek admission to nursing programs. Focusing on stated program outcomes rather than on specific skills puts faculty into a better position to make decisions about what are reasonable accommodations for students who are disabled or have other special needs. Failure of an institution to make reasonable accommodations for a student who is disabled is considered discrimination (Helms, Jorgensen, & Anderson, 2006), and the institution and faculty may be sued for failing to make reasonable accommodations.

Implications for Nursing Education

By law, students have the responsibility to notify the institution regarding a disability and the need for accommodation (Helms et al., 2006). While disclosure of disabilities is voluntary and not legally required, students who have a disability and require accommodation are encouraged to share this information with the institution's office for students with disabilities. However, many students will not share information regarding their disabilities for fear of rejection (Maheady, 2005).

Barriers to student success may be related more to faculty attitudes rather than to student ability (Nichols & Quaye, 2009; Scullion, 2010; Sowers & Smith, 2004a, 2004b). Sowers and Smith (2004a) explored the impact of in-service training on faculty members' attitudes regarding nursing students with disabilities. One hundred and twelve faculty members participated in a 2-hour training program. The program was developed based on survey results from a study of nursing faculty attitudes and knowledge regarding disabilities (Sowers & Smith, 2004b). Faculty who participated in the in-service

training had more favorable attitudes toward and more knowledge about students with disabilities compared to faculty who participated in the survey that formed the basis of the in-service program. Education for faculty related to providing accommodations and understanding the possibilities for achievement among students with disabilities is key for students' academic success. Helping staff in clinical agencies to understand that nursing is more than hard physical labor is also key to accommodating students with disabilities (Neal-Boylan & Guillet, 2008).

When a student makes known the presence of a disability, upon student consent, course faculty are notified about the disability that requires accommodation. Even when student consent is given to share information with faculty, the nature of the disability is not disclosed to faculty unless the student decides to disclose it. Box 4-1 is an example of a statement of services provided for students with disabilities.

Faculty are not allowed to inquire about the nature of the disability. In fact, decisions regarding whether accommodation is possible must be made after the student has been admitted, unless essential abilities are published and *all* students are asked before admission whether they possess the abilities needed for academic success (Helms et al., 2006).

BOX 4-1 Services for Persons with Disabilities

Students who need adaptations in their learning environment may obtain help through the services located in the Student Academic Services Center. Services include assistance in accessing recorded textbooks or readers for the blind and learning disabled. This office also arranges for note-takers or signers for hearing impaired persons. Alternate testing procedures may be arranged as needed. Services for persons with disabilities are based on individual needs and the University's intent to offer appropriate accommodations according to the student's documentation of need for same. These services are coordinated by the Student Support Services Grant Program. It is recommended that persons with disabilities visit Indiana State University prior to making a decision to enroll.

Courtesy Indiana State University Undergraduate Catalog, 2011–2012.

However, most lists of essential abilities focus, in part, on physical abilities such as lifting. Recent initiatives call into question such requirements (American Nurses Association [ANA], n.d.).

When considering the admission of a student who has a disability, admission committees in schools of nursing must consider the following questions:
- Disregarding the disability, is the individual otherwise qualified to be admitted to the program?
- What reasonable accommodations can the school make to enable the student to be successful in the pursuit of becoming a nurse who can deliver safe patient care?

Although institutions are not expected to lower or alter academic or technical standards to accommodate a student with a disability, they are expected to determine what accommodations would be reasonable for a student who is disabled. Examples of reasonable accommodations include altering the length of test taking times or methods, providing proctors to read tests or write test answers, allowing additional time to complete the program of study, providing supplemental study aids such as audiotapes of texts, providing note takers, or altering the method of course delivery. The same considerations must be given to students who become disabled during their enrollment in a nursing program. Questions to be asked include the following:
- Disregarding the disability, is the student otherwise qualified to continue in the nursing program?
- What reasonable accommodations can be made to allow the student to continue?

When considering accommodations, "Accumulating precedents, however, suggest that accommodations to curricula and to some testing methods may not be required if there are good pedagogical reasons that substantiate prevailing practices" (Helms et al., 2006, p. 193). For example, testing methods, such as multiple-choice questions, could be required for pedagogical reasons (Helms et al., 2006).

Faculty should consider in their decision making that just because a student has a disability, he or she is not necessarily ill, and the type of support needed is not the type needed to cure an illness, but to support health (Sin, 2009). Furthermore, how those with a disability are viewed is a result of

social constructs (Marks, 2000; Nichols & Quaye, 2009). Whether a person's limitations are viewed as a disability is defined by society rather than by the actual abilities of the person involved. Thus making the decision regarding what is a reasonable accommodation for a person with a disability is a complex process influenced as much by faculty attitudes as by actual student abilities. Marks further suggested that referring to those with disabilities as those with "special needs" invites discrimination against persons with disabilities.

As the impact of the ADA on nursing education continues to unfold in the courts and in the workplace, nurse educators must keep current with legal developments that relate to the education of individuals with disabilities who are pursuing degrees in the health professions. Some suggestions for increasing faculty awareness of the needs of students with disabilities include periodic continuing education sessions related to the legal implications of educating such students and the use of consultants who are experts in working with students with disabilities. Most institutions of higher education have an office dedicated to assisting and supporting students with disabilities who are enrolled on campus. This office can provide resources and expert advice to faculty and students. Another source of information may be individuals with disabilities who have successfully developed a career in nursing. These successful nurses can help nursing faculty understand the issues involved in educating students with disabilities and they can serve as mentors to students with disabilities who are pursuing a nursing education (Maheady, 2003, 2006).

Nursing faculty should begin to separate the truly essential components of nursing education from the merely traditional nursing curricula and teaching strategies. Bohne (2004) and Carroll (2004) have suggested that nursing faculty need to consider such philosophical issues as whether nursing education might be extended to those individuals who will never practice bedside nursing in an acute care setting. Such nursing jobs might include staff development, infection control, case management, or a variety of jobs in the community settings where nursing care is delivered. A study of admission and retention practices of California nursing schools (Persaud & Leedom, 2002) shows that nursing faculty struggle with what are reasonable accommodations that balance student access with patient safety. In making admission and progression decisions, faculty need to balance student rights, safety, and abilities with issues of patient safety and university responsibility for providing appropriate accommodations according to the ADA (Watkins & Kurz, 1997). Having an ongoing evaluation plan that shows how making appropriate accommodations affects student outcomes in terms of graduation and subsequent employment is essential (Watkins & Kurz, 1997). One note of caution, however: Faculty may need to seek alternative placements for disabled students if clinical agencies,

despite ADA regulations, are reticent to work with a particular student (Andre & Manson, 2004).

Some schools of nursing, as well as other professional schools, have identified in writing the abilities students need to possess to be successful in their chosen educational program. The essential abilities that students need to possess for successful progression through the nursing program at one school of nursing are presented in Box 4-2. Faculty should note that the delivery of holistic nursing care relies more on the use of complex cognitive processes than on physical labor.

BOX 4-2 Essential Requirements

The Indiana University School of Nursing faculty have specified essential abilities critical to the success of students enrolled in any Indiana University nursing program. Students must demonstrate the following essential abilities (technical standards) with or without reasonable accommodations to meet all progression criteria:

ESSENTIAL ABILITIES POLICY

The School of Nursing faculty have specified essential abilities critical to the success of students in the IU nursing program. Students must demonstrate these essential abilities to succeed in their program of study. They are expected to meet all progression criteria, as well as these essential abilities with or without reasonable accommodations. Each student who enters the program must sign an Essential Abilities form, which will be kept in the student's permanent file.

- **Essential judgment skills** to include: ability to identify, assess, and comprehend conditions surrounding patient situations for the purpose of problem solving around patient conditions and coming to appropriate conclusions and/or courses of action.
- **Essential physical/neurological functions** to include: ability to use the senses of seeing, hearing, touch, and smell to make correct judgments regarding patient conditions and meet physical expectations to perform required interventions for the purpose of demonstrating competence to safely engage in the practice of nursing. Behaviors that demonstrate essential neurological and physical functions include, but are not limited to observation, listening, understanding relationships, writing, and psychomotor abilities consistent with course and program expectations.
- **Essential communication skills** to include: ability to communicate effectively with fellow students, faculty,

patients, and all members of the health care team. Skills include verbal, written, and nonverbal abilities as well as information technology skills consistent with effective communication.
- **Essential emotional coping skills:** ability to demonstrate the mental health necessary to safely engage in the practice of nursing as determined by professional standards of practice.
- **Essential intellectual/conceptual skills** to include: ability to measure, calculate, analyze, synthesize, and evaluate to engage competently in the safe practice of nursing.
- **Other essential behavioral attributes** to include: ability to engage in activities consistent with safe nursing practice without demonstrated behaviors of addiction to, abuse of, or dependence on alcohol or other drugs that may impair behavior or judgment. The student must demonstrate responsibility and accountability for actions as a student in the School of Nursing and as a developing professional nurse consistent with accepted standards of practice.

Students questioning their ability to meet the essential abilities criteria are encouraged to speak with an Academic Counselor. Students failing to meet these criteria at any point in their academic program may have their progress interrupted until they have demonstrated these essential abilities within negotiated time frames.

Students will be dismissed from their program of study if the faculty determine students are unable to meet these essential abilities even if reasonable accommodations are made. Students failing to demonstrate these essential abilities may appeal this adverse determination in accordance with Indiana University's appeal procedures.

From Indiana University School of Nursing Essential Abilities Policy U-VI-A-15. Used with permission.

The Nursing Student with a Learning Disability

Fifteen percent of the United States population has some form of learning disability (LD Online, n.d.). Learning disabilities are the most common type of student disability found on college campuses (Eliason, 1992), with approximately 2% of undergraduates having some form of learning disability (Vickers, 2010). Learning disabilities include dyslexia and attention deficit hyperactivity disorder (ADHD) (Bradshaw, 2006). Frequently students begin college with learning disabilities undetected. However, persons with learning disabilities are presumed to have lifelong difficulties with learning, whether the disabilities are diagnosed or not (Selekman, 2002). In nursing education learning disabilities are commonly first uncovered when faculty notice striking differences between a student's classroom performance and clinical performance. The student may display an adequate knowledge base and competent skills during clinical experiences but be unable to demonstrate the same degree of knowledge when taking tests in the classroom. Such disparities in performance lead to much frustration and stress for the student and, not uncommonly, academic failure. Faculty should have an understanding of the characteristics of learning disabilities so they can refer students for the appropriate assistance from counselors.

Definitions of learning disabilities vary, but generally learning disabilities are considered neurological disorders of the brain that affect the way a person learns or processes oral or written language and/or mathematical concepts and reasoning (LD Online, n.d.). A person with a learning disability may struggle academically even in adulthood.

Characteristics of Learning Disabilities

Learning disabilities may manifest as a number of characteristics, each necessitating a different treatment and accommodation. Eighty percent of those with diagnosed learning disabilities have trouble with basic reading skills (LD Online, n.d.). Memory difficulties, such as trouble remembering details and sequencing, commonly lead to reading and spelling difficulties. Poor handwriting, distractibility with difficulty concentrating, a history of poor academic performance, difficulty meeting deadlines, anxiety, and low self-esteem are also signs of a learning disability (Bradshaw, 2006; McCleary-Jones, 2008). Students with learning disabilities may have difficulty following verbal instructions and difficulty organizing ideas in writing or may be unable to articulate ideas verbally but be able to articulate them in writing. Students may also have auditory processing deficits that have an impact on their ability to recite from memory (Selekman, 2002). Time management may also be a problem for these students (Kolanko, 2003).

Learning disabilities are highly individualized and each student manifests a different grouping of characteristics (Selekman, 2002). Students with learning disabilities have average or above average intelligence and should be expected to meet the same academic standards as other students (McCleary-Jones, 2008).

Evidence supports the fact that despite sometimes facing overwhelming odds, students with learning disabilities can achieve success in nursing programs. Kolanko (2003) used a case study method to study nursing students with learning disabilities. She discovered that these students had to work harder to achieve passing grades. Students expressed anxiety and frustration and lack of confidence, which interfered with their ability to process information. Once students understood what facilitated their learning, they were able to better deal with the rigors of the curriculum. For example, students needed to learn personalized test taking skills so they could be successful on tests. For some students, sitting in classes for long periods hampered their concentration. Those students had to take breaks and move around every hour.

Performing in the classroom presents one set of challenges for those with learning disabilities. Success in the clinical arena presents another set. Price and Gale (2006) interviewed 10 British female nursing students with dyslexia, a form of learning disability, and 10 students who did not have dyslexia. Whereas both groups had some similar experiences, such as difficulty with understanding medical terminology and coping with a changing care environment, the dyslexic students had special issues. The dyslexic students often had difficulty with doing things rapidly, such as charting, and with remembering names. Students coped by practicing spelling over and over in order to chart without errors. Although both groups of students experienced some difficulty with keeping up with change-of-shift reports, those with dyslexia had more troubles. Dyslexic students were also more concerned with safety, because they knew they had to check their work more thoroughly than did the other students. The key to the dyslexic students' success was to develop strategies to keep them on track. Several research participants mentioned that they wrote everything down or used colored stickers to highlight important details of their work and keep themselves more organized.

Morris and Turnbull (2006) studied 18 British nursing students with dyslexia. Five themes were identified: disclosure, self-managing strategies, need for more time, emotional aspects of being a dyslexic nursing student, and choice of future work setting. Six of the 18 students did not disclose their dyslexia to clinical staff. Twelve believed that disclosure leads to the potential for discrimination against them, but six saw disclosure as a way to receive more help.

Like students in Price and Gale's (2006) study, these students also developed coping strategies. Some used reminder pads and others used a voice recorder to keep track of activities. Practicing clinical skills repeatedly facilitated learning for them. Students were keenly aware of the potential for making errors so they had drug calculations checked by others. They also knew that they needed more time than others to maintain safe patient care practices. Because of this, these students knew that they more than likely would not choose to work in a fast-paced acute care environment. Those who lacked self-confidence had trouble with accepting criticism and letting others know what they needed. However, the majority of the participants did not view themselves as disabled.

ADHD is closely linked with learning disabilities (Bradshaw, 2006; Bradshaw & Salzer, 2003). Students who have ADHD also have difficulty with academic performance. Most are diagnosed as children and their symptoms may persist into adulthood (Bradshaw & Salzer, 2003). Student nurses who have this disorder exhibit some of the same symptoms as those with learning disabilities, such as dyslexia and difficulties with memory and organization of work. Bradshaw and Salzer (2003) suggest that faculty members develop a trusting relationship with students whom they believe have ADHD but have not disclosed such, encouraging these students to receive accommodations, if needed, in the learning environment to help them succeed. They note, however, that if the student fails despite accommodations having been made or fails because ADHD was not disclosed and thus no accommodations were made, then the student must accept responsibility for his or her own actions.

Accommodating Learning Disabilities

When faculty believe that a student, previously undiagnosed, may have a learning disability, the initial action is to refer the student to an expert in learning disabilities for assessment. After the diagnosis is made, a plan for accommodation of the disability can be developed. Counseling may also help a student with learning disabilities gain self-confidence in the learning environment. As stated earlier, if the student chooses, the faculty can be made aware of the disability and what accommodations are required. Faculty members who are made aware of a student's disability are not allowed to discuss that information with other faculty members unless the student gives permission.

Depending on the type of learning disability, a variety of accommodations may be appropriate for the student. Students who have memory difficulties may have difficulty with remembering details and taking notes but will be able to grasp concepts. These students find learning to be a tiring experience and will usually experience greater success with learning activities that incorporate "hands-on" and observation experiences in the teaching strategies (Eliason, 1992). Simulation experiences help students to rehearse clinical skills in a safe environment (Ashcroft et al., 2008). Skills such as time management, prioritization, and dealing with multiple stimuli can be practiced over and over until students feel comfortable with the skills before entering the "real world." These students may need specific step-by-step instructions for tasks and help with time management (Selekman, 2002).

Students may also benefit from the assistance of an in-class note taker. This allows students to concentrate on classroom discussion without the distraction of trying to take notes. Some students have difficulty processing multiple stimuli at once. Students who have difficulty reading, and as a result read slowly, often find this disability to be the greatest barrier to their academic success. Faculty can help students overcome this difficulty by providing an audio recording of textbooks and other readings and providing them with the required reading assignments early in the semester, or helping them identify the key sections of reading assignments. Findings from a research study by Tee et al. (2010) suggested that reading aloud to students and using simple words to describe medical terms may help students to learn better. For example, beginning by stating that high blood pressure is equivalent to hypertension may be useful. Tee et al. (2010) also suggested helping students build confidence early on.

Students with learning disabilities may also need accommodations for testing because slow reading skills can affect the student's ability to complete a test within the time allowed. Questions that are grammatically complex or contain double negatives, although difficult for all students, can be particularly challenging for students with learning disabilities and should be avoided. Providing the student with an extended testing time and a quiet room free of distractions may also be necessary (Bradshaw & Salzer, 2003). A test proctor who either reads the test to the student or writes and records the student's dictated answers to the test questions may also be helpful.

An additional strategy that faculty can use to assist students with learning disabilities is to incorporate a multimedia approach, such as computer-assisted instruction (McCleary-Jones, 2008; Selekman, 2002). Other strategies can benefit both students with learning disabilities and students without them. These include providing copies of Power-Point slides or other notes before class, placing visual cues within class notes, and checking nursing notes before placing them on the patient charts (Ijiri & Kudzma, 2000; Selekman, 2002). Use of a pocket speller in the clinical area may also be beneficial (Ijiri & Kudzma, 2000). The use of smart phones with appropriate applications may also be helpful for all students, but particularly those with learning disabilities. Another strategy that benefits all students, including those with learning disabilities, is to meet with students on a regular basis to ensure that learning goals are being set appropriately and are then being achieved.

Part-time study is another option (Selekman, 2002). Accommodation does not mean that academic standards are lowered but that multiple ways to achieve those standards are provided for all students, including those with learning disabilities. Any one classroom contains students with multiple learning styles. By structuring classes to take into account different learning styles and by providing a variety of learning aids, nurse educators will also help accommodate those with diagnosed learning disabilities (Ijiri & Kudzma, 2000). Successful students with learning disabilities, and perhaps all other disabilities, are those who are cognizant of their learning needs and always focus on patient safety and meeting academic standards (Ashcroft et al., 2008).

Campus Support Services

As previously mentioned, most institutions of higher education have established an office responsible for providing support services to students who identify themselves as learning disabled. Use of these services is voluntary, and they are usually available at little or no cost to the student. Services vary among institutions but typically include assessment and diagnosis of learning disabilities, identification of appropriate accommodations for the student, guidance counseling, and development of study and test taking skills. Faculty education about students with learning disabilities is another service commonly provided by these offices.

Another resource for faculty might be a center for teaching and learning or some similar campus office. Those in such a center can assist faculty in using principles of universal design in the preparation of online course materials. When used, these principles facilitate the learning of those with a variety of disabilities, including those with learning disabilities (Crow, 2008). For example, when designing materials for students with learning disabilities, faculty should keep pages uncluttered, avoid a lot of flashing graphics, and use a larger font (Crow, 2008).

Accommodations for the National Council Licensure Examination

Nurse educators need to be familiar with the accommodations provided for students with disabilities in their states when taking the National Council Licensure Examination (NCLEX). Accommodations are offered to individuals with learning disabilities in accordance with the ADA (National Council of State Boards of Nursing, n.d.). Each state individually determines the degree of accommodation offered to students on a case-by-case basis. Educators should investigate and verify the accommodations offered to students in their respective state and encourage students with disabilities to seek appropriate accommodations. One of the most common accommodations has to do with time allotted for the examination. Regulations do change, and the student and faculty are encouraged to check with the National Council of State Boards of Nursing website (www.ncsbn.org) or the individual state board of nursing for further information. The student must provide documentation as to what accommodations have been made during his or her course of study before arriving at the testing center.

The Student with Physical Disabilities

Required abilities that schools use to exclude students may include hearing, seeing, and lifting. The United States Supreme Court ruled more than 30 years ago that a prospective nursing student with a hearing impairment could be denied admission because of the potential for lowering educational standards (*Southeastern Community College* v. *Davis*, 442 U.S. 397 [1979]). Since that time there have been published reports of students with hearing impairments who have achieved success in nursing programs and in subsequent employment (Maheady, 2003). Many aids, such as amplified stethoscopes, are now available, and an interpreter could be used for auscultation (Association of Medical Professionals with Hearing Losses, n.d.). Through the use of note takers and tape recorders, many students with hearing impairments have little difficulty participating in the classroom. Pagers and cell phones that vibrate may help students keep in contact with others in the clinical setting.

Some students with impaired vision may be accommodated (Murphy & Brennan, 1998). In one report, a nurse with impaired vision successfully graduated from a baccalaureate nursing program and went on to a successful career (Maheady, 2006). Providing alternative learning environments and enabling students to work with preceptors may be accommodations that can reasonably be made. For example, a student with a visual impairment might need a magnifier to help with reading printed matter or a computer with large fonts.

Lifting restrictions may not be a barrier because many hospitals and nursing homes are striving for an environment that minimizes lifting (ANA, n.d.; Nelson & Lentz, 2003). Teaching students how to use lifting equipment while in school may prevent injury on the job. Videman, Ojajarviä, Riihimakiä, and Troup (2005) and Mitchell et al. (2009) found that many nurses either began nursing school with a history of back pain or developed low back pain while in school. Employed nurses have successfully functioned in wheelchairs, and with some creativity students could as well (Maheady, 2003, 2006; Nettina, 2003).

Students may become disabled during their time in school, and thus reasonable accommodations for students with physical disabilities may include time extensions for assignments and the assignment of an "incomplete" grade for courses that may not be completed on time. Maheady (2003) relates a case study of a nursing student who became wheelchair bound as a result of an accident. The student successfully completed her program and went on to obtain a master's degree in nursing and gainful employment. Fleming (2006) reported that she has been successful in completing a nursing program and is a successful registered nurse despite having only one hand. She has her basic RN preparation from a diploma program and has gone on to get her bachelor's and master's degrees and now is working on her doctoral degree (S. Fleming, personal communication, January 6, 2011). One might ask whether she can perform basic nursing skills such as starting an intravenous infusion and doing CPR. The answer is "yes" (S. Fleming, personal communication, January 6, 2011).

Students may have disabilities that are less readily apparent. Dailey (2010) conducted a phenomenological study of 10 students with various chronic illnesses such as multiple sclerosis, diabetes, adrenal hyperplasia, and asthma. Students reported they were determined to finish their programs of study despite feeling ill much of the time. Students expressed a desire to appear normal and they feared being penalized for excessive absences so they often placed their own health, and perhaps those of their patients, in jeopardy by attending class and clinical experiences when perhaps they should not have done so. Dailey (2010) recommended that faculty accommodate students by providing short rest periods during clinical experiences; promoting group work for learning activities, so that the load for all students was lessened; and incorporating self-care strategies into the curriculum that would benefit all students, not just those with chronic illnesses.

Creative clinical placements may help students achieve the required program outcomes, including delivering safe patient care (Andre & Manson, 2004). According to Moore (2004), if educators look upon disabilities as differences rather than impairments, all students can be helped to practice nursing according to the ANA Code of Ethics and achieve the core essentials of nursing, which include the ability to "practice with compassion and respect for the inherent dignity and uniqueness of every individual, unrestricted by considerations or social or economic status, personal attribute, or the nature of the health problems" (Fowler, 2008, p. 1). Essential abilities for basic nursing programs, however, may be different from those required in specialty graduate programs. For example, Helms and Thompson (2005) suggest that nurse anesthetists and nurse anesthetist students must be able to work in a fast-paced environment using complex information that is translated into immediate action. Nurse anesthetists must also be able to work closely with team members, so those who have any impairments that affect their ability to work in groups might not be suited for nurse anesthetist roles.

When students with physical disabilities graduate, their successful employment may depend on nurse managers' experience in working with nurses who are disabled. A study by Wood and Marshall (2010) revealed that nurse managers rated disabled nurses' performance as outstanding 22% of the time and rated them as below average only 11% of the time. Most would surmise that disabled nurses' job performance mirrors that of nondisabled nurses.

The Nursing Student with Substance Abuse

Determining the number of nursing students who may be impaired by drug or alcohol use is difficult. However, substance abuse has been found in college students. Johnston, O'Malley, Bachman, and Schulenberg (2005) estimated that 7.2% of college-age men and 1.8% of college-age women drink daily. Forty-nine percent of college-age men and 38% of college-age women had had five or more drinks at a time in the previous 2 weeks. O'Malley and Johnston (2002) estimated that two thirds of college students had had at least one drink within a 30-day period. They also noted that 20% of college students had used marijuana.

Other studies have confirmed the extent of college student substance abuse. The college environment does provide students with easy access to alcohol and drugs, including prescription stimulants, such as Ritalin, and can expose students to situations in which alcohol and drug use is considered an acceptable activity. Johnston et al. (2005) reported a national survey that showed 36% of college students reported illicit drug use.

Teter, McCabe, Cranford, Boyd, and Guthrie (2005) surveyed students at the University of Michigan by sending a random sample of 9161 undergraduates an invitation to participate in a web-based survey regarding illicit use of stimulants such as Ritalin. Forty-seven percent responded. Using prescription stimulants prescribed for those other than themselves was reported by 8.1% of the respondents. The students reported they took stimulants to remain alert, to concentrate, and to get high. Eighty-eight percent took the drugs for the sole purpose of experimentation. Male and white students reported the most use. The authors attributed the illicit use to the need to stay awake for long periods of time and to increase performance in school. An additional finding was that those using the stimulants had higher general drug and alcohol use.

Given the number of college students who abuse drugs and alcohol, it is not surprising that nurses who are substance abusers often cite that they began alcohol or drug abuse while they were students (Kenna & Wood, 2004). All college students experience academic pressures, and nursing students have additional stressors. The psychological stressors associated with caring for acutely ill clients while still acquiring the clinical knowledge and skills necessary to do so are considerable (O'Quinn, 1996). Students may also feel powerless to relieve the suffering they see their clients experiencing.

Baldwin, Bartek, Scott, Davis-Hall, and De Simone II (2009) published data gathered from 14 Midwestern schools of nursing in 1999. They found that, during the prior year, 6.8% had used marijuana and almost 29% reported excess alcohol use. Kenna and Wood (2004) surveyed pharmacists, nurses, and pharmacy and nursing students in one Northeastern state and at one university in the Northeast to examine the rates of substance abuse in these groups. The response rates were as follows: 73.3%

for nurses, 71.7% for pharmacists, 45.5% for pharmacy students, and 26.7% for nursing students. Marijuana was the most common drug used during the nurses' and pharmacists' lifetime. More nursing than pharmacy students had used marijuana during their lives and nursing students had higher monthly marijuana use compared to students in the general college population. Pharmacists, however, had used opiates more than nurses and, compared to the general population, pharmacists used more opiates, stimulants, and anxiolytics. Most students had used alcohol in their lifetime. The top predictor of substance abuse was family history. Other predictors included access to drugs and use of alcohol and tobacco in the past month. Kenna and Wood (2004) found that extensive use of opiates and anxiolytics was reported among both pharmacy and nursing students. Because substance abuse is often underreported, the rates for substance abuse among those sampled may, indeed, not be accurate (Kenna & Wood, 2004).

Even students attending faith-based nursing programs have reported substance abuse. In fact, Gnadt (2006) reported that 24% of the students in her sample reported substance use and 15% indicated that they may have had a substance abuse problem.

Characteristics of Students with Chemical and Alcohol Impairments

The potential for substance abuse obviously exists among nursing students. This substance abuse, if not dealt with, can affect a student's professional practice upon graduation. Dunn (2005), for example, noted that 10% of nurses have a substance abuse problem and more than 6% have impaired practice.

Faculty need to have an understanding of this issue so they may assist students in receiving the appropriate professional support necessary to treat their problem. Faculty also have a responsibility to ensure that students deliver safe patient care, which includes protecting clients from the actions of a potentially unsafe student whose clinical performance and judgment may be impaired because of substance abuse (Bugle, Jackson, Kornegay, & Rives, 2003). Faculty should be aware of the characteristics of students who may be chemically dependent, knowledgeable about the policies and procedures within their institution that relate to students

who are chemically dependent, and familiar with the support services that are available to students who have a chemical dependency problem.

Dunn (2005) and Talbert (2009) identified the following behavioral, personality, and physical characteristics that may be present in nurses, which would include nursing students, who abuse alcohol and drugs: being fearful and having panic attacks, decreased social interaction, impaired cognition, social isolation, frequent illnesses, mood swings, gastrointestinal distress, elevated blood pressure, bloodshot eyes, slowed or slurred speech, poor hygiene, and blackouts. Nursing students with substance abuse problems may also have excessive tardiness and absenteeism in both clinical and classroom settings.

Faculty Responsibilities Related to Students with Impairments

What are the responsibilities of faculty if they suspect that a student is displaying characteristics that are indicative of chemical dependency? Faculty have ethical responsibilities toward the student and the student's clients and therefore should not ignore or make excuses for such behavior. While the ADA considers substance abuse a disability, unsafe clinical practice is not protected under the law (Menendez, 2010).

Bugle et al. (2003) surveyed nursing faculty nationwide (response rate 37%) and found that faculty believe they should assist students in dealing with substance abuse, but were unsure of their ability to detect substance abuse in students. Faculty also felt that state boards of nursing should assist students in achieving licensure if students self-disclose substance abuse. Qualitative comments from this same study revealed four major themes: emotional/intellectual responses, responsive actions, other influences on attitudes, and beliefs about chemically dependent individuals (Kornegay, Bugle, & Rives, 2004). Quotations from these themes showed that faculty were supportive of students who were dealing with substance abuse. One faculty member noted, however, that a student was put on medical leave while undergoing rehabilitation. This action reflects the disease model of addiction, which does not promote disciplinary action against a student (Baldwin et al., 2009; Monroe, 2009).

Before taking any measures, faculty need to clearly understand the policies and procedures for assisting chemically dependent students that are in place within their institution. Behavior must be documented, and it is helpful if it is documented by more than one faculty member (Clark, 1999). A faculty member might have to take immediate action if, for example, a student appears impaired in the clinical area. Faculty have reported removing students from clinical rotation if they exhibited signs and symptoms of substance abuse (Kornegay et al., 2004). In cases in which the student does not impose an immediate danger to clients but is suspected of substance abuse, an appointment might be made with the student for the purpose of making the student aware of institutional policies regarding substance abuse. Clark (1999) suggested that, in addition to the faculty member who has identified the problem, someone else, such as a department chair and/or the director of student affairs, should be present. Having two persons, in addition to the student, present helps ensure more accurate documentation of the meeting.

Written policies about chemical impairment that include the institution's definition of chemical dependency, the nursing faculty's philosophy on chemical dependency, and student and faculty responsibilities related to suspected chemical dependency should be clearly stated in the student handbook. Without such policies faculty may not be legally supported if they implement actions against a student for chemical impairment (Clark, 1999). Furthermore, adhering to the institution's established policies helps ensure that the student's right to due process is not denied.

The American Association of Colleges of Nursing (1998) provides guidelines for policy development for the management of substance abuse. These guidelines include recommendations for education, identification of students with substance abuse problems, intervention, treatment, and reentry into the program if the student must enter into treatment and take a break from the educational course of study. The guidelines emphasize the use of professional resources for students instead of the use of faculty as counselors. Many colleges and universities offer treatment programs and support groups for students who are chemically impaired. It is highly recommended that faculty maintain a listing of effective counselors and programs located within the campus vicinity that can be used for student referrals. Another resource for faculty may be their respective state board of nursing Peer Assistance of Impaired Professionals program. In fact, at its 2002 convention, the National Student Nurses Association passed a resolution that encouraged state boards of nursing to extend their peer assistance programs to student nurses (Murphy-Parker, Kronenbitter, & Kronenbitter, 2003). Monroe (2009) developed such a program in conjunction with the Board of Nursing in Tennessee.

Some schools of nursing have formulated their own intervention program for nursing students who are impaired. The following are key considerations: (1) ensuring the confidentiality of students who access the program; (2) clarifying the responsibilities of individuals associated with the program (i.e., faculty, students, administrators, alumni, counselors, and substance abuse professionals); and (3) orienting the student population to the purpose, activities, and responsibilities of the program (Monroe, 2009).

Whether or not a school institutes a policy for random drug testing is controversial. While athletes are subject to random testing and most agencies have preemployment drug screening, the extent to which nursing students are required to undergo random screening is unknown, even though the American Association of Colleges of Nursing (1998) published a position paper on the subject of dealing with substance abuse. Drug testing was suggested as one part of a proposed comprehensive policy on substance abuse. One participant in the study by Kornegay et al. (2004) did speak about required drug testing, but no other studies mentioned required drug testing for nursing students.

Although schools may not have policies requiring drug testing, students should be made aware that clinical agency policies may require blood or urine testing of individuals, including students, suspected of chemical dependency. Levine and Rennie (2004) question the value of preemployment drug screening in promoting patient safety; they note that exhaustion from long hours worked may contribute more to medical errors than does substance abuse. Nevertheless, some schools are instituting policies for drug screening because of clinical agency requirements (Rockford College, 2010). Much more research is needed to determine the extent and nature of drug screening policies within nursing programs. Even state boards of nursing have policies about drug testing, albeit mostly for those nurses who have been reported to the boards because of impaired practice (Sheets, n.d.).

Many colleges and universities are attempting to deal with this problem by increasing student awareness of the effects of substance abuse through campus educational programming. Incorporating information about substance abuse among health care professionals into the nursing curriculum may raise nursing students' awareness of the significance of the problem (O'Gara & Strang, 2005).

Nursing Students with Mental Health Problems

Even though nursing students may be considered to be at risk for developing mental health problems due to the high levels of stress that are generally reported among nursing students, little research has been conducted on interventions to alleviate mental health problems in nursing students. What research exists has been primarily descriptive and has focused on behaviors, such as signs of anxiety, stress, and anger. One study by Patton and Goldenberg (1999) suggested that nursing students with higher degrees of hardiness can handle personal stress better than students with lower degrees of hardiness. Even though their research is more than a decade old, it remains timely as more students with severe mental illness are enrolled in higher education (Storrie, Ahern, & Tuckett, 2010). Mental health issues include anxiety, depression, eating disorders, and obsessive compulsive behavior (Storrie et al., 2010). Some nursing students may have mental health problems before enrolling in nursing school, which may have led them to be attracted to a "helping" profession. Students who experience mental health problems may need assistance in identifying and addressing these problems.

Undergraduate and graduate nursing students have many fears and worries about their ability to succeed in their program of studies. Jimenez, Navia-Osorio, and Diaz (2010) reported a study of 357 Spanish nursing students. Students identified clinical, academic, and external stressors. Students stated that clinical practice caused them to be anxious. Students were stressed by seeing patients suffering and due to differing expectations from instructors. Clinical practice caused more stress than academic or external factors (defined as daily life). An interesting finding was that more experienced students were more stressed academically.

Using a grounded theory approach, Higginson (2006) studied the fears and worries of five first-year nursing students. He discovered that first-year students worried not only about what they would experience in the clinical area, such as dealing with bodily fluids and death and dying, but also about personal finances and classroom examinations. Students also worried about how they were developing as a nurse. One student asked, "How should a nurse feel?" (Higginson, 2006, p. 45). Higginson concluded that the process of becoming a nurse is complex and students need the opportunity to discuss their fears and worries.

Part-time students may experience unique stressors (Nicholl & Timmons, 2005; Timmons & Nicholl, 2005). Seventy part-time Irish BNS students (equivalent in the United States to RN to BSN students) were surveyed. Balancing work and studies was the primary concern for these students. Attending classes and getting off from work did not seem problematic. However, completing assignments, taking examinations, and dealing with theoretical knowledge contributed to these students' stress (Nicholl & Timmons, 2005). Students recognized the need for additional education in order to get job promotions (and perhaps felt pressure in this regard).

Graduate students also experience stress while undertaking their program of studies. Maville, Kranz, and Tucker (2004) used grounded theory to explore stress in nurse practitioner students. Although students knew that becoming a nurse practitioner would increase their skill level and grant them more autonomy in their practice, students expressed the fact that the high demands of their courses and having to be independent in their learning caused high levels of stress. Like the students in Nicholl and Timmons' (2005) study, time management and financial concerns were sources of stress. Students were able to identify what faculty could do to help decrease the stress in their lives. Students stated that more lectures and greater supervision during clinical learning experiences would help. Because many graduate programs are now offered online, faculty teaching in those programs might want to consider how to provide audio and/or video streaming when presenting materials. In addition, faculty might want to explore how technology, such as Skype or other similar video conferencing software programs, could be used to provide more clinical supervision for those students who want and need this supervision.

Because of their close interaction with students, nursing faculty are often the first to note the signs of mental health problems, such as stress and anxiety, in nursing students. Some behavioral indicators, either in the classroom or in the clinical setting, may include fatigue, poor concentration, change in outward appearance, frequent absenteeism, disruption of logical thought patterns, and a decrease in the quality of work (Lambert & Nugent, 1994; Phimister, 2009). Instituting interventions early on can help ameliorate stress and anxiety felt by nursing students. Sharif and Armitage (2004) conducted a quasi-experimental study to test the effect of psychological and educational counseling on anxiety reduction in nursing students. A total of 100 second- and fourth-year Iranian baccalaureate nursing students were randomly assigned to a control group or an experimental group that participated in a 12-week program that included 2-hour sessions on anxiety reduction exercises, time management, and study skills. Focus groups were conducted before and after tests. Anxiety was measured using the Hamilton Anxiety Rating Scale, translated into Persian, and self-esteem was measured by the Coopersmith Self-Esteem Inventory, also translated into Persian. The experimental group had a statistically significant reduction in anxiety at the follow-up after one semester, which was confirmed by the focus groups. The control group also had a statistically significant reduction of anxiety at follow-up, which the authors attributed to skill development. The experimental group, however, had a higher grade point average. At follow-up, the experimental group had a statistically significant improvement in self-esteem as compared to the control group.

Kanji, White, and Ernst (2006) conducted a randomized clinical trial to test the effect of autogenic training on British nursing students. Autogenic training includes a series of six calming exercises. Ninety-three students were randomized into three groups. One group received the 20-minute intervention once a week for 8 weeks, one group received laughter therapy, and the control group received no intervention. The intervention group had a statistically significant reduction in trait and state anxiety as measured by the Spielberger State-Trait Anxiety Inventory. Burnout, as measured by the Maslach Burnout Inventory, was no different between the groups following the training. However, systolic and diastolic blood pressures were lower in the experimental group. At 5 months, 8 of 14 students were still using the training, and at 14 months, 4 were still using the training. The authors concluded that, in the short run, the training was helpful in reducing anxiety and that students could continue to use the skills learned if needed.

Kang, Choi, and Ryu (2009) tested mindfulness meditation as a strategy to decrease stress, anxiety, and depression. Forty-one nursing students were randomly assigned to experimental and control groups. The experimental group participated in 90- to 120-minute sessions for 8 weeks. Before randomization, both groups attended a lecture about stress management. Following the intervention, students in the experimental group had decreased anxiety and stress. However, the amount of depression was not significantly different between the two groups. While specific training can help students learn to control their anxiety, the role of faculty and peer mentoring cannot be overlooked.

Hughes et al. (2003) randomized junior nursing students into two groups. One group received an intervention in one semester and the other group in the second semester. All incoming students were involved in the study which involved three data collection points. Fifty-eight percent participated in all of the data collection. The intervention consisted of meeting in a group of 9 to 12 students and one faculty mentor. One of the main purposes of the groups was to model caring and healing behavior and to develop trusting behaviors. A variety of outcome measures were used including the Rosenberg Self-Esteem Scale, the Spielberger State-Trait Anxiety Inventory, and the Nurse Role Self-Efficacy Scale. The students were also asked to describe their experiences of participating in the groups. All students showed increases in anxiety and depression and decreases in self-esteem over the academic year's time. However, group attrition may have contributed to the non-significant findings. Many, but not all, students found attending the sessions impinged on their time and scheduling the group meetings became cumbersome. Those students who did attend more sessions expressed more benefit and stated the sessions allowed them to develop relationships with the faculty mentor and their peers. They also described their peers as more caring.

Hughes et al. (2003) recommended that faculty develop interventions that promote positive learning environments. One strategy to promote a positive learning environment is the use of peer mentors in the clinical setting. Sprengel and Job (2004) designed a peer mentoring project for the purpose of decreasing anxiety in 30 freshman baccalaureate nursing students. Sophomore students were paired with freshmen who were in their initial clinical course. Both mentor and mentee were oriented to their roles and worked together on the clinical unit. Before the initial clinical experience, freshmen completed the Kleehammer, Hart, and Keck Clinical Experience Assessment Form. Eight of the 16 items were rated as anxiety producing: fear of making mistakes, procedures, equipment, talking to physicians, being observed by instructors, evaluation by faculty, patient teaching, and initial clinical experience. Items that were not anxiety producing included talking to patients, asking questions of faculty, and being late. Freshmen and sophomores then evaluated the mentoring experience using an investigator-designed instrument. Both groups of students were enthusiastic in their response to the experience. Comments indicated that freshmen felt at ease and sophomores gained self-confidence.

Appropriate use of humor can also lesson anxiety (Moscaritolo, 2009). Humor can lesson anxiety, help increase self-esteem, and contribute to an overall positive learning environment. A more positive learning environment may lead to better student learning outcomes.

Another strategy that has been tested to decrease stress and increase academic performance is the use of a home hospital program (Yucha, Kowalski, & Cross, 2009). The home hospital program involved keeping nursing students, in so far as possible, at the same clinical agency throughout their program of study. Nurses in the hospitals served as the clinical instructors. The program was predicated on the fact that familiarity with the clinical agency can decrease stress and, as a side benefit, be used as a recruiting tool for the agencies involved. Yucha et al. (2009) used a quasi-experimental study to test their model. Students were divided into two groups, with half participating in the home hospital program. The results of the study were based on 78 students in the home hospital group and 79 students in the control group. Findings showed that the experimental group had a significant reduction in perception of academic load and

state anxiety (as measured by the Spielberger State Anxiety Inventory). However, there was no relationship between academic performance and stress and anxiety, as academic performance did not differ between the two groups. The authors noted that small sample size and the fact that even some clinical assignments in the experimental group were outside of the home hospital may have affected the results.

Faculty Responsibilities Related to Students with Mental Health Problems

Mental health issues range from anxiety and stress to severe depression and other mental illnesses. The process used to assist students with suspected mental health problems is similar to the approach used with any student whose academic progress is jeopardized by unsatisfactory performance. First, the ADA prohibits discrimination against individuals who are mentally impaired. Second, all actions taken by faculty must be congruent with existing institutional policies and afford students the due process that is their right. When mental health issues interfere with student behavior, keeping detailed anecdotal notes that describe the events of concern, sharing these notes and concerns with the individual student, and informing administrators of these concerns are all appropriate steps to be taken by the faculty members involved (Lambert & Nugent, 1994). Those with specific diagnoses may need some accommodation, such as permission to take tests in an alternate setting, more time to complete assignments, and written contracts for completing assignments (Job Accommodation Network, 2010).

Students should be made clearly aware of the behavior adversely affecting their academic performance and what they need to do to correct this behavior. A learning contract may be used in this instance to indicate what the student needs to do to improve the behavior and the time frame in which this must be accomplished. Faculty may need to encourage students with mental health issues to seek professional help (Morrissette, 2004). Many university campuses offer this service to students free or for a reduced fee. Nursing faculty may be tempted to counsel students on their own, but separating the student–faculty relationship from the student–counselor relationship is more effective and indeed safer (Brooke, 1999). If, despite these interventions, the behavior does not improve and the student is unable to perform effectively or patient safety is compromised, administrative withdrawal or dismissal from the program may be necessary. As always, the student who is administratively withdrawn or dismissed has the right to pursue the grievance and appeal process in place within the institution (Lambert & Nugent, 1994).

Mental health issues may manifest themselves in a variety of ways. One common way is in the form of test anxiety. Although nursing students' level of anxiety may be no different than that of their university peers, their level of test anxiety has been found to be significantly higher (Brewer, 2002). Because test anxiety can interfere with cognitive processing, students must learn to control their anxiety so performance is not compromised (Edelman & Ficorelli, 2005). For nursing students, passing tests is crucial to program success and ultimately to licensure success. Although test anxiety may not always affect a student's level of success in the program, faculty need to help students cope with their anxiety. Brewer (2002) has noted that often faculty are very abstract and conceptual in their thinking, whereas students are more concrete and pragmatic. This difference in thinking patterns may cause cognitive dissonance within the student that, in turn, may lead to stress and anxiety when trying to comprehend classroom presentations.

Edelman and Ficorelli (2005) used a phenomenological methodology to study the experience of test anxiety in eight nursing students. Three themes were elicited from the participants: "the reality of an anxiety episode; the academic implications of test anxiety; and effective measures of dealing with anxiety" (Edelman & Ficorelli, 2005, p. 57). Anxiety was so high in one student that she felt disconnected from her body. Students knew the stakes were high for them and coped by using stress management techniques and developing techniques for self-control such as listening to loud music before a test. Students also learned that they need to endure the anxiety to be successful. Edelman and Ficorelli (2005) suggest that faculty educate students about stress management as a way to promote academic success.

Mental health issues may also display themselves in the form of student incivility in the classroom and ultimately in anger within the student–faculty relationship. Lashley and de Meneses (2001) reported on a national survey of nursing programs. Of the 408 responding schools, 100% reported instances of incivility. In addition to students' tardiness and repeated absences, 24.8% reported that there was objectionable physical contact from students and 42.8% reported that students verbally abused or yelled at instructors in the clinical area (Lashley & de Meneses, 2001).

Luparell (2004) also surveyed faculty for the purpose of describing faculty response to student incivility. She used a semistructured interview technique to elicit critical incidents of incivility. Twenty-one faculty members reported 36 encounters of student incivility. From these interviews, themes were placed within a wartime framework. Themes included incivility as a battle, before the confrontation–escalating tensions and events, diplomatic efforts, on the battlefield, ambush, the attacks, battlefield emotions, calling in reinforcements–medic, the aftermath–missing in action, and costs of war. The findings clearly suggested that faculty were negatively affected by their experiences and often felt lack of administrative support in dealing with students.

Faculty concern about student incivility and violence is such a major concern that the National League for Nursing held a panel on this issue at the 2005 Faculty Summit (Kolanko et al., 2006). Sadly, anger and incivility can be taken to the extreme, which occurred at the University of Arizona when a nursing student shot and killed three nursing faculty members (Rooney, 2002). Thomas (2003) provides guidelines on how to deal with angry students. First, recognizing signs and risk factors for potential violence may help avert tragedy. Second, violent students tend to be males in their thirties and forties who may have had a previous history of violence (Thomas, 2003). Third, depression is often a precursor to violence, and anger and violence are more likely to occur in times of high stress, such as at examination time or program dismissal (Thomas, 2003). Fourth, having policies and procedures in place for dealing with potential violence is important. Threats should be promptly reported to campus security. All schools should have a procedure for dealing with student complaints and that procedure should be publicized to all students and faculty (Clark, 2009). Finally, if a faculty member is in a situation in which a student is extremely angry, the student should be asked to make an appointment and discuss the issue when tempers are less heated. If the faculty member thinks that the student may become violent, security should be notified. Having a third party to mediate disputes is sometimes helpful. In addition, a respectful proactive strategy that faculty can use is to put classroom behavioral expectations in the course syllabus and to role model appropriate communication when rudeness occurs in the classroom (Ehrmann, 2005). Students with mental illness must realize that their disability doesn't excuse inappropriate behavior.

Criminal Background Checks

In addition to mental health issues, which can compromise patient safety, the student who has a record of criminal activity can also compromise patient safety. Patient safety is a major concern for state boards of nursing and health care accreditation agencies. The Joint Commission (TJC) (2008) states, "Staff, students and volunteers who work in the same capacity as staff who provide care, treatment, and services, would be expected to have criminal background checks verified when required by law and regulation and organization policy" (para 1). Therefore nursing programs often require criminal background checks. Some states, including Louisiana, for example, require applicants applying for a license to practice to have an FBI and/or a state criminal background check (Tate & Moody, 2005). The Louisiana board of nursing requires that students self-disclose a criminal background before enrollment in clinical courses. Students must submit a written explanation and certified court documents if they disclose a criminal background. All of this documentation is then sent to the board of nursing for a ruling regarding whether a student has the ability to deliver safe nursing care. One might wonder to what extent students may have been involved in criminal activity. Tate and Moody (2005) stated that between 1995 and 2003, a total of 588 students submitted documents to the board of nursing.

Given the TJC regulation and state licensure requirements, how many schools require criminal background checks? Certainly that number is changing and is influenced by state law. As of 2007, a total of 33 states required criminal background checks before licensure, 8 states did checks based on self-disclosure, and 6 states were in the process of implementing regulations, with an additional 2 states having pending legislation (Jones & Weninger, 2007). Farnsworth and Springer (2006) conducted a stratified random sample of licensed practical, associate degree, and baccalaureate programs to determine how many schools required criminal background checks and the nature of those checks. Two hundred and fifty-eight of 398 schools responded. At the time of the survey, 41% of the total sample did not require checks, 7% were planning on doing checks, 14% required disclosure, and 38% did formal background checks.

Whether or not a school requires a criminal background check before admission, faculty have a duty to warn students that, although they may have successfully completed the nursing program, licensure could be denied if a student has a criminal background. Additionally, clinical agencies, as noted above, may have requirements for background checks and may refuse clinical placements based on the results of the criminal background check. For an example of criminal background check policy, see the Indiana State University College of Nursing Criminal Background Check Policy (www.indstate.edu/nursing/pdfs/handbook-docs/criminal-background-check.pdf).

Denying admission based on the results of a criminal background check requires careful consideration. Decisions need to be made in line with state law and clinical agency policy. Guidelines for making decisions need to be readily available to all faculty and students. When admission decisions are made, faculty need to consider the nature of the criminal conviction and how long ago the offense occurred, and afford due process for those denied admission (Jones & Weninger, 2007).

The areas of criminal background checks and drug testing continue to evolve and nursing faculty will need to keep apprised of changes in health care agency policies and state laws. The National Council of State Boards of Nursing has published a position paper and a resource packet, including model statutory language for state boards of nursing to use in crafting laws regarding criminal background checks (National Council of State Boards of Nursing, 2006a, 2006b). The National Council of State Boards of Nursing continues to update its policy recommendations.

SUMMARY

This chapter has provided information about the legal and educational issues related to teaching students with disabilities and other special needs. The needs of students with learning disabilities, chemical dependency, and mental health problems are presented, along with faculty responsibilities associated with teaching these students. Interventions are identified for assisting students to cope with a disability or impairment that can be used for all students to promote academic success.

Nursing faculty are responsible for creating a learning environment that supports the teaching–learning process for all students. Working with students who have disabilities or impairments brings special challenges to the student–faculty relationship. No specific rules say what level of disability or impairment prevents admission to a nursing program. However, faculty who are knowledgeable about the legal issues related to students with disabilities or impairments, their institution's and school's policies and procedures related to students with these special needs, and the interventions designed to help students maintain their self-esteem and be successful will find themselves capable of meeting these challenges in a caring, facilitative manner. Viewing persons with disabilities through a nonmedical paradigm paves the way for lessening the discrimination those persons often face in the educational environment and in the workplace (Marks, 2000; Sin, 2009).

Furthermore, if faculty are open to working with students who have disabilities, students might be more inclined to disclose, without fear of adverse consequences, that they have a need for accommodations (Maheady, 1999). Developing strong partnerships with clinical agencies may also be a key to successfully integrating those students with disabilities into the nursing program (Maheady, 2006). Educating nursing students about various disabilities will also help future generations of nurses and nursing faculty to view disabilities as differences rather than deficiencies (Moore, 2004). As Ashcroft et al. (2008) have noted, learning to work with nursing students, and practicing nurses for that matter, who are disabled is a journey—a journey that could benefit from additional research to support the best strategies to facilitate learning and practice for those with disabilities.

Those with disabilities will continue to seek enrollment in nursing programs. Faculty may need to consult resources that give guidance on how to accommodate those with disabilities. In addition to the resources available on individual campuses, the following websites contain much information regarding how to accommodate students with disabilities:

www.exceptionalnurse.com: This website contains many resources for those with disabilities and links for faculty that teach students with disabilities.

http://askjan.org/media/nurses.html#Info: The Job Accommodation Network provides resources for nurses with disabilities. The site is funded by the Office of Disability Employment Policy, U.S. Department of Labor.

www.amphl.org: This website for the Association of Medical Professionals with Hearing Losses contains case studies and other resources to aid faculty who have students who are hearing impaired.

www.ohsu.edu/oidd/CSD/index.cfm: This website for the Center on Self Determination at Oregon Health & Science University contains resources of interest to those who have various disabilities or care for such persons.

http://nursingworld.org/MainMenuCategories/ThePracticeofProfessionalNursing/workplace/ImpairedNurse.aspx: The American Nurses Association's Impaired Nurses Resource Center provides resources for nurses with substance abuse problems.

The following is a video that depicts a nurse with a disability performing a complex clinical skill. The video presents a discussion about nurses with disabilities:

Blythe, M. (Cameraman). Dupler, A. (Author), Fleming, S., (Author), Maheady, D. (Author), & Reynolds, J. (Producer). (In production). *Disabilities in nursing: Legal implications and skills demonstrations* [Motion picture]. (Available from Washington State University, College of Nursing, PO Box 1495, Spokane, WA 99210.)

A YouTube video also depicts one the film's authors (Susan Fleming).

Fleming, S. & Maheady, D. (2008). Nursing with the hand you are given [Video file]. Retrieved from http://www.youtube.com/watch?v=d3AfRRNxLWg&feature=related.

CASE STUDIES FOR FUTURE DISCUSSION

Case Study 1

Charlie was a 49-year-old construction worker who fell while building an addition to a hospital. He sustained a severe head injury and was in a coma and suffered hemiplegia. With aggressive rehabilitation, Charlie regained full movement of all extremities and was able to pursue a new career. He enrolled in an associate degree nursing program because he felt he needed to redirect his work life. He was able to successfully complete the program in 4 years and to pass the NCLEX. Accommodations made during his program of study that contributed to his achievement included allowing his testing to take place in isolation from other students, having tests read to him if needed to promote understanding of what was asked, and permitting additional time to complete tests. As well, he was permitted, as were all students, to pursue part-time study. Support from faculty was crucial to his success. One faculty member in particular had experienced a head injury and was able to help Charlie improve his reading comprehension skills by teaching him to place transparent colored film over and a line above the text he was reading.

Case Study 2

Paula was a nursing student who had a hearing impairment before enrollment. Only one instructor knew of her hearing impairment, and Paula was able to self-accommodate by sitting in the front in class and walking up and down hospital hallways to detect which direction alarms came from because her hearing loss was on one side. In her junior year she injured her back and had to drop out for a year. When she returned to the program, she had a lifting restriction, which she did not share with the faculty. She again self-accommodated by asking for lifting help or ignoring the restriction. She was able to successfully complete her program and gain employment that did not require lifting. During the program, however, she believed that other students and some faculty resented her disabilities (D. Maheady, personal communication, August 23, 2003).

REFLECTING ON THE EVIDENCE

1. Case studies indicate that nursing students with various disabilities can succeed academically and get jobs. What types of jobs do these graduates get and how successful are they on the job? How do these nurses handle issues of patient safety?

2. There is evidence that some schools of nursing require drug testing of students. How many schools require drug testing? What happens if a student tests positive on a random drug test?

3. Student incivility is an important issue when faculty try to maintain a positive learning environment. What kinds of support do faculty need to deal effectively with aggressive students?

4. What accommodations should faculty make in the learning spaces in order to maximize learning for all students, both nondisabled and disabled?

REFERENCES

American Association of Colleges of Nursing. (1998, November). *Policy and guidelines for prevention and management of substance abuse in the nursing education community* (Position statement). Retrieved from http://www.aacn.nche.edu/

American Nurses Association. (n.d.). *Ergonomics/handle with care*. Retrieved from http://www.nursingworld.org

Americans with Disabilities Act, 42 U.S.C. § 12111 et seq. (1990). Retrieved from http://www.ada.gov/pubs/ada.htm

Andre, K., & Manson, S. (2004). Students with disabilities undertaking clinical education experience. *Collegian*, *11*(4), 26–30.

Arndt, M. E. (2004). Education nursing students with disabilities: One nurse educator's journey from questions to clarity. *Journal of Nursing Education*, *43*(5), 204–206.

Ashcroft, T. J., Chernomas, W. M., Davis, P. L., Dean, R. A. K., Seguire, M., Shapiro, C. R., & Swiderski, L. M. (2008). Nursing students with disabilities: One faculty's journey. *International Journal of Nursing Education Scholarship*, *5*(1), Art 18. doi:10.2202/1548-923X.1424

Association of Medical Professionals with Hearing Losses. (n.d.). *Stethoscope information* (Online forum). Retrieved from http://www.amphl.org/stethoscopes.php

Baldwin, J. N., Bartek, J. K., Scott, D. M., Davis-Hall, R. E., & Desimone II, E. M. (2009). Survey of alcohol and other drug use attitudes and behaviors in nursing students. *Substance Abuse, 30*(3), 230–238. doi:10.1080/08897070903040964

Bohne, J. M. (2004). Valuing differences among nursing students. *Journal of Nursing Education, 43*(5), 202–203.

Bradshaw, M. (2006). The nursing student with attention deficit syndrome. *Annual Review of Nursing Education, 4*, 235–250.

Bradshaw, M. J., & Salzer, J. S. (2003). The nursing student with attention deficit hyperactivity disorder. *Nurse Educator, 28*(4), 161–165.

Brewer, T. (2002). Test-taking anxiety among nursing and general college students. *Journal of Psychosocial Nursing, 40*(11), 23–29.

Brooke, C. P. (1999). Feelings from the back row: Negotiating sensitive issues in large classes. In S. M. Richardson (Ed.), *Promoting civility: A teaching challenge* (pp. 23–33). San Francisco, CA: Jossey-Bass.

Bugle, L., Jackson, E., Kornegay, K., & Rives, K. (2003). Attitudes of nursing faculty regarding nursing students with a chemical dependency: A national survey. *Journal of Addictions Nursing, 14*(3), 125–132.

Carroll, S. M. (2004). Inclusion of people with physical disabilities in nursing education. *Journal of Nursing Education, 43*(5), 207–212.

Clark, C. M. (1999). Substance abuse among nursing students: Establishing a comprehensive policy and procedure for faculty intervention. *Nurse Educator, 24*(2), 16–19.

Clark, C. M. (2009). Faculty guide for promoting civility in the classroom. *Nurse Educator, 34*(5), 194–197.

Colon, E. J. (1997). Identification, accommodation, and success of students with learning disabilities in nursing education programs. *Journal of Nursing Education, 36*(8), 372–377.

Crow, K. L. (2008). Four types of disabilities: Their impact on online learning. *TechTrends, 52*(1), 51–55.

Dailey, M. A. (2010). Needing to be normal: The lived experience of chronically ill nursing students. *International Journal of Nursing Education Scholarship, 7*(1), 1–23. doi:10.2202/1548-923X.1798

Dunn, D. (2005). Substance abuse among nurses—Intercession and intervention. *AORN Journal, 82*(5), 775–799.

Edelman, M. A., & Ficorelli, C. (2005). A measure of success: Nursing students and test anxiety. *Journal for Nurses in Staff Development, 21*(2), 55–59.

Ehrmann, G. (2005). Managing the aggressive nursing student. *Nurse Educator, 30*(3), 98–100.

Eliason, M. J. (1992). Nursing students with learning disabilities: Appropriate accommodations. *Journal of Nursing Education, 31*(8), 375–376.

Farnsworth, J., & Springer, P. J. (2006). Background checks for nursing students: What are schools doing? *Nursing Education Perspectives, 27*(3), 148–153.

Fleming, S. E. (2006). Am I handicapped? Nursing with one hand. In D. C. Maheady (Ed.), *Leave no nurse behind: Nurses working with disabilities* (pp. 26–31). New York, NY: iUniverse.

Fowler, M. D. M. (Ed.). (2008). *Guide to the code of ethics for nurses.* Silver Spring, MD: American Nurses Association.

Gnadt, B. (2006). Religiousness, current substance abuse, and early risk indicators for substance abuse in nursing students. *Journal of Addictions Nursing, 17*(3), 151–158. doi:10.1080/1088-1600600862103

Helms, L., Jorgensen, J., & Anderson, M. A. (2006). Disability law and nursing education. *Journal of Professional Nursing, 22*(3), 190–196. doi:10.1016/j.profnurs.2006.03.005

Helms, L. B., & Thompson, E. S. (2005). Nurse anesthesia students with disabilities: A legal and academic review of potential professional standards. *AANA Journal, 73*(4), 265–269.

Higginson, R. (2006). Fears, worries and experiences of first-year pre-registration nursing students: A qualitative study. *Nurse Researcher, 13*(3), 32–49.

Hughes, L. C., Romick, P., Sandor, M. K., Phillips, C. A., Glaister, J., Levy, K., & Rock, J. (2003). Evaluation of an informal peer group experience on baccalaureate nursing students' emotional well-being and professional socialization. *Journal of Professional Nursing, 19*(1), 38–48.

Ijiri, L., & Kudzma, E. C. (2000). Supporting nursing students with learning disabilities: A metacognitive approach. *Journal of Professional Nursing, 16*(3), 149–157.

Jimenez, C., Navia-Osorio, P. M., & Diaz, C. V. (2010). Stress and health in novice and experienced nursing students. *Journal of Advanced Nursing, 66*(2), 442–455. doi:10.1111/j.1365-2648.2009.05183.x

Job Accommodation Network. (2010). *Accommodation and compliance series: Nurses with disabilities.* Retrieved from http://askjan.org/media/downloads/Nurses.pdf

Johnston, L. D., O'Malley, P. M., Bachman, J. G., & Schulenberg, J. E. (2005). *Monitoring the future: National survey results on drug use, 1975–2004: Volume II, College students and adults ages 19–45 (NIH Publication No. 05-5728).* Bethesda, MD: National Institute on Drug Abuse. Retrieved from http://monitoringthefuture.org/pubs/monographs/vol2_2004.pdf

Joint Commission, The. (2008, November). *Requirements for criminal background checks.* Retrieved from http://www.jointcommission.org/

Jones, M. M., & Weninger, R. A. (2007). Student criminal background checks: Considerations for schools of nursing. *Journal of Nursing Law, 11*(3), 163–169.

Kang, Y. S., Choi, S. Y., & Ryu, E. (2009). The effectiveness of a stress coping program based on mindfulness meditation on the stress, anxiety, and depression experienced by nursing students in Korea. *Nurse Education Today, 29*(5), 538–543. doi:10.1016/j.nedt.2008.12.003

Kanji, N., White, A., & Ernst, E. (2006). Autogenic training to reduce anxiety in nursing students: A randomized control trial. *Journal of Advanced Nursing, 53*(6), 729–735.

Kenna, G. A., & Wood, M. D. (2004). Substance use by pharmacy and nursing practitioners and students in a northeastern state. *American Journal of Health-System Pharmacy, 61*(9), 921–930.

Kolanko, K. M. (2003). A collective case study of nursing students with learning disabilities. *Nursing Education Perspectives, 24*(5), 251–256.

Kolanko, K. M., Clark, C., Heinrich, K. T., Olive, D., Serembus, J. F., & Sifford, K. S. (2006). Academic dishonesty, bullying, incivility, and violence: Difficult challenges facing nurse educators. *Nursing Education Perspectives, 27*(1), 34–43.

Kornegay, K., Bugle, L., & Rives, K. (2004). Facing a problem of great concern: Nursing faculty's lived experience of encounters with chemically dependent nursing students. *Journal of Addictions Nursing, 15*(3), 125–132.

Lambert, V. A., & Nugent, K. E. (1994). Addressing the academic progression of students encountering mental health problems. *Nurse Educator, 19*(5), 33–39.

Lashley, F. R., & de Meneses, M. (2001). Student civility in nursing programs: A national survey. *Journal of Professional Nursing, 17*(2), 81–86.

LD Online. (n.d.). *LD basics: What is a learning disability?* Retrieved from http://www.ldonline.org/

Levine, M. R., & Rennie, W. P. (2004). Pre-employment urine testing of hospital employees: Future questions and review of current literature. *Occupational and Environmental Medicine, 61*(4), 318–324.

Luparell, S. (2004). Faculty encounters with uncivil nursing students: An overview. *Journal of Professional Nursing, 20*(1), 59–67.

Maheady, D. C. (1999). Jumping through hoops, walking on egg shells: The experiences of nursing students with disabilities. *Journal of Nursing Education, 38*(4), 162–170.

Maheady, D. C. (2003). *Nursing students with disabilities change the course.* River Edge, NJ: Exceptional Parent Press.

Maheady, D. C. (2005). Teaching nursing students with disabilities. In L. Caputi (Ed.), *Teaching nursing: The art and science* (Vol. 3, pp. 209–231). Glen Ellyn, IL: College of DuPage Press.

Maheady, D. C. (Ed.). (2006). *Leave no nurse behind: Nurses working with disabilities.* New York, NY: iUniverse.

Marks, B. A. (2000). Commentary: Jumping through hoops and walking on egg shells or discrimination, hazing, and abuse of students with disabilities. *Journal of Nursing Education, 39*(5), 205–210.

Maville, J. A., Kranz, P. J., & Tucker, B. A. (2004). Perceived stress reported by nurse practitioner students. *Journal of the Academy of Nurse Practitioners, 16*(6), 257–262.

McCleary-Jones, V. (2008). Strategies to facilitate learning among nursing students. *Nurse Educator, 33*(3), 105–106.

Menendez, J. B. (2010). Americans with Disabilities Act—Related considerations: When an alcoholic nurse is your employee" When is a nurse legally considered a "direct threat" to patient safety. *JONA's Healthcare Law, Ethics, and Regulation, 12*(1), 21–24.

Mitchell, T., O'Sullivan, P. B., Smith, A., Burnett, A. F., Straker, L., Thornton, J., & Rudd, C. J. (2009). Biopsychosocial factors are associated with low back pain in female nursing students: A cross-sectional study. *International Journal of Nursing Studies, 46*, 678–688.

Monroe, T. (2009). Addressing substance abuse among nursing students: Development of a prototype alternative-to-dismissal policy. *Journal of Nursing Education, 48*(5), 272–278. doi:10.9999/01484834-20090416-06

Moore, C. (2004). Disability as difference in the nursing profession. *Journal of Nursing Education. 43*(5), 197–201.

Morris, D., & Turnbull, P. (2006). Clinical experiences of students with dyslexia. *Journal of Advanced Nursing, 54*(2), 238–247.

Morrissette, P. J. (2004). Promoting psychiatric student nurse well-being. *Journal of Psychiatric and Mental Health Nursing, 11*(5), 534–554.

Moscaritolo, L. M. (2009). Interventional strategies to decrease nursing student anxiety in the clinical learning environment. *Journal of Nursing Education, 48*(1), 17–23.

Murphy, G. T., & Brennan, M. (1998). Nursing students with disabilities. *Canadian Nurse, 94*(10), 31–34.

Murphy-Parker, D., Kronenbitter, S., & Kronenbitter, R. (2003). USA National Student Nurses Association passes resolution: In support of nursing school policies to assist and advocate nursing students experiencing impaired practice. *The Drug and Alcohol Professional, 3*(2), 9–14.

National Center for Education Statistics. (n.d.). *Table 231: Number and percentage distribution of students enrolled in postsecondary institutions, by level, disability status, and selected student and characteristics: 2003–04 and 2007–08* [Data file]. Washington, DC: Author. Retrieved from http://nces.ed.gov/programs/digest/d09/tables/dt09_231.asp

National Council of State Boards of Nursing. (n.d.). *2010 NCLEX examination candidate bulletin.* Retrieved from http://www.ncsbn.org/

National Council of State Boards of Nursing. (2006a). NCSBN 2006 annual meeting: Section 2. *The threshold of regulatory excellence: Taking up the challenge* (pp. 107–135). Retrieved from http://www.ncsbn.org/pdfs/II_BB_2006_Section_2a_Recom.pdf

National Council of State Boards of Nursing. (2006b). *Using criminal background checks to inform licensure decision making.* Retrieved from http://www.ncsbn.org/pdfs/Criminal_Background_Checks.pdf

Neal-Boylan, L. J., & Guillet, S. E. (2008). Nurses with disabilities: Can changing our educational system keep them in nursing. *Nurse Educator, 33*(4), 164–167.

Nelson, A., & Lentz, K. (2003). Safe patient handling and movement. *American Journal of Nursing, 103*(3), 32–43.

Nettina, S. (2003, May). The untapped nursing workpool: Nurses with disabilities. *Medscape Today.* Retrieved from http://www.medscape.com/viewarticle/452605

Nicholl, H., & Timmons, F. (2005). Programme-related stressors among part-time undergraduate nursing students. *Journal of Advanced Nursing, 50*(1), 93–100.

Nichols, A. H., & Quaye, S. J. (2009). Beyond accommodation: Removing barriers to academic and social engagement for students with disabilities. In S. R. Harper & S. J. Quaye (Eds.), *Student engagement in higher education* (pp. 39–60). New York, NY: Routledge.

O'Gara, C., & Strang, J. (2005). Substance misuse training among psychiatric doctors, psychiatric nurses, medical and nursing students in a South London psychiatric teaching hospital. *Drugs: Education, Prevention and Policy, 12*(4), 327–336.

O'Malley, P. M., & Johnston, L. D. (2002). Epidemiology of alcohol and other drug use among American college students. *Journal of Studies on Alcohol, 63*(Suppl. 14), 23–39.

O'Quinn, J. L. (1996). Chemical abuse in nursing students: A retrospective view. *Journal of Addictions Nursing, 8*(3), 94–98.

Patton, T. J., & Goldenberg, D. (1999). Hardiness and anxiety as predictors of academic success in first-year, full-time and part-time RN students. *Journal of Continuing Education in Nursing, 30*(4), 158–167.

Persaud, D., & Leedom, C. L. (2002). The Americans with Disabilities Act: Effect on student admission and retention. *Journal of Nursing Education, 41*(8), 349–352.

Phimister, D. (2009). Pressure too much? *Nursing Standard, 22*(33), 61.

Price, G. A., & Gale, A. (2006). How do dyslexic nursing students cope with clinical practice placements? The impact of the dyslexic profile on the clinical practice of dyslexic nursing students: Pedagogical issues and considerations. *Learning Disabilities: A Contemporary Journal, 4*(1), 19–36.

Rehabilitation Act, 29 U.S.C. 794 § 504 et seq. (1973). Retrieved from http://uscode.house.gov/download/pls/29C16.txt

Rockford College. (2010). *Nursing dept. background checks and drug screening.* Rockford, IL: Author. Retrieved from http://www.rockford.edu/

Rooney, M. (2002, November 8). Student kills 3 U. of Arizona professors. *Chronicle of Higher Education.* Retrieved from http://www.chronicle.com

Scullion, P. A. (2010). Models of disability: Their influence in nursing and potential role in challenging discrimination. *Journal of Advanced Nursing, 66*(3), 697–707. doi:10.1111/j.1365-2648.2009.05211.x

Selekman, J. (2002). Nursing students with learning disabilities. *Journal of Nursing Education, 41*(8), 334–339.

Sharif, F., & Armitage, P. (2004). The effect of psychological counselling in reducing anxiety in nursing students. *Journal of Psychiatric and Mental Health Nursing, 11*(4), 386–392.

Sheets, V. (n.d.). *Criminal background checks (CBCs) as a regulatory tool (Poster).* Retrieved from https://www.ncsbn.org/ICN_Poster%2815_CBC%29.pdf

Sin, C. H. (2009). Medicalising disability? Regulation and practice around fitness assessment of disabled students and professionals in nursing, social work and teaching professions in Great Britain. *Disability and Rehabilitation, 31*(18), 1520–1528.

Southeastern Community College v. Davis, 442 U.S. 397 (1979).

Sowers, J., & Smith, M. (2004a). Evaluation of the effects of an inservice training program on nursing faculty members' perceptions, knowledge, and concerns about students with disabilities. *Journal of Nursing Education, 43*(6), 248–252.

Sowers, J., & Smith, M. (2004b). Nursing faculty members' perceptions, knowledge, and concerns about students with disabilities. *Journal of Nursing Education, 43*(5), 213–218.

Sprengel, A. D., & Job, L. (2004). Reducing anxiety by clinical peer mentoring with beginning nursing students. *Nurse Educator, 29*(6), 246–250.

Storrie, K., Ahern, K., & Tuckett, A. (2010). A systematic review: Students with mental health problems—A growing problem. *International Journal of Nursing Practice, 16*(1), 1–6. doi:10.1111/j.1440-172X.01813.x/full

Summary of key provisions: EEOC's notice of proposed rulemaking (NPRM) to implement the ADA Amendments Act of 2008 (ADAAA). (n.d.). Retrieved from http://www.EEOC.gov/laws/regulations/upload/adaaa-summary.pdf

Talbert, J. A. J. (2009). Substance abuse among nurses. *Clinical Journal of Oncology, 13*(1), 17–19.

Tate, E. T., & Moody, K. (2005). The public good: Regulation of nursing students. *JONA's Healthcare Law, Ethics, and Regulation, 7*(2), 47–53.

Tee, S. R., Owens, K., Plowright, S., Ramnath, P., Rourke, S., James, C., & Bayliss, J. (2010). Being reasonable: Supporting disabled nursing students in practice. *Nurse Education in Practice, 10,* 216–221. doi:10.1016/j.nepr.2009.11.006

Teter, C. J., McCabe, S. E., Cranford, J. A., Boyd, C. J., & Guthrie, S. (2005). Prevalence and motives for illicit use of prescription stimulants in an undergraduate student sample. *Journal of American College Health, 53*(6), 253–262.

Thomas, S. P. (2003). Handling anger in the teacher–student relationship. *Nursing Education Perspectives, 24*(1), 17–24.

Timmons, F., & Nicholl, H. (2005). Stressors associated with qualified nurses undertaking part-time degree programmes—Some implications for nurse managers to consider. *Journal of Nursing Management, 13*(6), 477–482.

Vickers, M. Z. (2010, March). *Accommodating college students with learning disabilities: ADD, ADHD, and dyslexia.* Raleigh, NC: John W. Pope Center for Higher Education Policy. Retrieved from http://www.popecenter.org/

Videman, T., Ojajarviä, A., Riihimakiä, H., & Troup, J. D. G. (2005). Low back pain among nurses: A follow-up beginning at entry to the nursing school. *Spine, 30*(20), 2334–2341.

Watkins, M. P., & Kurz, J. M. (1997). Managing clinical experiences for minority students with physical disabilities and impairments. *The ABNF Journal, 8*(4), 82–86.

Wolf, L. E., Brown, J. T., & Bork, G. R. K. (2009). *Students with Asperger syndrome: A guide for college personnel.* Shawnee Mission, KS: Autism Asperger.

Wood, D., & Marshall, E. S. (2010). Nurses with disabilities working in hospital settings: Attitudes, concerns, and experiences of nurse leaders. *Journal of Professional Nursing, 26*(3), 182–187. doi:10.1016/j.profnurs.2009.12.001

Yucha, C. B., Kowalski, S., & Cross, C. (2009). Student stress and academic performance: Home hospital program. *Journal of Nursing Education, 48*(11), 631–637. doi:10.3928/01484834-20090828-05

5 Curriculum Development: An Overview

Nancy Dillard, DNS, RN
Linda Siktberg, PhD, RN

In today's world there are multiple factors affecting and challenging institutions of higher education, such as shifting resources; internal influences, including changing faculty and student demographics and institutional mission and governance; and external forces, such as health care reform, change of focus from national health to global health, changing societal demographics, market and employment, discipline and professional associations, and accrediting bodies. One major external force affecting curriculum, the Institute of Medicine (IOM, 2003), established competencies for health professions education that were adapted to nursing education, including patient-centered care, informatics, teamwork and collaboration, evidence-based practice, quality improvement, and safety. Redesign of the work environment of nurses began in 2003 with Transforming Care at the Bedside (TCAB), funded by the Robert Wood Johnson Foundation, with four main components: safe and reliable care, vitality and teamwork, patient-centered care, and value-added care processes. Finkelman and Kenner (2009) discussed the relevance and integration of the competencies to nursing education with development of competencies in knowledge, skills, and attitudes.

Creative, innovative methods of curriculum delivery are being used in an effort to provide cost-effective, quality programming to an increasingly diverse population of students. Flexible curricula are being developed that allow universities to provide programs that quickly respond to the needs of the local, regional, and national constituencies to which they are accountable, including the doctorate in nursing practice (DNP) and clinical nurse leader (CNL). Benefits and risks of changing nursing roles are being discussed and debated (Bargagliotti, 2006; Benner, Sutphen, Leonard, & Day, 2010; Chase & Pruitt, 2006; Cronenwett et al., 2007; Hathaway, Jacob, Stegbauer, Thompson, & Graff, 2006; IOM, 2003; Ironside, 2006; Lancaster, 2006; Lattuca & Stark, 2009; Long, 2004; McCabe, 2006; Porter-Wenzlaff & Froman, 2008; TCAB, 2008). Some authors have asserted that the quickest way to contain university costs and alleviate financial strain is to maintain quality courses yet limit the number of electives offered or to eliminate selected programs of study. At risk is the costly clinical nursing education with a 1:10 faculty-to-student ratio (Fitzpatrick, 2006; IMPAC, 2001).

As institutions of higher education reevaluate how to best achieve their stated missions and position themselves for the future, it is apparent that sweeping changes in higher education are affecting the development and delivery of curricula. Nurse educators in academia also need to be actively involved in exploring cost-effective, comprehensive curricula (American Association of Colleges of Nursing [AACN], 2006; Diefenbeck, Plowfield, & Herrman, 2006; Diekelmann, Ironside, & Gunn, 2005; Fitzpatrick, 2006; Tanner, 2006a, 2006b).

Traditionally, faculty autonomy has been closely tied to curriculum; in fact, faculty are considered to "own" the curriculum. This means faculty are accountable for assessing, implementing, evaluating, and changing the curriculum to assure quality in programs. Monitoring of the "processes and outcomes" to verify currency of the content is a responsibility of the faculty, who must identify problems and offer ideas to resolve the problems.

The authors acknowledge the work of Juanita Laidig, EdD, RN, in the previous edition(s) of the chapter.

Expert faculty are responsible for mentoring new faculty in the process of teaching curriculum; new faculty are responsible for recognizing whether the program and teaching philosophies are a cultural fit for them. Faculty roles are changing and increasing as curriculum involves more than content, including development of collegiality and integrity among students, establishing clinical partnerships, and advancing with technological changes. A strong knowledge of health care systems is necessary as faculty plan clinicals, provide student supervision, and plan preceptorships in acute care and community-based agencies.

To enhance the success of what has unfortunately become a content-laden curriculum, faculty are becoming more engaged with nurse colleagues in creating evidence-based scenarios and practice opportunities for students to learn the processes of collaboration, inquiry, and "knowing" that are needed to provide safe patient care. Faculty are assuming new teaching roles as high-fidelity simulators, mobile devices, online distance education, and virtual environments accelerate the pace with which students make more sophisticated decisions about complex care. Some faculty are undoubtedly uncomfortable with using these new technologies, not having had previous experience with integrating technology into their teaching practices. Due to rapidly changing societal forces and limited economic resources, faculty will continue to play an important role in curriculum redesign in order to keep curricula contemporary and relevant to practice (Allen & Seaman, 2010; AACN, 2009; Belleck, 2006; Benner et al., 2010; Courey, Benson-Soros, Deemer, & Zeller, 2006; Diekelmann et al., 2005; Frank, Adams, Edelstein, Speakman, & Shelton, 2005; Giddens & Brady, 2007; Jones & Wolf, 2010; Keating, 2006; Larson, 2006; Morris & Hancock, 2008; Nelson et al., 2006; Phillips, Shaw, Sullivan, & Johnson, 2010; Ruth-Sahd & Tisdell, 2007; Skiba, 2006a; Tanner, 2007).

An increase in student diversity provides opportunities and challenges for curriculum development. Students are seeking faster and more economical means of earning a degree in higher education. An increased number of adult students are entering nursing programs as job displacement increases and students have become dissatisfied with their original jobs. The adult students begin the nursing programs highly motivated,

goal directed, and expecting to be respected and recognized for their previous successes. An increased number of students with diverse racial and ethnic backgrounds are seeking degrees in nursing and present with diverse learning needs. Universities and nursing programs that expect to survive must respond to the needs of consumers and communities. Curricula must be flexible to accommodate work schedules; offer diversity in courses and programs, including distance education and environments; teach management of culturally diverse people, as well as delegation and negotiation skills; enhance verbal, written, speaking, and information technology skills; and enhance the decision-making skills needed for this increasingly complex world (Allen & Seaman, 2010; AACN, 2009; Belleck, 2006; Doll, 1996; Jones & Wolf, 2010; Morris & Hancock, 2008; Phillips et al., 2010).

Distance education through the Internet has gained popularity as students across the country share ideas in virtual chat rooms, complete discussion board assignments, send electronic papers, and complete quizzes and examinations in online courses without ever seeing the faces of their professors and their colleagues. Educators focus on opening new courses to students; responding to basic and adult students' learning needs; providing student support resources; and providing well-developed, cost-effective learning materials to distance education students. Potential students compare programs offered through the Internet to determine which will be the best, shortest, and most cost effective (Allen & Seaman, 2010; Cangelosi & Whitt, 2006; Hodson Carlton, Siktberg, Flowers, & Scheibel, 2003; Jones & Wolf, 2010; Melton, 2002; Miklancie & Davis, 2005; Phillips et al., 2010).

To develop relevant nursing curricula for the future, faculty must consider the following questions:

- Are students prepared to practice in a complex and changing health care environment, understanding that they will be required to engage in lifelong learning so they can have a sustained nursing career?
- Are students prepared as professionals, learning to think, make clinical decisions based on a culture of patient safety, collaborate interprofessionally, and demonstrate integrity in their practice within a legal and ethical framework,

as well as demonstrate other requisite knowledge and skills?

- Are students learning essential multicultural and holistic concepts for culturally sensitive patient care?
- Are faculty working dynamically and productively to design curricula that will most effectively help prepare students for the workforce, including the design of innovative clinical models of instruction?
- Is a major focus of the curricula on evidence-based research and practice, promoting faculty and student collaboration in inquiry?
- Are curricula meeting the needs of the elderly, women, the culturally diverse, and other vulnerable populations?
- Are curricula being delivered using active learning strategies, such as unfolding case studies, scenarios, and interactive technologies that require students to engage with the topics and apply their knowledge?
- Does the university provide programs that are high quality, accessible, and economically affordable, as compared to other peer institutions?
- Is the curriculum meeting the needs of their communities and other relevant stakeholders?
- Does the curriculum foster use of current and emerging instructional and patient care technologies, and are faculty adequately prepared to integrate these new technologies into their teaching?

These and other questions challenge nursing faculty to critically review current curricula and methods of instruction with the goal of preparing graduates for the future.

The rapid development of technology has also affected curriculum development, and faculty must be cognizant of the implications of technology in education. How is the development of curricula being affected by the technology explosion? Which programs can be, and should be, offered through the use of online methodologies and other distance-accessible means? The Internet is playing an increasingly larger role in higher education, and students expect the technology to be incorporated into their courses, allowing them flexibility with their coursework that complements their work and family responsibilities. The use of technology also enhances professional education, as enrollment in certification programs that offer advanced knowledge and skills and "just-in-time" opportunities to learn new information will continue to increase and attract learners. Faculty are developing new technology skills to be used for course delivery, testing, curriculum design, and networking among professionals (Benner et al., 2010; Commission on Collegiate Nursing Education [CCNE], 2009; Courey et al., 2006; Diekelmann et al., 2005; Hodson Carlton et al., 2003; Lindeman, 2000).

How are professional curricula, such as nursing and health care, being affected and what are the implications for faculty in redesigning a content-laden curriculum? Restructuring and reforms in the health care system are rapidly changing the focus of nursing curricula, as graduates must learn to deliver care within a health care environment that is focusing more and more on transitional care and the primary health care needs of individuals. Nursing practice must be safe and cost effective across patient care settings. Of course, nursing education must continue to maintain standards and meet the requirements of state boards of nursing and national accrediting agencies while responding to these health care and institutional changes. Nursing curricula need to include the concepts of patient safety, coordination of care, self-management, and health literacy, with emphasis on the burden of health problems on patient and family, strategies to decrease the gap between practice and evidence-based practice, and strategies that are generalizable across populations (Finkelman & Kenner, 2009). Also important to nursing curricula are goals from *Healthy People 2020*, including a focus on reducing disparities, preventable diseases, disability, injury, and premature death in improving health care for all (*Healthy People 2020*, n.d.). Forbes & Hickey (2009) reviewed the literature related to nursing curriculum reform, including the effects of the National Council Licensure Examination–Registered Nurse (NCLEX-RN) test blueprint. The NCLEX- RN blueprint is changed every 3 years based on practice surveys, interviews, and other data. As knowledge and practice patterns change, faculty add to the already content-laden curriculum. Forbes and Hickey (2009) noted that the "'lag' between current practice and revised examination content contributes significantly to the widening gap between academia and practice" (p. 8).

A decade ago, Lenburg (2002) challenged nurses and nurse educators to consider the following changes that affect the profession and curriculum:

(1) Rapid knowledge expansion and use of changing information technology; (2) necessity for documented practice-based competencies; evidence-based practice; (3) sociodemographic, cultural, economics, political influences on healthcare, education, community; (4) community-based, collaborative, interdisciplinary healthcare and education; (5) consumer-oriented society and impact on healthcare and education; (6) ethics and bioethical issues, dilemmas; biotechnology, biogenetic advances; (7) shortage of qualified nurses, teachers, and other healthcare personnel; aging; (8) increasing professional and personal responsibility and accountability; required continuing competency; (9) diversity, flexibility, mobility, and delivery of education; changing methods for learning and assessment of competence for practice; and (10) increasing reality of terrorism in various forms; fear, preparedness, consequences (pp. 6–7).

Lenburg's challenges to the nursing profession are still pertinent today. Nursing education faces a great transformation as faculty strive to adapt curricula to prepare graduates at all levels of education for an increasingly complex workforce that has greater practice expectations and a heavier reliance on the use of advanced technologies (Benner et al., 2010; Commission on Collegiate Nursing Education, 2009). Faculty remain challenged to reconsider curricula with a focus on strengthening student inquiry and teaching concepts across settings (Giddens & Brady, 2007; Tanner, 2007). Traditions in higher education and nursing are changing as faculty progress to more interactive curriculum models that involve students and faculty actively collaborating in the learning process.

Definition of Curriculum

The term *curriculum* was first used in Scotland as early as 1820 and became a part of the education vernacular in the United States nearly a century later. Over time, curriculum—derived from the Latin word *currere*, which means "to run"—has been translated to mean "course of study" (Wiles & Bondi, 1989). Ronald Doll (1996) defined curriculum as the "formal and informal content and process by which learners gain knowledge and understanding, develop skills, and alter attitudes, appreciations, and values under the auspices of that school" (p. 15). William Doll (2002) described curriculum in relation to a shifting paradigm, moving from a formal definition to a focus on one's multiple interactions with others and one's surroundings. He defined curriculum using the following five concepts:

1. *Currere*: "To run a course . . . a process or method of 'negotiating passages'—between ourselves and the text, between ourselves and the students, and among all three" (pp. 45–46).
2. *Complexity*: "Looking at curriculum . . . as a complex and dynamic web of interactions evolving naturally into more varied interconnected forms is a formidable task that will require vision and perseverance" (p. 46).
3. *Cosmology*: Viewing the curriculum as alive, combining "the rigorousness of science . . . the imagination of story . . . the vitality and creativity of spirit" (p. 48).
4. *Conversation*: "Teachers and students respect, honor, and understand their own humanness . . . the 'otherness' of each other . . . [and] the texts studied and the ways of thinking inscribed in them" (pp. 49–50).
5. *Community*: "An extension of community beyond self," which will include "ecological, global, and cosmological issues within which all humans are enmeshed" (pp. 51–52).

Because of the amorphous nature of the term *curriculum*, it has a variety of definitions. Educators prefer particular definitions based on individual philosophical beliefs and the emphasis placed on specific aspects of education. A review of literature revealed that common components in the definition of curriculum include the following (Beauchamp, 1968; Doll, 1996; Longstreet & Shane, 1993; Ornstein & Hunkins, 1993; Wiles & Bondi, 1989):

- Preselected goals and outcomes to be achieved
- Selected content with specific sequencing in a program of study
- Processes and experiences to facilitate learning for traditional and adult learners
- Resources used
- The extent of responsibility for learning assumed by the teacher and the learner
- How and where learning takes place

Curriculum can be viewed from a variety of perspectives, ranging from narrow and circumscribed to broad and encompassing. Oliva (1992) and others offered additional varied interpretations of curriculum as follows (Doll, 1996; Erickson, 1995; Klein, 1995):

- Knowledge organized and presented in a set of subjects and courses
- Modes of thought
- Cognitive and affective content and process
- Instructional set of outcomes and performance objectives
- Everything planned by faculty in a planned learning environment
- Interschool activities, including extracurricular activities, guidance, and interpersonal relationships
- Individual learner's experience as a result of schooling

Curriculum Development in Nursing

Curriculum in nursing has also been viewed from a number of perspectives. Heidgerken, a respected nurse educator in the 1940s and 1950s, believed that curriculum entailed all planned and day-to-day learning experiences of the students and faculty, including both organized instruction and clinical experiences (Diekelmann, 1993). Taba (1962), a curriculum expert whose work influenced nursing education, defined curriculum as the following:

> All curricula, no matter what their particular design, are composed of certain elements. A curriculum usually contains a statement of aims and of specific objectives; it indicates some selection and organization of content; it either implies or manifests certain patterns of learning and teaching, whether because the objectives demand them or because the content organization requires them. Finally, it includes a program of evaluation of the outcomes (p. 11).

Building on curriculum as a plan, Beauchamp (1968), another expert in curriculum development, viewed curriculum as a written document depicting the scope and arrangement of a projected educational program for a school.

For the past 25 years, nurse educators have been greatly influenced by the work of Bevis. The definition of curriculum used in her earlier writings reflected her allegiance to the Tyler behaviorist, technical model of curriculum development, an orientation supported by most nurse educators at the time. In 2000 Bevis defined curriculum as "those transactions and interactions that take place between students and teachers and among students with the intent that learning takes place" (p. 72). Bevis challenged nurse educators to move from what she termed the *Tylerian/behaviorist curriculum development paradigm* to one that focuses on human interaction and active learning. Relative to this new paradigm, Bevis proposed that the definition of curriculum be changed to incorporate students' and teachers' interactions and the transactions that occur (Bevis, 1989, 2000).

Other nurse educators have attempted to broaden Bevis' definition of curriculum. To capture the personal meaningfulness of curriculum, Nelms (1991) defined the term as intensely personal learning within a transpersonal interaction, stating that curriculum is "the educational journey, in an educational environment in which the biography of the person (the student) interacts with the history of the culture of nursing through the biography of another person (the faculty) to create meaning and release potential in the lives of all participants" (p. 6).

The nursing curriculum is often based on current practice, accreditation standards, regulation requirements, and faculty interests, which leads to lack of standardization of curricula. Dialogues among nursing educators about the conceptualization of curriculum include challenges to traditional ways of designing curricula in which curricula often follow practice. "It is the responsibility of nursing education in collaboration with practice settings to shape practice, not merely respond to changes in the practice environment" (AACN, 1999, p. 60). New opportunities abound to foster collaborative debate and dialogue on a number of issues, including how to accomplish the following:

- Enhance students' delegating, supervising, prioritizing, clinical decision making, and leadership skills to effect change.
- Focus on health promotion, disease prevention, and health care disparities across health care settings.
- Enhance student–faculty–preceptor interactions in the learning process.
- Design clinical models that allow for student immersion in the practice setting.
- Use "anticipatory–innovative learning" rather than "maintenance learning" (Watson, 2000, pp. 40–41).
- Use evidence-based research and nursing practice.

- Integrate culture of safety concepts in specifically designed interdisciplinary practices.
- Focus on quality, cost-effective patient-centered care.
- Expand culturally sensitive nursing practice in community-based agencies.

Although various curriculum models are found in the literature, most authors in nursing education agree that for learning to be successful and satisfying, an ongoing, responsive relationship between curriculum and instruction is essential (Baldwin & Nelms, 1993; Benner et al., 2010; Commission on Collegiate Nursing Education, 2009; Keating, 2006; Morris & Hancock, 2008; Morse & Corcoran-Perry, 1996; Wink, 2003).

Types of Curricula

Regardless of the interpretation of curriculum, several curricula may occur concurrently. The *official curriculum* includes the stated curriculum framework with philosophy and mission; recognized lists of outcomes, competencies, and learning objectives for the program and individual courses; course outlines; and syllabi. Bevis (2000) stated that the "legitimate curriculum . . . [is] the one agreed on by the faculty either implicitly or explicitly" (p. 74). These written documents are distributed to other faculty members, students, curriculum committee members, and accrediting agencies to document what is taught.

The *operational curriculum* consists of "what is actually taught by the teacher and how its importance is communicated to the student" (Posner, 1992, p. 10). This curriculum includes knowledge, skills, and attitudes emphasized by faculty in the classroom and clinical settings.

The *illegitimate curriculum*, according to Bevis (2000), is one known and actively taught by faculty yet not evaluated because descriptors of the behaviors are lacking. Such behaviors include "caring, compassion, power, and its use" (p. 75).

The *hidden curriculum* consists of values and beliefs taught through verbal and nonverbal communication by the faculty. Faculty may be unaware of what is taught through their expressions, priorities, and interactions with students, but students are very aware of the "hidden agendas" (curriculum), which may have a more lasting impact than the written curriculum. The hidden curriculum includes the way faculty interact with students, the teaching methods used, and the priorities set (Bevis, 2000; Posner, 1992; Schubert, 1986).

The *null curriculum* (Bevis, 2000; Eisner, 1985; Schubert, 1986) represents content and behaviors that are not taught. Faculty need to recognize what is not being taught and focus on the reasons for ignoring those content and behavior areas. Examples include content or skills that faculty think they are teaching but are not, such as critical thinking. As faculty review curricula, all components and relationships need to be evaluated.

The idea of an interrelationship between curriculum and instruction is also supported by other educators, and is not a new concept. In 1996, Lempert advocated that a new approach to education and curriculum must be developed, one in which faculty were active participants and guides in learning, not lecturers. Lempert urged an increased involvement in the community, with the university becoming responsible and accountable to the needs of the community. He also favored a curriculum that recognized and accepted individual differences to enhance multiculturalism. He believed that curriculum and learning should be focused on acquiring skills, not just factual knowledge. After all, knowledge should be measured by the ability of the students and graduates to perform, not recite facts. Therefore he argued that the most effective learning occurs by experience, not just by passively learning facts. These thoughts, while introduced more than 15 years ago, are still pertinent to the design of nursing curricula today.

General education and nursing curricula are becoming more integrated, with classroom and workplace joining to meet learning goals set by diverse groups of students. Students must develop the ability to communicate across cultures; understand and respect others' views and lives; and learn teamwork skills, including management, delegation, and negotiation. The curriculum should offer activities to enable students to gain actual experiences and learn to work collaboratively with other disciplines in seeking solutions to problems (Balakas & Sparks, 2010; Benner et al., 2010; Dacey, Murphy, Anderson, & McCloskey, 2010; Porter-Wenzlaff & Froman, 2008). The concept of service learning, which embodies these principles, is further discussed in Chapter 12.

Curriculum Components

Components of the curriculum that are used by faculty in the review, restructuring, and development of contemporary curricula include foundations; philosophy and mission; designs; organizing frameworks; outcomes, competencies, and objectives; educational activities; and evaluation (Doll, 1996; Keating, 2006). These curriculum components are briefly discussed in this overview with further elaboration in following chapters.

Foundations

The foundations of curriculum set the external boundaries for a given field of study, whereas historical perspectives provide a view of the evolving content and roots of the discipline. In nursing, historical perspectives enable students to learn of the development of nursing as a profession, nursing education, and nursing research. Review of sociological and political forces also provides a historical perspective of the effects of various legal actions; economics; and events, such as wars, on the nursing profession. Psychological foundations of curriculum have formulated teaching and learning aspects of nursing education, including evaluation and curriculum revisions (Bevis, 2000; Doll, 1996; Keating, 2006; Longstreet & Shane, 1993; Ornstein & Hunkins, 1993). Forces and issues that are currently influencing the development of nursing curricula are discussed in Chapter 6.

Philosophy and Mission

The program must integrate the philosophy and mission of the university or college and the program itself within the curriculum. The mission of the university or college varies with the social forces that affect faculty, students, and curricula. For example, institutional missions must address the knowledge and technology explosion, critical thinking, problem solving, multiculturalism, and communication in response to the multiple changes occurring in today's workplace. Students learn what to value as they receive a foundation for specialized content and skills.

The philosophy provides the framework for curriculum choices that are made. Most curricula are formulated and based on several philosophies, not just a single one (Keating, 2006). The values and beliefs on which curricula are founded provide coherence, shape, and consistency for a program. The beliefs set the criteria from which to develop, teach, and evaluate the learning of concepts, such as the concepts of nursing (Bevis, 2000).

Educational philosophies include perennialism, essentialism, progressivism, reconstructionism, and existentialism (Bevis, 2000; Ornstein & Hunkins, 1993; Wiles & Bondi, 1989). In *perennialism* (grounded in realism) the curriculum is based on knowledge and conservative, inflexible, traditional content, including mathematics, grammar, languages, sciences, and strong moral and spiritual teachings. Goals of the curriculum include character training and development of reasoning abilities, and faculty are considered the authorities and experts at developing the content, which is taught primarily by lecture. Students' opinions are not useful in curriculum development because students, as passive recipients, are not able to adequately judge what must be learned. Further studies in realism would include Aristotle and the writings of Thomas Aquinas, Harry Broudy, and John Wild (Ornstein & Hunkins, 1993; Schubert, 1986; Wiles & Bondi, 1989).

Essentialism is another conservative philosophy grounded in idealism and realism, with traditional content and teachings. Students are viewed as having "spongelike" minds that absorb new content provided. The curriculum should be the same across student populations; however, students should be allowed to learn at an individual pace based on ability. Such a philosophical base would be viewed as costly in the contemporary environment if the curriculum was offered on campus and the teacher, a model of ideal behavior, continued to be viewed as the authority (Ornstein & Hunkins, 1993; Wiles & Bondi, 1989). Essentialism can be studied further in works on idealism (e.g., by Plato, Hegel, Fredrich Froebel, and J. Donald Butler) and realism.

Both perennialism and essentialism can be considered outdated in a rapidly changing world in which the teacher and student learn from each other. The application of just one of these philosophies implies a lack of flexibility in the curriculum, which is a necessity in today's dynamic and complex U.S. health care system.

Progressivism, rooted in pragmatism, views problem-solving skills, scientific inquiry, and critical thinking as essential to the curriculum. The teacher's role is more participative, and the emphasis is on teaching students how to learn and how to problem-solve rather than on the content of a specific subject. Traditional course content is replaced by a set of activities and experiences that encourage group participation and teamwork. Further study on the history of pragmatism is offered in the writings of John Dewey and William James (Bevis, 2000; Ornstein & Hunkins, 1993).

The philosophy of *reconstructionism,* also grounded in pragmatism, focuses education on the needs of society rather than the individual. Social and cultural issues are primary areas of the curriculum, which is viewed as constantly changing. A major goal is that teachers and students will become change agents in a world of crises and controversy. The works of Alvin Toffler and Theodore Brameld can be studied to enhance the understanding of reconstructionism (Ornstein & Hunkins, 1993).

Existentialism focuses on individualism and self-fulfillment, teaching about choices one has to make, freedom of choice, the meaning of choice, and the responsibility one has for choice. There is no established curriculum other than the focus on choices and the human condition. Established standards, authority, and group norms are rejected and replaced by self-expressive activities, experiments, emotions, feelings, and insights. Teachers and students learn by dialogue and discussion in the development of choices. The origin of existentialism can be further studied with a review of the works of Søren Kierkegaard and other existentialist philosophers (Ornstein & Hunkins, 1993; Sartre, 1974; Schubert, 1986; Wiles & Bondi, 1989).

As discussed, various complex philosophical beliefs exist within curricula. Philosophies are being reevaluated by educators as curriculum restructuring occurs. Further discussion of philosophy and mission statements, including how to develop them, can be found in Chapter 7.

Designs

Curricula today need to incorporate opportunities for students to problem-solve, think critically about issues of the day, and communicate in the real world. Ratcliff (1997) stated that curricula must be coherent to stimulate creativity among students as they prepare for the workplace. He believed that curricula must be designed to encourage students to consider divergent ideas and differences among people. Learning about different cultures and considering a variety of beliefs and ideas fosters questioning and intellectual development. In a prescribed curriculum such as nursing, graduates should be better prepared and equipped to work within a changing society if both the general studies core courses and the clinical courses require students to learn about multicultural peoples and global issues. The prescribed goals and outcomes of a professional program such as nursing should prepare graduates for opportunities for divergent thinking.

Will design change with the complexities of nursing practice and technology? Benner et al. (2010) "suggest faculty and students make four shifts in their thinking and approach to nursing education:

1. From a focus on covering decontextualized knowledge to an emphasis on teaching for a sense of salience, situated cognition, and action in particular clinical situations;
2. From a sharp separation of classroom and clinical teaching to integrative teaching in all settings;
3. From an emphasis on critical thinking to an emphasis on clinical reasoning and multiple ways of thinking that include critical thinking; and
4. From an emphasis on socialization and role taking to an emphasis on formation" (p. 89).

Curricula today are changing rapidly because of the technology explosion. However, more and more students are entering higher education with greater technological literacy than the faculty. The addition of high-fidelity simulators and mobile devices enable use of virtual patient simulations to increase decision making not always available in clinical settings, increase speed of data access, and foster a new level of questioning that enhances use of critical thinking skills (Barron et al., 2006; Childs & Sepples, 2006; Farrell, 2006; Larew, Lessans, Spunt, Foster, & Covington, 2006; Miller et al., 2005; Nehring & Lashley, 2004; Thompson, 2005; Walton, Childs, & Blenkinsopp, 2005). Faculty must have access to training and equipment, including various types of digital media, which enables them to increase their computer literacy to meet students' needs and adequately address students' different learning styles. The costs of higher education by means of technology-mediated instruction will need to be evaluated to determine whether electronic education is more or less cost effective than traditional classroom education. Technology-mediated education is more consumer oriented with regard to the timing of course offerings and the decreased time and costs for students who otherwise would have to drive to and from school. Electronic resources are available for faculty and students around the clock, and students can easily access library holdings and databases when seeking evidence-based research, decreasing the time required for searches and for extracting journals from a variety of settings (Courey et al., 2006; Eland, 2006; Simpson, 2006; Skiba, 2006b; Walton et al., 2005).

Because of these and other influences, curricula of the future will by necessity be flexible. Chapter 8 provides further discussion of undergraduate and graduate curriculum designs used in nursing education.

Organizing Frameworks

An organizing framework provides faculty with a means of delivering a cohesive curriculum that provides students with the learning experiences necessary to achieve the desired educational outcomes. There are a number of ways to design an organizing framework for a curriculum, and faculty must carefully consider the implications of the framework they have implemented. As an example from general education literature, Ratcliff (1997) opposed general education curricula programs in which students are permitted simply to choose among arts, humanities, social sciences, life and physical sciences, and mathematics courses. He believed that this approach to general education did not build on the students' abilities, reasoning skills, and intellectual development and leads to failure of students with lesser abilities and lack of stimulation of intellectual development in successful students.

Ratcliff (1997) also suggested the use of a variety of coursework sequences, rather than a single set curriculum pattern, with assessment measures to evaluate progress and performance as students work toward meeting degree requirements. He asserted that multiple core curricula for general education could be tailored to students' abilities and content majors as the overall organizing frameworks are redesigned.

Whatever organizing framework is used, assessment of outcomes is an essential component of curriculum development. Assessment data must be used to determine whether students have learned and to evaluate the effects of curriculum changes.

Assessment findings should be given to students in a timely manner to enable them to evaluate their own learning. The development and assessment of organizing frameworks for nursing education are further discussed in Chapter 9.

Outcomes, Competencies, and Objectives

Outcomes, competencies, and objectives are derived from the philosophical beliefs that create the framework of the curriculum. Learning outcomes became prevalent in the mid-1980s in higher education as accrediting agencies focused on measuring student and graduate performance, holding faculty and institutions of higher learning accountable for student learning (Diamond, 1998; Keating, 2006; Keith, 1991).

Lempert (1996) stated that outcomes of curriculum and learning would be stretched beyond the walls of the traditional classroom and focus on building skills for the real world through connecting various disciplines. He stated that the outcome of curricula should be to build better citizens who are productive in the workforce and in the community. As competition for education dollars increases, legislators and other external forces have a greater influence over curriculum development by mandating review of outcomes. The focus on preparation of graduates for the workforce has increased in importance as societal changes have occurred. If educational systems are to continue to maintain accreditation, questions that must be answered include not only how many students graduated, but also how long it took them to complete degree requirements, how many graduates were employed upon graduation, and whether or not employers are satisfied with the graduates' readiness for the workforce.

Traditional outcomes and competencies in nursing and other areas of health care are being challenged and pressured to change. Nurse educators are being challenged to recognize and further define the various levels of nursing programs and to promote academic progression between the levels (IOM, 2010; National League for Nursing [NLN], 2011).

Outcomes must incorporate the increasing diversity and technological explosion in the sequence of learning experiences that will prepare the graduate to survive within the workforce (Benner et al., 2010). Institutions will be held accountable for students' performance and will be assessed by how well students meet course outcomes and competencies. Many states are now defining performance indicators that are used to influence funding decisions for public institutions. Faculty need to evaluate the learning that occurs in classroom and clinical settings to verify that outcomes are being met. The use of classroom assessment techniques (CATs) provides faculty and students with information about strengths and weaknesses in the students' learning. Faculty and students can adapt teaching strategies midcourse to increase students' learning in the semester (Angelo & Cross, 1993; Cross & Steadman, 1996). A further discussion of selecting outcomes and competencies is provided in Chapter 9. Classroom assessment techniques are discussed further in Chapter 16.

Educational Activities

Learning activities provided to enhance students' knowledge and inquisitiveness must also prepare the graduate for real-world experiences. Creativity, oral and written communication, problem solving, managing diverse groups of people, and negotiation are among the outcomes that have been identified in general education for undergraduate curricula (Ratcliff, 1997). Learning activities can be planned to encourage collaboration and enhance progressive learning, starting with less difficult activities and progressing to activities that require students to synthesize complex concepts. For example, problem-based learning enables students to engage in complex situations to determine what they need to learn and what skills are needed to arrive at solutions. The teamwork associated with problem-based learning strengthens students' communication, negotiation, and social skills; creative and critical thinking skills; and clinical reasoning abilities (Savin-Baden, 2000).

Learning should be assessed and feedback given to students in a timely manner, enabling them to see their progress and make decisions about their learning. Clinical experiences, while still including the traditional acute care setting, need to be redesigned so that the use of community-based agencies increases, thus requiring students to demonstrate clinical reasoning skills in unstructured settings and flexibility in problem-solving patient care issues with interdisciplinary health care teams. Immersion experiences in clinical settings will strengthen program outcomes (Diefenbeck et al., 2006; Frank et al., 2005; Freeman, Voignier, & Scott, 2002; Kotecki, 2002; Massey, 2001; Matteson, 2000; Wink, 2003).

Poirrier (2001) and others have stressed the importance of service learning using community-based partnerships to provide educational activities focused on health promotion and prevention in communities. Including an emphasis on service learning in the curriculum broadens the students' view of nursing, addressing collective human needs in addition to individual patient needs. The curriculum focus can include such activities as the promotion of a healthy lifestyle; the care of underserved, vulnerable populations; environmental concerns; and cultural diversity. Service learning enhances the student's role as a citizen with health care, social justice, and policy responsibilities. Environmental, global health, and bioterrorism issues can also be addressed in these experiences (Bailey, Carpenter, & Harrington, 2002; Hamner & Wilder, 2001; Leonard, 2001; Redman & Clark, 2002; Reece, Mawn, & Scollin, 2003; Reising, 2006; Reising, Allen, & Hall, 2006a, 2006b; Seifer & Vaughn, 2002; Veenema, 2001, 2002; Wink, 2003; Wright, 2003). Designing service learning activities is discussed in depth in Chapter 12.

Finally, as part of curriculum restructuring, increasing the involvement of alumni and other professionals in curriculum design—for example, by integrating their ideas for useful educational activities—should increase curriculum relevance to the workplace. The selection and design of learning activities are further discussed in Chapter 10.

Evaluation

As stated previously, universities and faculty are increasingly being evaluated on the basis of how well students and graduates perform, including student retention and graduation rates, and funding decisions are associated with these performance indicators. Outcome measures for nursing programs include entry and graduation rates, licensure (NCLEX pass rates) and certification of graduates, and postgraduation employment rates (CCNE, 2009; National League for Nursing Accrediting Commission, n.d.; U.S. Department of Labor, 2010). Evaluation of program outcomes, including the curriculum, is discussed in detail in Chapter 28.

Curriculum Development as a Process

Many global changes are occurring and these changes affect curriculum development in higher education. Faculty must remain responsive to the needs of society and students and design curricula that reflect these changes. Faculty in higher education across the nation are engaging in curriculum revision and development in an effort to provide curricula that will produce graduates who possess the skills necessary for success in the workplaces of the twenty-first century.

Curriculum development is an ongoing deliberative process that takes concentrated time, effort, and faculty commitment, not simply an isolated event that occurs periodically (Bevis & Murray, 1990; Civian, Arnold, Gamson, Kanter, & London, 1997; Diamond, 1998; Hord, Rutherford, Huling-Austin, & Hall, 1987; Lindquist, 1997; Oliva, 1992). According to Oliva (1992) and others, curriculum change begins at the level of its current state and continues as a process of making choices from a number of alternatives. If curricula are to continue to exist, change is inevitable because of the effects of external change agents, such as community pressure, policy changes, and funding sources (Doll, 1996; Fullan, 1991; Wiles & Bondi, 1989).

Curriculum development, which may consist of changes ranging from simple substitutions or alterations of content from course to course to a complete restructuring of the entire curriculum, should be a cooperative group activity. However, change results only as people alter their thoughts and patterns of behavior. Significant curriculum change is associated with ambiguity, ambivalence, and uncertainty; therefore smooth implementation is often a sign that little change has occurred. Relearning is at the heart of change and may be a powerful inhibitor of change (Oliva, 1992). Faculty engaging in curriculum development will benefit from scanning their environment for facilitators and barriers to curriculum development, working collaboratively to maximize the facilitative aspects and minimize the barriers. According to Diamond (1998), "An effective curriculum provides multiple opportunities to apply and practice what is learned" (p. 85).

Facilitators of Curriculum Development

Ritchie (1986) and McNeil (1990) offered suggestions to promote an effective curriculum change process, including faculty development workshops and focus groups. The group of faculty involved initially in the change must be key faculty members who understand the problem and can effectively evaluate strategies for problem solving. Faculty serving on a curriculum committee need to perceive that their contributions will be heard and have an impact on the outcome of decisions. Faculty also need to believe that their contributions will be recognized and rewarded and be assured that their contributions will promote a greater good for the organization. Mutual respect must be present among participants of the committee, fostered by trust, honesty, and confidence between the committee leader and faculty. Recognition of the components of effective change can help ensure that the change process will produce the desired outcomes (Carmon, Hauber, & Chase, 1992; Doll, 1996; Fullan, 1991; Lindquist, 1997; Oliva, 1992). However, curriculum change takes time. In today's uncertain world, curriculum changes must occur carefully but quickly for nursing schools to survive. Several examples of the process of curriculum change are found in nursing literature (Hamner & Wilder, 2001; Mawn & Reece, 2000; Webber, 2002).

Barriers to Curriculum Development

Real change causes conflict, and the idea of conflict leads to fear in many faculty members (Erickson, 1995; Mawn & Reece, 2000; McNeil, 1990). In many institutions of higher education and in many nursing programs, real changes need to be made so that the necessary contemporary curricula can be developed. For example, faculty need to be flexible, adaptable, and open to experiential learning if the curriculum is to change to meet workforce and community needs. In the past, any experiential learning was typically viewed as an "add-on" to the curriculum, not an integration of learning that would increase creativity and individual initiative. Because of the complexity and acuity of patient care, changes in health care reimbursement, movement of care to home and community, and advances in new technologies, curricula need to be evaluated and redesigned for nursing programs.

According to Belleck (2006), new graduates are required to perform complex procedures and make complex decisions that previously were expected of experienced and expert nurses. As changes occur, more content is added to what the student "needs to know" rather than attending to competencies and what is salient for safe patient care at the novice nurse level. Changes in health care and community needs are not reflected in the NCLEX test plan, which is primarily based on hospital and acute care nursing. This viewpoint is no longer compatible with society's needs. Students should actively be involved in real-world activities throughout the curriculum, not only during an internship at the end of the program (Lempert, 1996). Working with community leaders and cultural groups enables students to learn to work in the real world and enhances communication and decision-making skills beyond those learned from the textbook and in the classroom (Erickson, 1995). Hamner and Wilder (2001) identified the need to determine possible obstacles to curriculum implementation early so that faculty could address the issues.

To make the changes necessary to integrate experiential learning throughout the curriculum, faculty are required to conceptualize curriculum development differently than they have in the past. Faculty may be uncertain about how to effectively incorporate such changes into the curriculum, with this uncertainty manifesting itself in reluctance or refusal to change.

Thus, as this example illustrates, one of the major barriers to curriculum development is the fear of change itself. Faculty who resist change often lack the flexibility, adaptability, and vision to combine theory and workplace skills. Ritchie (1986) described these barriers and others and identified the following 13 reasons, which are still valid today, as to why curriculum change is resisted by faculty:

1. Fear of losing control of the curriculum
2. Misunderstanding due to lack of information or confusion about new vocabulary and jargon
3. Perception of lack of ability to progress because of new time and energy demands
4. Different views about what needs to be done
5. Lack of motivation to study the change
6. Lack of perception of a need for change (*If it ain't broke, don't fix it.*)
7. Too many changes and too many demands related to the change process
8. Desire to be vindictive and make the leader look bad
9. Idea that *no one can tell me what to do*
10. Threat to current social support systems
11. Lack of resources
12. View that formal methods used to facilitate change are a barrier rather than a help
13. Lack of rewards

Because of these potential barriers, the leader, organizational culture, and students are key players in successful curriculum change (Fullan, 1991; Middlewood, 2001; Ritchie, 1986; Wiles & Bondi, 1989). For example, nursing is faced with many uncertainties as technology and the U.S. health care system undergo rapid and dramatic changes; faculty are challenged to predict future health care needs and trends and align the curricula to prepare graduates to meet these needs. As external changes occur, leadership characteristics become extremely important. Faculty observe the manner in which the leader (1) responds to critical incidents and crises; (2) supervises, evaluates, praises, handles conflict resolution, directs changes, and represents the organization; and (3) executes rewards and assigns, promotes, and terminates employees.

The leader must acknowledge potential barriers to change and understand that faculty have differing beliefs and opinions about change. When a change is proposed, faculty members may each react differently because the change will affect them individually. For example, teaching styles may need to be altered for some faculty members, whereas others already use the needed strategies. Also, courses may be removed from the curriculum or moved to a different location within the curriculum pattern. Faculty may then experience a need to teach new courses, face employment changes, or deal with the challenges associated with teaching a different level of students. Effective leadership is important in the change process; if the leader's vision and goals differ greatly from those of the faculty, desired outcomes likely will not occur (Fullan, 1991; Middlewood, 2001).

Curriculum Development as Planned Change

A plan should be developed for a regular review of the curriculum. Diamond (1998) stated that curriculum change must be planned: "The needs for . . . improvement are too great and resources too limited to allow us to be inefficient or ineffective in the way we address our curricular problems. We cannot afford to leave things to chance" (p. 15). This also means that curriculum changes should be evidence-based and not driven by the special interests of individual faculty. It is expected that faculty will routinely update individual courses with the latest developments in the given field. As individual courses are changed, however, the overall curriculum may change without faculty awareness, leading to redundancy or gaps in content or skills. Faculty must plan to evaluate the curriculum on a regular basis to avoid this pitfall.

The organizational culture must facilitate the innovative ideas of faculty in curriculum change. Administrative support of faculty innovations is important. Creativity may lead to a better product, or graduate, than originally planned. Faculty must also view the opportunity to participate on the curriculum committee as a means for program improvement and innovation rather than as a hindrance or inconvenience. By fostering an environment that supports the review of the curriculum on a regular basis, continuous open dialogue about needed changes, and the incorporation of planned changes, leaders can help faculty become more comfortable with the change process. The results will be a curriculum that remains on the leading edge, meeting the needs of the students, community, and society.

SUMMARY

Rapid changes in today's world mandate review and restructuring of the curricula across the university setting, including health care. Faculty must cope with transition from tradition to an era of information explosion led by massive changes in technology, economics, and the development of multiculturalism. In the past, curricula in higher education were designed to teach students how to inquire, how to perform in a specialty field, and how to do research, with the professor being the central figure (Gaff, 1997). Faculty felt comfortable with this authority, this belief, and this practice.

Significant curricula change is now necessary to lower the cost of education and increase productivity while maintaining high-quality curricula based on sound educational principles. According to Gaff (1997) and others, faculty and administrators who are restructuring curriculum must do the following:

- Use technology in the classroom and beyond the four walls.
- Design interdisciplinary studies.
- Develop more holistic, experimental, and integrative models of learning.
- Incorporate cultural diversity.
- Develop academic majors that will cultivate writing and critical thinking skills and integrate theoretical and practical knowledge.
- Internationalize the curriculum.
- Assess student learning, provide feedback, and provide supplemental instruction to help at-risk students achieve high academic standards.
- Use collaborative group work to enhance the learning of students and faculty together.

Administrative personnel need to be visionary in providing leadership and coordination of activities across departments as the restructuring process occurs. Curriculum change must be accompanied with faculty change as student learning outcomes become the focus of contemporary higher education (Curry & Wergin, 1997; Doll, 1996; Gaff, 1997; Lindquist, 1997; McNeil, 1990).

This chapter provides an overview to curriculum development. Definitions of curriculum are provided, and curriculum components are reviewed. The discussion of how to approach curriculum changes briefly describes the process, barriers, and facilitators of change in curriculum development. The impact of social, economic, and technological forces are also described.

REFLECTING ON THE EVIDENCE

1. What type of organizational culture is most likely to facilitate innovative and successful curriculum change?

2. What are some strategies that will ensure that faculty engage in evidence-based curriculum change?

3. Is it important that faculty be aware of the "hidden curriculum" in their program curricula? If so, how can faculty most effectively identify and influence the "hidden curriculum" in their program?

REFERENCES

Allen, I. E., & Seaman, J. (2010). *Class differences: Online education in the United States, 2010.* Babson Survey Research Group.

American Association of Colleges of Nursing. (1999). A vision of baccalaureate and graduate nursing education: The next decade. *Journal of Professional Nursing, 15*(1), 59–65.

American Association of Colleges of Nursing. (2006). *The essential clinical resources for nursing's academic mission.* Retrieved from http://www.aacn.nche.edu

American Association of Colleges of Nursing. (2009). *Nursing shortage [Fact Sheet].* Retrieved from http://www.aacn.nche.edu/

Angelo, T. A., & Cross, P. K. (1993). *Classroom assessment techniques* (2nd ed.). San Francisco, CA: Jossey-Bass.

Bailey, P. A., Carpenter, D. R., & Harrington, P. (2002). Theoretical foundations of service-learning in nursing education. *Journal of Nursing Education, 41*(10), 433–436.

Balakas, K., & Sparks, L. (2010). Teaching research and evidence-based practice using a service-learning approach. *Journal of Nursing Education, 49*(12), 691–695.

Baldwin, D., & Nelms, T. (1993). Difficult dialogues: Impact on nursing education curricula. *Journal of Professional Nursing, 9*(6), 343–346.

Bargagliotti, L. A. (2006). The DNP: Historical parallels and persistent questions. *Nursing Education Perspectives, 27*(4), 174.

Barron, W. M., Reed, R. L., Forsythe, S., Hecht, D., Glen, J., Murphy, B., & Concklin, M. (2006). Information technology: Implementing computerized provider order entry with an existing clinical information system. *Joint Commission Journal on Quality and Patient Safety, 32*(9), 506–516.

Beauchamp, G. A. (1968). *Curriculum theory* (2nd ed.). Wilmette, IL: Kagg Press.

Belleck, J. P. (2006). Recalibrating prelicensure education. *Journal of Nursing Education, 45*(11), 435–436.

Benner, P., Sutphen, M., Leonard, V., & Day, L. (2010). *Educating nurses: A call for radical transformation.* San Francisco, CA: Jossey-Bass.

Bevis, E. O. (1989). *Curriculum building in nursing.* New York, NY: National League for Nursing Press.

Bevis, E. O. (2000). Nursing curriculum as professional education. In E. O. Bevis & J. Watson (Eds.), *Toward a caring curriculum: A new pedagogy for nursing* (pp. 74–77). New York, NY: National League for Nursing Press.

Bevis, E. O., & Murray, J. P. (1990). The essence of curriculum revolution: Emancipatory teaching. *Journal of Nursing Education, 29*(7), 326–331.

Cangelosi, P. R., & Whitt, K. J. (2006). Accelerated nursing programs: What do we know? *Nursing Education Perspectives, 26*(2), 113–116.

Carmon, M., Hauber, R. P., & Chase, L. (1992). From anxiety to action. *Nursing & Health Care, 13*(7), 364–368.

Chase, S. K., & Pruitt, R. H. (2006). The practice doctorate: Innovation or disruption? *Journal of Nursing Education, 45*(5), 155–161.

Childs, J. C., & Sepples, S. (2006). Clinical teaching by simulation: Lessons learned from a complex patient care scenario. *Nursing Education Perspectives, 27*(3), 154–158.

Civian, J. T., Arnold, G., Gamson, G. F., Kanter, S., & London, H. B. (1997). In J. G. Gaff, J. L. Ratcliff et al. (Eds.), *Handbook of the undergraduate curriculum* (pp. 647–660). San Francisco, CA: Jossey-Bass.

Commission on Collegiate Nursing Education (2009, April). Standards for accreditation of baccalaureate and graduate degree nursing programs. Retrieved from http://www.aacn.nche.edu/

Courey, T., Benson-Soros, J., Deemer, K., & Zeller, R. A. (2006). The missing link: Information literacy and evidence-based practice as a new challenge for nurse educators. *Nursing Education Perspectives, 27*(6), 320–323.

Cronenwett, L., Sherwood, G., Barnsteiner, J., Disch, J., Johnson, J., Mitchell, P., . . . Warren, J. (2007). Quality and safety education for nurses. *Nursing Outlook, 55*(3), 122–131.

Cross, P. K., & Steadman, M. H. (1996). *Classroom research: Implementing the scholarship of teaching.* San Francisco, CA: Jossey-Bass.

Curry, L., & Wergin, J. F. (1997). Professional education. In J. G. Gaff, J. L. Ratcliff et al. (Eds.), *Handbook of the undergraduate curriculum* (pp. 341–358). San Francisco, CA: Jossey-Bass.

Dacey, M., Murphy, J. I., Anderson, D. C., & McCloskey, W. W. (2010). An interprofessional service-learning course: Uniting students across educational levels and promoting patient-centered care. *Journal of Nursing Education, 49*(12), 696–699.

Diamond, R. M. (1998). *Designing and assessing courses and curricula: A practical guide.* San Francisco, CA: Jossey-Bass.

Diefenbeck, C. A., Plowfield, L. A., & Herrman, J. W. (2006). Clinical immersion: A residency model for nursing education. *Nursing Education Perspectives, 27*(2), 72–79.

Diekelmann, N. L. (1993). Behavioral pedagogy: A Heideggerian hermeneutical analysis of the lived experiences of students and teachers in baccalaureate nursing education. *Journal of Nursing Education, 32*(6), 245–250.

Diekelmann, N. L., Ironside, P. M., & Gunn, J. (2005). Recalling the curriculum revolution: Innovation with research. *Nursing Education Perspectives, 23*(2), 70–77.

Doll, R. C. (1996). *Curriculum improvement: Decision making and process* (9th ed.). Boston, MA: Allyn & Bacon.

Doll, W. E., Jr. (2002). Ghosts and the curriculum. In W. E. Doll, Jr. & N. Gough (Eds.), *Curriculum visions* (pp. 23–70). New York, NY: Peter Lang.

Eisner, E. W. (1985). *The educational imagination* (2nd ed.). New York, NY: Macmillan.

Eland, J. (2006). Electronic information and methods for improving education: Realities and assumptions. In P. S. Cowen & S. Moorhead (Eds.), *Current issues in nursing* (7th ed., pp. 134–138). St. Louis, MO: Mosby.

Erickson, H. L. (1995). *Stirring the head, heart and soul: Redefining curriculum and instruction.* Thousand Oaks, CA: Corwin.

Farrell, M. (2006). Learning differently: E-learning in nurse education. *Nursing Management, 13*(6), 14–17.

Finkelman, A., & Kenner, C. (2009). *Teaching IOM: Implications of the Institute of Medicine reports for nursing education* (2nd ed.). Silver Spring, MD: American Nurses Association.

Fitzpatrick, J. J. (2006). The cost and quality agenda comes to higher education. *Nursing Education Perspectives, 27*(6), 297.

Forbes, M. O., & Hickey, M. T. (2009). Curriculum reform in baccalaureate nursing education: Review of the literature. *International Journal of Nursing Education Scholarship, 6*(1), Article 27.

Frank, B., Adams, M. H., Edelstein, J., Speakman, E., & Shelton, M. (2005). Community-based nursing education of prelicensure students: Settings and supervision. *Nursing Education Perspectives, 26*(5), 283–287.

Freeman, L. H., Voignier, R. R., & Scott, D. L. (2002). New curriculum for a new century: Beyond repackaging. *Journal of Nursing Education, 41*(1), 38–40.

Fullan, M. G. (1991). *The new meaning of educational change* (2nd ed.). New York, NY: Teachers College Press.

Gaff, J. G. (1997). *New life for the college curriculum: Assessing achievements and furthering progress in the reform of general education.* San Francisco, CA: Jossey-Bass.

Giddens, J. F., & Brady, D. P. (2007). Rescuing nursing education from content saturation: The case for a concept-based curriculum. *Journal of Nursing Education, 46*(2), 65–70.

Hamner, J., & Wilder, B. (2001). A new curriculum for a new millennium. *Nursing Outlook, 49*(3), 127–131.

Hathaway, D., Jacob, S., Stegbauer, D., Thompson, C., & Graff, C. (2006). The practice doctorate: Perspectives of early adopters. *Journal of Nursing Education, 45*(12), 487–496.

Healthy People 2020. (n.d.) Retrieved from http://healthypeople.gov/2020/TopicsObjectives2020/pdfs/HP2020_brochure.pdf

Hodson Carlton, K. E., Siktberg, L. L., Flowers, J., & Scheibel, P. (2003). Overview of distance education in nursing: Where are we now and where are we going? In M. H. Oermann & K. T. Heinrich (Eds.), *Annual review of nursing education* (pp. 165–189). New York, NY: Springer.

Hord, S. M., Rutherford, W. L., Huling-Austin, L., & Hall, G. E. (1987). *Taking charge of change.* Austin, TX: Southwest Educational Development Laboratory.

IMPAC Annual Report 2000–2001. (2001, March). *Nursing* [Summary of Identified Issues]. Retrieved from http://www.cal-impac.org/RESOURCES/AnnualReport01/AnnualReport01_Nursing.htm

Institute of Medicine. (2003). *Health professions education: A bridge to quality.* Washington DC: The National Academies Press.

Institute of Medicine. (2010). *The future of nursing: Leading change, advancing health.* Washington, DC: The National Academies Press.

Ironside, P. M. (2006). Reforming doctoral curricula in nursing: Creating multiparadigmatic, multipedagogical researchers. *Journal of Nursing Education, 45*(2), 51–52.

Jones, D. P., & Wolf, D. M. (2010). Shaping the future of nursing education today using distant education and technology. *Journal of Association of Black Nursing Faculty, Inc, 21*(2), 44–47.

Keating, S. B. (2006). *Curriculum development and evaluation in nursing.* Philadelphia, PA: Lippincott Williams & Wilkins.

Keith, N. Z. (1991). Assessing educational goals: The national movement to outcomes evaluation. In M. Garbin (Ed.), *Assessing educational outcomes* (pp. 1–23). New York, NY: National League for Nursing Press.

Klein, M. F. (1995). Alternative curriculum conceptions and designs. In A. C. Ornstein & L. Behar (Eds.), *Contemporary issues in curriculum* (pp. 30–35). Boston, MA: Allyn-Bacon.

Kotecki, C. N. (2002). Community-based strategies: Incorporating faith-based partnerships into the curriculum. *Nurse Educator, 27*(1), 13–15.

Lancaster, J. (2006). DNP discussion continues. *Journal of Nursing, 45*(8), 295–296.

Larew, C., Lessans, S., Spunt, D., Foster, D., & Covington, B. G. (2006). Innovations in clinical simulation: Application of Benner's theory in an interactive patients care simulation. *Nursing Education Perspectives, 27*(1), 16–21.

Larson, L. (2006). Who will teach the nurses we need? *Hospitals & Health Networks, 80*(12), 52–58.

Lattuca, L. R., & Stark, J. S. (2009). Shaping the college curriculum: Academic plans in context. (2nd ed.). San Francisco, CA: Jossey-Bass.

Lempert, D.H. (1996). *Escape from the ivory tower.* Jossey-Bass: San Francisco.

Lenburg, C. B. (2002). Changes that challenge nursing education. *Alabama Nurse, 29*(4), 6–7.

Leonard, B. J. (2001). Quality nursing care celebrates diversity. *The Online Journal of Issues in Nursing, 6*(2), 3.

Lindeman, C. A. (2000). The future of nursing education. *Journal of Nursing Education, 39*(1), 5–12.

Lindquist, J. (1997). Strategies for change. In J. G. Gaff, J. L. Ratcliff et al. (Eds.), *Handbook of the undergraduate curriculum* (pp. 633–646). San Francisco, CA: Jossey-Bass.

Long, K. A. (2004). RN education: A matter of degrees. *Nursing, 34*(3), 48–51.

Longstreet, S. & Shane, H.G. (1993). *Curriculum for a new millennium* Allyn & Bacon: Boston.

Massey, C. M. (2001). A transdisciplinary model for curricular revision. *Nursing and Health Care Perspectives, 22*(2), 85–88.

Matteson, P. S. (2000). Preparing nurses for the future. In P. Matteson (Ed.), *Community-based nursing education* (pp. 1–7). New York, NY: Springer.

Mawn, B., & Reece, S. M. (2000). Reconfiguring a curriculum for the new millennium: The process of change. *Journal of Nursing Education, 39*(3), 101–108.

McCabe, S. (2006). What does it take to make a nurse? Considerations of the CNL and DNP role development. *Perspectives in Psychiatric Care, 42*(4), 252–255.

McNeil, J. D. (1990). *Curriculum: A comprehensive introduction* (4th ed.). Glenview, IL: Scott, Foresman.

Melton, R. (2002). *Planning and developing open and distance learning.* New York, NY: Routledge Falmer.

Middlewood, D. (2001). Leadership of the curriculum: Setting the vision. In D. Middlewood & N. Burton (Eds.), *Managing the curriculum* (pp. 107–117). Thousand Oaks, CA: Sage.

Miklancie, M., & Davis, T. (2005). The second-degree accelerated program as an innovative educational strategy: New century, new chapter, new challenge. *Nursing Education Perspectives, 26*(5), 291–294.

Miller, J., Shaw-Kokot, J. R., Arnold, M. S., Boggin, T., Crowell, K. E., Allegri, F., . . . Berrier, S. B. (2005). A study of personal digital assistants to enhance undergraduate clinical nursing education. *Journal of Nursing Education, 44*(1), 19–26.

Morris, T., & Hancock, D. (2008). Program exit examinations in nursing education: Using a value added assessment as a measure of the impact of a new curriculum. *Education Research Quarterly, 32*(2), 19–29.

Morse, W. A., & Corcoran-Perry, S. (1996). A process model to guide selection of essential curriculum content. *Journal of Nursing Education, 35*(8), 341–347.

National League for Nursing. (2011). *Academic progression in nursing education.* New York, NY: Author.

National League for Nursing Accrediting Commission, Inc. (n.d.). *NLNAC 2008 standards and criteria.* Retrieved from http://www.nlnac.org/

Nehring, W. M., & Lashley, F. R. (2004). Using the human patient simulator in nursing education. *Annual Review of Nursing Education, 2,* 163–181.

Nelms, T. (1991). Has the curriculum revolution revolutionized the definition of curriculum? *Journal of Nursing Education, 30*(1), 5–8.

Nelson, R., Meyers, L., Rizzolo, M. A., Rutar, P., Proto, M. B., & Newbold, S. (2006). The evolution of educational information systems and nurse faculty roles. *Nursing Education Perspectives, 27*(5), 247–253.

Oliva, P. (1992). *Developing the curriculum* (3rd ed.). New York, NY: HarperCollins.

Ornstein, A. C., & Hunkins, F. P. (1993). *Curriculum: Foundations, principles and issues* (2nd ed.). Boston, MA: Allyn & Bacon.

Phillips, B., Shaw, R. J., Sullivan, D. T., & Johnson, C. (2010). Using virtual environments to enhance nursing distance education. *Creative Nursing, 16*(3), 132–135.

Poirrier, G. P. (2001). *Service-learning: Curricular applications in nursing.* Sudbury, MA: Jones & Bartlett.

Porter-Wenzlaff, L. J., & Froman, R. D. (2008). Responding to increasing RN demand: Diversity and retention trends through an accelerated LVN-to-BSN curriculum. *Journal of Nursing Education, 47*(5), 231–235.

Posner, G. J. (1992). *Analyzing the curriculum.* New York, NY: McGraw Hill.

Quality and Safety Education for Nurses (QSEN). (n.d.). [Website]. Retrieved from http://www.qsen.org/

Ratcliff, J. L. (1997). Quality and coherence in general education. In J. G. Gaff, J. L. Ratcliff et al. (Eds.), *Handbook of the undergraduate curriculum.* San Francisco, CA: Jossey-Bass.

Redman, R. W., & Clark, L. (2002). Service-learning as a model for integrating social justice in the nursing curriculum. *Journal of Nursing Education, 41*(10), 446–449.

Reece, S. M., Mawn, B., & Scollin, P. (2003). Evaluation of faculty transition into a community-based curriculum. *Journal of Nursing Education, 42*(1), 43–47.

Reising, D. L. (2006). Service-learning in undergraduate curricula. *Journal of Nursing Education, 45*(2), 95.

Reising, D. L., Allen, P. N., & Hall, S. G. (2006a). Student and community outcomes in service learning: Part 1: Student perceptions. *Journal of Nursing Education, 45*(12), 512–515.

Reising, D. L. Allen, P. N., & Hall, S. G. (2006b). Student and community outcomes in service learning: Part 2: Community outcomes. *Journal of Nursing Education, 45*(12), 516–518.

Ritchie, J. B. (1986). Management strategies for curriculum change. *Journal of Dental Education, 50*(3), 97–101.

Ruth-Sahd, L. A., & Tisdell, E. J. (2007). Intuition in novice nurses: A phenomenological study. *Adult Education Quarterly, 57*(115), 115–140.

Sartre, J. P. (1974). *Between existentialism and Marxism.* New York, NY: Pantheon Books.

Savin-Baden, M. (2000). *Problem-based learning in higher education: Untold stories.* Buckingham, UK: SRHE and Open University Press.

Schubert, W. H. (1986). *Curriculum: Perspective, paradigm, and possibility.* New York, NY: Macmillan.

Seifer, S. D., & Vaughn, R. L. (2002). Partners in caring and community: Service learning in nursing education. *Journal of Nursing Education, 41*(10), 437–439.

Simpson, R. L. (2006). See the future of distance education. *Nursing Management, 37*(2), 42–51.

Skiba, D. (2006a). Think spots: Where are your learning spaces? *Nursing Education Perspectives, 27*(2), 103–104.

Skiba, D. (2006b). Web-based education. In P. S. Cowen & S. Moorhead (Eds.), *Current issues in nursing* (pp. 139–144). St. Louis, MO: Mosby.

Taba, H. (1962). *Curriculum development: Theory and practice.* New York, NY: Harcourt, Brace & World.

Tanner, C. (2006a). Changing times, evolving issues: The faculty shortage, accelerated programs, and simulation. *Journal of Nursing Education, 45*(3), 99–100.

Tanner, C. (2006b). The next transformation: Clinical education. *Journal of Nursing Education, 45*(4), 99–100.

Tanner, C. (2007). The curriculum revolution revisited. *Journal of Nursing Education, 46*(2), 51–52.

Thompson, B. W. (2005). The transforming effect of handheld computers on nursing practice. *Nursing Administration Quarterly, 29*(4), 308–314.

Transforming Care at the Bedside (TCAB). (2008). [Website]. Retrieved from http://www.ihi.org/IHI/Programs/StrategicInitiatives/TransformingCareAtTheBedside.htm

United States Department of Labor, Bureau of Labor Statistics. (2010). *Occupational outlook handbook 2010–11 edition.* Retrieved from http://www.bls.gov/

Veenema, T. G. (2001). An evidence-based curriculum to prepare students for global nursing practice. *Nursing and Health Care Perspectives, 22*(6), 292–298.

Veenema, T. G. (2002). Chemical and biological terrorism: Current updates for nurse educators. *Nursing Education Perspectives, 23*(2), 62–71.

Walton, G., Childs, S., & Blenkinsopp, E. (2005). Using mobile technologies to give health students access to learning resources in the UK community setting. *Health Information & Libraries Journal Supplement, 22*(2), 51–65.

Watson, J. (2000). A new paradigm. In E. O. Bevis & J. Watson (Eds.), *Toward a caring curriculum: A new pedagogy for nursing* (pp. 37–49). New York, NY: National League for Nursing.

Webber, P. B. (2002). A curriculum framework for nursing. *Journal of Nursing Education, 41*(1), 15–23.

Wiles, J., & Bondi, J. (1989). *Curriculum development: A guide to practice* (3rd ed.). Columbus, OH: Merrill.

Wink, D. M. (2003). Community-based curricula at BSN and graduate levels. In M. H. Oermann & K. T. Heinrich (Eds.), *Annual review of nursing education* (pp. 3–25). New York, NY: Springer.

Wright, D. J. (2003). Collaborative learning experiences for nursing students in environmental health. *Nursing Education Perspectives, 24*(4), 189–191.

6

Forces and Issues Influencing Curriculum Development

Linda M. Veltri, PhD, RN
Joanne Rains Warner, PhD, RN, FAAN

Leaders in the nursing profession must remain vigilant to the forces and issues influencing the direction of professional education. In any dynamic organization, curriculum change is not a choice but a requirement. Noted change expert Jack Welch posits "when change is happening on the outside faster than on the inside, the end is in sight" (as cited in Leverich, 2010, para. 13). The magnitude, pace, and intensity of change within the health care arena have astonished providers, consumers, and financers of health care. Sweeping health care reforms affect everyone, including the nursing profession. As a result, nurse educators are continually challenged to develop relevant curricula aimed at preparing and equipping practitioners for their new roles and responsibilities. Curriculum does not occur in a vacuum but is instead a contextual representation of global trends, national circumstances, advancements in science and technology, professional priorities, academic forces, the school's mission, and faculty values. As such, it is imperative for curriculum to be congruent with this social context, the interrelated conditions, and other factors in the venue in which nurses practice and are educated. Without a fit between the curriculum and the broad practice environment, nurses would not have the relevant knowledge, skills, and attitudes necessary to provide patient-centered care, effectively intervene in contemporary health care challenges, or advocate for improved delivery of health care.

The context of interrelated forces and issues that influence the development and direction of curriculum is complex and ever changing. Some of these forces and issues are external to the nursing profession, including the political climate, societal patterns, demographic trends, and economic characteristics that shape the general environment. Some are current forces within higher education, including issues of affordability, access, and accountability. Some forces and issues are specific to the nursing profession, including workforce trends, practice competencies, and nursing leadership. Other forces, such as health policy trends, changing health care needs and patient characteristics, or work redesign, are internal and external to the nursing profession (Andre & Barnes, 2010; Hegarty, Walsh, Condon, & Sweeney, 2009).

This influential socioeconomic context is dynamic and involves interrelating factors that are regularly prompting change. To remain relevant, curriculum and educators charged with its development must keep abreast of and be responsive to these changes. The ability to plan and develop meaningful curricula, and thus prepare graduates for their future roles within a changing health care environment, requires faculty to consider, closely examine, and analyze various forces providing direction for curriculum change (Hegarty et al., 2009). Faculty need assessment strategies and tools to monitor the pulse of the curriculum context. These tools should assist faculty to monitor the strength and regularity of the signs coming from the practice environment and suggest times and ways for curriculum adaptation.

This chapter describes the current social context for curriculum development, including issues and forces in the environment external to the nursing profession, the higher education environment, and the profession's internal environment. This chapter also describes four strategies to identify the forces and issues that significantly influence nursing practice and education. Faculty can use these tools to develop curricula that match the populations needing care, the leading health challenges, and the skills and abilities needed to promote health and prevent illness. Faculty with intimate and current knowledge of the forces and issues influencing nursing curricula are better positioned to navigate the political processes of building consensus and obtaining approval by all significant stakeholders.

Forces and Issues in the Current Curriculum Context

The issues that are currently influencing curriculum development can be explicated. In attempting to describe a time so proximate, faculty run the risk of either overlooking what will become an enduring feature of the time or underestimating the difficulty in winnowing the significant issues from the irrelevant ones. However, faculty do not have the luxury of waiting until history tells the story of our times. They must be proactive developers of a dynamic curriculum, one that will provide students with knowledge, skills, and competencies necessary to lead and successfully practice in today's changing and global society.

In an effort to describe the current setting and environment for curriculum development, the following issues are discussed: issues external to the nursing profession, issues in higher education, and issues specific to the nursing profession. Each section is by no means an exhaustive discussion of the topic but rather an identification of major current and projected themes.

Issues External to the Nursing Profession

Increasingly, health issues are related to the sociopolitical and economic characteristics of the communities where people live, work, and play. Curriculum must acknowledge the broad determinants of health to prepare practicing nurses to effectively intervene in complex problems such as bioterrorism, climate change, global and domestic violence, economic recession, homelessness, teen pregnancy, emerging infectious diseases, and increasing drug-resistant organisms.

These issues external to nursing relate to curriculum in several ways. First, they provide the setting for the world in which nurses practice and learn. Collectively, they describe the current states of humanity and health. Second, they comprise the risk factors for health and disease and contribute to the complex web of causation. Nurses need to have a working knowledge of these issues as they strive to prevent health problems and promote

wellness. From both of these perspectives, issues external to nursing provide a crucial foundation for nursing's understanding of societal needs and characteristics and therefore form an essential piece of the foundation necessary for contemporary curriculum development.

Five trends capture significant developments and concerns for society and are presented as the broad sociopolitical and economic context of nursing practice and education. These trends are global violence and the threat of violence, demographic revolutions, the technological explosion, globalization and the rise of the global economy, and environmental challenges. Although these trends are discussed separately, their interconnectedness is undeniable.

Global Violence, Threat of Violence, and Other Disasters

On September 11, 2001, hijacked airplanes hit the World Trade Center towers in New York City and the Pentagon near Washington, DC. A fourth plane crashed in rural Pennsylvania. These attacks marked an end to a sense of national invulnerability and left behind feelings of uncertainty about national security as well as the impact they would have on economies of the U.S. and the global community (Jackson, 2008). A decade later, these events continue to play significantly into the current sociopolitical, economic, and cultural landscape of the nation and the word *terrorism* is part of our nation's daily lexicon.

The societal reverberations of the 9/11 attacks have been many, including two immediate economic consequences: the events aggravated the economic downturn of 2001 and they shifted national spending toward security and antiterrorism strategies and away from social programs and human needs (Wiener & Tilly, 2002). Since that fateful September day there continues to be historic growth in defense spending in the U.S. and the first ever national health care reform bill was signed into law (Eisman, n.d.). The health implications from both of these consequences, along with the emergence of new infectious diseases and the aftermath of such natural disasters as the Indian Ocean tsunami in 2004, Hurricane Katrina in 2005, and the Haiti earthquake in 2010 are tremendous. In response, the health care system has focused resources on disaster and mass trauma preparedness, bioterrorism responses, and a multitude of strategies to prepare for unpredictable and diverse catastrophic events (Lewis, 2009). As a result, nurses must possess skills and knowledge in order to help create emergency response systems and work within the public health infrastructures characterized by community-wide collaboration, communication, and appropriate public policy. Nurses also need clinical knowledge related to biological agents, as well as skills to address the emotional stresses related to vulnerability and loss (Norman & Weiner, 2011).

The Demographic Revolution

The United States is getting more populous, older, and more racially and ethnically diverse (Institute of Medicine [IOM], 2010; Shrestha, 2006). In 2009 the older population, persons 65 years or greater, numbered 39.6 million and represented 12.9% of the U.S. population. By 2030 it is estimated there will be 72.1 million people age 65 and older and that these older Americans will represent 19.3% of the population. Additionally, by 2020 the age 85 and older population is projected to number 6.6 million, which represents a 15% increase in this age group (U.S. Department of Health & Human Services, Administration on Aging, 2010). "Population aging, especially when baby boomers reach ages 85 and older, signals a likely surge in the use of long-term care services" (Johnson, Toohey, & Wiener, 2007, p. iv). Other aging "boomers" will enter assisted living facilities or be cared for by their families and communities.

Regardless of the venue in which the aging population receives care, issues surrounding geriatric health have obvious curricular implications because educators must prepare nurses to promote health and self-care and prevent disease and disability in the large aging population. The responsibility to prepare future nurses in this manner is in keeping with a vision for health care recently proposed by the committee on the Robert Wood Johnson Foundation Initiative on the Future of Nursing (IOM, 2010). This vision calls for a system in which quality care is accessible, wellness and disease prevention is intentionally promoted, and compassionate care is provided across the life span (IOM, 2010). Not only will nursing care's emphasis be shifted from acute to chronic illnesses, but it will increase in complexity for the ongoing management of multiple disabilities and diseases. Initiatives such as those of the Hartford Institute for Geriatric Nursing are excellent examples of bringing best practices and resources to improve the health care of older adults.

End-of-life issues also loom large for the profession. In 2000 the Robert Wood Johnson Foundation began funding the End-of-Life Nursing Education Consortium (ELNEC) administered by the American Association of Colleges of Nursing (AACN) and the City of Hope National Medical Center. To date more than 11,650 nurses and other health care professionals, representing the 50 U.S. states and 65 international countries, have received ELNEC training and are using this innovative strategy to equip the nursing workforce with needed skills and knowledge (AACN, 2010b).

The disproportionate growth of the aged population is juxtaposed to a slower growth in the working population age cohort. After its peak in the 1970s, "the growth rate of the labor force has been decreasing with each passing decade and is expected to continue to do so in the future" (Toossi, 2006, p. 19). The projected workforce shortage is also predictive of a shortage of health care providers, particularly nurses, to care for elderly patients. The declining labor workforce coupled with the second economic recession within a decade also results in fewer individuals contributing to federal and state tax resources necessary to support social programs (Buerhaus, Auerbach, & Staiger, 2009; Toossi, 2006). Additionally, soaring health costs have imposed enormous pressures on public budgets and private individuals, especially older Americans (Penner & Johnson, 2006). Collectively, these issues require difficult policy discussions relative to resource allocation. Therefore curricula should include opportunities to develop the political advocacy skills needed to influence public policy decisions relative to the allocation of resources toward health and human needs.

Another demographic phenomenon in the United States is the growth of immigrant populations. The net immigration rate, which occurs when in-migration exceeds out-migration, "will continue to be an important component of population growth in the United States through 2050" (Shrestha, 2006, p. 10). As immigration patterns change, the composition of the country (currently an Anglo-European majority) turns into a microcosm of the world's peoples. Such racial and ethnic diversity presents policy challenges in a number of areas including assimilation, income disparities, and poverty (Shrestha, 2006). The conflict and controversy that accompany this significant demographic shift are exacerbated by the economic insecurity and volatility of our times. Multicultural diversity and ethnic understanding have major curriculum implications. Recruitment and retention of faculty and students who reflect the diversity of the population being served are also significant issues for schools of nursing.

Whether the demographic shifts include age, diversity, or other population features, there are implications for health and the resources needed to promote health. Future nurses need "the skills to influence policy formulation and the development of creative solutions to respond to changing demographics and the ageing chronically ill" (Hegarty et al., 2009, p. 5). Preparation of tomorrow's nursing practitioners requires attention to all demographic revolutions of both developed and developing areas of the globe, including patterns of growth, migration, and ethnic or racial composition.

Technological Explosion

America's transition from a resource-based, industrial economy characterized by semiskilled factory workers and raw materials to a knowledge-based, information age economy has been reshaping society for decades. Currently, "information and communication technology (ICT) continue to change us and the world we live in" (Abbott & Coenen, 2008, para. 1) while new technological possibilities continue to revolutionize life. As a result, issues in biotechnology, genetic engineering, information management ethics, and robotics that accompany the technological progress each carry multiple implications for nursing practice and education.

Access to education and knowledge is access to wealth, which can widen the gap between the rich and the poor. Technological advancements offer "new opportunities to enhance and broaden learning experiences" (Flynn & Vredevoogd, 2010, p. 7) and prepare students who are working within complex care environments to be decision makers (IOM, 2010). As technology evolves, increased numbers of nursing programs have found that e-learning, simulation, and mobile devices offer much potential for nursing education (IOM, 2010). Web-enhanced or online learning in particular provides opportunity for practicing nurses to pursue educational programs in conjunction with busy lives (IOM, 2010; Salyers, 2005). Simulation allows students to learn and practice in a safe environment, while the use of mobile devices teaches students real-life skills (IOM, 2010). The use of technology in this manner provides educational mobility, 24/7 access to education and knowledge, and enhanced opportunities for teaching and learning or career advancement and contributes to the availability of a qualified nursing workforce (IOM, 2010).

Globalization and the Rise of the Global Economy

National boundaries are becoming less relevant in an era of instantaneous telecommunications, free trade, and multinational corporations. The globe operates as a single worldwide production system, and the important skills are investing, strategic planning, and securing a market presence. The consequences of globalization are staggering and depend, in part, on a country's state of development.

The health implications of globalization are both positive and negative. In the positive sense, globalization results in trade expansion, which in turn increases living standards and improves social and economic status. When the wealth of a nation improves, so does the health of the nation. Globalized knowledge exchange also allows for the spread of health knowledge regarding treatment and causes of disease between countries and health systems (Abbott & Coenen, 2008). However, advances in globalization have also served to negatively affect health. For example, adoption of unhealthy Western habits and lifestyles has resulted in increased obesity and chronic disease. Additionally, open borders and access allow for rapid transmission of infectious agents and disease (Abbott & Coenen, 2008).

Nursing curriculum should acknowledge the realities of a market-driven or demand-driven health care system based increasingly on a global economy. Curriculum should also acknowledge that health care is a significant industry whose profit margins, stock prices, and bottom lines influence salaries and employment opportunities. Curriculum should help nurses understand the influence of globalization on the transmission and treatment of disease. Nurses best prepared for changes due to economic forces understand the significance of globalization and the global economy.

Environmental Challenges

Just as currency more readily crosses borders, so can environmental and epidemiological hazards. Besides health issues across the globe, there are concerns regarding sustainable development, energy availability, pollution-free water, and climate change, to name a few issues. Environmental health involves understanding how the environment influences human health and disease (National Institute of Environmental Health Sciences, 2005). It also involves an awareness of the impact that environmental conditions have on the health of individuals and populations and of interventions that can improve the impact nurses and others have on the environment and the impact the environment has on the health of the people (National Institute of Environmental Health Sciences, 2005; Shaner-McRae, McRae, & Jas, 2007).

Increasingly, Americans are becoming aware that the threats to public health and life are found in the frailty of our earth and our delicate interdependence. Therefore it is important for nurses to be aware that the environment affects our health and that actions in our professional and personal lives can and do make a difference. Nursing curricula should address the content and competencies related to environmental health as well as environmentally responsible clinical practice. Additionally, curricula should encourage and prepare nurses to factor environmental issues into the web of disease causation and to intervene to improve environmental health. The implications of global warming provide an excellent platform for students to discuss the ethics of protecting the environment as well as ways to conserve resources and make educated choices among products that are environmentally friendly.

Summary

These recurring issues from the broad sociopolitical and economic setting have current and future influence on the practice of nursing. Curriculum needs to acknowledge the possibilities and implications of global violence; demographic revolutions in number, age, and ethnic composition of populations; the technological explosion; the globalization of the economy and health; and the increasing awareness of environmental fragility.

Issues in Higher Education

Institutions of higher education sit at an interesting juncture of at least two global themes: the technological explosion and globalization. As learning, knowledge, and skills become the primary resources of a country, the public and private financing of quality higher education becomes more challenging. Colleges and universities, faced with shrinking resources, technological advances, and increased enrollments must strive to find a balance between innovation and tradition if they are to remain relevant and current in an ever-changing and evolving world (Flynn & Vredevoogd, 2010). Therefore affordability, access, and accountability continue to be three key issues facing higher education. Each issue affects the other, for affordability determines access and, as public concerns related to these issues mount, there are increasing calls for accountability. These challenges must be met in the face of shrinking public higher education budgets. Institutions often deal with the question of whether they can "do more with less" or whether they will be forced to "do less with less."

Affordability

The concern for affordability, noted as early as 1947, persists today as economic and societal factors promote an increased value of a college degree in labor markets. Higher education is considered an avenue to a livable wage or to a salary to support a middle-class lifestyle. Higher education is also associated with better health and positive effects on civic engagement, including voting (Brock, 2010).

Today, higher education faces many challenges due to the current economic situation, increasing student enrollment, and rising expectations for quality and equity (Flynn & Vredevoogd, 2010; Heyneman, 2006). Cuts in federal and state funding have affected publicly funded institutions while fluctuations in the stock market have contributed to the declining value of endowments. In short, higher education "will be asked to do more with less" (Flynn & Vredevoogd, 2010, p. 6).

Because of societal concern for a living wage, the financing of higher education becomes a crucial public policy debate. Within that debate, the academy should prepare persuasive arguments for the merits of education beyond salary, society's obligation to invest in human infrastructure, and the importance of public commitment to higher education.

The specific charge for schools of nursing is to articulate the cost-effective contribution that nursing makes to the improvement of the health of the nation.

Access

Another issue with historical roots that persists today is access to higher education. The issue of access is important considering society's transformation from an industrial economy to an information-based, global economy because college graduates have "substantially better prospects in the labor market than peers who stop their formal education after high school" (Brock, 2010, p. 110). While access to higher education has increased substantially for women, Hispanics, Asians, and Pacific Islanders, other racial and ethnic groups, such as American Indians and Alaskan Natives, remain underrepresented (Brock, 2010).

In the twenty-first century all Americans must be provided with the "skills they need to succeed in the global economy and lead satisfying, productive lives. Our people and our nation will be poorer and weaker if we fail to provide real opportunities for all Americans to fulfill their potential and succeed in higher education" (National Commission on Accountability in Higher Education, 2005, p. 6). The ability of more Americans to take advantage of the multiple benefits and opportunities that higher education affords requires public policies and political will that support access as well as higher education institutions that make real those opportunities. As administrators of nursing schools pursue robust enrollments of diverse and talented students, affordability and access are crucial considerations for the profession.

Accountability

Worldwide, governments and taxpaying publics are questioning the allocation of scarce public resources. The concept of high-quality, affordable public education is threatened by the competition for funding of other public needs. This, along with rising fear about the deterioration of the U.S. higher education system, low completion rates, and poor preparation of a workforce ready and able to compete in a global marketplace, led to the formation of the Spelling Commission. The purpose of this commission was to recommend a national strategy for postsecondary education reform, with an emphasis on "how well colleges and universities are preparing students for

the 21st century workforce" (Floyd & Vredevoogd, 2010, p. 19).

Several forces prompt this increased accountability for higher education. In times of cost cutting and corporate downsizing, business and private sector management looks to education, and its products, for competitive strategies. Also, drastic state budget cuts have caused policy makers and taxpayers to require justification for higher education funding. Legislatures have tended to disallow tuition hikes and request internal moves toward efficiency. Additionally, "publicly funded institutions must be accountable to their principal stakeholder—the public" (Floyd & Vredevoogd, 2010, p. 10). Each of these forces promotes increased public scrutiny and higher expectations.

Accountability, therefore, becomes a multidirectional force. Institutions of higher education depend on the government for funding and are therefore highly accountable to the public for academic productivity and fiscal prudence. Schools of nursing are accountable to state legislatures, Congress, and the public regarding the preparation of adequate numbers of competent nurses. Governments, in response to their perceived accountability to the public, act to regulate and reform higher education. Accountability will continue as a significant theme in higher education.

Summary

Institutions of higher education are affected by major trends in the environment and very specifically by the need to create an educated and skilled workforce and by the financial challenges of doing so. The financial challenges include both private costs from individuals and families and public expenditures from state tax budgets. There is a potential for dissonance because the public both desires education and scrutinizes public expenditures in light of other societal needs. Increased accountability will be required of higher education in terms of measurable outcomes for quality education.

Issues Specific to the Nursing Profession

This chapter began by looking through the lens of the broad socioeconomic and sociopolitical issues that shape our world and influence contemporary life. Within that context, forces in higher education influence the education of the present and future nursing workforce. This section focuses the lens more specifically on the profession, highlighting issues of particular consideration within the profession. It is a false dichotomy to separate issues as internal and external to the profession, for it denies an interactive exchange between issues. Included are the context of nursing care delivery, the nursing and nurse faculty shortage, new and reemerging degrees, and competencies for the twenty-first century.

Context of Nursing Care Delivery

The nursing profession influences and is influenced by the health care delivery system, which provides a context for nursing services. The 2010 American Hospital Association Environmental Scan provides insight into several trends affecting the health care field, five of which have great implications for nursing practice and education: science and technology, rising costs, health policy, quality of care and patient safety, and human resources (O'Dell & Runy, 2009).

Science and Technology

Science and technology continues to revolutionize the health care possibilities. For example, the Human Genome Project presents a multitude of individualized genetic therapies, as well as ethical quandaries. As a result, nurses must be able to identify, understand, and support patients facing genetic decisions (Forbes & Hickey, 2009). The American Nurses Association's *Essentials of Genetic and Genomic Nursing: Competencies, Curricula Guidelines, and Outcome Indicators* (2008) details basic competencies nurses should posses in order to "deliver competent genetic and genomic focused nursing care" (Forbes & Hickey, 2009, p. 9).

In 2009 more than one half of Americans aged 18 to 64 went online to look up health information (Cohen & Stussman, 2005). Through the Internet consumers have become armed with and have access to information previously available only to clinicians. Today's health care consumer knows what they should expect from their health care providers and expect to participate in decisions affecting their health care (Hegarty et al. 2009; Heller, Oros, & Durney-Crowley, n.d.). Internet-savvy health care consumers often approach providers with extensive information, requesting treatments or drugs and expecting quality ratings on provider and institution report cards. Therefore nursing needs to appreciate these empowered consumers

and "respect, affirm, and share decision-making with increasingly knowledgeable patients" (Hegarty et al., 2009, p. 6).

In addition, electronic health records and telehealth technologies demand that nurses acquire significant technological proficiencies while schools are challenged to use sophisticated simulations for skill acquisition and critical thinking development (IOM, 2010; O'Dell & Runy, 2009). The health care industry is following the lead of the aviation industry in providing increased education and assessment using simulation technology, particularly in this era of scarce and complex clinical sites for training. Informatics education within schools of nursing assists students to understand data, combine data and knowledge, and make decisions, often through the use of technology (Forbes & Hickey, 2009; Heller, Oros, & Durney-Crowley, n.d.; Hegarty et al., 2009; IOM, 2010). Collectively, these advances in science and technology make it imperative that nurses of the twenty-first century possess "knowledge and skills for practice in a complex, emerging technologically sophisticated, consumer-centric, global environment" (Warren & Connors, 2007, p. 58).

Rising Costs

The second trend involves the continued surge in health costs and the need for hospitals and providers to manage care more efficiently within finite budgets. Hospital budgets will be challenged by declining charitable donations and investment income; increasing numbers of Medicare, Medicaid, and self-pay clients; labor shortages; and increased pharmaceutical and supply costs (O'Dell & Runy, 2009). Research that documents nursing's contribution to efficient, quality care is needed to advocate in budget negotiations and hospital changes.

Health Policy

Health policy, the third trend, becomes an increasingly significant strategy to shape, finance, and regulate the health care system. With the cost of national health expenditures anticipated to rise from 16% to 20% of the gross domestic product (GDP) by 2017, state and federal policies seek to regulate costs, shift care to less expensive settings, and use market forces to control costs when possible (Henry J. Kaiser Family Foundation, 2009; O'Dell & Runy, 2009). Ensuring that everyone in the U.S. has health insurance is one strategy that would help reduce health care expenditure to only 18.5% of the GDP (O'Dell & Runy, 2009).

The U.S. Census Bureau (2010) reported that in 2009 the number of uninsured Americans rose to 50.7 million (16.7%) and that for the first time since 1987 the number of people with health insurance decreased. In particular, the number of people covered by private health insurance dropped while increasing numbers received coverage by government health insurance. On March 23, 2010, the Affordable Care Act was signed into law by President Barack Obama. This historic health reform legislation represents great progress toward making health care available to and affordable for all Americans. The ability to implement this health care reform act requires the effective production and use of the nursing workforce as well as participation by nursing leaders who possess the ability to understand the complexities of our health and education systems and can readily apply evidence-based solutions to health reform (Rother & Lavizzo-Mourey, 2009).

Nurses are poised to participate in the transformation of this nation's health care system (Nursing's Rx for Health Care Reform, 2009). Participation requires nurses to possess political advocacy skills to campaign at both state and national levels so that nursing's voice is brought to the policy debates and will play a meaningful role in policy development.

Quality of Care and Patient Safety

A need exists to improve patient safety and provide quality care (Forbes & Hickey, 2009). While the quality of care has improved steadily over the past 14 years, further improvement continues at a low pace. In addition, health care quality is suboptimal, patient safety is lagging, and there remains a significant geographic variation in quality of care (U.S. Department of Health & Human Services, Agency for Healthcare Research and Quality, 2008; O'Dell & Runy, 2009). Given the loud call from several authorities, including the IOM, the Robert Wood Johnson Foundation, and the Agency for Healthcare Research and Quality, in tandem with the key role that nurses play in protecting patient safety and providing quality health care, there exists a need to better prepare today's nurses for professional practice. To this end, the AACN identified the following essential core competencies for nurses related to ensuring high quality and patient safety: critical thinking, health care systems and policy, communication, illness and disease management, ethics, and information and health care technologies (AACN, 2006; Forbes & Hickey, 2009). Teaching strategies and concrete examples of learning activities that nurse educators can use to teach these competencies can be found at the Quality and Safety Education for Nurses (QSEN) website at www.qsen.org.

Human Resources

Human capital becomes a significant trend with nursing and physician shortages and the unionization of health care providers. In February 2009 three nursing unions merged to form the United American Nurses–National Nurses Organizing Committee. The legislative priorities of this union, which has 150,000 members, include a push for nurse staffing ratios, workplace safety rules, and a national pension for registered nurses (RNs) (O'Dell & Runy, 2009).

Retention of satisfied employees will be the goal of viable organizations, which is related to the creation and maintenance of healthy and safe work environments. Creation of "workplace cultures that can attract and retain health care workers" will be an important element of hospitals of the future given the "average voluntary turnover rate of new hospital nurses is 27%" during their first year on the job (Joint Commission, 2008, p. 29). In part, respecting human capital means attention to the work environment and relationships as well as sanctions against verbal abuse by physicians, patients, and nurse colleagues; sexual harassment; and workplace violence, including horizontal violence or hostile behaviors within a group of nurse colleagues (Felblinger, 2008; Joint Commission, 2008).

These trends inform educators as they determine what and how to teach the next generation of nurses. Additionally, educators should assist students to understand the proactive steps that the nursing profession is taking within this changing health care environment to define nursing practice and educate the public on nursing's role in quality care. Seeking "Magnet" recognition as an institution by fulfilling and demonstrating the 5 model components and 14 "forces of magnetism" (Box 6-1) is a powerful example of nursing action that students should understand.

Future practitioners will need knowledge and abilities to assist informed health care consumers, understand science, use technology, stem rising

---

BOX 6-1 ANCC Magnet Model—Model Components and Associated Forces of Magnetism

I. TRANSFORMATIONAL LEADERSHIP

- Visionary, knowledgeable nursing leadership
- Participative management style

II. STRUCTURAL EMPOWERMENT

- Organizational structures with unit-based, decentralized decision-making
- Personnel policies and programs that support competitive salaries, flexible staffing, and healthy work environment
- Strong partnerships to impact health of community
- Perception of the organization that nurses are an integral part of essential patient care services
- Professional growth and development fully supported for competency-based clinical advancement

III. EXEMPLARY PROFESSIONAL PRACTICE

- Professional models of care where nurses are accountable and responsible for care provision

- Availability of adequate consultation and other resources
- Autonomous nurse practice, using independent judgment within an interdisciplinary team approach
- Incorporation of teaching in all aspects of nursing practice
- Positive and mutually respectful interdisciplinary relationships

IV. NEW KNOWLEDGE, INNOVATION, AND IMPROVEMENTS

- Structures and processes exist to support quality improvement

V. EMPIRICAL QUALITY RESULTS

- Quality of care valued by nurses and nursing leaders, and supported within the environment

Adapted from American Nurses Credentialing Center. (2008). A new vision for Magnet. Retrieved from http://www.nursecredentialing.org/Magnet/ProgramOverview/New-Magnet-Model.aspx

---

costs, provide quality health care and protect the safety of patients, advocate for effective health policy, actively participate in the process of health care reform, and work to create a health care system with competent, empowered human capital. In short, "nurses will need to take leadership roles in ensuring quality health care" (Nursing, 2010, p. 11).

Nursing Shortage

The United States is "in the midst of a shortage of RNs that is expected to intensify" (AACN, 2010e, para.1). The shortage of nurses and nursing faculty along with the aging of practitioners and educators pose a threat to patient safety and the quality of health care delivery and present significant challenges to the profession, practice settings, and nursing programs (AACN, 2010d, 2010e; Rother & Lavizzo-Mourey, 2009).

The December 2007 economic depression served to temporarily ease the nursing shortage in many parts of the country. Despite this, a long-term shortage of RNs is still predicted to occur in the U.S. within the next 10 years (AACN, 2010e; Buerhaus et al., 2009). Not only is the profession witnessing a shortage in absolute numbers but in

the ethnic, gender, and cultural reflections of the greater society (AACN, 2005). For example, Buerhaus et al. (2009) assert that men and Hispanics are a rich yet virtually untapped segment of the population as a readily available source of prospective nurses and that their entry into the profession would do much to ease the nursing shortage. However, the stigma of nursing as a white, female-dominated profession along with the lack of mentors and role models serve to discourage men and Hispanics from considering a career in the profession. Additionally, educational and financial barriers work to discourage Hispanics from becoming RNs.

Multiple factors contribute to these complex phenomena, including fewer persons entering nursing, more career options for bright men and women that compete with the choice of nursing, the aging workforce, negative work environment, job dissatisfaction, and the exit of nurses from the profession (AACN, 2010e; Buerhaus et al., 2009; Sims, 2009). Collectively, these factors can hinder retention and recruitment into nursing. Inadequate staffing, inadequate support staff, heavy workload, employer expectation to work overtime, inadequate wages, and the rigors of treating increasingly ill patients, as well as issues mentioned previously related to verbal abuse and workplace violence, collectively contribute to job dissatisfaction, emotional exhaustion, and increased stress within the profession. These factors are known by most within the profession and must be articulated to policy makers, physicians, hospital administrators, and society at large.

The nursing shortage is further exacerbated by the nurse faculty shortage. Schools of nursing simply cannot accept all qualified applicants into their programs due, in part, to an insufficient number of faculty (AACN, 2010d, 2010e; National League for Nursing, 2010; Sims, 2009). The faculty shortage begins with a deficit; there are simply not enough nurses holding a master's degree or earned doctoral degree, which is the academic norm (Allen, 2008; AACN, 2010d; Sims, 2009). Add to the equation the "graying professoriate," the narrowing pipeline of baccalaureate and master's prepared nurses, the older age of nurses completing their doctorate, lucrative salaries luring nurse educators away from teaching, and the severity of the shortage expands (Allen, 2008; AACN, 2010d; Cleary, Bevill, Lacey, & Nooney, 2007; IOM, 2010; Sims, 2009). At risk is not only a restriction in nursing school enrollments during a time of increased need but also reduction in scientific knowledge generation from nurse scholars and fewer professional leaders shaping policy and bringing a nursing voice to interdisciplinary discussions.

The nurse educator shortage is an invitation for creative and innovative solutions: forging partnerships that share, among other things, faculty and rethink faculty roles, academic resources, and teaching methods; creating ways in which retired yet vibrant faculty can contribute their wisdom and expertise in flexible, part-time projects; supporting senior faculty with resources and rewards to prolong productivity; and recruiting individuals into doctoral programs at a younger age.

The nurse and nurse faculty shortages therefore present opportunities and challenges. Nursing professionals are taking steps to seize the opportunity to create nursing programs that will adequately prepare future practitioners for societal health needs and care settings that optimize the contribution that nursing makes to the health of the nation. The challenges are undertaken in partnership with nursing colleagues within service and education, policy makers and business leaders, the media, and

society in general. As with the shortage of practicing nurses, strategies that promote graduate education, encourage and mentor students to consider a career in teaching, and increase funding and support for nurses pursuing advanced degrees will do much to address the nurse faculty shortage (Cleary et al., 2007; Sims, 2009).

New and Reemerging Degrees

Two graduate degrees, the clinical nurse leader (CNL) and the doctorate in nursing practice (DNP), have recently been created. In 2000, considering declining nursing enrollment among other professional issues, the AACN determined that changes must be made in education, practice, licensure, and credentialing. The AACN recommended a new educational model for a master's entry, the CNL, to improve patient care and maximize patient safety (AACN, 2007). Programs to educate CNLs require ongoing partnership between practice and education so that both arenas shape the learning and graduates enter practice environments designed to use their skill set. By 2009 the national movement to advance the CNL role had gained momentum as seven new programs opened, student enrollment was up by 9.6% (1,808 students), and almost 500 (6.9%) CNLs graduated from this generalist master's program (AACN, 2010a).

In 2004 the AACN voted to move the current level of preparation necessary for advanced nursing practice from the master's degree to the doctorate level by 2015. This move shaped two terminal nursing degrees: the research-focused PhD and the clinically focused DNP. The drive to create the DNP was the complexity of current health care and curriculum creep that results in some advanced practice degree programs far exceeding the credit hours of a usual master's degree. The AACN's membership vote that education for all advanced practice nurses will transition to the DNP prompted some schools to create new doctoral programs consistent with the DNP essentials and standards from the particular specialty focus of the program. As a result, by 2009 there were 120 DNP programs available in 35 states with an additional 161 programs in the planning stage (AACN, 2010a). In contrast, other schools perceive budgetary, regulatory, or philosophical barriers to this transition and have not moved to the DNP and will likely continue to offer master's degree advanced practice education as the nursing profession further addresses graduate level education issues related to advanced practice nursing.

The CNL and DNP are two examples of efforts within the profession to create roles and curriculum to match changing societal needs for health care.

Competencies for the Twenty-First Century

The profession needs not only robust workforce numbers, but also practitioners with requisite knowledge, abilities, and work behaviors to meet the health demands of the population as well as nurses who possess leadership skills. Educators are challenged to prepare individuals who, upon graduation, can lead as well as deliver competent and compassionate care and have the ability to navigate future changes in the system and acquire future abilities associated with evolving roles. Box 6-2 represents eight leadership competencies suggested by Hutson (2008) as essential for the 2020 nurse leader.

More than a decade ago, Bellack and O'Neil (2000) discussed the recommendations from the Pew Health Professions Commission's fourth and final report, which represented a continuing effort to support the health professions' education reform and align educational programs more fully with the health needs of the population. They presented five recommendations for all health professions schools, including nursing. Despite being issued more than 10 years ago, these recommendations continue to provide excellent guideposts for nurse educators as they pursue the preferred future via the current reality. The first general recommendation prompted educators to recognize the characteristics of the new health care system and cease preparation for "yesterday's health care system" (p. 15). Included is the advice to form creative and reciprocal relationships with clinical partners and to be an active agent in the creation of "tomorrow's" system.

The second recommendation was an imperative for a diverse workforce, noting that the configuration of diversity varies by region. While great strides have occurred in "recruiting and graduating nurses that mirror the patient population, more must be done before adequate representation becomes a reality" (AACN, 2010c, para. 1). A diverse workforce allows consumers of health care to see practitioners who share their diversity and presupposes greater resources in addressing the challenges of our most vulnerable populations.

Interdisciplinary competence, the third recommendation, requires that professions dismantle the "silos" that isolate practitioners and inhibit the sharing of perspectives and potential solutions (Flynn & Vredevoogd, 2010; Thompson & Tilden, 2009). In an effort to improve the delivery of safe, quality health care, the IOM (2003) proposed that health professions education ensure "all health professionals should be educated to deliver patient-centered care as members of an interdisciplinary team" (p. 121). Since that time, the concept of interprofessional education has been endorsed by health professions educators worldwide as a way to improve the quality of health care (Center for Interprofessional Education, 2009). Interdisciplinary competence does not diminish individual professions but rather provides health care professionals with the "knowledge and skills of how to work collaboratively to improve patient care and outcomes" (Goldman, Zwarenstein, Bhattacharyya, & Reeves, 2009, p. 151).

The fourth recommendation, an emphasis on ambulatory practice, is compatible with interdisciplinary competence. Community-based care experiences benefit from creative partnerships between the community, agencies, and educational programs.

The fifth recommendation emphasizes the value of community service and suggests that it is an integral component of the educational process. Service-learning experiences benefit the learner

---

BOX 6-2 2020 Essential Nurse Leader Competencies

1. A global perspective or mindset of healthcare and professional nursing issues
2. A working knowledge of technology
3. Expert decision-making skills that are evidence based
4. Ability to create organization cultures that permeate quality healthcare and patient/worker safety
5. Political astuteness
6. Possess collaborative and team-building skills
7. Ability to balance authenticity with performance expectations
8. Be visionary and proactive in response to a health care system that is fraught with change and chaos

Adapted from Hutson, C. (2008). Preparing nurse leaders for 2020. *Journal of Nursing Management*, 16, 905–911. doi:10.111/j.1365-2834.2008.00942.x.

and the community partner. As faculty model service through their community engagement, they enrich themselves, the community, and student learning.

In many respects, nursing education is still grappling with developing educational models that successfully address the Pew Commission's recommendations from 2000. Most recently, the IOM (2010) released the report *Future of Nursing: Leading Change, Advancing Health,* which offers a new set of recommendations that call for significant changes in how we educate and prepare nurses for practice in an era of health care reform. The four key messages delivered in the *Future of Nursing* report are that nurses should: (1) be able to practice to the full scope of their educational preparation; (2) seek higher levels of educational preparation, and be able to do so in seamless academic progression systems; (3) function as full partners in interdisciplinary teams to redesign health care delivery; and (4) benefit from improved data collection and information infrastructures. The IOM report promises to be influential in focusing attention on solutions to the barriers that have kept nurses from being as influential as they can be in leading and advocating for changes in health care.

Summary

Through intentional efforts and collaboration with other stakeholders, nursing has worked within the societal and higher education contexts to advance health and continually refine the process that produces tomorrow's workforce. Nursing has shaped and is shaped by the context of care and by the challenges of the nursing shortage; nursing remains mindful of the competencies needed for twenty-first-century practice.

Strategies to Identify Influential Forces and Issues

To develop a curriculum that is relevant and current, faculty must continually monitor the environments internal and external to the institution and the profession. This section presents four strategies that faculty can use separately or in combination to identify influential forces and issues: environmental scanning, forecasting, epidemiology, and survey research and consensus building.

Environmental Scanning

"Strategic planning is critical to the survival of health care organizations in today's turbulent environment" (Layman & Bamberg, 2005, p. 200). Environmental scanning, a component of strategic planning, involves various activities that monitor and evaluate information from the external environment (Layman & Bamberg, 2005). The goal of environmental scanning is for leaders and managers to become aware of general trends and events affecting health care and higher education generally and nursing specifically. Information from the environment can be acquired in various ways, including careful review of scientific and professional journals as well as lay literature and newspapers and attendance and networking at professional meetings. Information gathered from these activities becomes "the basis of future initiatives" (Layman & Bamberg, 2005, p. 200).

Environmental scanning continues to be successfully used by colleges and universities to determine the context of the forces affecting curriculum development. For example, use of strategic environmental scanning led one southeastern university to develop a non–nurse practitioner program designed to prepare nurses for other types of advanced practice roles. Following review of program evaluations and assessment of graduates and other nursing leaders in the community, the Master of Science in Nursing in Advanced Care Management and Leadership program was developed with the goal of preparing nurse leaders who are "equipped to manage and improve client care outcomes" (Aduddell & Dorman, 2010, p. 171).

In curriculum development, environmental scanning allows faculty to be simultaneously reactive and proactive. Through awareness and acknowledgment of significant trends (reactive), faculty can more actively choose a future direction for nursing education and curriculum (proactive). The use of environmental scanning as a strategy to obtain a broad scope of information and evaluate its relevance to nursing is the foundation of the other strategies that follow.

Forecasting

Forecasting is a process of producing likely futures on the basis of factual information about the present. Dunn (2004) described three forms of forecasting: projection, prediction, and conjecture. The forms can be differentiated by the basis of their forecast. Projection is based on current and previous trends taken into the future. Using projection and inductive reasoning, nursing faculty can extrapolate from present data (e.g., morbidity rates or census data) what a future rate will be. Prediction is based on explicit theoretical assumptions. Using prediction and deductive reasoning, nursing faculty can forecast the future using laws, propositions, or theories. Conjecture is based on subjective judgments about the future and applies retroductive reasoning. In this form of reasoning, nursing faculty rely on insights, creativity, and tacit knowledge to present a claim about the future. The claim is related back to, and supported by, information and assumptions. These three forms of forecasting show that descriptions of a future can be created using current or previous data, theory, or subjective judgments and that the reasoning can be inductive, deductive, or retroductive.

Forecasting is not an exact science but is an art that includes judgments and assumptions. Errors can occur with incomplete data, superficial analysis, and flawed communication about the data. Even with the limitations inherent in the art and science of forecasting, it is a tool for nursing faculty to develop a curriculum that prepares students for the future.

Epidemiology

Epidemiology is the study of the distribution and determinants of states of health and illness in human populations. Epidemiology provides nursing faculty with systematic ways to understand patterns of disease, characteristics of people at high risk for disease, environmental factors, and shifts in demographic characteristics of the population. Using epidemiological data with groups or populations, nurses understand and document the need for programs and policies to reduce risk and promote health. Epidemiology can therefore be seen as a method for planned change.

In the same way, nursing faculty responsible for the development of curriculum can use epidemiological data and methods to understand factors affecting the health of populations and trends occurring in health and illness states. Epidemiology provides faculty with methods for understanding that part of the context that involves the broad determinants of health and patterns of disease and disability in the population.

Survey Research and Consensus Building

Another tool at the disposal of faculty is survey research. Surveys involve systematically collecting information from individuals and deriving statistical statements, such as some measure of central tendency, or consensus statements from groups of experts or involved individuals. If the design is iterative and involves a series of surveys, feedback, and more surveys, it is considered a form of Delphi technique.

Surveys and consensus-building processes provide an opportunity to sample the perspectives of various stakeholders and knowledgeable persons, for example, employers or consumers. They facilitate tapping the rich diversity of group wisdom related to complex issues.

The strategies of environmental scanning, forecasting, epidemiology, and survey research and consensus building have utility in preparing for curriculum development or revision. Using some combination of the four strategies presented here, faculty can be equipped to develop curriculum compatible with the current and projected issues influencing nursing and health care.

SUMMARY

The forces and issues that influence and are influenced by nursing curriculum originate in the external, higher education, and internal environments. Educators sensitive to major sociopolitical and economic trends can develop curriculum that matches global characteristics. Educators aware of prevailing higher education issues can assist schools of nursing to be leaders in the academy. Educators attuned to prevailing and visionary thinking within the profession can shape the future through progressive curriculum and pedagogy. Nursing deserves curriculum that is both compatible with the contemporary health care context and flexible enough to be relevant for emerging circumstances and needs.

REFLECTING ON THE EVIDENCE

1. How is your curriculum relevant to the broad societal changes, issues, or health care reform? In what new ways can it become more relevant to broad societal changes, issues, or health care reform?

2. How does your curriculum prepare students to be engaged citizens in society whose practice matches current issues and trends?

3. How is your curriculum compatible with new developments in the discipline?

4. In what ways does your school incorporate new input and acknowledge new influences on curriculum development? How do people respond to those voices of change?

5. How is your curriculum preparing students to lead and become leaders?

REFERENCES

Abbott, P. A., & Coenen, A. (2008). Globalization and advances in information and communication technologies: The impact on nursing and health. *Nursing Outlook, 56*(5), 238–246.e2. doi:10.1016/j.outlook.2008.06.009

Aduddell, K. A., & Dorman, G. E. (2010). The development of the next generation of nurse leaders. *Journal of Nursing Education, 49*(3), 168–171. doi:10.3928/01484834-20090916-08

Allen, L. (2008). The nursing shortage continues as faculty shortage grows. *Nursing Economics, 26*(1), 35–40.

American Association of Colleges of Nursing. (2005). *Report of the Task Force on Education and Regulation for Professional Nursing Practice I.* Retrieved from http://www.aacn.nche.edu/

American Association of Colleges of Nursing. (2006). *Hallmarks of quality and patient safety.* Retrieved from http://www.aacn.nche.edu/

American Association of Colleges of Nursing. (2007). *White paper on the education and role of the clinical nurse leader.* Retrieved from http://www.aacn.nche.edu/

American Association of Colleges of Nursing. (2010a). Amid calls for more highly educated nurses, new AACN data show impressive growth in doctoral nursing programs. Retrieved from http://www.aacn.nche.edu/

American Association of Colleges of Nursing. (2010b). End of life nursing education consortium. Retrieved from http://www.aacn.nche.edu/

American Association of Colleges of Nursing. (2010c). Fact sheet: Enhancing diversity in the nursing workforce. Retrieved from http://www.aacn.nche.edu/

American Association of Colleges of Nursing. (2010d). Nursing faculty shortage fact sheet. Retrieved from http://www.aacn.nche.edu/

American Association of Colleges of Nursing. (2010e). Nursing shortage fact sheet. Retrieved from http://www.aacn.nche.edu/

Andre, K., & Barnes, L. (2010). Creating a 21st century nursing workforce: Designing a bachelor of nursing program in response to the health reform agenda. *Nurse Education Today, 30*(3), 258–263. doi:10.1016/j.nedt.2009.09.011

Bellack, J. P., & O'Neil, E. H. (2000). Recreating nursing practice for a new century: Recommendations and implications of the Pew Health Professions Commission's final report. *Nursing and Health Care Perspectives, 21*(1), 14–21.

Brock, T. (2010). Young adults and higher education: Barriers and breakthroughs to success. *The Future of Children, 20*(1), 109–132.

Buerhaus, P. I., Auerbach, D. E., & Staiger, D. O. (2009). The recent surge in nurse employment: Causes and implications. *Health Affairs, 28*(4), w657–w668. doi:10.1377/hlthaff.28.4.w657

Center for Interprofessional Education. (2009). *Why interprofessional education?* Retrieved from http://www.ipe.umn.edu/

Cleary, B., Bevill, J. W., Lacey, L. M., & Nooney, J. G. (2007). Evidence and root causes of an inadequate pipeline for nursing faculty. *Nursing Administration Quarterly, 31*(2), 124–128.

Cohen, R. A., & Stussman, B. (2005, February). Health information technology use among men and women aged 18–64: Early release of estimates from the National Health Interview survey, January–June 2009. Health E-Stats, National Center for Health Statistics. Retrieved from http://www.cdc.gov/nchs/

Dunn, W. N. (2004). Public policy analysis: An introduction. Englewood Cliffs, NJ: Prentice-Hall.

Eisman, D. (n.d.). Obama proposes another surge in military spending. *AOLNews.* Retrieved from http://www.aolnews.com/

Felblinger, D. M. (2008). Incivility and bullying in the workplace and nurses' shame responses. *Journal of Obstetrics, Gynecology, and Neonatal Nurses, 37*(2), 234–242.

Flynn, W. J., & Vredevoogd, J. (2010). The future of learning: 12 views on emerging trends in higher education. *Planning for Higher Education, 38*(2), 5–10.

Forbes, M. O., & Hickey, M. T. (2009). Curriculum reform in baccalaureate nursing education: Review of the literature. *International Journal of Nursing Education Scholarship, 6*(1), 1–16.

Goldman, J., Zwarenstein, M., Bhattacharyya, O., & Reeves, S. (2009). Improving the clarity of the interprofessional field: Implications for research and continuing interprofessional education. *Journal of Continuing Education in the Health Professions, 29*(3), 151–156.

Hegarty, J., Walsh, E., Condon, C., & Sweeney, J. (2009). The undergraduate education of nurses: Looking to the future. *International Journal of Nursing Education Scholarship, 6*(1), 1–11.

Heller, B. R., Oros, M. T., & Durney-Crowley, J. (n.d.). *The future of nursing education: Ten trends to watch.* Retrieved from http://www.nln.org/

Henry J. Kaiser Family Foundation. (2009). Health care costs: Key information on health care costs and their impact. Menlo Park, CA: Author. Retrieved from http://www.kff.org/

Heyneman, S. P. (2006). Global issues in higher education. Retrieved from http://www.america.gov/st/econ-english/2008/June/20080608095226xjyrreP0.6231653.html&distid=

Hutson, C. (2008). Preparing nurse leaders for 2020. Journal of Nursing Management, 16, 905–911. doi:10.111/j.1365-2834.2008.00942.x

Institute of Medicine. (2003). Health professions education: A bridge to quality. Retrieved from http://www.ipe.umn.edu/

Institute of Medicine. (2010). The future of nursing: Leading change, advancing health. Washington, DC: National Academics Press.

Jackson, O. A. (2008). The impact of the 9/11 terrorist attacks on the US economy. Retrieved from http://www.journalof-911studies.com/

Johnson, R. W., Toohey, D., & Wiener, J. M. (2007). Meeting the long-term care needs of the baby boomers: How changing families will affect paid helpers and institutions. Washington, DC: Urban Institute.

Joint Commission. (2008). Health care at the crossroads: Guiding principles for the development of the hospital of the future. Retrieved from http://www.jointcommission.org/

Layman, E. J., & Bamberg, R. (2005). Environmental scanning and the health care manager. Health Care Manager, 24(3), 200–208.

Leverich, J. P. (2010). Building leaders key to success. Retrieved from http://www.leverich.com/Article_building_leaders.htm

Lewis, K. L. (2009). Emergency planning and response. In G. Roux & J. A. Halstead (Eds.), Issues and trends in nursing: Essential knowledge for today and tomorrow (pp. 261–285). Sudbury, MA: Jones & Bartlett.

National Commission on Accountability in Higher Education. (2005, March 10). Accountability for better results: A national imperative for higher education. Retrieved from http://www.sheeo.org/

National Institute of Environmental Health Sciences. (2005). What is environmental health? Retrieved from http://www.niehs.nih.gov/

National League for Nursing. (2010). 2010 NLN nurse educator shortage fact sheet. Retrieved from http://www.nln.org/governmentaffairs/pdf/NurseFacultyShortage.pdf

Norman, L. & Weiner, E. (2011). Emergency preparedness and response for today's world. In B. Cherry & S. Jacob (Eds.), Contemporary Nursing: Issues, Trends, and Management (5th ed., pp. 317-332). St. Louis, MO: Elsevier.

Nurses Association. (2008). Essentials of genetic and genomic nursing: Competencies, curricula guidelines, and outcome indicators (2nd ed.). Silver Spring, MD: Author.

Nursing. (2010). Q & A with Kathy Rideout Associate Dean for Academic Affairs. Rochester, NY: School of Nursing, University of Rochester Medical Center.

Nursing's Rx for Health Care Reform. (2009). Retrieved from http://www.rwjf.org/

O'Dell, G. J., & Runy, L. A. (2009). 2010 AHA environmental scan. Hospitals and Health Networks, 83(9), 36–41.

Penner, R. G., & Johnson, R. W. (2006). Health care costs, taxes, and the retirement decision: Conceptual issues and illustrative simulations. Washington, DC: Urban Institute. Retrieved from http://www.urban.org/

Rother, J., & Lavizzo-Mourey, R. (2009). Addressing the nursing workforce: A critical element for health reform. Health Affairs, 28(40), w620–w624. doi:10.1377/hlthaff.28.4.w620

Salyers, V. L. (2005). Web-enhanced and face-to-face classroom instructional methods: Effects on course outcomes and student satisfaction. International Journal of Nursing Education Scholarship, 2(1), 1–11.

Shaner-McRae, H., McRae, G., & Jas, V. (2007). Environmentally safe health care agencies: Nursing's responsibility, Nightingale's legacy. Online Journal of Issues in Nursing, 12(2), 1–13. Retrieved from http://www.nursingworld.org/MainMenuCategories/ANAMarketplace/ANAPeriodicals/OJIN/TableofContents/Volume122007/No2May07/EnvironmentallySafeHealthCareAgencies.aspx

Shrestha, L. B. (2006). The changing demographic profile of the United States. Congressional Research Service, The Library of Congress. Retrieved from http://www.ncseonline.org/

Sims, J. M. (2009). Nursing faculty shortage in 2009. Dimensions of Critical Care Nursing, 28(5), 221–223.

Thompson, S. A., & Tilden, V. P. (2009). Embracing quality and safety education for the 21st century: Building interprofessional education. Journal of Nursing Education, 48(12), 698–701. doi:10.3928/01484834-20091113-13

Toossi, M. (2006, November). A new look at long-term labor force projections to 2050. Monthly Labor Review, 19–39. Retrieved from http://www.bls.gov/

U.S. Census Bureau. (2010). Income, poverty, and health insurance coverage in the United States: 2009. Retrieved from http://www.census.gov

U.S. Department of Health & Human Services, Administration on Aging. (2010). Aging statistics. Retrieved from http://www.aoa.gov/

U.S. Department of Health & Human Services, Agency for Healthcare Research and Quality. (2008). National healthcare quality report. Retrieved from http://www.ahrq.gov/

Warren, J., & Connors, H. (2007). Health information technology can and will transform nursing education. Nursing Outlook, 55(1), 58–60.

Wiener, J. M., & Tilly, J. (2002). Population ageing in the United States of America: Implications for public programs. International Journal of Epidemiology, 31(4), 776–781.

Philosophical Foundations of the Curriculum

Theresa M. Valiga, EdD, RN, ANEF, FAAN

7

Beautiful words. Admirable values. Published prominently on websites and in catalogues, student handbooks, and accreditation reports. The philosophy of a school of nursing is accepted by faculty as a document that must be crafted to please external reviewers, but for many it remains little more than that. Far too often the school's philosophy remains safely tucked inside a report but is rarely seen as a living document that guides the day-to-day workings of the school.

In reality, the philosophy of a school of nursing should be referenced and reflected upon often. It should be reviewed seriously with candidates for faculty positions and with those individuals who join the community as new members. It should be discussed in a deliberate way with potential students and with students as they progress throughout the program. And it should be a strong guiding force as the school revises or sharpens its goals, outlines action steps to implement its strategic plan, and makes decisions about the allocation of resources.

This chapter will explore the significance of reflecting on, articulating, and being guided by a philosophy; examine the essential components of a philosophy for a school of nursing; and point out how philosophical statements guide the design and implementation of the curriculum, as well as the evaluation of its effectiveness. The role of faculty, administrators, and students in crafting and "living" the philosophy will be discussed, and the issues and debates surrounding the "doing of philosophy" (Greene, 1973) will be examined. Finally, suggestions will be offered regarding how faculty might go about writing or revising the school's philosophy.

What Is Philosophy?

The educational philosopher Maxine Greene (1973) challenged educators to "do philosophy." By this she meant that we need to take the risk of thinking about what we do when we teach and what we mean when we talk of enabling others to learn. It also means we need to become progressively more conscious of the choices and commitments we make in our professional lives. Greene also challenged educators to look at our presuppositions, to examine critically the principles underlying what we think and what we say as educators, and to confront the individuals within us. She acknowledged that we often have to ask and answer painful questions when we "do philosophy."

In his seminal book, *The Courage to Teach*, Parker Palmer (2007) asserted that "though the academy claims to value multiple modes of knowing, it honors only one—an 'objective' way of knowing that takes us into the 'real' world by taking us 'out of ourselves'" (p. 18). He encouraged educators to challenge this culture by bringing a more human, personal perspective to the teaching–learning experience. Like Greene, Palmer suggested that, in order to do this, educators must look inside so that we can understand that "we teach who we are" (p. xi) and so that we can appreciate that such insight is critical for "authentic teaching, learning, and living" (p. ix).

Philosophy, then, is a way of framing questions that have to do with what is presupposed, perceived, intuited, believed, and known. It is a way of contemplating, examining, or thinking about what is taken to be significant, valuable, or worthy of commitment. As well, it is a way of becoming self-aware and thinking of the everyday as "problematic" so that questions are posed about what we do and how we do it, usual practices are challenged and not merely accepted as "the way things are," and positive change can occur. Indeed, Sartre asserted that each of us needs to develop—as a fundamental practice of being—going beyond the reality we confront, refusing to accept it as a given and, instead, viewing life as a reality to be created.

These perspectives on "doing philosophy" focus primarily on individuals—as human beings in general or as teachers in particular—reflecting seriously on their beliefs and values. There is no question that such reflection is critical and is to be valued and encouraged. However, "doing philosophy" must also be a group activity when one is involved in curriculum work. In crafting a statement of philosophy for a school of nursing, the beliefs and values of all faculty must be considered, addressed, and incorporated as much as possible. In fact, the very process of talking about one's beliefs and values—while it may generate heated debates—leads to a deeper understanding of what a group truly accepts as guiding principles for all it does.

Philosophical Statements

A philosophy is essentially a narrative statement of values or beliefs. It reflects broad principles or fundamental "isms" that guide actions and decision making, and it expresses the assumptions we make about people, situations, or goals. As noted by Bevis (1989, p. 35), the philosophy "provides the value system for ordering priorities and selecting from among various data."

In writing a philosophical statement, we must raise questions, contemplate ideas, examine what it is we truly believe, become self-aware, and probe what might be . . . and what should be. It calls on us to think critically and deeply, forge ideas and ideals, and become highly conscious of the phenomena and events in the world.

We also must reflect on the mission, vision, and values of our parent institution and of our school itself, as well as on the values of our profession. Figure 7-1 illustrates how a school's statement of philosophy is related to but different than these other sources. A *mission statement* describes unique purposes for which an institution or nursing unit exists: to improve the health of the surrounding community, to advance scientific understanding or contribute to the development of nursing science, to prepare responsible citizens, or to graduate individuals who will influence public policy to ensure access to quality health care for all. A *vision* is an expression of what an institution or nursing unit wants to be: the institution of choice for highly qualified students wishing to make a positive difference in our world; the leader in innovative integration of technology in the preparation of nurses; or a center of synergy for teaching, research, professional practice, and public service. Institutions and schools of nursing often also articulate a set of *values* that guide their operation: honesty and transparency, serving the public good, excellence, innovation, or constantly being open to change and transformation.

As stated, a *philosophy statement* is the narrative that reflects and integrates concepts expressed in the mission, vision, and values of the institution or profession; it serves to guide the actions and decisions of those involved in the organization. Educational philosophy is a matter of "doing philosophy" with respect to the educational enterprise as it engages the educator. It involves becoming critically conscious of what is involved in the complex teaching–learning relationship and what education truly means. The following statements about education, many by well-known individuals, provide examples of different philosophical perspectives:

The secret of education is respecting the pupil.
—Ralph Waldo Emerson

If the student is to grow, the teacher must also grow.
—Confucius

I think [education] refines you. I think some of us have rough edges. Education is like sanding down a piece of wood and putting the varnish to it.
—Suzanne Gordon (1991, p. 131)

Education is not the filling of a pail but the igniting of a fire.
—William Butler Yeats

The whole act of teaching is only the act of awakening the natural curiosity of young minds.
—Anatole France

The teacher learns from the student just as the student learns from the teacher with their encounters as examples of mutual openness to each other's needs.
—Nili Tabak, Livne Adi, and Mali Eherenfeld (2003, p. 251)

INTERRELATION OF CURRICULAR ELEMENTS

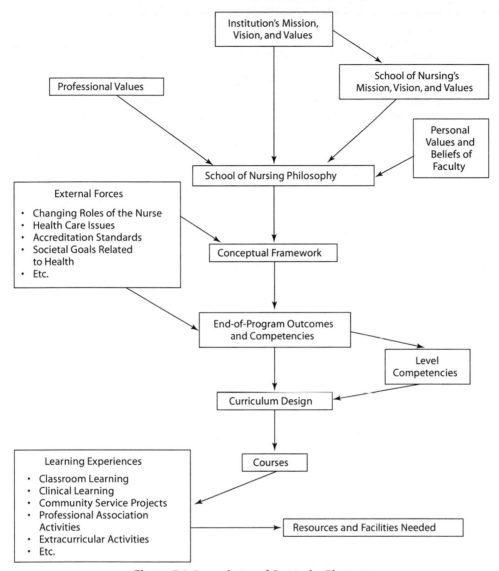

Figure 7-1 Interrelation of Curricular Elements

Philosophy as It Relates to Nursing Education

As noted earlier, "doing philosophy" must move from individual work to group work when engaged in curriculum development, implementation, and evaluation. Faculty need to reflect on their own individual beliefs and values, share them with colleagues, affirm points of agreement, and discuss points of disagreement. Table 7-1 summarizes many of the philosophical perspectives expressed through the years, and faculty are encouraged to explore the meaning and implications of each as they engage in developing, reviewing, or refining the philosophical statement that guides their work. A discussion of three basic educational ideologies is

TABLE 7-1 Summary of Philosophical Perspectives

Philosophical Perspective	Brief Description
Behaviorism	Education focuses on developing mental discipline, particularly through memorization, drill, and recitation. Since learning is systematic, sequential building on previous learning is important.
Essentialism	Since knowledge is key, the goal of education is to transmit and uphold the cultural heritage of the past.
Existentialism	The function of education is to help individuals explore reasons for existence. Personal choice and commitment are crucial.
Hermeneutics	Since individuals are self-interpreting beings, uniquely defined by personal beliefs, concerns, and experiences of life, education must attend to the meaning of experiences for learners.
Humanism	Education must provide for learner autonomy and respect their dignity. It also must help individuals achieve self-actualization by developing their full potential.
Idealism	Individuals desire to live in a perfect world of high ideals, beauty, and art, and they search for ultimate truth. Education assists in this search.
Postmodernism	Education challenges convention, values a high tolerance for ambiguity, emphasizes diversity of culture and thought, and encourages innovation and change.
Pragmatism	Truth is relative to an individual's experience; education, therefore, must provide for "real-world" experiences.
Progressivism	The role of learners is to make choices about what is important, and the role of teachers is to facilitate their learning.
Realism	Education is designed to help learners understand the natural laws that regulate all of nature.
Reconstructionism	Education embraces the social ideal of a democratic life, and the school is viewed as the major vehicle for social change.

Adapted from Csokasy, J. (2009). Philosophical foundations of the curriculum. In D. M. Billings & J. A. Halstead, *Teaching in nursing: A guide for faculty* (pp. 105–118). St. Louis, MO: Saunders.

presented here to point out how differences might arise if each person on a faculty were to approach education from her or his own belief system only.

One basic educational ideology is that of *romanticism* (Jarvis, 1995). This perspective, which emerged in the 1960s, is highly learner-centered and asserts that what comes from within the learner is most important. Within this ideological perspective, one would construct an educational environment that is permissive and freeing; promotes creativity and discovery; allows each student's inner abilities to unfold and grow; and stresses the unique, the novel, and the personal. Bradshaw (1998, p. 104) asserted that "this 'romantic' educational philosophy underpins current nurse education"; however, those who acknowledge our current "content-laden curricula" in nursing (Diekelmann, 2002; Diekelmann & Smythe, 2004; Giddens & Brady, 2007; Tanner, 2010) would disagree and posit that while a "romantic" philosophy is embraced as an ideal, it is not always evident in our day-to-day practices.

A second educational ideology, that of *cultural transmission* (Bernstein, 1975), is more society- or culture-centered. Here the emphasis is on transmitting bodies of information, rules, values, and the culturally given (i.e., the beliefs and practices that are central to our educational environments and our society in general). One would expect an educational environment that is framed within a cultural transmission perspective to be structured, rigid, and controlled, with an emphasis on the common and the already-established.

The third major educational ideology has been called *progressivism* (Dewey, 1944; Kohlberg & Mayer, 1972), where the focus is oriented toward the future and the goal of education is to nourish the learner's natural interaction with the world. Here the educational environment would be designed to present resolvable but genuine problems or conflicts that "force" learners to think so that they can be effective later in life. The total development of learners—not merely their cognitive or intellectual abilities—is emphasized and enhanced.

Increasingly, education experts agree that development must be an overarching paradigm of education, that students must be central to the educational enterprise, and that education must be designed to empower learners and help them fulfill their potentials. Beliefs and values such as these surely would influence expectations faculty express regarding students' and their own performance, the relationships between students and teachers, how the curriculum is designed and implemented (see Figure 7-1), and the kind of "evidence" that is gathered to determine whether the curriculum has been successful and effective.

There is no doubt that a statement of philosophy for a school of nursing must address beliefs and values about education, teaching, and learning. However, it also must address other concepts that are critical to the practice of nursing, namely human beings, society and the environment, health, and the roles of nurses themselves. These major concepts have been referred to as the metaparadigm of nursing, a concept first introduced by Fawcett in 1984.

Central Concepts in a School of Nursing's Philosophy

In preparing or revising the school of nursing's statement of philosophy, faculty must articulate their beliefs and values about *human beings*, including the individual patients for whom nurses care, their families, and the communities in which they live and work; students; and one another. It is inconsistent to express a belief that patients and families want to be involved in making decisions that affect them and then never give students an opportunity to make decisions that will affect them. Likewise, it is admirable to talk about respecting others, treating others with dignity, and valuing differences among people, but when faculty then treat one another in disrespectful ways or insist that everyone teach in the same way and do exactly the same thing, the validity of those expressed values must be questioned. Consider the following statements about human beings that might be expressed in your school's philosophy, keeping in mind that "human beings" refers to students, faculty, and administrators, as well as patients:

- Human beings are unique, complex, holistic individuals.
- Human beings have the inherent capacity for rational thinking, self-actualization, and growth throughout the life cycle.
- Human beings engage in deliberate action to achieve goals.

- Human beings want and have the right to be involved in making decisions that affect their lives.
- All human beings have strengths as well as weaknesses, and they often need support and guidance to capitalize on those strengths or to overcome or manage those weaknesses or limitations.
- All human beings are to be respected and valued.

Faculty also need to reflect on their beliefs and values related to *society or environment*, its effect on human beings, and the ways in which individuals and groups can influence their environments or society. The following statements may be ones to consider as faculty write or refine the philosophy of their school of nursing:

- Human beings interact in families, groups, and communities in an interdependent manner.
- Individuals, families, and communities reflect unique and diverse cultural, ethnic, experiential, and socioeconomic backgrounds.
- Human beings determine societal goals, values, and ethical systems.
- Society has responsibility for providing environments conducive to maximizing the health and well-being of its members.
- While human beings often must adapt to their environments, the environment also adapts to them in reciprocal ways.

Since the goal of nursing is to promote *health* and well-being, faculty must consider the values and beliefs they hold about health. Which of the following are congruent with what you and your faculty colleagues believe?

- Health connotes a sense of wholeness or integrity.
- Health is a goal to be attained.
- Health is the energy that sustains life, allows an individual to participate in a variety of human experiences, and supports one's ability to set and meet life goals.
- Health is a dynamic, complex state of being that human beings use as a resource to achieve their life goals; it is, therefore, a means to an end rather than an end in itself.
- Health can be promoted, maintained, or regained.
- Health is a right more than a privilege.
- All human beings must have access to quality health care.

Finally, it is critical for faculty to discuss their beliefs about *nurses* and *nursing* since this is the essence of our programs. In doing so, it may be important to reflect on what the current and evolving roles of the nurse are, what the purpose of nursing is, the ways in which nurses practice in collaboration with other health care professionals, and how one's identity as a nurse evolves. The following statements may stimulate thinking about beliefs and values related to nurses and nursing:

- Nursing is a human interactive process.
- The focus of nursing is to enhance human beings' capacity to take deliberate action for themselves and their dependent others regarding goals for optimal wellness.
- Nursing is a practice discipline that requires the deliberate use of specialized techniques and a broad range of scientific knowledge in order to design, deliver, coordinate, and manage the care for complex individuals, families, groups, communities, and populations.
- Nurses are scholars who practice with scientific competence, intellectual maturity, and humanistic concern for others.
- The formation of one's identity as a nurse requires deep self-reflection, feedback from others, and a commitment to lifelong learning.
- Nurses must be educated at the university level.
- Nurses must be prepared to provide leadership within their practice settings and for the profession as a whole.
- Nurses collaborate with patients and other professionals as equal yet unique members of the health care team.
- Nurses are accountable for their own practice.

Box 7-1 provides examples of actual statements of philosophy regarding these components of the metaparadigm. These examples illustrate the beliefs of various groups of faculty, some of which may express vastly different perspectives and some of which express essentially the same idea but through different words.

Purpose of a Statement of Philosophy

Given that "doing philosophy" is hard work, takes time, and may lead to substantial debates among faculty, one may ask, "Why bother?" Perhaps part of the answer to that question lies in a statement made by Alexander Astin, a noted educational scholar whose seminal study (1997) of more than 20,000 students, 25,000 faculty members, and 200 institutions helped educators better understand who our students are; what is important to them; what they value; what they think about teachers; how they change and develop in college; and how academic programs, faculty, student peer groups, and other variables affect students' development and college experiences. Although Astin's original research was completed more than 10 years ago and focused on traditional-age students enrolled, typically, on a full-time basis—thereby not fully reflecting today's student population—the following comment has relevance for this discussion of why faculty need to "bother" with philosophy: "The problems of strengthening and reforming American higher education are fundamentally problems of *values*" [*emphasis added*] (Astin, 1997, p. 127).

Engaging in serious discussions about beliefs and values—about human beings, society and environment, health, nurses and nursing, and education—challenges faculty to search for points of congruence, brings to the surface points of incongruence or difference, and highlights what is truly important to the group. In a time when nursing faculty are struggling to minimize content overload and focus more on core concepts, gaining clarity about what is truly important can be helpful in deciding "what to leave in and what to leave out" of the curriculum.

Such exercises also help faculty minimize or avoid what is often referred to as the "hidden curriculum" (Adler, Hughes, & Scott, 2006; D'eon, Lear, Turner, & Jones, 2007; Gofton & Regehr, 2006) by ensuring that faculty are fully aware of and committed to upholding certain beliefs and values in how they interact with and what they expect of students and one another. Such agreement and consistency is likely to avoid having three components to the curriculum: "what is planned for the students, what is delivered to the students, and what the students experience" (Prideaux, as cited in Ozolins, Hall, & Peterson, 2008, p. 606). When what is delivered to and experienced by students does not match what was planned for them, confusion can reign, due process can be challenged, and the relationships between students and teachers can be irreparably damaged. Thus having clear statements of values to which all faculty agree to subscribe can serve a most practical, as well as philosophical, purpose.

BOX 7-1 Examples of Statements of Philosophy from Current Schools of Nursing

We believe that nursing is a dynamic, challenging profession that requires a synthesis of critical thinking skills and theory based practice to provide care for individuals, families, and communities experiencing a variety of developmental and health–illness transitions. Caring, which is at the heart of the nursing profession, involves the development of a committed, nurturing relationship, characterized by attentiveness to others and respect for their dignity, values, and culture. We believe that nursing practice must reflect an understanding of and respect for each individual and for human diversity.

Transitions involve a process of movement and change in fundamental life patterns, which are manifested in all individuals. Transitions cause changes in identities, roles, relationships, abilities, and patterns of behavior. Outcomes of transitional experiences are influenced by environmental factors interacting with the individual's perceptions, resources, and state of well-being. Negotiating successful transitions depends on the development of an effective relationship between the nurse and client. This relationship is a highly reciprocal process that affects both the client and nurse.

Clayton State University, School of Nursing, Morrow, GA. Retrieved from http://nursing.clayton.edu/nursstud/Program_Information/phil.htm

The Philosophy of the College of Nursing is in accord with the Philosophy of Villanova University as stated in its Mission Statement. While the Philosophy is rooted in the Catholic and Augustinian heritage of the university, the College of Nursing is welcoming and respectful of those from other faith traditions. We recognize human beings as unique and created by God. The faculty believes that human beings are physiological, psychological, social and spiritual beings, endowed with intellect, free will, and inherent dignity. Human beings have the potential to direct, integrate, and/or adapt to their total environment in order to meet their needs.

The faculty believes that education provides students with opportunities to develop habits of critical, constructive thought so that they can make discriminating judgments in their search for truth. This type of intellectual development can best be attained in a highly technologic teaching–learning environment that fosters sharing of knowledge, skills, and attitudes as well as scholarship toward the development of new knowledge. The faculty and students comprise a community of learners with the teacher as the facilitator and the students responsible for their own learning.

Villanova University College of Nursing, Villanova, PA. Retrieved from http://www.villanova.edu/nursing/about/mission/philosophy.htm

The focus of professional nursing is the promotion, maintenance, and restoration of a person's health. A **PERSON** is defined as a biological, psychosocial, spiritual, holistic

being with potential for growth and change, who achieves **HEALTH** by meeting universal health care requisites. Individuals are capable of making decisions and taking independent actions to achieve optimal health for themselves or dependents. Individuals exist in a complex **ENVIRONMENT** consisting of constantly changing internal and external factors which influence their self-care requisites and abilities.

HEALTH is a state of integrated structural and functional wholeness which allows for successful responses to physical, psychological, cultural, spiritual, and economic life events. Individuals achieve this state through continuous, deliberate self-care actions. A change in any of the factors that affect health can overwhelm a person's self-care agency and result in self-care deficits that produce a state of illness which generates a need for nursing interventions.

Bergen Community College, Paramus, NJ. Retrieved from *2010/2011 Nursing Student Handbook* (p. 6), http://www.bergen.edu/documents/nursing/pdf/Nursing%20Student%20Handbook%20FA%202010%20SP%202011.pdf

The faculty is committed to an educational philosophy that emphasizes competency assessment and learning at a distance. The faculty supports programs that are designed to meet the educational goals of a diverse population of adult learners who bring varied lifelong knowledge and experience to the learning encounter. The faculty views adult independent learning as a process of knowledge acquisition attained through exposure to varied planned educational strategies, unconstrained by time and/or place.

The faculty is responsible for determining what must be learned; how learning can be supported; and how learning is assessed. The faculty believes that adult learners have the capability to create their own learning experiences guided by each program's curricular framework. The ability to learn, readiness to learn, motivation to learn, and responsibility to learn are seen as characteristics of the adult learner rather than of the faculty or the educational institution providing the degree.

Excelsior College School of Nursing, Albany, NY. Retrieved from *School of Nursing Handbook* (p. 2), http://www.excelsior.edu/c/document_library/get_file?uuid=cd58ff27-7254-4755-a8c4-6dcfe39d78a0&groupId=78666

ENVIRONMENT

Environment is the context within which anything internal and external to an individual influences that person. The individual and the environment are continuously exchanging matter and energy along the life continuum. The environment includes one's self, family, home, work setting, community, and a rapidly changing world.

Continued

BOX 7-1 Examples of Statements of Philosophy from Current Schools of Nursing—cont'd

HEALTH

Health is a dynamic state of being influenced by the individual's potential for self-determination, self-actualization, and the ability to function within the environment. As individuals move along the life continuum, they experience changes that affect their ability to function independently in their environment at any given point in time. The perception of health is highly individualized and is influenced by multiple contextual variables.

From: University of Oklahoma College of Nursing, Oklahoma City, OK. Retrieved from *College of Nursing Bulletin 2007–2009* (pp. 31–32), http://nursing.ouhsc.edu/Current_Students/documents/Bulletin%202007-2009%20updated%2011-16-10.pdf

---

Developing or Refining the School of Nursing's Statement of Philosophy

Developing or refining the school's statement of philosophy, while important and valuable, is far from easy. It takes time and effort and is not to be taken lightly. But just how does a group of faculty go about developing a philosophical statement for the school and getting "buy-in" on it? As expected, there are no formulas or step-by-step guidelines on how to go about doing this work, but some suggestions for a process may be helpful.

One approach to engaging in this work may include reflecting on the nursing theories that have been developed to determine if any of them capture the essence of faculty beliefs. For example, if faculty are in agreement that human beings are self-determining individuals who want to take responsibility for their own health and need specific knowledge, skills, and attitudes to do whatever is required to maintain, regain, or improve their health, then Orem's (1971) self-care nursing model may be evident in that school's statement of philosophy. Likewise, Roy's (1980) adaptation model may be reflected in another school's philosophical statement where the faculty believe that a central challenge to individuals and families is to adapt to their environments and circumstances, and that the role of the nurse is to facilitate that adaptation. Finally, if the concept of caring is essential to a third group of faculty, their philosophy may clearly be congruent with Watson's (1979) theory of human caring.

Whether or not to acknowledge a single nursing theory in a school's statement of philosophy (and then use that theory to develop the school's conceptual framework, end-of-program outcomes or competencies, and other curriculum elements) has been debated in recent years. Those in favor of such an approach argue that it provides students with a way to "think nursing" and approach nursing situations in a way that clearly is nursing-focused, not medical model–focused, and that provides an opportunity to contribute to the ongoing development of the theory and, therefore, the science of nursing. Those against such an approach argue that it limits students' thinking and engages them with language and perspectives that are not likely to be widely encountered in practice, thereby making it difficult for graduates to communicate effectively with their nursing and health care team colleagues. Obviously, there is no one right answer to this debate. The key question to consider is whether the concepts that are central to a theory—nursing or otherwise—truly are congruent with the beliefs and values of the majority of faculty, since that is what a statement of philosophy must reflect.

Another approach that can be most useful to faculty when developing or refining their philosophical statement is inductive in nature. All faculty may be asked to list no more than five bullet items that express what they believe about each concept in the metaparadigm: human beings, society and environment, health, nurses and nursing, and education and teaching–learning. The responses in each category could be compiled and faculty—perhaps in small groups—could then engage in an analysis of the items listed for each. These working groups might be asked to note the frequency with which specific ideas were mentioned, thereby identifying those points where there was great agreement and those where only one or a few faculty identified an idea. The fact that only a single faculty member or few faculty identified a particular belief or value, however, would not necessarily mean that it should be discarded. It is possible that other faculty simply did not think of that idea as they were creating their own lists, or it is possible that other faculty did identify the idea but did not include it because they were limited to five bullet items. The compilation from each working group could then be shared with the entire faculty. At this point, a discussion about the meaning and significance of the statements in each category could ensue, or faculty could be asked to review each list, select the three to five statements they believe are most critical to include in the philosophy, and then engage in dialogue about why they selected the statements they did, what those statements mean to individuals, and so on. A draft statement of philosophy could then be written by an individual or small group and circulated to faculty for comment and further discussion.

Using a more deductive approach can also be effective in developing or refining a statement of philosophy. When no such statement exists, an individual faculty member—one who is viewed as a leader in the group, who is respected and trusted by her or his peers, who has good writing skills, and who is knowledgeable about curriculum development—may be asked to talk to faculty about their beliefs about human beings and so on, and use that input to draft a statement of philosophy that incorporates what faculty had expressed. This draft could then be circulated to all faculty for comment, editing, and revision. The original writer would then revise the statement based on feedback from colleagues and present the new statement to the group for discussion and dialogue. This back-and-forth process would continue until there is consensus about what to include in the statement.

In either of these scenarios, or when a philosophical statement already exists but is being reviewed for possible updating and revision, "clickers" or simple online, anonymous surveys can be used to get a sense of faculty agreement or endorsement. With this approach, each sentence in the draft (or existing) philosophy would be listed as a separate item and faculty asked to indicate the extent to which they agree with it (e.g., Strongly Agree, Agree, Disagree, or Strongly Disagree). Instead of using the entire sentence as the item to be responded to, it may be more helpful to use phrases or major concepts within each sentence as the item. Regardless of the degree of detail in each item, the anonymous responses could then be compiled, the results shared with the entire faculty, and discussions held to explore the meaning of the data obtained.

Finally, the entire process—whether it involves starting from an existing philosophy or creating a new one—can be prompted or stimulated by the thinking of those outside the school of nursing. For example, faculty may be assigned to review major contemporary documents or reports—for example, the Carnegie study (Benner, Leonard, Day, & Sutphen, 2009), the *Future of Nursing* report (Institute of Medicine, 2010), accreditation standards, or published articles about employers' assessment of what new graduates can and cannot do. In reviewing those reports, faculty might identify values that are expressed or implied, beliefs about patients and nurses, or societal expectations related to health and health care. Those values and beliefs could then be compiled and faculty asked to reflect on the extent to which they are aligned with the beliefs expressed by others. Through an iterative process such as one of those described above, the group could craft its own statement of philosophy, one that has been informed by the larger context in which our educational programs exist.

Regardless of the process used, it is critical that all faculty be involved and that adequate time and safe environments be provided for faculty to disagree, struggle, contemplate, rethink, debate, and "do philosophy." Ending the process prematurely is not likely to be wise. It also is important to remember that this is an iterative process that will continue, to some extent, throughout all subsequent steps of curriculum development. For example, the statement of philosophy may have been endorsed and approved-in-concept by faculty, but as various groups work on developing course syllabi, they may generate questions about "what we really meant" by something in the philosophy. Should this occur, it would be worthwhile to revisit the philosophical statement and make revisions to it, if such revisions will lead to greater clarity about its meaning.

The preceding discussion has focused exclusively on the role of faculty in the creation or revision of the school's philosophy. It is assumed that school administrators (e.g., dean, program chair) are faculty who also must be involved in this process. Additionally, consideration should be given to including students in dialogue about beliefs and values; however, in the end, the final document must reflect what faculty believe and are guided by regarding human beings, society and environment, health, nurses and nursing, and education and teaching–learning.

The final statement of philosophy should be clearly written, internally consistent, easily understood, and give clear direction for all that follows. It should be long enough to clearly express the significant beliefs and values that guide faculty actions but not excessively detailed, as expressions of detail (rather than fundamental beliefs) often are more congruent with the work that must be done in formulating the conceptual framework, end-of-program outcomes or competencies, and curriculum design. Since chapters that follow this one will explore all of those subsequent curriculum development steps in detail (see Figure 7-1), only a few examples of how the philosophy gives direction to the development, implementation, and evaluation of the curriculum will be offered here.

Implications of the Philosophical Statement for the Development, Implementation, and Evaluation of the Curriculum

If the statements included in the school of nursing's philosophy reflect what the faculty truly believe— and are not merely words on a page to "get the task done"—then those values should be evident in how the curriculum is designed, how it is implemented, and how it is evaluated. Examples of this influence are presented in Box 7-2 as if–then statements.

It is hoped that these examples, combined with the detail provided in subsequent chapters, reinforce the importance of the philosophy. Faculty aim

---

BOX 7-2 Examples of If–Then Statements Regarding Implications of the Philosophical Statement for the Development, Implementation, and Evaluation of the Curriculum

If the philosophical statement says . . .	*Then* one would expect to see . . .
We believe that human beings should have choices regarding what they do . . .	Free, unrestricted elective courses in the curriculum, or choice among several courses to meet a degree requirement (e.g., English)
We believe that human beings engage in deliberate action to achieve goals . . .	Opportunities throughout the curriculum for students to write their own learning goals and collaborate with faculty or clinical staff to design unique learning experiences to achieve those goals
We believe that individuals reflect unique and diverse cultural, ethnic, experiential, and socioeconomic backgrounds . . .	Face-to-face or virtual experiences with a wide variety of patient populations and within communities having a range of resources and challenges
We believe that health can be promoted, maintained, or regained . . .	Equally distributed clinical learning experiences in wellness settings, with patients and families who are managing chronic illnesses, and in acute care settings
We believe that nurses are scholars who practice with scientific competence and intellectual maturity . . .	Courses and learning experiences that expose students to the concept of scholarship, what it means to be a scholar, and how one develops and maintains scientific competence
We believe that nurses must be prepared to provide leadership within their practice settings and for the profession as a whole . . .	Courses and learning experiences that help students appreciate the differences between leadership and management, study nursing leaders, and reflect on their own path toward becoming a leader
We believe that nurses collaborate with patients and other professionals as equal yet unique members of the health care team . . .	Face-to-face or virtual experiences where nursing students learn with students preparing for other professional roles, dialogue with or interview members of other health care professions, or undertake projects that call for interprofessional collaboration to meet the health needs of a patient population or community
We believe that the goal of teaching is to awaken the learner's natural curiosity . . .	Problem-based learning experiences where students must identify what it is they need to know in order to address a problem, seek out that information, judge its quality, ask questions about established practices, and so on
We believe that education involves nurturing students and pulling them forth to a new place . . .	A program evaluation plan that incorporates open forums with students about the extent to which they feel nurtured, supported, and challenged by faculty; dialogue with graduates about how their educational experience changed them as human beings; and surveys of students and alumni regarding the contributions they have made in their practice settings and to the profession

to establish positive relationships with students, clinical partners, alumni, administrators, and each other; one way to achieve that goal is to be clear about the values we share and, more importantly, to "live" those values in everything we say and do.

SUMMARY

As noted earlier, "doing philosophy" is hard work. However, it is important and valuable work that has implications for faculty and our practice as teachers, as well as for our students.

"Doing philosophy" may prompt us to attend more deliberately to affective domain learning and identity formation as we design learning experiences and interact with students, a focus that is likely to enhance their educational experience. It may challenge us to ask new questions about our practice as teachers and seek answers to those questions through rigorous pedagogical research efforts, an effort that can contribute to the development of the science of nursing education. It also may direct us to seek out new teaching strategies and evaluation methods that better facilitate student learning, an outcome that may serve to maintain the joy in teaching as we see students become excited about their formation as nurses.

One can conclude that the philosophical foundations of the curriculum extend far beyond mere program designs and course syllabi. Reflections on and clarity regarding those philosophical foundations can help us better understand who we are and how we can best help our students, our colleagues, and ourselves to grow and continue to learn.

REFLECTING ON THE EVIDENCE

1. While faculty share a commitment to the values of the profession, they are likely to have varied beliefs about the implications of those and other values, particularly in relation to how they "play out" in the educational arena. What impact can such differences have on students? How can such differences be resolved?

2. How can faculty "track" congruence of beliefs, values, and significant concepts from mission, vision, and values to philosophy to framework to end-of-program outcomes and competencies and on through specific learning experiences that are designed for students? As well, how can they assess the congruence of these beliefs and values with their own personal beliefs?

3. What are some signs that a "hidden curriculum" is operating? What implications might such signals have for reexamining the school's philosophical underpinnings?

REFERENCES

Adler, S. R., Hughes, E. F., & Scott, R. B. (2006). Student "moles": Revealing the hidden curriculum. *Medical Education, 40,* 463–464.

Astin, A. W. (1997). *What matters in college? Four critical years revisited.* San Francisco, CA: Jossey-Bass.

Benner, P., Leonard, V., Day, L., & Sutphen, M. (2009). *Educating nurses: A call for radical transformation.* San Francisco, CA: Jossey-Bass.

Bernstein, B. (1975). *Class, codes and control: Volume III— towards a theory of educational transmission.* New York, NY: Routledge.

Bevis, E. O. (1989). *Curriculum building: A process* (3rd ed.). New York, NY: National League for Nursing.

Bradshaw, A. (1998). Defining "competency" in nursing (part II): An analytic review. *Journal of Clinical Nursing, 7,* 103–111.

D'eon, M., Lear, N., Turner, M., & Jones, C. (2007). Perils of the hidden curriculum revisited. *Medical Teacher, 29,* 295–296.

Dewey, J. (1944). *Democracy and education: An introduction to the philosophy of education.* New York, NY: The Free Press.

Diekelmann, N. (2002). "Too much content . . ." Epistemologies' grasp and nursing education (Teacher Talk). *Journal of Nursing Education, 41*(11), 469–470.

Diekelmann, N., & Smythe, E. (2004). Covering content and the additive curriculum: How can I use my time with students to best help them learn what they need to know? (Teacher Talk) *Journal of Nursing Education, 43*(8), 341–344.

Fawcett, J. (1984). The metaparadigm of nursing: Present status and future refinements. *Image: The Journal of Nursing Scholarship, 16*(3), 84–86.

Giddens, J. F., & Brady, D. P. (2007). Rescuing nursing education from content saturation: The case for a concept-based curriculum. *Journal of Nursing Education, 46*(2), 65–69.

Gofton, W., & Regehr, G. (2006). What we don't know we are teaching: Unveiling the hidden curriculum. *Clinical Orthopaedics and Related Research, 449,* 20–27.

Gordon, S. (1991). *Prisoners of men's dreams: Striking out for a new feminine future.* Boston, MA: Little, Brown.

Greene, M. (1973). *Teacher as stranger: Educational philosophy in a modern age.* Belmont, CA: Wadsworth.

Institute of Medicine. (2010). *The future of nursing: Leading change, advancing health.* Washington, DC: The National Academies Press.

Jarvis, P. (1995). *Adult and continuing education*. London, UK: Routledge.

Kohlberg, L., & Mayer, R. (1972). Development as the aim of education. *Harvard Educational Review, 42*(2), 449–496.

Orem, D. (1971). *Nursing: Concepts of practice*. New York, NY: McGraw-Hill.

Ozolins, I., Hall, H., & Peterson, R. (2008). The student voice: Recognizing the hidden and informal curriculum in medicine. *Medical Teacher, 30*, 606–611.

Palmer, P. (2007, 10th anniversary edition). *The courage to teach: Exploring the inner landscape of a teacher's life*. San Francisco, CA: Jossey-Bass.

Robinson, F. P. (2009). Servant teaching: The power and promise for nursing education. *International Journal of Nursing Education, 6*(1), Article 5.

Roy Sr., C. (1980). The Roy adaptation model. In J. P. Riehl & C. Roy (Eds.), *Conceptual models for nursing practice* (pp. 179–188). Norwalk, CT: Appleton, Century Crofts.

Tabak, N., Adi, I., & Eherenfeld, M. (2003). A philosophy underlying excellence in teaching. *Nursing Philosophy, 4*, 249–254.

Tanner, C. A. (2010). Transforming prelicensure nursing education: Preparing the new nurse to meet emerging health care needs. *Nursing Education Perspectives, 31*(6), 347–353.

Watson, J. (1979). *Nursing: The philosophy and science of caring*. Boston, MA: Little, Brown.

Curriculum Designs

Donna L. Boland, PhD, RN, ANEF
Linda M. Finke, PhD, RN

Curriculum, by its very nature, holds a different element of promise for different groups of stakeholders. Traditionally, curriculum is a product to be delivered. For stakeholders focusing on consumerism, curriculum is a product that should be available for purchase at a fair market value with explicit outcomes noted. There are also those with a gestalt view who believe that curriculum is to be experienced and that what is learned can be interpreted only from the perspective of the learner and that is the true value of the educational experience. No matter how one defines curriculum, the concept should be "sufficiently inclusive and dynamic to account for the many innovations that involve instruction methods, sequencing, and assessments as well as instructional goals and content, all of which have been implemented to improve learning" (Dezure, 2010).

A well-conceived curriculum is critical to the preparation of practicing nurses at all levels. Curricula in general and undergraduate curricula specifically have been under scrutiny for the last decade. There have been a number of reports since the 1980s that have been critical of higher education, suggesting that reform is needed if graduates are to meet the expectations of business and industry (Dezure, 2010). These calls for reform led to four major initiatives of the 1990s that included the introduction of learning outcomes in the language of competencies, emphasis on integration of learning experiences, focus on enhancing learning, and growth in learning from a more global perspective (Dezure, 2010). Today the priority for learning is not so much on *what* is learned, as much as it is on what graduates can *do* with their learning. For nursing, the curriculum must prepare graduates to function in a dynamic and increasingly complex environment.

O'Neil (2009) speaks to transformational changes that will require students to learn how to apply knowledge in emerging care systems that are and will continue to be ill defined. The challenge facing nurse educators is how to reenvision curriculum to prepare nurses to practice in a system that will continue to change and evolve well into the future. Tanner (2010) suggests that the critical questions that curricula design need to address are what must be taught, how to teach it effectively and efficiently, and where teaching and learning occur to achieve the best outcomes. Dezure (2010) indicates that the curriculum shifts that shape curricula today are the move to broad learning competencies from a narrower focus on mastery of learning specific content, a shift to more integrative learning experiences from those that emphasize specific skill sets, and an exploration of innovative teaching practices beyond the traditional pedagogical approaches designed to deliver subject matter.

Regardless of the view held about general education or professional education, the underlying theme is that curriculum must be designed to be responsive to the needs of today's and tomorrow's society. Within the nursing profession, curricula design must reflect the current health care system and be fluid and flexible. These curriculum changes follow Bevis' (1988) original call for a curriculum transformation. Bevis called for a:

> [R]evolution that attacks the basic tenets of nursing curriculum development; that deinstitutionalizes the Tyler curriculum model and its mandated products; that makes nursing philosophy, research, and education congruent; that distinguishes between learning that is training and

learning that is education; that alters our perception of teaching and the role of teacher; that abandons the industrial metaphor; that restructures the relative roles of classroom and clinical practice; that de-emphasizes curriculum development and concentrates on faculty development; that develops a national strategy for change; and, above all, that provides new guideposts for a new age (pp. 27–28).

More recently, the profession has faced continued calls for radical curriculum transformation to best prepare nurses who are equipped to practice and lead in evolving health care systems (Benner, Sutphen, Leonard, & Day, 2010; Institute of Medicine [IOM], 2010). This transformative process needs to focus on how to design or revise curricula without using an additive process that continues to overload the curriculum with content (Benner et al., 2010).

Faculty have historically viewed curriculum revisions that meet student learning needs from a content perspective rather than a context perspective. As new technologies emerge, new evidence is discovered, and new best practices are identified, they are packed into a curriculum structure that is already saturated with content. Curricula in most nursing programs today are at the breaking point. Instead of simply continuing to add content to the curriculum, the challenge for faculty is to determine what students need to know to survive and prosper in a dynamic health care system driven by uncertainties and shifting priorities, and how best to design learning experiences that will facilitate acquisition of those competencies. According to O'Neil (2009), nursing faculty will need to revise curricula to accommodate a "shift from hospital based care to community based care" (p. 319). This shift will require faculty to redefine what we have identified as traditional competencies critical to the practice of nursing "within the context of community-based and consumer responsive care services" (p. 319). This process of envisioning and rethinking nursing curricula will require us to generate new models of educating the next generation of nurses.

This chapter discusses the issues of undergraduate and graduate education that have historically had an impact on program and curriculum designs, as well as current designs for all levels of nursing programs. It is important to have a sense of the issues that have shaped and continue to shape nursing curricula as faculty make decisions about the design of curriculum in their programs.

Undergraduate Education in Nursing

Constituencies Invested in Undergraduate Curriculum Design

Traditionally, undergraduate nursing curricula are assumed to set the stage for entry into nursing practice and to provide a foundation essential to graduate education and advanced nursing practice. However, as transformative discussions continue, there is increasing concern as to what level of educational preparation is needed to prepare nurses for an evolving health care system. Designing curricula that facilitate the academic progression of the nursing workforce (National League for Nursing [NLN], 2011a) will be imperative to achieve the recommendations set forth in the IOM (2010) report on the future of nursing that call for increasing numbers of baccalaureate and advanced degree–prepared nurses. Emerging from these conversations is the need for expanding knowledge and skill sets to meet increasing responsibilities and complexities related to work and work settings.

The increase in public accountability has expanded the visibility of nursing education at the national, state, and local levels, which has ultimately increased stakeholder involvement in the education and practice of nurses. Given the many different constituencies that are invested in the outcomes and products of undergraduate nursing programs, there has been an increase in the number of often competing controls on the development, implementation, and evaluation of undergraduate curricula. As a professional educational degree program, nursing is seemingly among the most regulated educational enterprises on campuses of higher education today. One advantage of regulation for nursing programs is the high level of scrutiny to which they are subjected. A disadvantage to this level of control is the perceived decrease in latitude to be unique and creative in the design and delivery of the curriculum. Some of this regulation stems from the high level of accountability to produce graduates with the knowledge and skills required to practice and the pressures to produce more nurses in a quicker and more efficient manner in the face of shrinking resources. In this reality the emphasis is on outcomes achieved, not the process leading to those outcomes.

State Boards of Nursing

The first constituents interested in nursing education programs and curricula are the individual state boards of nursing. Early in the history of state boards of nursing, rules and regulations were set for programs that often specified content areas that must be covered, minimum hours that must be spent by all students in specified health care areas, and competencies or skills that all students must possess at the completion of a nursing program leading to licensure. Although these rules and regulations have tended to become less prescriptive, they are still state specific and varied. Today, state boards are also involved in issues related to evolving teaching pedagogies being driven by technological advances, the constitution of clinical learning experiences, faculty credentialing, and advanced practice nursing. However, state rules and regulations are still primarily focused on overseeing the implementation of undergraduate nursing curricula. The establishment of state regulations stems from the need to hold licensed health care personnel to standards of social responsibility and public accountability for actions taken on behalf of others. It can be argued that the education of nurses is and should be independent of regulatory licensure agencies, whose sole interest should be the protection of the consumer of nursing services, but many state boards of nursing continue to hold significant regulatory control over undergraduate programs. It is apparent that these regulatory controls can be perceived to affect the creativity and flexibility that nursing faculty have within nursing programs, especially with regard to undergraduate curricula. Some state boards are actively engaged in conversations as to what constitutes acceptable alternative learning experiences and how much of these alternative learning experiences are acceptable within the curricula. These alternative experiences include preceptor and simulated experiences. It is anticipated that the growth in the creation of alternative or nontraditional learning experiences will continue as faculty seek innovative ways of delivering learning to an increasingly diverse population of learners.

Accrediting Bodies

Other constituents interested in nursing education programs are accrediting bodies. The NLN historically served the role of the professional accrediting body for the evaluation of undergraduate nursing programs. Through the establishment and refinement of program assessment criteria, the NLN also affected the development, implementation, and evaluation of undergraduate nursing curricula across the country for a number of decades. These criteria, which address the mission and governance of the institution, faculty, students, curriculum, resources, and program effectiveness, had to be met by all programs seeking or renewing accreditation. The curriculum was developed by the nursing faculty and provided learning experiences consistent with the nursing unit's mission and stated outcomes of the program. The National League for Nursing Accrediting Commission (NLNAC) was established in 1996 to act as an independent body that would carry out the accreditation activities that were once controlled through the NLN. The NLNAC continues to accredit all levels of nursing curricula and has identified standards by which program effectiveness and student achievement can be measured. Today, student academic achievement is measured against graduation rates, performance on licensure examinations, job placement rates, and program satisfaction (NLNAC, 2008).

The Commission on Collegiate Nursing Education (CCNE) entered the arena of professional accreditation in 1997 and began accrediting baccalaureate and graduate nursing programs. Unlike the NLNAC, with its broad accreditation scope, the CCNE focuses its accrediting efforts on baccalaureate and higher degree programs exclusively. This commission has also identified standards for judging the degree to which nursing programs meet these published expectations. Student achievement is still very much a priority for this accreditation body and the focus of its updated *2009 Standards for Accreditation of Baccalaureate and Graduate Degree Nursing Programs* (CCNE, 2009).

Although accreditation criteria are not meant to be prescriptive, they are becoming more so as the U.S. Department of Education becomes more explicit in its emphasis on outcome data specified in its standards for accrediting professional accreditation associations (U.S. Department of

Education, 2010). Nursing faculty have a tendency to use professional standards in shaping curricula. Although this is not the explicit intent of accreditation criteria, it is a reality. Traditionally, the effect of accreditation standards can be seen in the balance between nursing and general education distribution credits, the sense of a need for theoretical frameworks on which to design curricula, the need for rationale for course sequencing, and credit hour limits. As an example, one can look to *The Essentials of Baccalaureate Education for Professional Nursing Practice* (American Association of Colleges of Nursing [AACN], 2008) as an example of how accrediting bodies are and will continue to influence program development and curricula design. See Chapter 28 for additional information about curriculum evaluation and Chapter 29 for a further discussion of the accreditation process.

Institutions of Higher Education

Historically, nursing has been viewed as having or needing regulatory oversight from those outside its discipline. Institutions of higher education that house nursing programs often actively influence the development and implementation of nursing curricula. This involvement takes many forms, including the development of general education requirements, procurement of clinical sites, hiring of teaching faculty, defraying the cost of undergraduate nursing education, supporting faculty practice, monitoring distance education offerings, and equipping learning resource centers to keep pace with the advances in technological support for teaching and learning. Higher education institutions have often based funding formulas on enrollment patterns. Historically, these funding formulas have led to increases in recruitment efforts, expansion of existing programs, and the addition of new programs. More recently, state funding decisions for higher education institutions are placing increasing emphasis on outcome productivity. This shift in priorities places more value on the retention and graduation of students in a timely fashion, the employment patterns (which includes numbers employed, time between employment and graduation, distribution of employed graduates), and employer satisfaction with graduates' abilities to meet stated expectations.

Curricula are also being transformed to meet the needs of more nontraditional students or students with unique needs, leading to more creativity and flexibility in curriculum construction and delivery. The expected outcome is to entice, retain, and graduate a diverse population of students.

Market Forces

The marketplace also has a strong voice in the design and implementation of nursing curricula. The first schools of nursing were hospital-based and generally administered by the director of the hospital, with direct supervision of the students being delegated to the nursing staff affiliated with the institution. Class content was identified and taught by medical staff members, who had a large investment in what these young nursing students were being prepared to do. This strong voice has changed in both tone and expression over the last 100 years. Today, nursing educators collaborate with their nursing practice counterparts in the design, implementation, and evaluation of nursing curricula. The challenge facing nursing educators and practicing nurses is to design and deliver curricula that meet expectations for those entering today's practice arena while equipping graduates with the skills and competencies necessary to adapt to anticipated demands of the future.

The marketplace is also affecting curriculum design and delivery as nursing faculty look for economical ways of preparing students. Consumers (students) are looking for quality education at an affordable price. Students no longer expect to fit into rigidly designed curricula but look for curricula that can be shaped around their needs as learners. There is recognition that students bring different experiences and interpretation of those experiences to the learning environment. These students, with their varied experiences and expectations, perceive more dissatisfaction with a highly structured curricula and a one-size-fits-all pedagogical approach to learning (Umbach & Kuh, 2006).

Organizational Forces

There are many organizational forces that affect undergraduate curricula. For example, professional organizations such as the American Nurses Association and AACN set forth professional standards that are used to guide undergraduate curriculum development. In another example of organizational influence, the American Organization of Nurse Executives' (AONE) (2004a) board of directors released the *AONE Guiding Principles for the Role of the Nurse in Future Patient Care Delivery Toolkit*, which outlined the work of the nurse in the future.

They envisioned the work of nurses as becoming increasingly complex and challenging and forecast that nurses would need to be educationally prepared for this increasing complexity. Given this view, the AONE membership supports the transition of educational preparation of nurses to the baccalaureate level, assuming that this level of education will "prepare nurses of the future to function as an equal partner, collaborator and manager of the complex patient care journey" (AONE, 2004b). The impact on undergraduate education means a revolution of the current educational structure and our approach to the education of our students. The AONE's guiding principles were updated in 2010 (AONE, 2010).

Another example of organizational influence is the IOM's 2001 report that called for a fundamental change in how health care is being delivered, indicating that the current health care system was not meeting the care needs of many. In this report the IOM asserted that to address systematic failings, the health care system must be focused on improving the safety of care; providing care that is grounded in scientific knowledge, patient-centered, focused on quality improvement, informatics-driven, and cost effective; delivering care in an acceptable time frame to avoid waste in time and energy; and demonstrating equity in distribution and quality of care (IOM, 2001). To meet these critical initiatives, the educational preparation of the workforce would need to be changed to incorporate new skills and competencies (IOM, 2003). In response to these initial IOM reports, the challenge to nursing programs was to adapt curricula to ensure that graduates were being prepared with these competencies.

Recently, the 2010 IOM report, *The Future of Nursing*, was released and is expected to have a major impact on both the practice and the education of nurses into this next decade. This report was released at a time when the United States is facing one of the largest health care reform movements of the last several decades. This reform movement is expected to shift the competencies nurses will need to practice in new and redesigned practice models.

Historical Implications for Understanding Undergraduate Curricula

Florence Nightingale has been credited as the founder of modern nursing. As a prolific writer who spoke in eloquent tones about the education and practice of nurses, Nightingale envisioned nursing as more than the understanding of disease. She is quoted as having said, "Pathology teaches the harm that disease has done. But it teaches nothing more" (Nightingale, 1969, p. 133). Her nursing orientation focused on health as a broad and encompassing concept that requires an understanding of human nature and the ability of that nature to affect individual health. Nightingale's thinking that nurses need to acquire an understanding of the science and art of human existence has continued to permeate undergraduate education from its original, hospital-based training programs to its current degree-granting educational programs.

Traditionally, nursing philosophy and theory are crucial to nursing curricula because philosophy and theory state what nursing is and what it should be. Salsberry (1994) stated that "philosophy of nursing identifies what is believed to be the basic or central phenomena of the discipline, relates nursing to a particular world view, and provides some information on how one may come to learn about the world" (p. 13). Nursing theorists, starting with Nightingale, have provided nursing with the theoretical foundation for educational philosophies, mission statements, curriculum models, and delivery of curriculum content. Despite differing beliefs posited among recognized nursing theorists, they, like the curriculum models that have been predicated on their thinking, have focused on the nature of humans, society, and nursing practice. It appears that the previous emphasis on the roles of nursing philosophy and theory in design of nursing curricula is decreasing as the emphasis has shifted to one that is more outcome-driven.

The focus on human beings and their society complements the aims of general education that date back to Hellenic times, when education examined both "human nature and the nature of society" (Brubacher & Rudy, 1976, p. 287). The desire to understand human nature and society is still a prevailing factor in shaping current undergraduate curricula, especially nursing curricula. However, the phenomenological lens is now being expanded to include the learner as we focus on understanding human nature. This broader focus encompasses the individual learner's desires and abilities to shape the learning experience through inquiry, reflection, and questioning assumptions about human nature and society (Cranton, 2006). It is this individual understanding that drives the learning process and through which nurses will filter their understanding of human nature and society as a liberally educated person. An example of how curriculum design can be used to foster an understanding of human nature and society can be found in Georgetown University's Bring Theory to Practice demonstration project, which has focused on infusing its undergraduate curriculum with community-based learning experiences around real-life issues that college students were facing (Riley & McWilliams, 2007).

Undergraduate Program Designs

The design and development of undergraduate nursing programs that reflect the mission of the university or college, the philosophy of the faculty, current and projected nursing practice trends, changes in the health care system (both real and theorized), changes in the demographics of the potential learner pool, and stakeholders' expectations require creativity, political savvy, negotiation skills, analytical rigor, psychic energy, and a modest amount of altruism. Faculty involved in designing programs and building curricula must possess a clear sense of purpose, a commitment to procuring resources, an understanding of market forces, the ability to anticipate health care trends of the future, and the ability to know when goals have been accomplished. Once programs are designed, curriculum building becomes a never-ending task that is indispensable to, but separate from, the acts of teaching and learning. Curriculum is a dynamic, evolving entity shaped by learner needs and faculty's beliefs about the science and art of nursing.

Factors Affecting Program Design

With the current emphasis on student learning and student engagement, it is important that curricula be designed to promote the development of individual students. This can be accomplished in part by encouraging interrelationships among the learners, faculty, and what is being learned. Additional factors affecting program design and student development include focusing on health and well-being of society; grounding learning in contemporary evidence; creating a learning environment that is infused with experientially and culturally based learning opportunities; and supporting individual creativity especially as it relates to inquiry, problem solving, and reflection.

When creating nursing curricula for the twenty-first century, Glasgow, Dunphy, and Mainous (2010) recommend that curricula be focused on the integration of science and research and the influences resulting from health care policies. These authors envision curricula that cut across various disciplines exposing students to interdisciplinary collaboration and teamwork. Curricula need to be "well grounded in disease prevention, health promotion and screening, and public health, aging and older adults, ethics, genetics, public speaking, and writing skills" (p. 356). Technology also plays a crucial role in the delivery of the curriculum.

Benner et al.'s (2010) work on transforming nursing education to some degree complements the recommendations of Glasgow et al. Grown out of her research efforts, Benner has identified four "shifts" that should guide curriculum design based on the evidence she has collected:

> a shift from a focus on covering decontextualized knowledge to an emphasis on teaching for a sense of salience, situated cognition, and action in particular situations;

> a shift from a sharp separation of clinical and classroom teaching to integration of classroom and clinical teaching;

> a shift from an emphasis on critical thinking to an emphasis on clinical reasoning and multiple ways of thinking that include critical thinking; and

> a shift from an emphasis on socialization and role taking to an emphasis on formation. (pp. 82–86)

Arhin and Cormier (2007) argue that a deconstruction approach to learning is more compatible with the postmodern generation of learners. The implications of this theoretical approach to curriculum design support the notion that curricula be less content weighted and more about the interpretation the learner searches for within the knowledge to which they are exposed.

The guiding principles that AONE identified are more prescriptive in nature than Benner et al. or Arhin and Cormier but also need to be taken into consideration when designing undergraduate curricula, especially those that lead to a baccalaureate degree. These guiding principles include the following (AONE, 2010):

- At the core of the work of nurses is knowledge and caring.
- Care is patient-centered and family oriented.
- Nurses need to know how to access knowledge and appropriately use that knowledge in the management of care.

- Accessed knowledge will need to be critically synthesized in the complex management of care.
- Nurses' knowledge will be grounded in the understanding of patient populations that include the concepts of generations, diversity, and interdependency.
- Nurses deliver care by creating relationships that include patients and interdisciplinary colleagues.
- Nurses will partner with patients in managing their care journey in the context of individual needs, desires, and resources.
- The concepts of quality and safety are core to the delivery of nursing care.

In translating some of the expectations of the IOM work into nursing curriculum operating principles, faculty will need to focus on improving the health and functioning of people; prepare students to deliver health care in a safe, effective, patient-centered, timely, efficient, and equitable fashion; and develop competencies to establish care benchmarks and evaluate the outcomes of care according to these benchmarks (IOM, 2001, 2010).

Various types of undergraduate nursing programs have been developed to allow multiple entry points into the profession. Generally there are many similarities among program designs, with variations occurring within the internal configuration of courses and course content. The three most common traditional program designs are the two-year associate degree, the four-year baccalaureate degree, and the three-year diploma program. In addition to these three educational models, there are accelerated baccalaureate programs, as well as accelerated graduate degree nursing programs for those students who hold a previously earned nonnursing degree. For example, students with previous nonnursing academic degrees may choose to pursue an accelerated or generic master's degree program, a clinical nurse leader program, or accelerated pathways leading to doctoral studies. Diploma, associate, and baccalaureate degree program designs are discussed in further detail in this section, as are licensed practical (vocational) nursing programs.

The doctorate in nursing practice (DNP) program and the PhD program are discussed in the graduate section of this chapter, as is the clinical nurse leader (CNL) program, which is currently being implemented primarily as a graduate program. As the nursing shortage continues to be of great concern, there is a national call to develop transitional or bridging programs that promote the academic progression of nurses from one educational degree level to another in an expedited fashion (IOM, 2010). These innovations share three main characteristics: a focus on decreasing the time to move from one academic degree to another, recognition for prior educational and practical or life experience, and the ability to transport educational credit.

Licensed Practical (Vocational) Programs

Licensed practical nursing (LPN) programs, also known as licensed vocational nursing (LVN) programs in some regions of the country, provide an opportunity for many individuals to first enter the nursing workforce. LPN programs are typically one year in length and are taught in community colleges and vocational schools. LPNs are employed in structured environments, with approximately 25% employed in hospitals, 28% in long-term care, and 12% in physician offices (U.S. Bureau of Labor Statistics, 2009). It is estimated that the demand for LPNs is expected to grow 21% between 2008 and 2018, mostly due to the anticipated increase in long-term care health care needs (U.S. Bureau of Labor Statistics, 2009). Individuals who are first licensed as LPNs frequently return to school to pursue licensure as registered nurses, thus increasing their levels of responsibility and accountability within the health care environment. Providing avenues of academic progression for LPNs that recognize their previous learning and experience will continue to be an important component of nursing education mobility programs.

Diploma Programs

Diploma programs represent the first curriculum model developed for training nurses in the late nineteenth and early to mid twentieth centuries. Initially affiliated with hospitals, many of today's diploma schools of nursing are also affiliated with institutions of higher education. Diploma programs prepare technical nurses who provide direct patient care in a variety of health care settings. Typically the curriculum is designed to be completed in three years and provides an emphasis on clinical practice. General education courses in the biological and social sciences are provided through affiliation with a local college or university. These college course credits can commonly be applied toward a baccalaureate degree in nursing if the student chooses to continue his or her education. With the shift of nursing education into colleges and universities, diploma schools have been gradually closing over the last 30 years, reconfiguring themselves as single-purpose institutions, or merging with existing colleges or universities. Diploma programs comprise less than 10% of nursing programs educating students at the entry level (AACN, 2010a).

Associate Degree Programs

Associate degree nursing (ASN, ADN) programs were first envisioned in 1952 by Mildred Montag in response to a critical nursing shortage. The intent of the associate degree programs, as originally conceived by Montag, was to prepare in two academic years a technical nurse who would provide direct patient care in acute care settings under the supervision of a professional nurse (Dillon, 1997). Despite the persistent call for increasing the level of preparation of the RN, associate degree programs continue to be very popular. In 2007–2008, 61% of the graduating prelicensure students were from associate degree nursing programs (NLN, 2011b). According to the National Advisory Council on Nurse Education and Practice (NACNEP) (2008), in 2004 approximately 33.7% of practicing nurses reported holding an associate degree as their highest nursing degree, while another 34.2% reported holding the baccalaureate as their highest nursing degree.

Associate degree programs are commonly located in community or vocational colleges but may also be located in four-year colleges and universities. The typical curriculum requires two academic years to complete and consists of approximately 30 credit hours of general education courses in the biological and social sciences and approximately 38 credit hours of nursing courses. It is interesting to note that associate degree students often take three or more years to complete their degree program for a number of personal or academic reasons.

The curriculum of associate degree programs commonly consists of nursing courses that include concepts and content related to the practice of medical–surgical, pediatric, maternity, and psychiatric–mental health nursing care. Some programs may also include management, community health, gerontology, and research (Ayers & Coeling, 2005). On completion of the program, graduates are prepared to practice in structured health care settings.

In response to future workforce needs and employment patterns, it is expected that faculty teaching in associate degree programs instill in their students a sense of lifelong learning and the expectation of advancing their initial education to at least the bachelor level. The recent IOM (2010) report on the future of nursing recommended that the profession move to increasing the proportion of practicing nurses with a baccalaureate degree to 80% by 2020. Facilitating the academic progression of associate degree–prepared nurses through innovative curriculum models will become a strategic goal of the profession over the next decade.

Baccalaureate Degree Programs

Baccalaureate degree (BSN, BS, BA) programs are traditionally offered by four-year colleges and universities. However, there are 16 states that have changed their regulations to allow community colleges to offer bachelor degrees (Community College Baccalaureate Association, 2008). The graduate of a baccalaureate nursing program is prepared to deliver care to individuals, families, groups, and communities in institutional, home, and community settings. In addition to content related to specific nursing areas, baccalaureate curricula also include concepts related to management, community health, nursing theory and research, group dynamics, and professional issues. Health promotion, illness prevention, and patient education may also be emphasized.

The baccalaureate curriculum offers a strong foundation of liberal arts and sciences in addition to nursing courses. The program may be designed to require students to take prerequisite courses in the sciences, arts, and humanities before admission to the nursing major, or students may be directly admitted to the nursing program and take these courses concurrently with nursing courses. Faculty must consider the issues related to each program design, their philosophical beliefs about education, the characteristics of the program's student population, and the institution's mission as decisions are made about the design of the curriculum.

It is imperative for the faculty to construct curricula that are flexible enough in adapting to changing practice expectations of baccalaureate-prepared nurses, especially as there is growing evidence and preference for the bachelor degree as entry into nursing practice (IOM, 2010). This growing evidence supports the need for more baccalaureate-prepared nurses in the workforce given the data showing increases in patient safety and patient care outcomes as a result of the practice of baccalaureate-prepared nurses. In order to develop contemporary curricula and meet the needs of the workforce, and consistent with the IOM's 2010 call for transformational partnerships, there will be a continuing need to stress the creation of academic–practice partnerships (Niederhauser, MacIntyre, Garner, Teel, & Murray, 2010). Faculty must maximize these partnerships as they develop revised program competencies that include but are not limited to such concepts as analytical reasoning, intellectual inquiry, inter- and intradisciplinary collaboration, negotiation, complexity thinking, efficient care management and coordination, change agency, evidence-based decision making, information technology, bioterrorism, genetics and genomics, gerontology, and care redesign. This is certainly not an exhaustive list of competencies but one that will evolve with the dynamics of a changing health care system.

Educational Mobility Options in Undergraduate Programs

Many undergraduate nursing program options have been developed to facilitate the educational mobility of learners within the profession. These programs—frequently called mobility or bridging programs—are designed to streamline the articulation of curricula between degree programs. Program designs vary and depend on the philosophy of the nursing faculty and the expectations of the parent institution. The most popular of these are the LPN to ASN (1–2 + 2) programs and the ASN to BSN (2 + 2) programs. Additionally, programs exist for diploma to BSN students and LPN to BSN students. Some accelerated, or second degree, nursing programs also exist for holders of nonnursing baccalaureate degrees to facilitate their acquisition of a bachelor's, master's, or even doctoral nursing degree. In light of the nursing shortage that is projected to continue into the next decade (Buerhaus, Auerbach, & Staiger, 2009), it is expected that nursing educators will continue to design educational options that facilitate educational transition for individuals coming from a nontraditional background. One example of an educational model that promotes academic progression is the NLN (2010) Education Competencies Model that identifies outcomes and competencies for all nursing programs from LVN (or LPN) programs to doctoral nursing programs and provides a seamless transition across

nursing programs. As a result, those wishing to pursue a nursing career will have many opportunities and choices among educational program offerings. Technology will continue to play a significant role in increasing access to regional and national program offerings. There are increasing numbers of online nursing degree programs that can be individualized by the student to meet his or her unique learning needs.

This richness has created challenges for nursing faculty and for the public who deal with the products of these educational programs. As noted previously, factors that affect a program choice are related to the type of degree being granted based on workforce needs and compatibility with the mission of the parent institution. This decision then dictates credit hours, program length, required courses, and types of learning experiences that need to be consistent with the degree being awarded. With educational mobility options, faculty must make decisions about how to recognize and credit previous learning experiences. This may be accomplished through articulation agreements, advanced placement opportunities, credit transfers, and validation of previous learning through testing and portfolios.

As the nursing profession seeks to increase the number of nurses prepared at the baccalaureate and advanced practice levels, mobility program offerings will continue to be a quality, cost-effective means of supporting career mobility and accomplishing this goal. Faculty will need to be creative and innovative as they design future programs. They must be willing to engage in experimentation as they find ways to produce and deliver quality, cost-effective programming. Curricula will need to consist of structured and unstructured learning experiences that build on prior knowledge and experiences of the learner. These nursing curricula will also be constructed to maximize the use of the latest technology that will support innovative teaching pedagogies and transformative learning environments.

Designing the Curriculum

Choosing a specific program design, such as an associate or a baccalaureate degree program, does not automatically dictate the design of that program's curriculum. Faculty should develop a curriculum structure that will support the type of program desired and the outcomes envisioned. Chapter 9 provides a discussion of developing program outcomes and competencies. After deciding on desired program outcomes and competencies, faculty are ready to provide additional structure to the curriculum.

There are a number of different ways to think about the construction of a curriculum design. The more traditional approach to designing curricula offers structured courses in a specific sequence. This approach identifies what the student is to learn, when the learning is to occur, and what the outcome of the learning should be. The delineation of nursing and support content, nursing skills, critical learning experiences, and evaluation methods for assessing learning outcomes are emphasized. These pieces are structured into any one of a number of curriculum patterns. Two common curriculum patterns, that of "blocking" course content and that of integrating or "threading" course content or concepts, are described.

Blocking Course Content

Patterns can be built on the premise of sequencing specific courses and corresponding clinical learning experiences. This approach assumes that there is a logical order to sequencing content that will facilitate learning. The courses usually consist of blocks or chunks of content that are structured around particular clinical specialty areas, patient population, pathology, or physical systems. Although each course or group of courses provides the foundation for the courses that follow, the content and focus of each course tends to be unique to that course.

A number of approaches can be used to organize the curriculum when blocking content. Content can relate to specific practice settings and content areas (e.g., medical–surgical nursing, mental health nursing, critical care nursing, pediatric nursing, maternity nursing, gerontological nursing, and community nursing). Faculty may also want to define, or block, content around developmental stages (e.g., birth, infancy, childhood, adolescence, adult, and older adult). Another potential conceptual blocking scheme is to construct courses around body systems (e.g., respiratory system, circulatory system, lymphatic system, regulatory system, digestive and elimination system, neurological system, and skeletal system).

The idea of blocking brings order or organization to both teaching and learning. It facilitates

faculty course assignments and complements faculty expertise because this approach to curriculum building allows faculty to teach in areas in which they are most knowledgeable. It is also relatively easy for faculty to trace placement of content within the curriculum; faculty can be reasonably assured that students have been presented the content at a particular point in the curriculum. However, the segregation or blocking of content into specific courses can often cause content to become isolated from previous or subsequent coursework and can impede the learner's ability to integrate knowledge and transfer concepts, information, and experiences from one course to another. By and large, this approach produces a curriculum that is highly structured, with little latitude for deviation from specified teaching and learning objectives and meeting individual learning needs.

Developing Concept-Based Curricula

In a more conceptual approach to curriculum design, selected nursing phenomena may be integrated throughout the curriculum. In this approach, faculty identify concepts considered core to nursing practice and then integrate, or thread, these concepts throughout the curriculum. For example, some undergraduate program curricula have been developed based on a particular nursing theory. In this approach, faculty engage students in thinking about how and why to use a specific nursing theory to help define concepts core to nursing practice. Faculty then develop and guide students through learning experiences that illustrate how the theoretical concepts are expressed in various patient populations in a variety of settings and how they are used to determine best nursing practice. Giddens and Brady (2007) described how concepts are used to provide an organizing framework for the curriculum, as well as become the foci for courses. They recommended that faculty engage students with the use of active learning strategies and use exemplar content to best illustrate the concepts being taught.

Another example of content integration may be seen in the following description. The concept of pain is one of many concepts that are commonly integrated, or threaded, into a curriculum design. In coursework early in the curriculum, students would first learn about the pathophysiology of pain, the causes of pain, the cardinal characteristics of pain, factors that shape or affect pain, and how to assess and evaluate the characteristics of pain. As students move through the curriculum, they would increase their understanding about the manifestations of and treatments for pain, review research related to the concept of pain, and identify appropriate therapeutic nursing interventions related to the care of the patient with pain, thus progressing from a global understanding of pain to a more specific, in-depth understanding of the concept. Eventually, students would learn about pain as it relates to acute and chronic health issues, to physical or nondisease-based causes, or to specific situations such as surgery and childbirth in various clinical populations. Students are able to grasp the relationships among concepts and can more easily transfer that knowledge from one patient care situation to another.

Other concepts that are commonly integrated through a curriculum include life span development, nutrition, and pharmacology. In a more conceptual or integrated approach to curriculum design, there are no boundaries to knowledge development and skill acquisition as noted in the blocking approach. Students use clinical experiences to learn the essence of those concepts identified and are encouraged to transfer their knowledge of those concepts to different settings and experiences. Problem-based learning (PBL), an approach that first gained roots in the 1960s, is an effective approach in "bridging the gap between theory and practice" for students (Raftery, Clynes, O'Neill, Ward, & Coyne, 2010, p. 210). Disadvantages to a more conceptual approach to curriculum design include difficulty in maintaining the integrity of the curriculum because of the lack of discrete boundaries for content and the potential for inadvertently eliminating from the curriculum key aspects of the concept. However, the counterargument is that students need to be users of knowledge and not "all-knowers" of knowledge. Another potential disadvantage is that student learning styles may favor a less conceptual approach to learning.

Summary

The more traditional approach to curriculum has focused on the identification of critical content, the sequencing of content, and the efficient delivery of content. In today's reality, a teacher-centered approach to learning is neither as effective as it needs to be nor as satisfying as it should be for the learners.

The traditional approach has led to an oversaturation of content as faculty have continued to add to the list of critical content needed to practice competently in a rapidly changing health care system. As noted earlier in this chapter, educational transformation calls for emphasizing learning and the learner, not teaching and the teacher. This shifting emphasis requires nothing less than a paradigm shift in how we, as faculty, view the education of our future nursing workforce.

One of the recommendations of the 2010 IOM report, *The Future of Nursing: Leading Change, Advancing Health*, is to "implement nurse residency programs to support transition-to-practice" (p. 3). It is assumed that these types of programs will not only smooth the transition from the education to the practice setting by some sort of proctored experience but also potentially increase retention of novice nurses while decreasing costs associated with early loss of novice nurses. Underlying this recommendation is the need for educational research that will identify best curricular models, the need for faculty to partner with practice to understand not only the drivers behind emerging health care delivery models but also what competencies graduates must have to work effectively within these models, the need to be part of the decision processes shaping health care policies and practices, and the need to conduct educationally oriented research on how learners best learn (Tanner, 2010).

Graduate Education in Nursing

Historical Development of Graduate Nursing Education

Graduate nursing education is going through a major paradigm shift in response to societal, scientific, and professional forces (Tri-Council for Nursing, 2010). The paradigm shift affects graduate education in nursing. An understanding of the development of graduate education provides a solid foundation for discussion of the current changes taking place. Graduate nursing education initially was developed in the early 1900s when nursing faculty, needing to be prepared at the graduate level, earned a graduate degree in a related field. The first doctoral program in nursing, an EdD, was offered at Teachers College, Columbia University, New York, in 1924 for the purpose of preparing educators and administrators of nursing schools (Peplau, 1966). Doctor of nursing science (DNS) programs were later developed as the need for nursing faculty prepared at the doctoral level grew. The DNS programs were seen as professional clinical degrees and as symbols of nursing's autonomy and control over the programs. Although the DNS programs had a strong research base, they grew primarily from the clinical base of nursing.

As the need for additional qualified nursing faculty continued to grow with the development of nursing's knowledge base, more educational programs that emphasized the strong clinical base of nursing were needed. Graduate nursing programs were developed to prepare nurses to meet the crucial shortage of nursing faculty and to promote the continued growth of the science of nursing. As the graduate programs in nursing multiplied, an increased need for researchers and not just educators became evident (Stevenson, 1988), thus leading to an increased number of PhD nursing programs across the country to prepare nurse researchers.

The rapid growth in the scientific knowledge base of nursing witnessed a corresponding increase in the number of doctoral programs. Although there was only an increase from 4 to 21 nursing doctoral programs in the United States from 1960 to 1980, there were 34 programs by 1985, and 64 programs by 1995 (AACN, 1995; Marriner-Tomey, 1990). There are currently just over 178 doctoral programs in nursing (AACN, 2010a). Many of these programs are PhD programs with a growing number of DNP programs.

The need for an advanced level of nursing practice, beyond baccalaureate preparation, to meet the health care needs of individuals and families was recognized in the 1960s and led to the development of master's degree programs. Rutgers University began a master's degree program to educate clinical specialists in psychiatric nursing. A nurse practitioner program that prepared pediatric nurse practitioners was founded at the University of Colorado in 1965 (Watson, 1995). In the 1990s there was an explosion of master's degree nursing programs.

Entrance to the twenty-first century came with several landmark publications concerning health care. *Crossing the Quality Chasm*, a report issued by the IOM (2001), called for the restructuring of the health care system to promote safe, effective, timely, efficient, and equitable health care. A second report by the IOM in 2003 recommended that all health professionals should be educated to deliver evidence-based, patient-centered care. The report further recommended that health care professionals function as an interdisciplinary team using quality improvement strategies and informatics. The third history-modifying report was issued by the National Research Council (2005), which suggested the development of a nonresearch practice doctorate to meet the critical need for clinical faculty to teach in nursing programs. The AACN responded to the recommendations of all three reports and others by issuing a Position Statement on the Practice Doctorate in Nursing (2004) and establishing a target date of 2015 to move advanced practice in nursing preparation from the master to doctoral level (AACN, 2006). According to this position statement, advanced practice preparation would now be the goal of the practice doctorate in nursing, the DNP.

The IOM (2010) *Future of Nursing* report acknowledges the fundamental role that nurses play and will play in the changing health care reform, and specifically calls for advanced practice nurses to function at their full scope of practice and, by 2020, for a doubling of nurses in the workforce who are prepared at the doctoral level. Achieving higher levels of education will allow nurses to be full partners in the redesign and implementation of a new health care environment.

Program Designs for Master's Education

The purpose of education at the master's level is to prepare advanced practice nurses. The roles of the advanced practice registered nurse include nurse practitioner, clinical nurse specialist, certified nurse midwife, and certified registered nurse anesthetist (American Nurses Association, 2004). The role of a master's-prepared nurse has evolved from being solely that of a practitioner, educator, administrator, or researcher to being a clinical nurse leader (CNL), a relatively new role (AACN, 2007). The practice of the CNL is to provide accountability for health care outcomes for a specific group of clients. The role of the CNL is based on a theory and research foundation that applies knowledge to the care of individuals, families, groups, and communities. A master's degree was not always a requirement for the preparation of advanced practice nurses. At the 1993 national convention of the NLN, a resolution was passed that the graduate degree be the minimal educational preparation for advanced practice in nursing (NLN, 1993). Although the clinical specialist had always been prepared at the master's level, the other roles were often prepared at the certificate level. At about the same time, the agencies that certify nurse practitioners and nurse anesthetists also adopted the requirement that nurses wishing to be certified in these roles complete a master's program in the appropriate specialty. The push by the AACN to move the preparation of advanced practice nurses to the doctoral level is being met with the sometimes unbending structure of academic units and the critical short supply of bedside and advanced practice nurses. CNL programs are replacing baccalaureate programs in some institutions, while the CNL is replacing the master's level preparation in other institutions. While many universities and colleges have moved to implement DNP programs if congruent with their institutional missions, many other institutions remain committed to offering master's degree programs for advanced practice nurses.

Program Characteristics

Master's level programs in nursing vary in length and focus. Most programs are two years in length, but some programs are 12 to 18 months in length. The length of the program is determined by a variety of factors, including the entry level of the student, curriculum design, credit hours per semester or quarter, and clinical hours required. Many students also enroll in part-time study, thus lengthening the program.

Most programs require an earned baccalaureate in nursing for entry. However, some programs have been developed for nonnurses with an undergraduate degree in another field. Mobility options are also available (e.g., RN to MSN programs) for nurses without a baccalaureate degree in nursing. Options also have been developed to meet the needs of nurses who already hold a master's degree in nursing but wish to pursue a different specialty. Strategies to facilitate the transition of nurses to CNL or DNP programs are being explored as nursing education across the country faces major curriculum revolution.

With health care reform, the need for advanced practice nurses has been recognized by the public and health care agencies, and the establishment of master's level nursing programs has boomed. The programs that have enjoyed the greatest growth are those established to prepare nurse practitioners (AACN, 2010a). While the majority of nurse practitioner programs are designed to prepare advanced practice nurses to meet frontline primary care health care needs, there are also specialties such as acute care nurse or neonatal nurse practitioner programs that are designed to meet acute care health care delivery needs.

The curriculum to prepare advanced practice nurses should be guided by the professional standards established for that specialty. For example, the National Organization of Nurse Practitioner Faculties (NONPF) (2006) has developed competencies of nurse practitioner practice, and programs that prepare nurse practitioners should prepare graduates that have those competencies. National certification is available and required for most specialties of advanced practice as well. NONPF (2008) has also endorsed the proposed *Consensus Model for APRN Regulation: Licensure, Accreditation, Certification, and Education*, which defines the four advanced practice registered nurse (APRN) roles and six population foci for practice of the APRN.

Faculty and Student Qualifications

The quality of graduate nursing education programs is maintained through the appointment and selection of well-qualified faculty and students. Fifty percent of the faculty teaching in a master's program in nursing must hold the doctorate. This is one of the criteria for program accreditation by the NLNAC (2008) and CCNE (2009). Faculty are expected to be certified in the nursing specialty in which they teach. They should also be active in advanced nursing practice or in nursing research.

Students admitted to a master's program should have the potential for academic success as indicated by past academic success, standardized tests such as the Graduate Record Examination (GRE), and references. Other common requirements for admission to a master's program are graduation from an NLN- or CCNE-accredited baccalaureate program, current licensure as an RN, a specified amount of work experience, completion of selected prerequisites such as health assessment and statistics courses, and participation in an admission interview. Potential students should also have the skills needed to provide leadership and practice in autonomous nursing roles.

Curriculum

From 1993 to 1995 the AACN worked with nursing faculty across the country to develop *The Essentials of Master's Education for Advanced Practice Nursing* (AACN, 1996). The *Essentials* are being reexamined and revised recommendations are in development (AACN, 2010a), with a new set of standards anticipated to be approved and implemented in 2011. The revised *Essentials* document will move away from a model that identifies specific roles for master's-prepared nurses to a role that addresses the changing health care system and is more global and based on scientific and technological advances, such as informatics and genomics. Graduates from a master's program in nursing will be prepared for direct care practice roles and more indirect roles such as those found in administration and education.

Accrediting Bodies

Master's degree programs in nursing and CNL programs have the choice of seeking accreditation through NLNAC or CCNE. Both have established accreditation criteria. A paradigm shift away from prescribed curricula to outcome-based assessment in the early 1990s opened the door for diversity and creativity in curriculum design. Master's level education in nursing is goal oriented and is guided today in a significant way by the requirements of the certifying agencies of advanced practice nurses. Accrediting agencies particularly focus on the number of clinical hours included in an educational program. Most certifying agencies establish minimums for clinical hours that must be met by nurses before taking the certification examination.

Program Designs for Doctoral Education

The first professional degree in nursing was the nursing doctorate (ND), which prepared graduates for general clinical practice (Fitzpatrick, Boyle, & Anderson, 1986). The ND curriculum assumed the need for nursing education to be at the postbaccalaureate level. This curriculum model was proposed by Schlotfeldt (1978) decades ago but was not widely adopted. All ND programs have transited to DNP programs because of the advancements in the science of nursing and evidence-based health care and the recommendation by the AACN to move nursing education to the postbaccalaureate level. PhD programs are research focused and DNP programs are practice focused.

While doctoral curricula are unique to each institution, PhD programs commonly include content related to theory construction; philosophy; development of research skills; nursing knowledge; and important social, political, and ethical issues affecting the profession (AACN, 2010b). Although many PhD programs require a master's degree in nursing for admittance, an increasing number will admit students with a baccalaureate degree in nursing (BSN to doctorate programs). Students who enter a doctoral program after earning the baccalaureate in nursing usually study full time for five years and complete a dissertation. Students who enter after they have a master's degree in nursing study full time for approximately three years and must also complete a dissertation. Many curricula are designed to allow part-time study. Traditional experiences such as a one-year residency requirement and qualifying examinations (oral, written, or both) following coursework are often part of the program; however, practices vary among institutions and in many cases are subject to the policies of the institutions' graduate schools in addition to any policies the nursing programs have adopted.

The DNP programs are rigorous and, through an intense practice immersion experience, prepare the graduate to provide leadership in the development and application of clinical knowledge (AACN, 2006). The AACN (2006) has established *The Essentials of Doctoral Education for Advanced Nursing Practice*. DNP programs have several points of entry (e.g., postbaccalaureate, post–master's degree, nonnursing degree) and provide a career ladder for nurse advancement. Graduates from DNP programs are expected to provide the leadership for implementing evidence-based practice and, with the appropriate preparation to assume a teaching role, could also be prepared as clinical faculty to teach in nursing programs.

There must be a critical mass of nursing faculty in a school or college who are active researchers to support a PhD program. Faculty must be not only excellent teachers but also scholars to guide and advise students in their development as researchers. As members of the scientific community, faculty disseminate their research findings through publication in peer-reviewed journals and presentations at scientific meetings. PhD students learn by participating with faculty in their research and dissemination of the findings. Faculty participating in the education of DNP students are likely to be more interdisciplinary, with a mix of some faculty having research expertise and others having practice expertise.

Accrediting Bodies

PhD programs in nursing are not accredited by a separate nursing body. Instead, the AACN (2001) published *Indicators of Quality in Research-Focused Doctoral Programs in Nursing*. Additionally, in 2010 the AACN (2010b) released a new position statement on research-focused doctoral programs that sets forth recommendations about the program elements needed to best meet the demand for nurse scientists who can develop the science and engage in interdisciplinary research and team science. PhD programs are also subject to institutionally required external reviews on regularly established timetables. These reviews typically focus on the program's curriculum, faculty and student qualifications and outcomes, and the adequacy of infrastructure and resources to support programs of research. Feedback obtained in the external review process is used by the institution and the faculty to engage in continuous quality improvement for the PhD program.

However, DNP programs are accredited by either the NLNAC or the CCNE. The AACN (2006) developed *The Essentials of Doctoral Education for Advanced Nursing Practice* to guide the evaluation of DNP programs. The *Essentials* document needs to be used in concert with the specialty content recommendations from specialty professional nursing organizations. Evaluation is always an important aspect of curriculum development. Feedback from the evaluation of program outcomes should lead to curriculum revision, implementation, and further evaluation of the doctoral curriculum.

Summary

Health care reform, with the increasing emphasis on advanced practice nurses as primary care providers who can provide quality, cost-effective, community-based health care, has led to increasing numbers of graduate nursing programs and a major paradigm shift to more advanced education. Nursing education has historically responded to the health care needs of our nation's citizens and again is making shifts to accommodate the future needs for health care.

Major issues related to the program design of graduate nursing programs will continue to revolve around maintaining quality standards for educational programs; recruiting and maintaining a culturally diverse student population reflective of our society's increasing multiculturalism; resolving certification and accreditation issues, especially in the area of advanced practice nursing; and developing flexible curriculum models that will facilitate the preparation of the large numbers of advanced practice nurses necessary to meet primary health care needs. Doctoral programs will need to continue to develop curriculum models that foster the development of nursing knowledge in the areas of clinical practice, research, and education. By vigorously addressing issues such as these, graduate education in nursing will continue to produce practitioners capable of meeting the demands of today's health care system and leaders to direct the development of new knowledge and the application of the evidence that already exists.

Future Trends in Nursing Education

Future trends in health care, nursing, and education will have a significant influence on how nursing education programs are designed and implemented over the next decade. The IOM (2010) *Future of Nursing* report clearly outlines the challenges currently facing the nursing profession as we reconceptualize how we academically prepare the next generation of nurses:

> Major changes in the U.S. health care system and practice environments will require equally profound changes in the education of nurses both before and after they receive their licenses. Nursing education at all levels needs to provide a better understanding of and experience in care management, and the reconceptualized roles of nurses in a reformed health care system. Nursing education should serve as a platform for continued lifelong learning and include opportunities for seamless transition to higher degree programs. Accrediting, licensing, and certifying organizations need to mandate demonstrated mastery of core skills and competencies to complement the completion of degree programs and written board examinations. To respond to the underrepresentation of racial and ethnic minority groups and men in the nursing workforce, the nursing student body must become more diverse. Finally, nurses should be educated with physicians and other health professionals as students and throughout their careers (p. 4-1).

There have been and will be continued changes that will prepare today's nurses with the skills required to safely and adequately care for tomorrow's patients. However, our greatest challenge likely lies in defining how the roles of nurses will transform to meet evolving and changing health care needs and translating these changes into educational goals that will shape the teaching–learning process for students and faculty.

To meet this challenge, future trends in nursing education will include an increase in the number of collaborative partnerships between nursing practice and education (NACNEP, 2008). Such efforts will focus on maintaining congruence between nursing curricula and contemporary nursing practice, developing initiatives that will help new graduates with the transition into nursing practice, and establishing mechanisms to retain and advance the education of experienced nurses in the workforce (IOM, 2010). There also will be an increased emphasis placed on collaboration between disciplines. There is support in the literature that interdisciplinary teamwork increases quality and safety in care (Dichter, 2003; Miller & LaFramboise, 2009). Faculty and students will be encouraged to participate on interdisciplinary practice and research teams that include a wide spectrum of disciplines.

The change in academia will include the increased development of educational products by nonacademic and for-profit organizations, especially in the area of teaching with technology. Tools and content that can be incorporated by faculty into their teaching will be available. Creative use of this content can assist with the faculty shortage that will continue. Students will also have increased technological resources at their fingertips to reach new levels of understanding.

Barriers to career mobility and articulation will continue to be removed, making articulation between degrees seamless and essentially hassle-free. Past barriers, such as the use of expensive, time-consuming validation examinations; duplication of learning; lack of flexibility; and difficulty with transferring credits, have all but disappeared. Today's articulation models are flexible in design, supported by broad course and credit transferability, and packaged to maximize the use of students' time. Distance learning technologies will continue to play a prominent role in successfully delivering education to geographically dispersed students. Faculty will seek new teaching strategies that will support distance learning using evolving technologies. These new strategies will play an important role in facilitating the learning of nontraditional students through curricula that will be taught more from an integrated conceptual orientation specially designed for the distance learner.

New educational models are being designed based on the premise that nurse educators must seek new ways of preparing the next generation of nurses. Nurse educators cannot hold on to the traditional models given the rapidly changing nature of health care and education and the massive infusion of technology in both environments. With strong education–practice partnerships, educators are designing new or modifying traditional curriculum models to ensure that graduates have the relevant skills to practice nursing in a complex and uncertain health care system.

The ways and means of educating the next generation of nurses must clearly be on the agenda at all nursing schools. Nurse educators must be able to step away from "what has been" to envision "what can be" (Boland, 2000). As new articulation and educational mobility models continue to emerge, traditional roles and responsibilities will become more obliterated, fueled by a continued drift toward a better qualified workforce. Faculty are exploring and will continue to explore the addition of internships and other types of intensive practicum experience either as part of a more formal curriculum design or in partnership with health care partners as part of an orientation program that bridges the gap between graduation and full nurse practice privileges (Tri-Council for Nursing, 2010). The influence and recommendations of the IOM (2001, 2003, 2010) and Benner et al. (2010) reports must also be considered as faculty redesign undergraduate curricula, as these recommendations continue to focus on best practices and future challenges for nursing.

Responding to a health care environment that focuses more on community-based health care between individuals who are well and those who have chronic illnesses, Wilkerson (1996) proposed the consideration of a curriculum that allows for differentiation and specialization of practice at the undergraduate level. Such role specialization has historically been reserved for graduate education, but with the increasing knowledge and technology explosion and the different skills and competencies required for caring for patients with acute illnesses, as opposed to the skills and competencies necessary for teaching health promotion, illness prevention, and caring for patients with chronic illnesses, this approach to undergraduate education warrants consideration.

Today, there are programs that make the distinction between these two patient populations. Preparing graduates at the undergraduate level who understand care transitions and are prepared to practice in such environments will become a priority.

Faculty and students can no longer attempt to "know it all and be able to do it all" in a two- to four-year span given the explosion of knowledge and technology involved in care delivery. The careful balance that must be achieved between theory and practice will continue to be an issue, with faculty making difficult decisions about which learning experiences are most essential to developing a competent practitioner and how much control the faculty need to have over the orchestration of these experiences. Although a set of basic competencies for the entering nurse will continue to be essential, the skill set for those functioning in acute health care settings will look different from those functioning in settings emerging outside traditional hospital structures. Advanced practice, however, will continue to focus on both acute and chronic health issues, especially those issues dealing with nurse-sensitive outcomes. Current health care legislation suggests an increasing role for the advanced nurse practitioner in the facilitation of health care, especially for the aging, which is consistent with the 2010 IOM recommendation that nurses practice to the full scope of their abilities and knowledge.

Professional education, by its very nature, faces several critical issues that faculty must continue to address at the undergraduate and graduate levels. These issues are of importance to all involved in professional education today, not just in the discipline of nursing. First, professional schools, such as professional schools of nursing, must continue to abide by the social contract that exists between them and society by producing competent practitioners. Increased consumerism has led to greater accountability. Accountability requires faculty to continue to design nursing programs that produce graduates with the knowledge, skills, and attitude necessary to function effectively and competently in a changing profession. Schools of nursing must also accept responsibility for providing continued professional development to help faculty maintain their competence as both educator and practitioner of nursing through research and practice.

Ongoing evaluation and assessment will be one of the most important tools faculty will use in developing future nursing curriculum models and in determining what teaching pedagogies produce the best learning experiences (Boland & Laidig, 2001). Evidence-based teaching practices will increase program effectiveness while helping to contain the costs associated with the educational process.

In the world of higher education, the nursing profession has long been the source of much educational innovation. The issues identified here are critical to the future of nursing education, but by no means are they an exhaustive listing of the issues that nursing faculty must consider as they design future nursing programs and curricula. The innovation and creativity that nursing faculty have demonstrated in the past will no doubt continue to identify them as leaders in professional and higher education into the future. If nurse educators are to become more collaborative in designing curricula at both the undergraduate and the graduate levels, then nursing faculty and administrators will need to take the lead in creating educational models that their academic colleagues will embrace.

SUMMARY

Nursing leaders have envisioned a future in which nurses play a predominant role in leading the delivery of health care instead of responding to the demands made by others. As nurses take an active role in developing health care delivery, nursing education will need to prepare graduates at all levels with appropriate leadership skills and an understanding of complexity and change. Nursing curricula will need to move away from rigid requirements to flexible learning opportunities to prepare nurses who are capable of managing large amounts of data-rich knowledge in technology-driven health care environments to make patient care decisions.

Designing curriculum provides an opportunity for faculty to use their scientific knowledge base, clinical competence, and creativity. Curriculum development at all levels is guided by the need to consistently include in the students' educational experiences opportunities to acquire the knowledge, skills, and competencies that are needed by graduates. Careful attention must be paid to accreditation requirements and preparation for licensure and certification examinations. Perhaps most important, students must be encouraged not only to learn new knowledge but also to enhance their metacognition and lifelong learning skills that will sustain their abilities to confidently meet the practice challenges they will face in their nursing careers.

REFLECTING ON THE EVIDENCE

1. Given the discussion in this chapter, what types of future innovations might be considered when designing educational models that will meet the contemporary needs of the nursing profession and students?

2. How has the proliferation of various educational mobility models influenced the quality of nursing education?

3. How does the history of graduate nursing education aid in projecting the future of graduate nursing education?

4. What critical factors should be considered by the faculty as a graduate program in nursing is developed or revised?

REFERENCES

American Association of Colleges of Nursing. (1995). *1994–95 special report on masters and post-masters nurse practitioner programs.* Washington, DC: Author.

American Association of Colleges of Nursing. (1996). *The essentials of master's education for advanced practice nursing.* Washington, DC: Author.

American Association of Colleges of Nursing. (2001). *Indicators of quality in research-focused doctoral programs in nursing.* Retrieved from http://www.aacn.nche.edu/

American Association of Colleges of Nursing. (2004, October). *AACN position statement on the practice doctorate in nursing.* Retrieved from http://www.aacn.nche.edu/

American Association of Colleges of Nursing. (2006). *The essentials of doctoral education for advanced nursing practice.* Washington, DC: Author.

American Association of Colleges of Nursing. (2007, February). *White paper on the education and role of the clinical nurse leader.* Retrieved from http://www.aacn.nche.edu/

American Association of Colleges of Nursing. (2008). *The essentials of baccalaureate education for professional nursing practice.* Retrieved from http://www.aacn.nche.edu

American Association of Colleges of Nursing. (2010a). *Nursing fact sheet.* Retrieved from http://www.aacn.nche.edu/

American Association of Colleges of Nursing. (2010b). *The research focused doctoral program in nursing: Pathway to excellence.* Retrieved from http://www.aacn.nche.edu/Education/pdf/PhDPosition.pdf

American Nurses Association. (2004). *Nursing: Scope and standards of practice.* Washington, DC: Author.

American Organization of Nurse Executives. (2004a). *AONE guiding principles for the role of the nurse in future patient care delivery toolkit.* Retrieved from http://www.aone.org/

American Organization of Nurse Executives. (2004b). *BSN-level nursing education resources.* Retrieved from http://www.aone.org/

American Organization of Nurse Executives. (2010). *AONE guiding principles for the role of the nurse in future patient care delivery toolkit.* Retrieved from http://www.aone.org/

Arhin, A. O., & Cormier, E. (2007). Using deconstruction to educate Generation Y nursing students. *Journal of Nursing Education, 46*(12), 562–567.

Ayers, D. M. M., & Coeling, H. (2005). Incorporating research into associate degree nursing curricula. *Journal of Nursing Education, 44*(11), 515–518.

Benner, P., Sutphen, M., Leonard, V., & Day, L. (2010). *Educating nurses: A call for radical transformation.* San Francisco, CA: Jossey-Bass.

Bevis, E. O. (1988). New directions for a new age. In P. M. Ironside (Ed.), *NLN curriculum revolution: Mandate for change.* New York, NY: National League for Nursing.

Boland, D. L. (2000). The future of nursing education: Helping to determine if nursing is to be or not to be. In N. Chaska (Ed.), *The nursing profession: Tomorrow and beyond* (pp. 867–880). Thousand Oaks, CA: Sage.

Boland, D. L., & Laidig, J. (2001). Assessment of student learning in the discipline of nursing. In C. Palomba & T. Banta (Eds.), *Assessing student competence in accredited disciplines* (pp. 71–95). Sterling, VA: Stylus.

Brubacher, J. S., & Rudy, W. (1976). *Higher education in transition: A history of American colleges and universities.* New York, NY: Harper & Row.

Buerhaus, P. I., Auerbach, D. E., & Staiger, D. O. (2009). The recent surge in nurse employment: Cause and implications. *Health Affairs, 28*(2), 124–128.

Commission on Collegiate Nursing Education. (2009). Standards for accreditation of baccalaureate and graduate degree nursing programs. Retrieved from http://www.aacn.nche.edu/Accreditation/pdf/standards09.pdf

Community College Baccalaureate Association. (2008). Baccalaureate conferring locations. Retrieved from www.accbd.org/resources/baccalaureate-conferring-locations/

Cranton, P. (2006). *Understanding and promoting transformative learning: A guide for educators of adults* (2nd ed.). San Francisco, CA: John Wiley.

Dezure, D. (2010). Innovations in the undergraduate curriculum. Retrieved from http://education.stateuniversity.com/pages/1896/Curriculum-Higher-Education.html

Dichter, J. (2003). Teamwork and hospital medicine: A vision for the future. *Critical Care Nurse, 43*(3), 8–11.

Dillon, P. (1997). The future of associate degree nursing. *Nursing & Health Care Perspectives, 18*(1), 20–24.

Fitzpatrick, J., Boyle, K., & Anderson, R. (1986). Evaluation of the doctor of nursing (ND) program: Preliminary findings. *Journal of Professional Nursing, 2*(6), 365–372.

Giddens, J., & Brady, D. (2007). Rescuing ourselves from content saturation: A case for a concept-based curriculum. *Journal of Nursing Education, 46*(2), 65–69.

Glasgow, M. E. S., Dunphy, L. M., & Mainous, R. O. (2010). Innovating nursing educational curriculum for the

21st century. *Nursing Education Perspectives, 31*(6), 355–357.

Institute of Medicine. (2001). *Crossing the quality chasm: A new health system for the 21st century.* Washington, DC: The National Academies Press.

Institute of Medicine. (2003). *Health professions education: A bridge to quality.* Washington, DC: The National Academies Press.

Institute of Medicine. (2010). *The future of nursing: Leading change, advancing health.* Washington, DC: The National Academies Press.

Marriner-Tomey, A. (1990). Historical development of doctoral programs from the Middle Ages to nursing education today. *Nursing and Health Care, 11*(3), 133–137.

Miller, C. L., & LaFramboise, L. (2009). Student learning outcomes after integration of quality and safety education competencies into a senior-level critical care course. *Journal of Nursing Education, 48*(12), 678–685.

National Advisory Council on Nurse Education and Practice. (2008, January). *Meeting the challenges of the new millennium: Challenges facing the nurse workforce in a changing health care environment* (6th Annual Report). Retrieved from ftp://ftp.hrsa.gov/bhpr/nursing/sixth.pdf

National League for Nursing. (1993). *Resolution of advanced nursing practice.* Paper presented at the Twenty-First Biennial Convention of the National League for Nursing, New York, NY.

National League for Nursing. (2010). *Outcomes and competencies for graduates of practical/vocational, diploma, associate degree, baccalaureate, master's, practice doctorate, and research doctorate programs in nursing.* New York, NY: Author.

National League for Nursing. (2011a). *Academic progression in nursing education.* New York, NY: Author.

National League for Nursing. (2011b). *Graduations from pre-licensure RN programs by program type, 2007–2008.* NLN DataView™. Retrieved from http://www.nln.org/research/slides/topic_graduations_rn.htm

National League for Nursing Accrediting Commission. (2008). *NLNAC 2008 standards and criteria.* Retrieved from http://www.nlnac.org/

National Organization of Nurse Practitioner Faculties. (2006). *Domains and competencies of nurse practitioner practice.* Washington, DC: Author.

National Organization of Nurse Practitioner Faculties. (2008). *Consensus model for APRN regulation: Licensure, accreditation, certification, and education.* Retrieved http://www.nonpf.com/associations/10789/files/APRNConsensus ModelFinal09.pdf

National Research Council of the National Academies. (2005). *Advancing the nation's health needs: NIH training programs.* Washington, DC: The National Academies Press.

Niederhauser, V., MacIntyre, R. C., Garner, C., Teel, C., & Murray, T. A. (2010). Transformational partnerships in nursing education. *Nursing Education Perspectives, 31*(3), 353–355.

Nightingale, F. (1969). *Notes on nursing.* New York, NY: Dover.

O'Neil, E. (2009). Four factors that guarantee health care change. *Journal of Professional Nursing, 25*(6), 317–321.

Peplau, H. (1966). Nursing: Two routes to doctoral degrees. *Nursing Forum, 5*(2), 57–67.

Raftery, S. E., Clynes, M. P., O'Neill, C., Ward, E., & Coyne, I. (2010). Problem-based learning in children's nursing: Transcending doubts to exceeding expectations. *Nursing Education Perspectives, 31*(3), 210–215.

Riley, J. B., & McWilliams, M. (2007). Engaged learning through curriculum infusion. *Peer Review, 9*(3), 14–17.

Salsberry, P. J. (1994). A philosophy of nursing: What is it? What is it not? In J. F. Kikuchi & H. Simmons (Eds.), *Developing a philosophy of nursing.* Thousand Oaks, CA: Sage.

Schlotfeldt, R. (1978). The professional doctorate: Rationale and characteristics. *Nursing Outlook, 26*(5), 302–311.

Stevenson, J. S. (1988). Nursing knowledge development: Into era II. *Journal of Professional Nursing, 4*(3), 152–162.

Tanner, C. A. (2010). 2010—A banner year for nursing education. *Journal of Nursing Education, 49*(6), 303–304.

Tri-Council for Nursing. (2010, May). Educational advancement of registered nurses: A consensus position. Retrieved from http://www.aacn.nche.edu/Education/pdf/Tricouncil EdStatement.pdf

Umbach, P. D., & Kuh, G. D. (2006). Student experiences with diversity at liberal arts colleges: Another claim for distinctiveness. *The Journal of Higher Education, 77*(1), 169–192.

U.S. Bureau of Labor Statistics. (2009). Occupational outlook handbook 2010–2011 edition. Retrieved from http://www.bls.gov/oco/ocos102.htm#outlook

U.S. Department of Education. (2010). *Accreditation in the United States.* Retrieved from http://www2.ed.gov

Watson, J. (1995). Advanced nursing practice and what might be. *Nursing and Health Care, 16*(2), 78–83.

Wilkerson, J. M. (1996). The C word: A curriculum for the future. *Nursing and Health Care: Perspectives on Community, 17*(2), 72–77.

9

Developing Curriculum: Frameworks, Outcomes, and Competencies

Donna L. Boland, PhD, RN, ANEF

The development of curricula has historically been the responsibility of faculty, as they are the experts in their respective disciplines and the best authorities in identifying the knowledge and competencies graduates need to have by graduation. As the emphasis for designing relevant curricula continues to increase, so does the need to involve a broader community of stakeholders in the curriculum development process. Practice disciplines such as nursing are actively engaging a diverse array of stakeholders in curriculum design, development, implementation, and evaluation. The desire to increase engagement can and does add to the complexity of the development process and the ability to alter curricula in a timely manner. To address the need to create or change curricula to be responsive to workforce expectations requires faculty to develop curricula that are flexible in design, open to broader interpretation as expectations change, and capable of being implemented using a variety of different methodologies. This chapter is therefore about the tale of two approaches to developing curriculum. Traditionally, curriculum development has been built on the concepts of frameworks, objectives, and closely orchestrated learning experiences. This approach envisions curriculum development as a logical, sequential process. The focus of the logic and sequencing is on what faculty believe students need to know and the content that faculty believe is critical to their ability to do (Diekelmann, Ironside, & Gunn, 2005). The more contemporary approach shifts the emphasis from an epistemological to an ontological orientation (Doane & Brown, 2011). Students in an ontological approach become the focus of curriculum development (Benner, Sutphen, Leonard, & Day, 2010). This approach "highlights the way in which meaning, interpretation, and the knowledge translation process are being shaped by the student" (Doane & Brown, 2011, p. 22). Knowledge is then shaped by the individual student in the context of the learning environment of the moment.

More than ever, today's curricula must prepare graduates to demonstrate how broadly they can apply their recently learned knowledge and skills to a dynamic and changing health care system. There is growing emphasis on college graduates being able to integrate knowledge and skills from a variety of disciplines and emerging from the educational experience with the worldview of both a citizen and a nurse.

In today's educational climate the value of education is measured against job marketability. In the discipline of nursing, emphasis has been placed on what knowledge and competencies graduates have on exit from their programs as it relates to the expectations of the roles into which they are hired. In response, nursing faculty have come to approach curriculum development from a product or outcomes perspective. This approach has been seen as a revolutionary departure from the traditional teaching process orientation used in the delivery of nursing curricula. Focusing on learning as the product, the emphasis is placed on what students know and can apply to changing and often uncertain situations. This approach assumes that both students and faculty have latitude in individualizing the learning experience and the processes used in creating that experience. Posner (1998) suggested that both process and product are critical to the development of curriculum by suggesting that there are "two necessary and complementary elements: curriculum development technique and curriculum conscience" (p. 96). He argued that curriculum development as a technique is a process that incorporates what we in nursing education see as the traditional approach that relies on theoretical models and frameworks. Curriculum conscience is described as the consequences of curriculum decisions made and assumes that the better decisions we make as faculty, the better the student outcome. The debate as to what curriculum is and should be most likely began with Plato (Grier, 2005) and it is not the intent of this author to challenge the prevailing thoughts. Therefore this chapter introduces faculty who are new to curriculum development to some of the classic building blocks as well as looking to the future of curriculum.

This chapter describes the use of curriculum frameworks for the purpose of conceptualizing and organizing the delivery of the knowledge, values, beliefs, and skills necessary for professional nursing practice. Various factors that shape the process of curriculum development are discussed. Because curriculum development begins with the need to conceptualize the discipline of nursing, a discussion of organizing frameworks is presented (Grier, 2005). Also addressed are historical factors that have affected the design of nursing curricula, and the chapter ends with a discussion of outcomes and competencies and how they are related to faculty's conceptualization of the discipline. Examples of outcomes and competencies illustrate the link between curricula, faculty expectations, and student learning.

Curriculum Defined

Although there are a number of definitions that fit an epistemological approach to curriculum, Glatthorn, Bosche, and Whitehead's (2006) definition of curriculum as "the plans made for guiding learning, usually represented in retrievable documents of several levels of generality" (p. 5) fits nicely with the notion of knowledge as a shared meaning. A major step in this planning is determining the desired learning outcomes that should occur as a result of this planning process. Therefore a pivotal question for faculty to ask is: "What should students know and do on completion of their educational experience?" Given today's environment of accountability, the issue of functionality is paramount. The need for accountability permeates all aspects of education, from primary through postdoctoral educational programs. Therefore it is critical to appropriately determine what competencies—in terms of knowledge, skills, and attitudes—students must successfully demonstrate

at the completion of a program that will meet the expectations of a dynamically changing health care system. Faculty must also decide what learning experiences will facilitate students' attainment of these competencies and how the attainment of these competencies will be evaluated (Boland, 2004). Accountability requires that curricula remain dynamic, especially as education faces the challenges of what seems like an exponential growth in knowledge, the impact of technology on how we teach and students learn, and the evolving and uncertain future of the health industry (Forbes & Hickey, 2009).

The more contemporary or ontological definition of curriculum is determining the learning processes that "support students to develop confident and competent practice within the shifting, complex terrain of contemporary health care milieus" (Doane & Brown, 2011, p. 22). Knowledge becomes the background as curriculum is focused on engaging students in identifying, interpreting, and using knowledge as they become competent practitioners.

Curriculum Frameworks as a Building Block

Curriculum frameworks provide faculty with a way of conceptualizing and organizing the knowledge, skills, values, and beliefs critical to the design of a coherent curriculum plan that facilitates student learning and their achievement of the desired educational outcomes. The value of curriculum frameworks is in their ability to provide the base for developing expected nursing competencies. Organizing or conceptual frameworks "allow students to apply what was learned to new situations and to learn related information more quickly" (Tanner, 2007, p. 52). This is critical, as the majority of nursing curricula today are overloaded, with students being overwhelmed by the amount of knowledge faculty expect them to entrust to memory.

Added to the complexity of curriculum development is the need to continue to address general education expectations and outcomes, which often are institutional specific. More and more emphasis is being placed on interdisciplinary learning and interprofessional collaboration and its impact on both undergraduate and graduate curricula. Today's higher education environment is reemphasizing a strong general education foundation for all undergraduate and graduate students, and this orientation is having an impact on professional curricula that are already pinched for space and time. An example of this effort is noted in the "standards for success," which were born out of a collaborative effort of the Association of American Universities and The Pew Charitable Trusts (2003). These standards tend to reflect lifelong learning skills that will continue to serve the learner as they move into a global workforce. These skills have been related to thinking critically, clearly expressing thoughts and ideas, clarifying their values, evaluating assumptions of self and others, and examining the evidence for thoughts and actions (Inderbitzin & Storrs, 2008).

The Institute of Medicine's (IOM) *Future of Nursing* report recommendations clearly speak to the need for more interprofessional educational didactic and practice learning experiences (IOM, 2010). The report challenges schools of nursing to integrate these collaborative learning opportunities into the curriculum. Also, nursing faculty cannot ignore the need to incorporate personal and social values along with the economics of an educated workforce in the development of curricula. As these external forces continue to prescribe critical elements that need to be included, nursing must find ways to meet expectations without continuing to add to already overloaded curricula.

In determining what needs to be taught and learned within the context of the phenomenon of nursing, nursing itself must first be defined. The faculty's philosophical beliefs about how teaching, learning, and the discipline of nursing should be viewed, described, and evaluated are often woven together into an organizing framework. This framework has historically guided the development of most nursing curricula (see Chapter 7). Organizing frameworks have been used in curriculum development to delineate the constructs embedded in a traditional philosophy statement that reflects the collective faculty belief. It is important that organizing frameworks not be construed as a permanent feature of a program but rather as a kaleidoscope of complex patterns related to what students need to know and how they will best learn it.

As faculty have moved away from developing formal philosophical statements, organizing frameworks have acted as a good substitute since they are conceptual in nature and reflect ideas and symbols inherent to the discipline of nursing. Their greatest utility is in providing faculty with a tool that turns mental images of nursing phenomena into visual schemes that represent the relationship of critical ideas and symbols to each other. This author would argue that this schematic conceptualization helps students understand the abstract nature of nursing. However, this conceptual level of abstraction has been a challenge for some students and faculty who view curriculum as a series of content units containing prescribed knowledge and technological skills that are to be taught. The focus on content blurs the essence of what nursing is.

Fawcett's (1989) classic work on conceptual models and frameworks can provide readers with a discussion of theories, models, and concepts that is beyond the scope of this chapter. Organizing frameworks can be a means for creating access to knowledge about the phenomena of interest or importance to the discipline. Organizing frameworks do provide a logical structure for cataloguing and retrieving knowledge. This structure is essential to the processes of teaching and learning as faculty guide students in the development of cognitive linkages among knowledge to which they are exposed "which allows them to see patterns, relationships or discrepancies that are not apparent to novices" (Tanner, 2007, p. 52). Additionally, organizing frameworks can assist the learner in building a context for storing and retrieving nursing knowledge and helping to promote an understanding and application of knowledge to new or dynamic practice situations.

Purposes of Organizing Frameworks in Curriculum Development

The purpose in constructing frameworks is to systematically design a mental picture that is meaningful to the faculty and students when determining what knowledge is important and has value to nursing today and how that knowledge should be defined, categorized, and linked with other knowledge. Today's critics of higher education are calling for the ability of graduates to be able to integrate knowledge and make application to complex and often uncertain situations. Ervin, Bickes, and Schim (2006) recognized that although the majority of nurses seek positions in acute care settings, there needs to be broader orientation to a continuum of care settings within a global context. This thinking is consistent with the recent IOM 2010 recommendation that tomorrow's nurse be prepared to practice across a broad range of care settings. Organizing frameworks need to reflect both concepts relevant to populations and settings. In summary, organizing curriculum frameworks provide a blueprint for determining the scope of knowledge (i.e., which concepts are important to include in the teachers' and learners' mental picture) and a means of structuring that knowledge in a distinctive and meaningful way for faculty and students.

A number of approaches are used in defining and shaping frameworks. However, an organizing framework must reflect the sphere of nursing practice, the phenomena of concern to nurses, and how nurses relate to others who are dealing with health concerns (Bevis & Watson, 1989; Warda, 2008). Organizing curriculum frameworks are the educational road maps to teaching and learning. As with any road map, multiple route options are available for arriving at a given destination or outcome.

As faculty move toward the adoption of an outcome orientation in curriculum building, organizing frameworks or models will continue to serve the same purposes noted earlier but will be driven by philosophical views and futuristic mental pictures regarding the evolving practice of nursing. An example of an organizing framework that is shaping recent outcomes in baccalaureate curricula stems from the Quality and Safety Education for Nurses (QSEN) project. Using its recommendations that "graduate nurses must have the *knowledge* to describe strategies for learning about outcomes of care, the *skill* to use quality measures, and the *attitude* to appreciate quality improvement" (Forbes & Hickey, 2009, p. 5), faculty are able to identify outcomes of the learning process for their institution. As increasing attention is being given to student learning, the emphasis on curriculum is transforming from teaching to learning. With this paradigm shift comes the need to look at theories and frameworks focused on learning. The concepts of emotional intelligence (Dekker & Fischer, 2008; Fischer et al., 2005) and transformational learning (Mezirow, 1991; Taylor, 2008) are now being considered by faculty as they develop curriculum.

Developing an Organizing Framework for Curriculum

It is not easy to decide on a specific organizing framework that will best serve a program. Faculty can use two traditional approaches in determining the kind of organizing framework they wish to construct. The first approach is to select a single, specific nursing theory or model on which to build the framework. The second approach is more eclectic: to select concepts from multiple theories or models. Both approaches are discussed further.

Developing a Single-Theory Framework

One traditional approach to constructing an organizing framework is to use a particular nursing theory or model to help shape the visual image that is consistent with the philosophy of the faculty. For example, if faculty believe that "health encompasses conditions known as disease and that it is an expansion of a person's consciousness" (Newman, 1997, p. 22), faculty will probably adopt Newman's theory of health as the vehicle for organizing knowledge for that particular nursing program. However, if faculty believe that caring is at the core of nursing, Watson's (1997) theory of caring might better serve when explaining the discipline to students and cataloguing knowledge about the discipline of nursing.

The advantage to building an organizing framework on a single theory or model is the ability to use a single image with a defined vocabulary that is shared by both the learner and the teacher. Drawing further on Watson's theory as an example, she says that "the transpersonal caring relationship and authentic presencing translate into *ontological caring competencies* of the nurse, which intersect with *technological medical competencies*" (Watson, 1997, p. 50). The image put forth in this description is "*transpersonal caring relationship*," which is at the core of Watson's theory. "*Ontological caring competencies*" and "*technological medical competencies*" evolve from this caring relationship. It is the development of these competencies that students would be expected to demonstrate in a program in which Watson's theory guided the knowledge to be learned and determined the expected performances of the program's graduates.

Using a single theory or existing conceptual model has limitations and poses challenges. One theory or model may not reflect everybody's visual image or view of nursing and nursing practice. This becomes problematic when faculty have developed or been educated in curricula that have used a different theory or orientation to the discipline (Webber, 2002). Forbes and Hickey (2009) suggest that the use of only one theory in a framework limits the ability of faculty to pull together all elements of their curriculum, which provides a rationale for moving away from this approach.

One of the more common challenges in using a theory is being able to take an ethereal explanation of reality and make it understandable for students being newly introduced to the discipline. The language of a theory also can pose challenges for faculty and students. Especially for beginning nursing students, the language of the theory and the definitions of the critical concepts may be too abstract to be helpful in promoting shared understanding and a common vision for learners and teachers. A good theory must also stand the test of time. Theories must continually be tested to determine relevance with current reality. As the practice of nursing is being transformed by a dynamic, evolving health care system, it is imperative to determine the degree to which any single theory is useful or practical. It is clear that nursing educators and practitioners will not, at least in the foreseeable future, agree on a single theory. Students educated in a curriculum driven by a single theory are likely to experience frustration and confusion when they find themselves in clinical practice settings that do not ascribe to the same theory, or to any theory for that matter.

Developing an Eclectic Framework

Given the challenges and limitations of using a single theory as an organizing framework, faculty choice does not have to be constrained by a single theory or model. Those who believe that a combination of many theories or concepts is more reflective of their beliefs about nursing may use an eclectic approach to developing a curricular framework. For example, an eclectic framework might include the concept of nursing as defined by Florence Nightingale, the concept of needs as defined by Maslow, the concept of self-care as defined by Orem, and the concept of a caring relationship as defined by Watson (Fawcett, 2000). All are critical concepts, but each concept comes from a different theory or theoretical orientation.

The use of a more eclectic approach when designing an organizing framework is not without its pitfalls. Some view this approach as an impediment to the development of a comprehensive nursing theory and the development of a body of knowledge that is uniquely nursing. The advantage to an eclectic approach is the ability to "borrow" concepts and

definitions that best fit the faculty's beliefs and values from nursing and nonnursing theories. However, if faculty develop an eclectic framework, where concepts and their definitions are "borrowed" from a number of theories, they need to ensure that in the act of borrowing they have not changed conceptual meaning. It is important to retain the original definitions and the characteristics or attributes used to explain or validate the existence of borrowed concepts in altered contexts.

For example, the concept of hope may be perceived as critical to the understanding of how individuals make decisions about self-care. If a person has hope that a certain self-care action will have positive results, he or she is more likely to perform that self-care behavior. A person without hope is less likely to initiate that self-care behavior. If a market analyst were to use the concept of hope in a model to predict sales trends, that analyst must determine whether hope has meaning that is altered by, or separate from, the current context in which it will be used. Borrowing concepts from other disciplines is acceptable as long as those doing the borrowing are cognizant of how, in the act of borrowing, the concept may have changed some of its characteristics. Therefore it is important to clarify the meaning of concepts that will be used in an organizing framework so that faculty and students are clear about the phenomena being studied.

Examples of Nontraditional Curricular Frameworks

Historically, accreditation standards and performance expectations have had a significant impact on many organizing frameworks as faculty have moved to incorporate or add into their organizing frameworks and curriculum models such concepts as critical thinking, problem solving, communication, caring, diversity, and therapeutic nursing interventions (McEwen & Brown, 2002). Although these concepts can be compatible with the essence of nursing, they are often not defined well enough to be consistently used by the teacher or applied by the learner. Faculty adopting an outcome orientation to curriculum must be able to construct the context and meaning that these outcomes will have in the curriculum structure. Critical thinking is one outcome that most undergraduate programs have adopted. A number of nationally normative tools have been created to measure critical thinking both on entry into and exit from a program. However, critical thinking as a cornerstone of an organizing curriculum framework is often not well defined, nor are its attributes identified for systematic and purposeful incorporation into nursing curriculum or assessment activities. Critical thinking is a skill, and without a nursing-oriented context to ground this skill, it is meaningless in and of itself. If the means is critical thinking, then faculty must determine the end in the development of the context. It is interesting to note that accreditation standards are moving away from prescribing expectations almost as quickly as these expectations were first embraced.

As faculty move away from the more traditional use of theory or theories in designing curriculum frameworks, a number of unique designs have been identified. One interesting approach to an eclectic curriculum design is the KSVME framework (Webber, 2002). This framework is constructed around five "conceptual cornerstones"— nursing knowledge, nursing skills, nursing values, nursing meanings, and nursing experience (Webber, 2002, p. 17)—and incorporates many of the recognized concepts present in today's nursing curricula.

The *healing web* is another example of a collaborative effort to design an organizing framework whose conceptual orientation is woven into a "collaborative clinical practice in a differentiated practice model" (Nelson, Howell, Larson, & Karpiuk, 2001, p. 404). The healing web draws components from Newman's health theory and Watson's caring theory to construct the essential building blocks of this "transformative model" (Nelson et al., 2001).

The *emancipatory curriculum*, designed to focus less on structure and content and more on the dynamic of learning through discovery, dialogue, and critical reflection, is yet another approach to creating a more meaningful educational experience (Diekelmann, Ironside, & Gunn, 2005; Schreiber & Banister, 2002). Although this curriculum design was conceived as the antithesis of the traditional structured curriculum designs, it is still anchored in philosophical conceptualizations from phenomenology, feminist theory, and critical social theory (Schreiber & Banister, 2002, p. 41). Challenges to a more individualized approach to curriculum structure can vary depending on individual faculty beliefs, experiences, and priorities.

The Quality and Safety Education in Nursing: Enhancing Faculty Capacity has developed a quality and safety framework that is being used to revise or is being incorporated into existing curriculum frameworks. This work began in 2005 through Robert Wood Johnson Foundation funding and the American Association of Colleges of Nursing (AACN) holding regional meetings designed to facilitate the incorporation of this framework into prelicensure programs (AACN, 2010). The Oregon Consortium for Nursing Education (OCNE) model is gaining in popularity across the country and has a number of elements believed to address some of the challenges in nursing education today (OCNE, 2006).

These eclectic approaches to thinking about curriculum frameworks appear to be driven by the need to make the education of nursing students relevant to tomorrow's practice of nursing. Relevancy is being defined around such concepts as differentiated practice, evidence-based practice, and care outcomes. As faculty and practitioners of nursing struggle to reenvision nursing practice for the next century, these concepts will assume center stage in the various curriculum dialogues. It is crucial that practice and education recognize and assume active roles in all future curriculum development activities. Without shared understanding and common goals there is little to ensure the relevancy of graduates beyond the skills they will develop in their educational programs. Although it is essential to build an undergraduate curriculum around the science of nursing, it is imperative to maintain the science of nursing knowledge in graduate programs, especially as faculty are reexamining graduate education with the doctorate in nursing practice (DNP) often replacing existing master's programs. Without a substantial and sustained commitment to the science of nursing, the practice of nursing will soon lose the guidance that frameworks offer.

Designing a Graphic of the Framework

Although it is unnecessary to accompany the description of the organizing framework with a graphic or model, it can be helpful for those trying to grasp concepts or ideas enfolded within the framework. A graphic can provide clarification, especially when the framework is complex or abstract. Simply put, the graphic facilitates how to see the association among concepts for the visual learner.

When developing organizing frameworks, faculty should be guided by a "less is better" approach. Faculty should remember that curriculum-organizing frameworks are roads to a specified destination, not the trip itself. If the framework is too complex, students and faculty spend more time trying to interpret and understand the framework than they do actually implementing and evaluating it. This trade-off is devastating because time is often perceived as the rarest of commodities in today's undergraduate and graduate nursing programs.

An example of a simplistic curriculum structure may include the concepts of health, person, and environment. As shown in Figure 9-1, if health has been defined as a continuum, with wellness at one end and illness at the other, the mental picture is very simple.

Adding the concept of person to this model requires that *person* first be defined. If a person is believed to have the ability to balance wellness and illness to achieve a high level of wellness, an additional dimension could be added to the model as depicted in Figure 9-2.

When the concept of environment is incorporated into the image, it creates additional complexity. If we define the environment as an external force that affects a person's ability to balance his or her state of wellness along the health continuum, shown in Figure 9-3, person and health occur within the context of an open environment, and the environment that is wrapped around the person

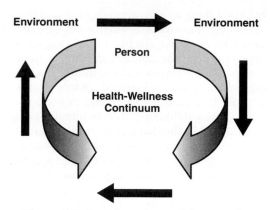

Figure 9-3 Complex conceptual framework.

affects the person's ability to balance his or her wellness state.

These examples demonstrate how busy a framework can become when concepts are added.

Again, with increasing emphasis on learning it is critical that the learner and learning become visible in curricular models or conceptual maps. As nurse educators we have spent the majority of our time attending to issues surrounding discipline-related knowledge. Today our lens must include the process by which learners are motivated to learn, how they construct what they are learning, and how they transport that learning into meaningful thoughts and actions (Taylor, Fischer, & Taylor, 2009).

Clancy, Effken, and Pesut (2008) describe complex systems as being constructed from a "highly connected network of entities from which higher order behavior emerges" that they believe has significant implications on how we think about learning and the practice of nursing (p. 249). The assumptions growing out of the work related to complex systems support the need to focus on learning and the integration of the student both in the knowledge being taught and in the process in which the knowledge is learned and used.

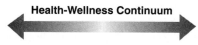

Figure 9-1 Simple conceptual framework.

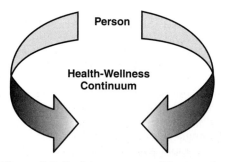

Figure 9-2 Evolving conceptual framework.

Summary

However faculty decide to approach the work of developing a framework for their curriculum, the framework eventually constructed must be consistent with the school's mission and philosophy statements, faculty values and beliefs, program goals, professional standards, state and federal regulations, and current and future nursing practice trends. Faculty should have broad-based agreement on the curriculum framework because such agreement is fundamental to the consistent interpretation, implementation, and evaluation of the curriculum in meeting the expected program goals and outcomes. This aspect of curriculum development can be time-consuming and is currently under some scrutiny within the profession because of the time associated with the process. It is critical to develop a framework that will prepare students to function in a dynamic and complex practice environment. If there is a disconnect among philosophy, values, program expectations, professional practice expectations and outcomes, and the framework, faculty need to raise significant questions as to the utility of the created framework.

Guiding Principles for Developing a Curriculum Framework

Although there are no specific steps or "how to's" for developing organizing frameworks for curriculum, there are some guiding principles to follow. The first principle is to choose those concepts that most accurately reflect the faculty's beliefs about the practice and discipline of nursing and how students learn. More contemporary approaches to learning, which stem from constructivism theory, are consistent with students and their learning being at the forefront of curriculum development. The concepts identified should also reflect or complement the philosophy, mission, and goals of the college or university in which the program is embedded. By creating an organizing framework that reflects concepts valued by both the discipline of nursing and the parent institution, faculty have begun to articulate the contributions their nursing program makes to all stakeholder entities. Mission statements, goals, or expected outcomes are the starting point for choosing concepts for inclusion in the curriculum framework. As higher education institutions focus on learning, it is important to incorporate the expression of this mission and goal as well.

Most traditional undergraduate curriculum frameworks minimally contain the concepts of health, person, environment, and nursing as they attempt to identify the essence of nursing. These four concepts, first collectively discussed by Florence Nightingale (1969), are still considered cornerstones of many nursing theoretical models even though they are defined differently by different theorists. Many philosophy and mission statements of schools of nursing still speak to these concepts from their own unique perspective. Faculty often expand their mission and philosophy statements to include such additional concepts as caring, self-care, diversity, growth and development, nursing process, adaptation, informatics, and evidence-based practice. However, there is no edict that faculty must follow when determining the concepts or configuration of concepts that will form the framework for the curriculum.

As noted earlier, some of the newer curriculum models have focused on nursing practice–related concepts and less on nursing discipline–related concepts. What is important in defining the concepts that tie the curriculum together is relevancy. This means that the concepts you choose need to be relevant to the future practicing nurse and consistent with the science of nursing. Again, it is critical to reach out to clinical partners or those hiring your graduates to help identify what is and will be relevant for tomorrow's practicing nurse. It is also important that the needs and desires of the students be taken into consideration, especially as their learning becomes a major focus. Requisite knowledge and competencies are categorized around what nurses do with knowledge gained through their education rather than on what nursing is. This refocusing will continue to be prevalent in the minds of both practitioners and educators of nursing who are being asked to articulate nursing's unique contributions to the health care and education systems in which nurses learn and work.

An updated view of a nursing framework can be seen in the complex adaptive system model proposed by Chaffee and McNeill (2007). For graduate education, the Nurse Educator Pathway Project is an example of competencies that faculty identified from their nurse educator program. These competencies are the "ability to demonstrate knowledge of and engagement with educational theories; fosters effective teaching and learning relationships; facilitates learning and creates effective learning environments; understands and works with multiple complexities related to learning; advances nursing professional practice; and demonstrates leadership abilities" (Young et al., 2010, p. 6).

The second principle is to clearly define these concepts. Consensus should be established in this process because it will fall to the faculty to articulate these concepts to the students. Concepts that are too obtusely, concretely, or narrowly defined are problematic, especially for undergraduate curricula that typically have espoused a "generalist" conception of nursing practice. If faculty wish to adopt a specific theory or theoretical orientation that they find congruent with their mission and philosophy, the concepts and definitions are derived directly from the theory or theoretical model. If faculty select a more open or eclectic approach, the definition of these concepts should reflect back to the philosophy, mission statement, or discipline in which the concepts were originally conceived.

There appears to be a rebirth of the integrative curriculum that gained popularity in the 1960s and 1970s. An integrative curriculum is designed to integrate knowledge from more than one discipline (Spelt, Biemans, Tobi, Luning, & Mulder, 2009). This curriculum approach focused on concepts perceived as critical to the practice of nursing. They often were drawn from a variety of theories or theoretical models and provided the foundation on which the curriculum was constructed. Today there is growing interest in core concepts as a focal point of curriculum construction (Giddens & Brady, 2007). The transformative curriculum is also gaining in popularity as more and more faculty are investing in learning. A transformative curriculum is based on the idea of students having a big-picture view of what they are learning (connective reality), having the opportunity to interact with the knowledge in a critical and reflective way (engagement), and being encouraged to construct meaning and actions appropriate to their learning (command of information). An example that supports the ideas of transformative curricula is embedded in the "learning centered curricula" proposed by Candela, Dalley, and Benzel-Lindley (2006), in which student learning becomes the focal point of the curriculum.

The third principle to attend to in this development process is to explain the linkages between and among the concepts identified. This is critical because the linkages are the basis for how students comprehend, apply, analyze, synthesize, and evaluate knowledge learned throughout the educational process. These principles are analogous to putting together a jigsaw puzzle in which the concepts are the puzzle pieces. Puzzles come in various numbers of pieces. Usually the greater the number of pieces

a puzzle has, the greater the challenge in its construction. The outline and coloring of the pieces are the definitions of the concepts. The more clearly the puzzle pieces are defined and the sharper the color delineations, the easier it is to fit the puzzle together. The linkages between the concepts can be related to the coupling of the puzzle pieces themselves into a picture that reflects a mental image that will be easily recognized. It is the picture puzzle that is emphasized in higher-order thinking that we wish students to be able to demonstrate at program completion.

Recognition of patterns is a critical outcome that one hopes faculty can achieve in the development of curriculum frameworks and students can obtain as they move through the program. The resulting framework or model must present a "gestalt" of the nursing theory or models from which the concepts are taken. It is critical that faculty and students grasp an understanding of the framework without an intensive investment of time and energy. Csokasy (2002) suggests that "to maintain curriculum integrity, it is critical that faculty design all curricular activities to reflect the selected philosophical framework" (p. 33). The cornerstones of all frameworks must be reviewed on a regular basis to ensure continued relevance to the education and practice of nurses. Lindeman (2000) suggests that "nurse educators must prepare nurses for the emerging health care system and not the system of the past or one that they wish were in place" (p. 7). This is truer today than ever as health care systems are operating in an uncertain, ambiguous, and changing environment. The National League for Nursing Education Advisory Council Competency Work Group (2010) has developed an integrated curriculum model that speaks to what is perceived as changes in education to complement the changes in a dynamic health care system.

The Role of Outcomes and Competencies in Curriculum Frameworks

In an outcomes-focused curriculum, faculty generally start by identifying the outcomes they feel are most relevant to expectations of practice. However, that does not negate the importance of looking at theoretical, conceptual, and scientific foundations for the outcomes chosen. The following discussion focuses on the process of choosing and developing outcomes for an outcomes-based curriculum.

If curriculum frameworks are the road maps to understanding the discipline of nursing, then outcomes can be equated with the trip's destination and competencies with the mileage markers seen along the way. Outcomes, then, take the place of what was generally called terminal objectives in that they are what students are expected to demonstrate at program completion. Competencies have been equated with course objectives. It is inappropriate to suggest that these terms are interchangeable.

Outcomes, in the simplest of terms, are those characteristics students should display at a designated time, most often at the completion of the curriculum. In 2006 Tardif (as cited in Goudreau et al., 2009) defined a competency as "a complex know-how based on the effective mobilization and combination of a variety of internal and external resources" (p. 22). Competencies may be either specific to the nursing discipline or more broad in nature (Goudreau et al., 2009). Competencies are those abilities that faculty want students to be able to do as they progress through the curriculum. The "know-how" is critical in being able to demonstrate outcomes at program completion. Competencies are specific for each outcome identified.

For higher education, outcomes have become the published measuring stick for public and professional accountability. This need for public accountability has grown out of a perception that the American educational system should be superior in educating students for the challenges of world leadership. The public has increasingly demanded that higher education be held accountable for the product produced and demonstrate that the cost of production is consistent with the quality of the product. Some think that the current emphasis on outcomes will improve both teaching and learning, keeping American education in a place of global prominence (Boland, 2004; Boland & Laidig, 2001; Glennon, 2006; Lindeman, 2000).

Identifying Curriculum Outcomes

The movement to an outcomes orientation has developed over time in nursing education. As early as 1993 there was an acknowledged need to move from a curriculum that is "politically correct to one

that is theoretically pluralistic; to incorporate caring and humanitarianism as core values rather than the dominations of technology; and the centrality of the student–teacher relationship over esoteric scholarship" (National League for Nursing [NLN], 1993, p. 11). As part of this curriculum reform, educators discussed the need to emphasize "critical thinking, skills in collaboration, shared decision making, social epidemiological viewpoint, and analyses and interventions at the systems and aggregate levels" (NLN, 1993, p. 13). These skills have served as the basis for outcome development in both undergraduate and graduate curricula. In higher education *The Futures Project*, a four-year investigation into trends shaping higher education in the twenty-first century, was at the forefront of outcome development. The outgrowth of this effort was *The Future of Higher Education: Rhetoric, Reality, and the Risks of the Market* by Newman, Couturier, and Scurry (2004). One of the premises growing out of this project was the need to ask the right questions. The questions identified that had relevancy to curriculum development included the following (pp. 148–149):

> What requisite knowledge needs to be acquired by students to be productive in the workforce?
>
> What knowledge and skills are needed by all graduates?
>
> What is the gap between current knowledge and skills and those that are needed in the future?
>
> What is the role of technology in facilitating the acquisition of these knowledge and skills?
>
> How do we deliver the curriculum in a way that will maximize the outcomes?

In response to these rather provocative questions, the NLN convened an advisory group to explore the skills needed at each educational program level. The outcome and competency report was released in the fall of 2010. This work has identified those outcomes and competencies for each level of current educational programming from LPN to doctorate (NLN, 2010).

Historically, curricula have been focused on learning behaviors that are appropriate to what was conceptualized by faculty as the "role of nurses." Faculty have moved from this rather dominant view of learning to the more outcomes-focused view with the assumption that nurses of tomorrow will work in less prescribed roles and settings. Changes in the health care system are also having a significant impact on viewing learning from the perspective of outcomes. These changes not only are shaping the outcomes themselves but also are shaping what those outcomes are designed to achieve in relation to current practice expectations. Current health care trends affecting curriculum development and program outcomes include the increasing severity of patients' illnesses in acute care settings, shifting emphasis from acute care settings to community-based settings, increasing consumer knowledge and interest in and control over health care, increasing demands from the public for high-quality health care at an affordable price, the increasing need to ground nursing in the latest evidence available, and the increasing emphasis on patient safety and quality assurance. In addition, the competencies that nurses need to develop for professional practice are being influenced by shifting demographics in the population; growing competition among traditional and new health care providers; increasing sensitivity to cultural differences and the impact of these differences on lifestyle and health care practices; spending limitations in the face of increasing health care costs; and continuing growth of health-related technology, accompanied by a decrease in affordability of this technology for everyone (IOM, 2001, 2003; NLN, 1993; Pew Health Professions Commission, 1995). See Chapter 6 for further discussion of these trends.

With the need for nursing educators to ensure that the curricula they design keep pace with the ongoing changes in health care and higher education, more emphasis will continue to be placed on the school's ability to demonstrate success. Outcome assessment has been seen as the key by which school programs can document strengths and weaknesses (National Institute of Education, 1984). A comprehensive assessment program can help faculty determine what works and what does not in achieving academic quality and producing the desired program outcomes (Aktan et al., 2009; Banta, 2001; Boland, 2004). This logic is a significant departure from the predominantly process-oriented Tylerian approach to curriculum and evaluation, in which the emphasis was placed on detailed course objectives, the identification of content needed to meet course objectives, and the appropriate pedagogical approaches to complement the type of content needing to be taught.

Outcome assessment emphasizes what students have actually learned in their educational experiences, not merely the knowledge and experiences that were designed with the intent of achieving these results (Boland, 2004; Keith, 1991; Wittmann-Price & Fasolka, 2010). These differences, which may seem like nuances to many, are at the core of the 1990s "curriculum revolution" in higher education and nursing education.

As discussed earlier in this chapter, the traditional approach to curriculum design has been to conceptualize the curriculum as a process that is constructed from a mission or philosophy statement; a conceptual model that reflects the mission and philosophy; a curriculum design woven by interlinking the concepts, often in intricate "grids" and knowledge maps; and a complex network of objectives leveled by course, semester, year, and end of program. These linkages are further developed by determining the content to be taught in each course, the required learning experiences, and the evaluation methods used. This beginning-to-end curriculum design approach dictates a systematic, logical, mechanistic sequencing of activities, each critical to the next activity, and has served nurse educators well for many years, ensuring program integrity. However, it requires full commitment of the faculty, takes a good deal of time and energy to develop and maintain, and requires even more energy to change. It also assumes that learning is a logical, sequential, orderly process in which faculty are able to exert control over the knowledge links identified, specified, and recreated in the learning environment. This traditional curriculum approach has led to "adding" content to courses as faculty identify new information that is critical to know. As noted by Diekelmann et al. (2005), this adaptive approach to curriculum development has resulted in overloaded or content-laden curriculum that pressures faculty and students. Faculty are expected to identify critical information ("must know") from interesting information ("nice to know") in assisting students in the learning process. Students, on the other hand, are stressed in trying to determine what content is necessary for an upcoming test. The end results often create learning that is fragmented and decontextualized for the student. There is also some speculation that our oversaturated curricula are leading to a disconnect between what practice expects of our graduates and what graduates are able to do in practice.

Today, the assumption that faculty have control over what and how students learn is being challenged. We know that learning is more chaotic in nature, although not without specific patterns for the individual learner, and that how students hear and retain information is shaped by their backgrounds and experiences (Benner et al., 2010). The focus is now on the learner, and as a result faculty need to develop curricula that focus on outcomes, acknowledging that individuals take different paths to reach these outcomes, which suggests that a generic, well-scripted curriculum structure loaded down with content may not meet every student's pattern of learning (i.e., gaining, retaining, retrieving, and using knowledge). Curricula need to reflect the essential nursing and general education knowledge, concepts, theories, and skills, which should be organized in such a way that students can connect them and demonstrate these connections in a nursing practice context (Feiman-Nemser, 2001). Students must be actively engaged in identifying what they already know and how they best learn given what they need to learn. It is critical that students develop lifelong learning skills, as well as the knowledge and competencies needed for graduation. In this paradigm, faculty facilitate students' access to knowledge and use of this knowledge in the context of promoting health and wellness.

When moving to a curriculum that is more centered on the development of outcomes relevant to nursing practice, it is often easier to think about curriculum development as starting at a program's end rather than its beginning. Goals then become the critical focus of curriculum development. This method of curriculum development places a different emphasis on the need for organizing frameworks as a starting point for curriculum development. Approaching curriculum development first from the outcome or what the student needs to know to be a skilled nurse and then working toward the beginning of the curriculum provides faculty with an opportunity to identify those essential outcomes and competencies that they wish to see their students demonstrate at the completion of the program. This approach often feels like faculty backing into curriculum development. The organizing framework is then shaped by the theories and concepts embedded in the outcomes and competencies. For example, if faculty believe that students need to

possess critical thinking, communication, or management skills, these concepts will shape the organizing framework. In an outcomes-focused curriculum, the driver of faculty conversations is not what content must be taught but rather what knowledge and skills students need to have to demonstrate ability to meet identified curriculum outcomes.

Before they can think about curriculum from the outcome, or end stage, faculty first must identify the desired program outcomes (Anderson & Tredway, 2009). They will need to discuss societal, economic, and political trends affecting health care and nursing practice; identify assumptions about the future of nursing practice as it changes in light of changing practice models; explore current evidence that is driving practice models; and examine both the institution's and the school's educational mission. In addition, faculty will need to call on various interest groups to help identify outcomes or crucial characteristics that are relevant to today's practice of nursing and to speculate on requisite knowledge and skills for tomorrow's nursing practice (Boland, 2000).

Outcomes should initially be viewed as core characteristics, or those qualities that faculty believe graduates need to demonstrate at time of graduation. One of the more frequent approaches to identifying outcomes is to use existing professional standards as a way of identifying the abilities and attitudes you wish students to demonstrate at the end of the program. If, for example, faculty used *The Essentials of Baccalaureate Education for Professional Nursing Practice* (AACN, 2008) as a guide in identifying essential qualities, that would define the graduates of their program; these qualities may include evidence-based provider of care, collaborator, participant in influencing health care practice and policies, patient care manager, fiscally responsible care provider, and competent information manager. These essential qualities would then guide the development of related outcomes and competencies.

Another example of core outcomes comes from the work of MacIntyre, Murray, Teel, and Karshmer (2009), who identified a minimal set of practice-related outcomes that include "satisfaction of students, staff nurses, faculty, and employers; professionalism and success in transition to practice; recruitment and orientation costs for employers; patient safety; and capacity of clinical sites to accommodate students" (p. 451). As these outcomes are visible in current accreditation criteria, they are an excellent reminder that faculty have a sense of current practice expectations, professional standards, regulatory body expectations, as well as educational expectations held by employers who tend to hire the majority of their graduates.

Once faculty have identified the core characteristics, or attributes, it is time for them to describe the context in which the characteristics are to be expressed. The process of concept clarification or analysis can be used by faculty with some modification to define the core characteristics believed to be critical to the professional nurse graduate of their program. In the process of concept clarification, as described in the classic work of Walker and Avant (1988), the first step is to describe the qualities that most clearly express the professional nurse. The next step is to describe the context of the qualities identified by linking the attributes in a meaningful way; this step is often guided by theory.

For example, if faculty decide that one quality of a professional nurse is that he or she is a critical thinker, and if faculty define critical thinking as having purpose, questioning, being evidence based, being conceptual, reaching solutions, being assumption based, and being based on perspective (Elder & Paul, 2006), then a program outcome might read as "a critical thinker is able to articulate the relevant questions and collect evidence that results in a reasoned solution." Faculty must link these behaviors to nursing practice outcomes. Specifically, by being a critical thinker a nurse can better frame care problems and seek care initiatives that decrease the length of hospital stays or decrease the number of complications. In today's reality, critical thinking is often aligned with diagnostic reasoning and clinical problem solving as it relates to application of evidence to guide practice decisions and actions. In this case, critical thinking becomes a tool that promotes the use of evidence to guide practice and not an end in itself.

As faculty identify outcomes, it is important to embed these outcomes in actions that promote the science and practice of nursing. Simply translated, outcomes should demonstrate the link between nursing practice and the application of science. Within the metacognition context, critical thinking is just one competency students need to have as they deal with complex issues. It is important that faculty not only clarify the concepts they wish to use in the development of outcomes but also ensure

that they have outcomes that are broad enough to incorporate all of the attributes desired.

In a more ontological approach to defining outcomes, the focus of core characteristics is on the perspective of the learner. For example, in the work of Doane and Brown (2011), students are expected to demonstrate "self-initiating, self-correcting and self-evaluating behaviors which they believe are at the core of skillful practitioners" (p. 24). The authors indicate that developing skills of communication is critical and that it is the learners' ability to identify what is not known that shapes the essential content within the curriculum.

Identifying Competencies

After the desired program outcomes have been established, the next step in the curriculum development process is to identify the competencies that students need to possess to attain these outcomes. Competency statements identify the knowledge, skills, and attitudes that students need to develop if they are to achieve the program outcomes. They are behaviorally anchored and student focused. Historically, faculty most often used Bloom's taxonomy in identifying the level of behavior at which competencies need to be demonstrated. Although there are other schemata that can be used to identify the level at which students must perform these competencies, Bloom's taxonomy addresses the cognitive, psychomotor, and affective domains that have traditionally resonated with the knowledge that nursing students need to have (Bloom, 1956). The learning emphasis in the cognitive domain is on knowledge. Knowledge skills in this domain are hierarchical in order of increasing complexity. From a nursing perspective it is important to emphasize higher-order cognitive skills. The expectation is that students be able to apply the knowledge they have gained to patient care situations. The aspects of this cognitive domain are illustrated in Figure 9-4.

The psychomotor domain deals with the development of manual or physical skills and is the domain that faculty use most often in competencies related to practice. Again, the learning is presented in ascending order of complexity of performance. As seen in Figure 9-5, students begin to learn skills through imitation and manipulation. As they move into clinical settings they are expected to gain the precision with which they demonstrate a skill. As new skills are added they then connect one skill to

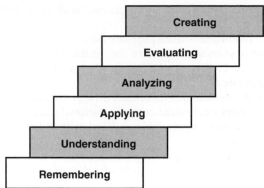

Figure 9-4 Cognitive domain.

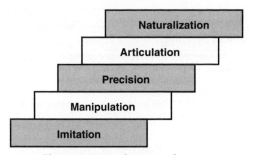

Figure 9-5 Psychomotor domain.

another in the formation of a skill set. The more experienced nurse, through consistent repetition, is able to internalize skills so that the performance becomes one that is natural and requires little conscious thought, like riding a bike or driving a car. Figure 9-5 demonstrates this increasing complexity of the abilities that reflect the psychomotor domain.

The affective domain of knowledge deals with knowledge from an emotional or feeling perspective. Faculty most often find this domain the most difficult to incorporate into learning and the most difficult to assess. There are five levels of learning identified by Bloom (1956). Receiving information is the lowest level and the learner needs only to be paying attention. The learner is passive and often functions at this level in listening to a traditional lecture. Responding requires not only listening but also the ability to use this information when questioned or when asked to respond in some fashion to the knowledge being received. As a learner moves up the pyramid, the level of involvement increases as the leaner now is required to attach a value to the knowledge and then be able to look at how this value fits with other determined values. This is demonstrated when a student is asked to identify what information is important in assessing a specific patient, or in comparing or contrasting information for worth. At the highest order of complexity we often ask students to examine their values in relation to an ethical issue or particular practice experience. This requires self-reflection and self-examination by the student. The affective domain is depicted in Figure 9-6.

Bloom and others have identified certain action verbs that reflect learning, and it is these verbs that many faculty use in writing competency statements. Table 9.1 gives some examples of these words.

Competency statements are important in assessing student learning because they become the foundation that drives evaluation. When identifying competencies, faculty should give attention to determining the right student, the right behavior, the right level of behavior, and the right context of the behavior. Here, *student* refers to the type of student from whom faculty are expecting these behaviors (e.g., prenursing, nursing sophomore,

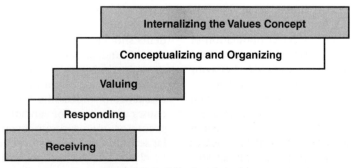

Figure 9-6 Affective domain.

TABLE 9-1 Examples of Action Verbs to Reflect Learning

Domains	Behaviors
COGNITIVE	
Knowledge	Define, list, label, select, locate, match
Understanding	Explain, describe, interpret, summarize, predict
Apply	Solve, apply, use, calculate, relate, change
Analyze	Compare, classify, differentiate
Evaluate	Reframe, critique, support, assess
Create	Design, compose, create, formulate, develop
PSYCHOMOTOR	
Imitation	Repeat, imitate, follow, show
Manipulation	Move, manipulate, demonstrate assemble, display
Precision	Consistent, precise
Articulation	Adapt, alter, change, connect, display
Naturalization	Create, revise, vary, alter
AFFECTIVE	
Receiving	Ask, choose, select, locate
Responding	Discuss, perform, recite, read, report
Valuing	Differentiate, form, justify, report, share
Organizing	Alter, arrange, formulate, order, synthesize
Characterizing	Consistent, revise judgment, change behavior, reorder priority

nursing senior); *level of behavior* refers to the level of learning or performance at which the behavior is to be demonstrated (this is where Bloom's taxonomy is helpful); and *context of the behavior* refers to the environment in which the behavior should occur. For example, if faculty believe that it is essential for students to exhibit a particular skill, knowledge, or attitude across a continuum of health care settings or with a select population of patients, then the competency statement should indicate the parameters in which the behavior should be expressed. It is equally important for faculty to remember not to be so specific as to "paint themselves into a corner" from which there is no escape (e.g., if faculty specify that a certain behavior will be demonstrated with postoperative patients in an outpatient surgical setting, all students must be guaranteed this type of experience

for faculty to make an accurate and consistent assessment).

The baccalaureate program outcomes and competency statements used by Indiana University School of Nursing (2004) faculty can be used to illustrate this process:

Program outcome: A critical thinker who demonstrates intellectual curiosity, rational inquiry, problem-solving skills, and creativity in framing problems

Senior-level competency: Evaluates decisions through logical organization, validation of information, and critical examination of assumptions underlying the processing of information and analyzes the conclusions drawn from the information (according to Bloom's taxonomy, this competency is written at the level of evaluation)

Junior-level competency: Validates care decisions with appropriate persons to determine the degree to which decisions are consistent with client–system information and environmental clues (according to Bloom's taxonomy, this competency is written at the level of analysis)

Sophomore-level competency: Participates in selected problem-solving exercises that promote critical examination of the professional nurse role (according to Bloom's taxonomy, this competency is written at the level of application)

In the above example, the identified competency related to critical thinking skills requires students to develop the ability to make reasoned decisions within the role of the nurse. This competency is designed to start to develop students' thinking as professional nurses. Sophomore students, who are relative novices at providing client care, could reasonably be expected to participate with other health care professionals in the decision-making process in selected care situations. To make good decisions, nurses must draw from various data sources. Students should begin to identify these informational sources and understand how these data are used to make decisions. Because these are sophomore students, it is expected that they would need some assistance in processing these data; this assistance comes in the form of validating with an instructor, preceptor, or an appropriate other within a particular setting. This competency may also be developed in classroom discussions with peers or through learning exercises that allow students to manage data sets in problem identification and application of information. A junior-level student would be expected to have developed some independence in gathering assessment data, using these data to make competent patient care decisions, and assuming responsibility to validate those decisions with appropriate individuals. By the end of the senior year, nearing graduation, students who are about to enter the workforce would be expected not only to exhibit evidence-based problem-solving skills that result in appropriate patient care decisions but also to demonstrate the ability to evaluate the quality of the decisions they have made. Faculty expect students to exhibit these identified competencies regardless of the health care setting assigned in specific courses; thus the "right" environment has not been explicitly identified in these examples. Faculty and students would use these competency statements to guide the development and implementation of appropriate learning experiences across the curriculum. The process by which students would achieve this competency has not been specified, allowing for flexible learning experiences and teaching pedagogies to be identified according to students' individualized learning needs. Learning experiences could be obtained through simulations, patient care settings, case studies, reflective journaling, and many other types of experiences that will provide students with the opportunity to develop this cognitive skill set.

Faculty have now completed the overarching curriculum structure with the identification of the outcomes and competencies. These competencies now need to be threaded through the courses that faculty will develop. To begin this process, faculty must consider the antecedents, or factors, that need to be in place for the outcomes and competencies to be achieved in each course in the curriculum. Antecedents are defined as the prerequisite knowledge needed to develop or foster the identified attributes or characteristics. It is assumed that each course within the curriculum will make a unique contribution to the ability of students to meet the identified competencies at each level of the program.

If faculty believe that one of the desired program outcomes for graduates should be critical thinking, then faculty need to identify the information and skills necessary for students to develop and refine their critical thinking abilities (see Table 9-2). Because structured learning tends to be grounded in developmental theories, students are expected to become more accomplished in applying knowledge to increasingly more complex or new situations as they move through the curriculum. Course competencies (course expectations) then should be written to reflect the placement of the course within the curriculum; expectations of learning for courses that precede, articulate, and follow each course; and how each course can contribute to the development of program competencies. See Table 9-3 for an

---

TABLE 9-2 Attributes and Antecedent Factors Related to Critical Thinking

Characteristic Values	Attributes of the Characteristic	Antecedent/Knowledge and Skills
• Critical thinking	• Creativity • Intellectual curiosity • Problem solving • Rational inquiry	• Ability to ask probing questions • Intellectual ability • Understanding of problem solving

---

TABLE 9-3 Leveling Competencies across Courses Using Critical Thinking

Medical-Surgical Nursing 1	Medical-Surgical Nursing 2	Pediatric Nursing	Nursing Research
Identifies a nursing intervention based on physical findings of a visual assessment of patient	Evaluates the effectiveness of nursing interventions related to compromised circulation	Adapts nursing interventions to the pediatric population with compromised mobility	Analyzes an identified patient care problem within the context of what is known through a literature review

example. Again, faculty have found Bloom's taxonomy to be helpful in writing course-specific competencies and expectations.

For faculty to develop an outcomes-focused, competency-based curriculum, they must emphasize the development of the knowledge and skills required to achieve a specified outcome. It is important to stress that outcomes-based education is designed for the acquisition of knowledge and should not be superimposed on an existing content-derived curriculum structure. Rather, this author believes that content should correspond to students' exposure to knowledge and skills needed to gain the identified competencies. Outcomes and competencies also should not, in and of themselves, dictate how faculty construct content, sequence courses, or determine best teaching pedagogies. Although some will argue that outcomes have not revolutionized nursing curricula (Diekelmann et al., 2005), it is this author's opinion that outcomes have provided faculty with a useful tool in looking at curriculum development from a quality assurance perspective. Outcomes will most likely continue to be important to curriculum, as public scrutiny and accountability are core indicators of performance among national and state oversight agencies.

Developing Outcomes and Competency Statements

Nursing faculty must approach curriculum development from the premise that nursing knowledge and skills are built on or interwoven with general education knowledge and skills. Outcomes and related competencies should reflect the "essential knowledge, skills, and attitudes students need to acquire" for their lifetime (Angelo, 1999; Association of American Colleges and Universities, 1994, p. ii). Outcomes should include those skills that are specific to the nursing discipline, as well as those skills that establish a foundation for lifelong learning (Boland, 2004; Lindeman, 2000). Outcomes for undergraduate education that have emerged from the early work of the Strong Foundation (Association of American Colleges and Universities, 1994, pp. iii–iv) suggested that students should do the following:

- Receive a generous orientation to the intellectual expectations, curriculum rationale, and learning resources of the institution.
- Acquire specific skills of thought and expression, such as critical thinking and writing, that should be learned "across the curriculum" and embedded within several courses.
- Learn about another culture and the diversity that exists within our own culture in terms of gender, race, ethnic background, class, age, and religion.
- Integrate ideas from across disciplines to illuminate interdisciplinary themes, issues, or social problems.
- Study some subjects—beyond their major—at an advanced, not just an introductory, level.
- Have an opportunity near the end of their course of study to pull together their learning in a senior seminar or project.
- Experience a coherent course of study, one that is more than the sum of its parts.

Much of this thinking is driving curricula today. Although these suggestions are not necessarily new to nursing education, faculty need to become clearer about how they are integrated into meaningful discipline-specific program outcomes and how the faculty will ensure that students are held to these outcomes throughout their educational experience. The latter takes both coordination and cooperation. This coordination effort is especially important for nursing programs that are housed in liberal arts schools, in schools where general education is the main mission or receives a strong emphasis, or in institutions that have established an undergraduate general education core curriculum.

Within this coordinated effort, nursing faculty should determine the role nursing education plays in the general education enrichment efforts of the college or university. The issue that faculty need to address is the contributions nursing programs make to the growth or development of students (Boland & Laidig, 2001). Nursing faculty are usually well prepared to meet this challenge because they tend to come from different disciplines and have been shaped by these interdisciplinary experiences. However, with the prevalence of doctoral nursing programs that are focused on nursing science and nursing practice, it is important to affirm a strong liberal education focus, especially at the undergraduate degree level. Nursing faculty are commonly leading the way in their respective higher education institutions and we need to keep this edge as a human practice discipline (Boland, 2004; Lindeman, 2000).

Guidelines for Writing Outcomes and Competency Statements

When writing outcome statements, nursing faculty need to have one foot firmly anchored in today's practice reality while the other foot seeks the future for nursing graduates. Faculty must be able to write outcomes and competencies that clearly focus on the transformation of nursing practice. Nursing faculty need to have the input of the practice sector when putting outcomes and competencies into words to ensure that what is being expressed relates to today's and tomorrow's reality as viewed by the practice experts.

As an example, competency with information technology is seen as a critical reality in today and tomorrow's practice environment. Technology is shaping both teaching and learning practices, it is a core concept to program outcomes, and it will continue to shape how we look at nursing practice. The 2007 Technology Informatics Guiding Education Reform (TIGER) is having an unprecedented impact on program outcomes and competencies, faculty development, and pedagogical approaches to teaching and learning (Fetter, 2009). The impact of information technology can be seen in electronic patient records and telehealth programs. As the health system is looking at cost-saving measures that are both safe and effective in meeting health care outcomes, the role of information technology will only increase in scope and sophistication.

Outcomes are general statements that refer to the characteristics that graduates must acquire by the end of the program. When writing outcome statements, faculty should determine the readiness of the learners to meet the outcomes identified and the length of time it will take the learners to demonstrate the characteristics. As faculty put outcomes and related competencies in writing, they should ask themselves the "why" question. The "why" or "what good is it" question helps faculty explain the importance of these outcomes and competencies as stated to various stakeholders. For example, why is it important that nursing students and graduates be able to think critically? It appears to be a value that is strongly held by nursing faculty, but to what end?

Outcome statements should be written to emphasize what is to be accomplished. For example, an outcome statement might read: "A competent care provider individualizes nursing care to maximize patient care outcomes." In this case the outcome is a competent care provider who can demonstrate the competency of individualizing nursing care to meet a valued expectation: maximization of patient care. To evaluate this outcome, the faculty need to observe and measure the students' ability to individualize care based on the uniqueness of each patient's needs. Faculty must then determine what skills and knowledge students need to have to be able to individualize care. What faculty must determine next are the competencies and behaviors that students must develop to be able to express this outcome. Once the competencies have been defined, faculty will identify what skills and knowledge are consistent with the development of these competencies and behaviors.

Students need to demonstrate their ability to meet outcome expectations to ensure a level of acceptable nursing practice at graduation. Outcomes, like objectives, are designed to communicate expectations and suggest appropriate means of measurement for judging student performance. However, in today's environment of public accountability, it is critical that faculty be able to collect data on actual outcomes achieved. Therefore faculty must not only identify curriculum outcomes but also clearly establish internal standards for outcomes identified throughout and at the end of the program. Graduate performance is not only compared with these internal standards but is often compared with state, regional, or national benchmarks. For example, the national pass rate on the National Council Licensure Examination for Registered Nurses (NCLEX-RN) is one benchmark that graduate performance is measured against on an annual basis. However, in an outcome orientation, performance on the NCLEX-RN needs to be linked to a specific program outcome. If the premise is that the NCLEX-RN is a measure of minimum level of knowledge to provide safe nursing care, then the program outcome would address the ability to provide safe nursing care. Courses throughout the curriculum would have competencies that would further define the concept of "safe nursing care" as it relates to the orientation of each course.

Precision is needed when writing outcome statements. The language of the competencies must reflect a continued sense of development. Development may take the form of increasing complexity, differentiation, delineation, or sophistication. Again, using the example of a "competent care provider" as an outcome, building this idea of development into course competencies might include the following:

- **Carries out procedures ordered for assigned patient**. This might be a realistic expectation for a beginning student. To develop this competency the student will need to be able to read a care plan to determine the interventions that are to be performed for the assigned client.
- **Modifies a standard plan of care consistent with desired patient care outcomes**. To achieve this competency the student is expected to do more than carry out procedures ordered for the patient. The student is now in control of modifying the care plan based on the assessment information collected. The student will have to demonstrate good decision-making skills in knowing how to use evaluation data to make corrections to obtain the desired outcomes.
- **Develops care plans that reflect the individual goals of the patient and desired medical treatment goals**. This competency requires a higher level of functioning than the previous competency statements because the student must again add to his or her skill mix. Individualizing care plans presumes that the student knows the most acceptable medical and nursing interventions for a specific patient and is able to use this information in conjunction with what is known about the patient to develop a plan of care that is consistent with both client desires and medical outcomes.

Note how each competency or skill identified leads to the eventual development of a competent care provider.

Leveling Competencies

In leveling, or specifying, competencies, faculty must recognize the level at which the knowledge and skills need to be demonstrated to obtain the outcome desired throughout the curriculum. The learning environment will need to be configured to enable the students to acquire knowledge at the level identified. Evaluation measures also need to be consistent with the level of learning identified to ensure consistency in evaluation from the time of input of information through the time of output of the behavior or skill required. Learning occurs at various levels, and the level of learning needs to be explicitly stated in the competencies faculty generate for each level within the curriculum.

Once competencies have been leveled to a year or semester or academic level, faculty must carefully examine these competencies and determine how particular courses can add to the ongoing development of these competencies. The behaviors embedded in each competency become the focus for writing course-level competencies. Not all competencies will or should be included in all courses that make up the curriculum. Competencies at the course level are more concrete and detail how the chosen competencies explicitly relate to the course (see Table 9-3). If, for example, faculty believe that the individualization of a standard care map is critical to student learning, then the course competency will reflect this behavior. The faculty will then need to identify what prerequisite and requisite knowledge and skills the students will need to possess to demonstrate this behavior. Faculty must also determine where, when, and how this knowledge and skill set will be developed. As part of course development, faculty must also identify how this competency will be assessed and what standard or benchmark will be established to note acceptable performance of this competency. These standards or benchmarks should be evident in the clinical evaluations used by clinically oriented courses and be visible in other evaluation tools used in didactic courses.

Benchmarking competencies is important because the use of this process generates information as to what skills and knowledge students are able to demonstrate from the beginning to the end of the program. These data are also valuable when trying to determine the impact the program had on the students' ability to develop all critical competencies chosen. Such data can also provide insight into resources needed for students to achieve an acceptable level of performance both within a course and across the curriculum.

SUMMARY

Organizing frameworks and outcomes should reflect the concepts most valued among the faculty, the professional community, and other identified stakeholders. Organizing frameworks, if used, should be designed to provide faculty and students with a tool to define, interpret, and communicate the essence of nursing. For some, organizing frameworks reflect a particular theoretical orientation. For others, organizing frameworks present a more eclectic theoretical view of nursing. However organizing frameworks are viewed, faculty should carefully consider the usefulness of the chosen framework in the face of a rapidly changing health care industry and the current movements within education toward more freedom of interpretation on the part of students and faculty. Faculty must also give thought to the outcomes and competencies that they believe students must demonstrate upon graduation for competent nursing practice. In the current environment of accountability and quality improvement, educational expectations are still core in assessing program effectiveness. However, the hallmark of today's curricula must be flexibility. Faculty will be called on to find ways of building dynamic, fluid curricula that reflect the values and beliefs of higher education and nursing in a world that embraces the explosion of knowledge and technology.

It is anticipated that there will continue to be an emphasis on learning and the learner. Based on this assumption, the idea of staging learning as it relates to leveling knowledge and skills to facilitate building competencies no longer fits the paradigm of transformational learning that is gaining in popularity within higher education

generally and nursing specifically. The process of integrative learning still requires that students have some command of basic information, but it is the ability to work with minimal data sets in making connections among information elements through inquiry, reasoning, reflection, synthesis, and evaluation that is core to learning. Learning will occur more through individual learning patterns and not neatly reflect preestablished levels of understanding and cognitive abilities. New outcome expectations emphasize the ability to be a system thinker, to use current and pertinent evidence to make decisions related to complex and often uncertain situations, to problem-solve efficiently and effectively in a complex dynamic system, to use technology in designing and implementing practice innovations, and to manage chronic health issues through collaboration, coordination, and cooperation. We know that teaching, learning, and the educational environment is changing and will continue to change, but we will continue to be held accountable for designing a context in which students can achieve the outcomes to which we and they will be held accountable.

REFLECTING ON THE EVIDENCE

1. How does a faculty know if a curriculum framework is providing adequate structure to support the decisions faculty are making regarding curriculum development and implementation?

2. What are some strategies that faculty can adopt to ensure that their program curricula remain fluid and dynamic?

3. What processes can faculty use to benchmark competencies of their students?

REFERENCES

Aktan, N. M., Bareford, C. G., Bliss, J. B., Connolly, K., DeYoung, S., Sullivan, K. L., & Tracy J. (2009). Comparison of outcomes in a traditional versus accelerated nursing curriculum. *International Journal of Nursing Education Scholarship*, *6*(1). doi:10.2202/1548-923X.1639

Anderson, G. L., & Tredway, C. A. (2009). Transforming the nursing curriculum to promote critical thinking online. *Journal of Nursing Education*, *48*(2), 111–115.

Angelo, T. A. (1999). Doing assessment as if learning matters most. *American Association for Higher Education Bulletin*, *51*(9), 3–6.

American Association of Colleges of Nursing. (2008). *The essentials of baccalaureate education for professional nursing practice*. Available from http://www.aacn.nche.edu/

American Association of Colleges of Nursing. (2010). *About QSEN education consortium*. Available from http://www.aacn.nche.edu/

Association of American Colleges and Universities. (1994). *Strong foundations: Twelve principles for effective general education programs*. Washington, DC: Author.

Association of American Universities and The Pew Charitable Trusts. (2003). *Standards for success*. Eugene, OR: Center for Educational Policy Research.

Banta, T. (2001). Assessing competence in higher education. In C. A. Palomba & T. W. Banta (Eds.), *Assessing student competence in accredited disciplines* (pp. 1–12). Sterling, VA: Stylus.

Benner, P., Sutphen, M., Leonard, V., & Day, L. (2010). *Educating nurses: A call for radical transformation.* San Francisco, CA: Jossey-Bass.

Bevis, E. O., & Watson, J. (1989). *Toward a caring curriculum: A new pedagogy for nursing.* New York, NY: National League for Nursing.

Bloom, B. S. (Ed.). (1956). *Taxonomy of educational objectives: The classification of educational goals.* New York, NY: Longman.

Boland, D. L. (2000). The future of nursing education: Helping to determine if nursing is to be or not to be. In N. Chaska (Ed.), *The nursing profession: Tomorrow and beyond* (pp. 867–880). Thousand Oaks, CA: Sage.

Boland, D. L. (2004). Program evaluation and public accountability. In M. Oermann & K. Heinrich (Eds.), *Annual review of nursing education.* New York, NY: Springer.

Boland, D. L., & Laidig, J. (2001). Assessment of student learning in the discipline of nursing. In C. Palomba & T. Banta (Eds.), *Assessing student competence in accredited disciplines* (pp. 71–95). Sterling, VA: Stylus.

Candela, L., Dalley, K., & Benzel-Lindley, J. (2006). A case for learning-centered curricula. *Journal of Nursing Education, 45*(2), 59–66.

Chaffee, M. W., & McNeill, M. M. (2007). A model of nursing as a complex adaptive system. *Nursing Outlook, 55*(5), 232–241.

Clancy, T. R., Effken, J. A., & Pesut, D. (2008). Applications of complex systems theory in nursing education, research, and practice. *Nursing Outlook, 56*(5), 248–256.

Csokasy, J. (2002). A congruent curriculum philosophical integrity from philosophy to outcomes. *Journal of Nursing Education, 41*(1), 32–33.

Dekker, S., & Fischer, R. (2008). Cultural differences in academic motivation goals: A meta-analysis across 13 societies. *The Journal of Educational Research, 102*(2), 99–110.

Diekelmann, N. L., Ironside, P. M., & Gunn, J. (2005). Recalling the curriculum revolution—Innovation with research. *Nursing Education Perspectives, 26*(2), 70–77.

Doane, G. H., & Brown, H. (2011). Recontextualizing learning in nursing education: Taking an ontological turn. *Journal of Nursing Education, 50*(1), 21–26.

Elder, L., & Paul, R. (2006). *The thinker's guide to analytic thinking* (2nd ed.). Dillon Beach, CA: The Foundation for Critical Thinking.

Ervin, N., Bickes, J., & Schim, S. (2006). Environments of care: A curriculum model for preparing a new generation of nurses. *Journal of Nursing Education, 45*(2), 75–80.

Fawcett, J. (1989). *Conceptual models of nursing.* Philadelphia, PA: F. A. Davis.

Fawcett, J. (2000). *Analysis and evolution of contemporary nursing knowledge: Nursing models and theories.* Philadelphia, PA: F. A. Davis Company.

Feiman-Nemser, S. (2001). From preparation to practice: Designing a continuum to strengthen and sustain teaching. *Teachers College Record, 103*(6), 1013–1055.

Fetter, M. S. (2009). Curriculum strategies to improve baccalaureate nursing information technology outcomes. *Journal of Nursing Education, 48*(2), 78–85.

Fischer, H. E., Klemm, K., Leutner, D., Sumfleth, E., Tiemann, R., & Wirth, J. (2005). Framework for empirical research on science teaching and learning. *Journal of Science Teacher Education, 16*(4), 309–349.

Forbes, M. O., & Hickey, M. T. (2009). Curriculum reform in baccalaureate nursing education: Review of the literature. *International Journal of Nursing Education Scholarship, 6*(1). doi:10.2202/1548-923X.1685

Giddens, J. F., & Brady, D. P. (2007). Rescuing nursing education from content saturation: The case for a concept-based curriculum. *Journal of Nursing Education, 46*(2), 65–69.

Glatthorn, A. A., Bosche, F., & Whitehead, B. M. (2006). *Curriculum leadership development and implementation.* Thousand Oaks, CA: Sage.

Glennon, C. (2006). Reconceptualizing program outcomes. *Journal of Nursing Education, 45*(2), 55–59.

Goudreau, J., Pepin, J., Dubois, S., Boyer, L., Larue, C., & Legault, A. (2009). A second generation of the competency-based approach to nursing education. *International Journal of Nursing Education Scholarshop, 6*(1). doi:10.2202/1548-923X.1685

Grier, A. S. (2005). Integrating needs assessment into career and technical curriculum development. *Journal of Industrial Teacher Education, 42*(1), 59–66.

Inderbitzin, M., & Storrs, D. A. (2008). Mediating the conflict between transformative pedagogy and bureaucratic practice. *College Teaching, 56*(1), 47–51.

Indiana University School of Nursing. (2004). *Baccalaureate program outcome statements.* Indianapolis, IN: Author.

Institute of Medicine. (2001). *Crossing the quality chasm: A new health system for the 21st century.* Washington, DC: The National Academies Press.

Institute of Medicine. (2003). *Health professions education: A bridge to quality.* Washington, DC: The National Academies Press.

Institute of Medicine. (2010). *The future of nursing: Leading change, advancing health.* Washington, DC: The National Academies Press. Retrieved from http://www.nap.edu/catalog/12956.html

Keith, N. Z. (1991). Assessing educational goals: The national movement to outcome evaluation. In M. Garbin (Ed.), *Assessing educational outcomes* (pp. 1–23). New York, NY: National League for Nursing.

Lindeman, C. A. (2000). The future of nursing education. *Journal of Nursing Education, 39*(1), 5–12.

MacIntyre, R. C., Murray, T. A., Teel, C. S., & Karshmer, J. F. (2009). Five recommendations for prelicensure clinical nursing education. *Journal of Nursing Education, 48*(8), 447–453.

McEwen, M., & Brown, S. C. (2002). Conceptual frameworks in undergraduate nursing curricula: Report of a national survey. *Journal of Nursing Education, 41*(1), 5–14.

Mezirow, J. (1991). *Transformative dimensions of adult learning.* San Francisco, CA: Jossey-Bass.

National Institute of Education. (1984). Involvement in learning: Realizing the potential of American higher education. Final report of the study group of the conditions of excellence in American higher education (ED246833). Washington, DC: Government Printing Office. Retrieved from http://www.eric.ed.gov:80/

National League for Nursing. (1993). *A vision for nursing education.* New York, NY: Author.

National League for Nursing Education Advisory Council Competency Work Group. (2010). *NLN education competencies model.* New York, NY: National League for Nursing. Retrieved from http://www.nln.org/

Nelson, M. L., Howell, J. K., Larson, J. C., & Karpiuk, K. L. (2001). Student outcomes of the healing web: Evaluation of a transformative model for nursing education. *Journal of Nursing Education, 40*(9), 404–413.

Newman, F., Couturier, L., & Scurry, J. (2004). *The future of higher education—Rhetoric, reality, and the risks of the market.* San Francisco, CA: Jossey-Bass.

Newman, M. (1997). Evolution of the theory of health as expanding consciousness. *Nursing Science Quarterly, 10*(1), 22–25.

Nightingale, F. (1969). *Notes on nursing.* New York, NY: Dover.

Oregon Consortium for Nursing Education. (2006). *OCNE curriculum.* Retrieved from http://ocne.org/

Pew Health Professions Commission. (1995). *Clinical challenges: Revitalizing the health professions for the twenty-first century.* San Francisco, CA: UCSF Center for the Health Professions.

Posner, G. F. (1998). Models of curriculum planning. In L. Beyer & M. W. Apple (Eds.), *The curriculum.* Albany, NY: SUNY Press.

Schreiber, R., & Banister, E. (2002). Challenges of teaching in an emancipating curriculum. *Journal of Nursing Education, 41*(1), 41–45.

Spelt, E. J. H., Biemans, H. J. A., Tobi, H., Luning, P. A., & Mulder, M. (2009). Teaching and learning in interdisciplinary higher education: A systematic review. *Educational Psychology Review, 21*, 365–378. doi:10.1007/s10648-009-9113-z

Tanner, C. A. (2007). The curriculum revolution revisited. *Journal of Nursing Education, 46*(2), 51-52.

Taylor, E. (2008). Transformative learning theory. *New Directions for Adult and Continuing Education, 119*, 5–15.

Taylor, M. A., Fischer, J. M., & Taylor, L. (2009). Factors relevant to the affective content in literature survey: Implications for designing an adult transformational learning curriculum. *Journal of Adult Education, 38*(2), 19–31.

Walker, L. O., & Avant, K. C. (1988). *Strategies for theory construction in nursing.* Norwalk, CT: Appleton & Lange.

Warda, M. R. (2008). Curriculum revolution: Implications for Hispanic nursing students. *Hispanic Health Care International, 6*(4), 192–199. doi:10.1891/1540-4153.6.4.192

Watson, J. (1997). The theory of human caring: Retrospective and prospective. *Nursing Science Quarterly, 10*(1), 49–52.

Webber, P. B. (2002). A curriculum framework for nursing. *Journal of Nursing Education, 41*(1), 15–24.

Wittmann-Price, R. A., & Fasolka, B. J. (2010). Objectives and outcomes: The fundamental difference. *Nursing Education Perspectives, 31*(4), 233–236.

Young, L., Frost, L. J., Bigl, J., Clauson, M., McRae, C., Scarborough, K. S., . . . Gillespie, F. (2010). Nurse educator pathway project: A competency-based intersectoral curriculum. *International Journal of Nursing Education Scholarship, 7*(1). doi:10.2202/1548.923X.2082

10 Developing Learner-Centered Courses

Diane M. Billings, EdD, RN, FAAN

Designing or redesigning courses for effective learning is an important aspect of the faculty role. Learner-centered courses are first and foremost designed based on a clear understanding of the students and their needs (Chapter 2). Thoughtful course design brings specificity to the school's mission and philosophy (Chapter 7) and program outcomes and curriculum design (Chapters 8 and 9), and sets the stage for choosing learning activities (Chapters 11 and 15) and assessment and evaluation strategies (Chapters 16 and 25). This chapter discusses a process that can be used to design learner-centered courses and explains how to develop a syllabus to communicate course expectations.

Learner-Centered Courses

In keeping with the shift from a focus on the teacher and teaching to a focus on the learner and learning, learner-centered courses focus on the needs of the student. Learner-centered courses are based on initial assessments of students' learning needs and are then designed to foster student inquiry, to facilitate students' learning as they construct their own knowledge, to promote interaction and collaboration, and to allow for choice in learning experiences and methods of assessment and evaluation.

Course Design Process

Course design follows a sequential process, starting with the broad program outcomes and ending with specific lesson plans (Candela, Dalley, & Benzel-Lindley, 2006; Diamond, 2008; Haas, Sheehan, Stone, & Hammer-Beem, 2009; Wiggins & McTighe, 2005). Although a sequential process is described here, the process is, in fact, iterative

as the course design or redesign unfolds. Courses may be designed by a faculty team or an individual with subject matter expertise. Instructional designers, a resource often available at teaching resource centers at many colleges, are an asset to the course development process.

Predesign

Course design begins by understanding the learning background and experience of the students who will enroll in the course, and then identifying how the course fits with overall academic program outcomes and competencies, the curriculum framework, and core concepts and competencies to be threaded within courses. During the predesign stage, faculty also should review, as needed, prerequisite, concurrent, or other courses if the course being developed is a part of a sequence. If the course has been taught previously, student course evaluations can provide additional insight for course development.

Prior to writing course outcomes, faculty also should review recommendations from national health care organizations; influential reports with recommendations for nursing education; and nursing organizations that make recommendations about essential competencies, concepts, and content as they relate to the course being developed. State and national accrediting agencies may also have prescriptive statements about course content and credit hour allocation.

Course Objectives, Outcomes, and Competencies

Course objectives, outcomes, and competencies are derived from end-of-program (terminal) and program-level (year or semester) outcomes and indicate what students should know, be able to do, and value at the end of the course, and how they will be evaluated and graded. Although faculty use terms in different ways, Wittman-Price & Fasolka (2010) suggest that the term *learning outcome* (as opposed to the term *objective*) is less restrictive and more appropriate in a learner-centered environment. Regardless of the term used, these "behavioral indicators" activate the curriculum, direct the choice of learning materials, guide the development of learning activities, and communicate to students what they are expected to learn and how they will be evaluated. Course learning objectives, outcomes, and competencies therefore must be written at appropriate levels of learning domains, for relevance to clinical practice, to be easily understood by students, and to guide evaluation of attainment.

Course Concepts and Content

Once learning outcomes are written, faculty can make decisions about the concepts and content to include in the course. Typically, faculty are selected to develop and teach courses because of their expertise with the content, and may be inclined to include all that is known about the subject; however, they also must design the course to fit within the curriculum and the level of practice for which the student is being prepared.

To prevent having a course burdened by content, Candela et al. (2006) recommend developing a process for making decisions about which content to retain and suggest including only content that is essential to meet program and course outcomes, that is required for safe practice, that needs to be reinforced and practiced, that is included in curriculum recommendations from professional nursing organizations, and that cannot be accessed easily when needed. Others (Davis, 2010; Diamond, 2008) recommend distinguishing between essential and optional material, considering core concepts versus details, and including only those topics relevant to practice or common existing problems. If the course is a part of a concept-based curriculum, the course designer must thread concepts and other broad outcomes and competencies, such as patient safety, communication, health information technology, or collaboration and teamwork, into the course (Giddens & Brady, 2007).

Organizing the Concepts and Content

Once core concepts and content are established, the next step is to organize them into units or lessons of related material. Courses can be organized in a variety of ways: using a logical sequence from beginning to end (for example, across the life span); following a sequential process (for example, the management process); by complexity (from simple to complex or from concrete to abstract); using a body systems approach; or, in the instance of case-based or problem-based learning, by inquiry about a particular problem. Regardless of how the concepts and content are organized, the structure should be evident to students and be consistent throughout the course.

Units and Lessons

By organizing the course into smaller units of study (modules, units, lessons), faculty provide additional direction for learning. For each unit or lesson, faculty should state the purpose, outcomes, assignments, learning activities, and evaluation strategies; this level of detail is particularly helpful for online or hybrid courses to provide necessary boundaries for unit or lesson activities (Chapter 23). Time limits must be considered when determining units of study; the time spent should be in proportion to the relative significance of the concepts and content and the students' ability to learn the material.

Learning Activities

Learning activities are selected to assist students in acquiring course learning outcomes (Chapter 11). They should be selected to provide opportunity for developing higher-order thinking and clinical decision-making skills (Benner, Sutphen, Leonard, & Day, 2010). Learning activities help students to synthesize content and concepts in context and connect the classroom to clinical practice (Benner et al., 2010). Learning activities should build from course to course, level to level, and be threaded throughout the course as they fit with the level and program outcomes. Learning activities can be designed to be completed as required assignments or as optional, supplemental, or remedial activities and can take place in class or be assigned as class preparation. Faculty should indicate how the learning activities will be used in the syllabus and provide information about how students will be given feedback or evaluated and graded.

Textbooks and Other Learning Resources

Faculty who are designing (or redesigning) courses have responsibility for choosing the course learning materials. These should be selected after faculty have determined the course outcomes, concepts and content, and learning activities. Students can also participate in the selection of learning materials, and faculty should design the course with sufficient options for students to choose resources that will meet their own learning needs.

When choosing learning materials, faculty should consider how these materials will align with course outcomes, fit with the course design, mirror faculty philosophy, and support students' learning needs. Faculty also should give careful consideration to how course materials will be used, for example, in class as a resource or as assigned readings as background for class participation. Faculty should avoid assigning excessive amounts of readings that do not respect the principle of effective use of time on task.

In many courses textbooks and other reading materials are the primary source of information. Beeson and Aucoin (2005) recommend that faculty focus on assigning essential content and focused reading assignments and building on the information from these readings during class.

Most textbook publishers offer ancillary study resources and web links, often at an additional cost. In one small study, researchers found that electronic textbook companion resources were not well used and that if faculty required students to purchase them, they should orient students to the materials available and integrate them into course learning activities (Missildine, Fountain, & Summers, 2009).

Another option for textbooks and readings is to create a custom-designed course pack with readings that include selected chapters from textbooks and reprints of required journal articles that are pertinent to the course. These can be deployed from publisher websites or to handheld devices or e-readers. Other faculty create course packs for print production or use e-reserve systems at the university library.

Regardless of the type and amount of course material, faculty must make course materials easy for students to access, provide directions about how and when to use them, and explain how the materials relate to course concepts and the evaluation and grading plan. This information should be included in writing in the syllabus.

Evaluation and Grading Plan

The final step of course design is to determine how student learning will be evaluated and how grades will be calculated and assigned (Chapters 16 and 25). Where possible, students should be able to choose among several options with regards to how their work will be evaluated and graded. The evaluation plan should be included in the syllabus to inform students of when and how evaluation will take place.

Course Syllabus

The syllabus communicates information about the course and specifies the responsibilities of both students and faculty (Clark, 2009; Davis & Schrader, 2009; Iwasiw, Goldenberg, & Andrusyszyn, 2009; O'Brien, Millis, & Cohen, 2008). A well-developed syllabus serves as a student guide to attaining course learning outcomes and explains how learning will be assessed, evaluated, and graded. Equally important, the syllabus sets the tone for the course by introducing the faculty and the faculty's philosophy, university, school, and course policies and norms for behavior to be demonstrated during the course; as such, it should be written in a welcoming style. The syllabus for a learner-centered course also explains the roles of the faculty and students in the teaching–learning process and conveys the attitudes and behaviors that will promote active and effective learning.

A course syllabus is developed for both on-campus and online courses. Additional information about using course management systems and course participation from a distance should be included in the syllabus for hybrid or blended and fully online courses.

A *full* course syllabus includes essential information about the course and information for students about how to implement the course. An *abbreviated* form of the syllabus may be developed as required by the university or school of nursing and contains basic information about course requirements; this abbreviated syllabus may also be required to be posted in the school or campus learning management system (LMS), and in this case may be limited to the style format of the LMS. Some schools publish the abbreviated syllabus on the website and offer full course information in electronic or print format at the beginning of the course.

A full course syllabus includes information about course implementation, university and school policies, and norms for behavior. The full course syllabus is described below. (See Boxes 10-1 and 10-2, and Box 14-2 in Chapter 14, for examples of course syllabi.)

Information about the Course

The following essential information should be included in the syllabus: title, purpose, description, prerequisites, corequisites, outcomes, teaching–learning strategies, learning activities, topical outline, policies and procedures, assessment and evaluation strategies, and the grading plan. In addition, faculty should list all dates for course meetings. If the course meets in varied places throughout the semester, such as online at synchronous or asynchronous times, in a learning resources center, or at a clinical agency, it is imperative to indicate this

---

BOX 10-1 Example of a Full Syllabus for an Undergraduate Nursing Course

B244 Comprehensive Health Assessment: Didactic Course Syllabus

COURSE INFORMATION

- 2 didactic credit hours
- Placement in Curriculum: Sophomore year, 3rd semester
- Prerequisites: N261 and all other Freshman year courses
- Co-requisites: B245, N217, B231, B232

FACULTY

XXXXX, Course Leader
Office: XXX Office Phone: XXXXXXX
Office hours: XXXX
Email: XXXX

COURSE DESCRIPTION

This course focuses on helping students acquire skills to conduct a comprehensive health assessment, including the physical, psychological, social, functional, and environmental aspects of health. The process of data collection, interpretation, documentation, and dissemination of assessment data will be addressed.

COURSE COMPETENCIES

At the completion of this course, the student will be able to:
1. Use the problem-solving process in the comprehensive nursing health and physical assessment of pediatric and adult clients.
2. Integrate biological, psychological, developmental, nutritional, and sociocultural theories and principles for health assessment and promotion of pediatric and adult clients.
3. Incorporate primary care principles related to disease prevention, early detection of health alterations, and education to maximize health and wellness for diverse pediatric and adult clients.

REQUIRED TEXT

Weber, J., & Kelley, J. (2009). *Health assessment in nursing* (4th ed.). Philadelphia: Lippincott, Williams & Wilkins. ISBN-13: 978-07817-81602 or ISBN-10: 0-7817-81604.

TEACHING STRATEGIES

Teaching strategies include lecture/discussion and supportive learning strategies for diagnostic reasoning, for example, audio- and videotapes, computer programs, models, and laboratory and clinical experiences.

EVALUATION

Evaluation consists of three (3) in-class examinations. Test #1 and Test #2 evaluate assessment of adult clients. Test #3 evaluates assessment of pediatric and adult clients. In addition to the three exams, students receive a score for taking the Kaplan Exam. Student must achieve a minimum final course grade of 73% for successful completion of the course. Exam scores are reported to the tenth place, e.g. 92.7 **and are not rounded up.** ONLY the final course grade will be rounded up. Grades at X.5 or above (examples 72.5 = 73 or 86.7 = 87), anything below a X.5 will not be rounded up (example 72.4 = 72 or 86.4 = 86). There is no extra credit offered in the BSN Program.

B244

Exam #1	100 points
Exam #2	100 points
Exam #3	100 points
Kaplan Exam	100 points
Total Points	400 points

Continued

BOX 10-1 Example of a Full Syllabus for an Undergraduate Nursing Course—cont'd

The following grading scale will be used:

97–100	A+	388–400 Points
93–96	A	372–387 Points
90–92	A–	360–371 Points
87–89	B+	348–359 Points
83–86	B	332–347 Points
80–82	B–	320–331 Points
77–79	C+	308–319 Points
73–76	C	292–307 Points
70–72	C–	280–291 Points
67–69	D+	268–279 Points
63–66	D	252–267 Points
60–62	D–	240–251 Points
59 or <	F	0–239 Points

ACADEMIC MISCONDUCT

Academic misconduct is a serious event that may result in an academic penalty or sanction. Misconduct includes cheating, fabrication, facilitation of cheating, unauthorized collaboration, interference, plagiarism, and violation of course rules. This includes, but is not limited to, assignments and examinations. Sanctions can result in a lower or failing grade on an assignment or exam. Sanctions can also result in probation or a course grade of "W" or "F". Additional sanctions may apply including dismissal from the nursing program. Refer to the Code of Student Rights, Responsibilities, and Conduct at http://www.iupui.edu/code.

SCHEDULE OF TOPICS

Orientation to B244 & B245, Assessment of Vital Signs & Assessment Techniques
Adult Health History
Assessment of Skin, Hair & Nails, and Pain Assessment
Assessment of Regional Lymphatics
Assessment of Breast, Testicle, and Genitalia
Assessment of Lungs & Thorax
Assessment of CV and PV systems
Assessment of Abdomen and GI System
Assessment of Musculoskeletal System
Assessment of Neurological System
Assessment of HEENT and Cranial Nerves
Assessment of the Newborn, Child, and Adolescent

SPECIAL NEEDS

***If you are an ENL (English as a New Language) student, please discuss this with your instructor prior to the first exam. If you need any special accommodation due to a disability, please contact Adaptive Educational Services at XXX or e-mail XXX. AES is located in XXXX.

Courtesy Dr. Rachel Walsh, with permission from Indiana University School of Nursing.

BOX 10-2 Example of a Syllabus for a Graduate-Level Course

Indiana University School of Nursing—Indianapolis Campus Department of Adult Health Master's Program Course Syllabus

COURSE NUMBER & TITLE	M559 Dynamics of Stress & Coping: Promoting Client Functioning
TOTAL CREDIT HOURS	2 credits—didactic 1 credit—clinical
NUMBER CONTACT HOURS	2 hours/week—didactic 5 hours/week—clinical
PLACEMENT IN CURRICULUM	Fall, 2010

FACULTY

Name, title, credentials XXXX
Office: XXX (hours by appointment)
Phone: XXXX
Secretary: XXX
Email: XXXX

COURSE DESCRIPTION

The course is designed to provide opportunities to analyze, synthesize, and apply knowledge of stress and coping. From observations, client and faculty interactions the student develops the ability to assess the stress experience of the person and make clinical judgments on the need for nursing intervention. Appropriate nursing interventions are based on emergent data within the framework of psychological and psychophysiological stress and related theories.

Therapeutic communication is inherent in the effective utilization of a conceptual framework of stress management in caring for persons experiencing stressful situations. Opportunities are provided for the student to become aware of how his/her communication patterns affect others in order to develop or increase competency in the therapeutic use of self with persons experiencing stress.

BOX 10-2 Example of a Syllabus for a Graduate-Level Course—cont'd

COURSE OBJECTIVES

Evidence of the student's achievement of the purposes of the course is reflected in the student's ability to:

1. Comprehend major psychological and psychophysiological theories of stress which provide a basis for nursing actions with persons experiencing psychological and/or psychophysiological stress.
   a. Identify correlational and causal theoretical relationships among concepts concerning psychological and psychophysiological stress.
   b. Compare and contrast theoretical relationships among stress and coping concepts.
   c. Identify research support for the theoretical relationships among concepts proposed to explain stress phenomena.
   d. Identify nursing implications from empirically supported theoretical relationships among stress concepts.
   e. Develop through use of theoretical and empirical data an operational framework for the assessment and diagnosis of stress and coping experiences.
2. Analyze clinical data obtained while caring for adults who are experiencing stress.
   a. Discern consistent patterns of psychological coping strategies and behaviors.
   b. Identify bio-psycho-social-familial interaction influences on the person's experience of stressors.
   c. Identify relationships between scope and intensity of stressor and the emergence of effective or ineffective coping strategies.
3. Synthesize theoretical and clinical data to formulate nursing diagnoses that identify potential problems, existing problems, and strengths as pertinent to the client's experience of stress and coping effectiveness.
   a. Formulate working diagnoses that are validated with the client.
   b. Utilize theoretical/operational frameworks which explain psycho-physiological-behavioral phenomena in stress-related experiences.
   c. Identify testable theoretical relationships among concepts that are inherent in derived nursing diagnoses.
4. Apply stress management interventions with persons who are experiencing stress.
   a. Initiate approaches to assist client to examine and evaluate the stress experience and coping effectiveness.
   b. Design with client appropriate nursing interventions taking into account client goals, health and/or illness care needs, social and familial interactions, and the nursing diagnosis.

   c. Modify interventions based on emergent data and other factors arising in the clinical situation.
   d. Identify testable theoretical relationships among concepts that are pertinent to the formulation of specific nursing interventions.
5. Evaluate effectiveness of nursing interventions with persons utilizing criteria jointly established by client and RN student.
   a. Evaluate outcomes of nursing intervention to assist client in lessening impact of stressors or in increasing coping effectiveness.
   b. Assess the value of the interpersonal stress management encounter for the client and formulate implications for future stress management interactions.
6. Accept responsibility in participating in overall plan of care of the client.
   a. As agreed to by client, communicate to appropriate staff members the assessment, nursing diagnosis, stress management plan, and outcomes of counseling relationship.
   b. Communicate to appropriate staff members recommendations for continued nursing approaches related to person's stress management.
   c. Participate in team conferences, group meetings, or other activities within the agency as necessary to carry out clinical activities.
   d. Examine own role in situational stress management counseling with clients who are experiencing stress.

TEACHING STRATEGIES

The primary teaching–learning strategies will include weekly seminar discussions; development of the student's own objectives; written assignments related to selected stress and coping theories/models; reflective learning journaling in student forum; clinical requirements include conducting stress counseling sessions with patients, participation in precepting group sessions, and completion of client data sheets; and completion of written self-evaluation.

COURSE REQUIREMENTS

1. *Weekly seminar discussions* in which students assume major participation responsibilities in analyzing, applying, and evaluating psychological and psychophysiological stress theories, research, and stress management strategies.
2. *Development of the student's own objectives* for personal and professional growth. In addition, one or more objectives can be written with respect to course content and/or client/patient experiences. A draft of these objectives is to be prepared for the *second week* of the semester. An evaluation of the extent to which the objectives were met needs to be included in the end of semester self-evaluation.

Continued

BOX 10-2 Example of a Syllabus for a Graduate-Level Course—cont'd

3. *Written Requirements:*
A. Three Concept Briefs: (**15% [5% each]** of final grade)
Each concept brief will be a 2–3 page paper 1) defining stress and coping concepts, 2) identification of implications for nursing assessment, and 3) discussion of measurability.
   A-1. Concept Brief #1—Stress, Demands, Resources, Threats
   • Define "stress".
   • Define "demands" including types of demands with examples, implications for assessment, and measurability.
   • Define "resources" including types of resources with examples, implications for assessment, and measurability.
   • Define "threat" with two examples.
   A-2. Concept Brief #2—Appraisal, Coping
   • Define "appraisal" including each type of appraisal and implications for assessment and measurability.
   • Define "coping" including each type of coping and implications for assessment and measurability.
   A-3. Concept Brief #3—Outcomes
   • Define "outcomes" including types of outcomes and implications for assessment and measurability.
B. Research Critique and Nursing Implications: (**15%** of final grade)
Research critique and nursing implication paper needs to focus on a research study focused on stress or stress management. Article will be assigned. *Consult the research critique/nursing* implications guidelines for M559 for the assignment.
C. Stress Counseling Synthesis Paper: (**20%** of final grade)
A written paper integrating Lazarus and Folkman's theory on stress and coping, and pertinent research, to your patient population. Paper will include critique of research findings and appropriateness to your patient population and implications for your practice. The paper should be 10 to 15 pages *using A.P.A. style for college papers.* A paper will be marked down one letter grade if it is not written with clarity; is not grammatically correct; has spelling errors; and/or does not follow APA format. (See guidelines for stress counseling paper)
4. *Clinical requirements:*
A. Stress counseling sessions (**20%** of final grade)
   1) Select a client population of particular interest to you. If you select a hospitalized population, take into consideration the need for a hospital stay that is long enough for you to have a chance to see the person at least 2–3 times in the hospital (home follow-up is also possible).
   2) Work with faculty and appropriate others to gain access to clients in the health care or other facility. If using a facility with which you are familiar, please identify appropriate persons to be contacted by faculty regarding your experience.
   3) Assume responsibility for obtaining written permission for audiotaping of sessions from the client and when necessary by hospital policy from the client's physician. (See permission to audiotape).
   4) Make contact with clients for the purpose of establishing a verbal contract for your sessions with them, including audiotaping.
   5) Conduct minimum of *five* stress counseling sessions with clients.
   6) Maintain collaborative relationships with appropriate staff in the hospital or other health care facility.
B. Precepting (validation) sessions
   1) Meet with faculty preceptor after each session with a client. This session is to precede the next session with the same client or a new client.
   2) Plan on *two to three hours* for each precepting group session, since multiple students will be sharing tapes during each session.
   3) Evaluate during precepting sessions the appropriateness and effectiveness of your own and other student's stress management communication and counseling skills in validating a working diagnosis, in planning nursing interventions, in evaluating coping responses and nursing interventions with clients.
C. Clinical Capstone Data Sheet: (**25%** of final grade)
Written analysis of stress counseling with client(s) that includes assessment, diagnosis, intervention plan, and evaluation of outcome.
M559 clinical data sheets are to be completed prior to the precepting group sessions, copied, and distributed to students and faculty in the precepting sessions. Data sheets will be initially reviewed by faculty during the precepting session and feedback given. These sheets may be hand written. Blank forms will be emailed to you using Oncourse. The **fifth** capstone data sheet will be used to determine the grade for this category.
Guidelines for counseling data forms:
   1) Identify context (see demographic information on data sheet).
   2) Identify client's stressor (threats) and challenges, emotions, coping responses, and coping resources.
   3) Derive nursing diagnoses regarding stress management needs.
   4) Develop nursing interventions to facilitate client's stress management.

BOX 10-2 Example of a Syllabus for a Graduate-Level Course—cont'd

5) Evaluate effectiveness of nursing interventions.
6) Identify theoretical and research basis for nursing diagnoses, and nursing interventions.
7) Identify "A" behaviors met on each data sheet.

NOTE: See guidelines for "A" behaviors for the M559 data sheets and for clinical requirements. The "A" behavior guidelines will be used by your preceptor for feedback and evaluation purposes.

5. Self-Evaluation (**5%** of final grade)
A. Written evaluation of your performance through the course includes:
1) Participation/contributions to weekly seminar/forum discussions.
2) Achievements/progress in meeting your own objectives/goals, which you established early in the course.
3) Achievements/progress through the course in gaining theoretical understanding of the stress experience (theories, research, stress management strategies).
4) Achievements/progress through the course in the application of theory, research and stress management strategies to your nursing practice.
5) Achievements/progress through the course in written assignments.
6) Achievements/progress in conduct of stress counseling sessions with clients. (Use "A" Behavior Guidelines for Situational Stress Management Counseling.)
7) Participation/contributions to precepting group sessions.
8) Achievements/progress in use of M559 Data Sheets. (Use "A" Behavior Guidelines for M559 Data Sheets)

B. Assign yourself a grade that you believe reflects your achievement in the course.
NOTE: not assigning yourself a grade results in not receiving a grade for this portion of the course.

REQUIRED TEXTS:

Burns, D.D. (1980). *Feeling good. The new mood therapy.* NY: New American Library.

Lazarus, R.S. & Folkman, S. (1984). *Stress, appraisal and coping.* NY: Springer.

Mckay, M., Davis, M. & Fanning, P. (1997). *Thoughts & feelings. Taking control of your moods & your life.* Oakland, CA: New Harbinger Publications.

CLINICAL EXPERIENCES:

Student completes 525 hours of supervised clinical practice as an Adult CNS major which includes 75 clinical hours in M559. Clinical time designated in each course is expected to directly relate to achievement of the specified clinical course competencies. Library work must be related to clinical outcomes and initiatives. Those wishing to count conference attendance must demonstrate to the course faculty how conference content directly relates to the attainment of CNS role competencies. Only content approved for continuing education contact hours will be considered. Faculty may require written or verbal reports about conference sessions or other clinical experiences as documentation of attainment of competencies. Final decisions regarding clinical preceptors, projects, and experiences are the responsibility of course faculty. Students should negotiate all clinical experiences with the faculty of record prior to the experience for which they are seeking clinical practice credit.

Courtesy Patricia Ebright, Jan Fulton, and Yvonne Lu, with permission from Indiana University School of Nursing.

information at the outset. Because the syllabus is an implied contract between the student and faculty, all involved must plan to adhere to the dates posted.

Information about the Faculty's Philosophy of Teaching and Learning

Faculty should include basic information such as name, rank, office hours, general availability, and contact information, with preferred way of contacting faculty. Faculty should also note their availability inside and outside of class. If providing telephone contact information, it is appropriate to set limits on when students can contact faculty and

for what reasons. In online courses, faculty may include more personal biographical information accompanied by a photograph or a short welcome video. Faculty should also provide a short description of their philosophy of teaching and learning to help students understand their particular point of view.

Course Materials and Resources

In this section faculty can provide information about required and supplemental readings such as textbooks, journal readings, and course pack information.

Course Requirements

A section of the full syllabus should include course requirements, including information about class attendance, clinical assignments, class participation, exams, and written work. Davis and Shrader (2009) found that students most wanted the syllabus to include information about how to complete the course requirements in an effective and efficient way. Faculty also should specify the consequences of not meeting course requirements and whether there are options for completing late or missed requirements, particularly in courses with clinical practica.

Course Grading Policies

In the full syllabus, faculty can provide detailed information about assignments and how they will be graded; rubrics facilitate clarity. Faculty should provide dates for assignments and tests, procedures for test makeup, information on the use of optional graded assignments, and procedures for late papers and projects, and should inform students when results from tests and papers will be available.

Study Assistance

If the campus or school provides resources to assist students with study and writing skills, this information can be noted in the syllabus. Faculty can also make suggestions for how students can learn the course material and how students can form their own study groups.

Course, School, and Campus Policies

Each school of nursing and campus has its own set of policies with specified consequences related to codes of conduct, academic honesty, incivility, criminal acts, student privacy, and resources for students with disabilities or special needs. This information can be provided in the syllabus with links to appropriate campus or school websites.

Course Norms

Course norms are guidelines for behavior in the classroom. Course norms can be written to describe expectations for individual and group participation and active learning within the class, when the use of computers and cell phones is acceptable, how to handle arriving late or leaving early, and how to prevent and manage other annoying or uncivil behavior (Chapter 14).

At the beginning of each course, faculty should spend time explaining and answering questions, soliciting input from the students, and modifying the syllabus as appropriate. Clark (2009) notes that clarifying expectations at the outset promotes desired classroom behavior. Faculty can ask students to commit to the behaviors specified in the syllabus in writing; in online courses, faculty can ask students to send an e-mail or post in the discussion forum indicating their agreement with the document. The syllabus then becomes a learning contract that can be reviewed and referred to throughout the course.

Evaluation of Course Design

Once the course and syllabus are sufficiently developed, and prior to their use with students, faculty can request internal and external review. Teaching colleagues can review the course for content accuracy, completeness, and fit with curricular threads. For additional and external review, faculty can consult curriculum and course design experts at the campus teaching center, if available. Ultimately, the course is submitted to the course review process of the curriculum committee as designated at the school of nursing and the college.

SUMMARY

Learner-centered courses are the bridge from general curriculum outcomes to specific concepts and content with associated learning activities that prepare the student for nursing practice. Developing or revising courses follows a systematic process that emphasizes student learning and attainment of course and curricular outcomes. A syllabus is used to communicate information about the course and expectations for learning and professional behavior during the course.

REFLECTING ON THE EVIDENCE

1. Review an existing course. What design elements exist? How were the course concepts and content determined? Is the organizing structure evident?

2. Review a course syllabus. Does it contain the elements necessary to communicate information about the course to the students? Evaluate the "tone" of the syllabus; does it welcome the student to the course?

REFERENCES

Beeson, S. A., & Aucoin, J. (2005). Assigning readings, faculty perceptions and strategies. *Nurse Educator, 30*(2), 62–64.

Benner, P., Sutphen, M., Leonard, V., & Day, L. (2010). *Educating nurses.* San Francisco, CA: Jossey-Bass.

Candela, L., Dalley, K., & Benzel-Lindley, J. (2006). A case for learning-centered curricula. *Journal of Nursing Education, 45*(2), 59–66.

Clark, C. M. (2009). Faculty field guide for promoting student civility in the classroom. *Nurse Educator, 34*(5), 194–197.

Davis, B. G. (2010). Preparing or revising a course. Retrieved from http://honolulu.hawaii.edu/intranet/committees/FacDevCom/guidebk/teachtip/prepcors.htm

Davis, S., & Schrader, V. (2009). Comparison of syllabi expectations between faculty and students in a baccalaureate nursing program. *Journal of Nursing Education, 48*(3), 125–130.

Diamond, R. M. (2008). *Designing and assessing courses and curricula* (3rd ed.). San Francisco, CA: Jossey-Bass.

Giddens, J. F., & Brady, D. P. (2007). Rescuing nursing education from content saturation: The case for a concept-based curriculum. *Journal of Nursing Education, 46*(2), 65–69.

Haas, B. A., Sheehan, J. M., Stone, J. A., & Hammer-Beem, M. J. (2009). Application of the Newell liberal arts model for interdisciplinary course design and implementation. *Journal of Nursing Education, 48*(10), 579–582.

Iwasiw, C. L., Goldenberg, D., & Andrusyszyn, M. (2009). *Curriculum development in nursing education.* Boston, MA: Jones & Bartlett.

Missildine, K., Fountain, R., & Summers, L. (2009). Textbook companion electronic study materials: Are students using them? *Nurse Educator, 34*(3), 107–108.

O'Brien, J. G., Millis, B. J., & Cohen, M. W. (2008). *The course syllabus: A learning-centered approach.* San Francisco, CA: Jossey Bass.

Wiggins, G., & McTighe, J. (2005). *Understanding by design.* Columbus, OH: Pearson/Merrill/Prentice Hall.

Wittman-Price, R. A., & Fasolka, B. J. (2010). Objectives and outcomes: The fundamental difference. *Nursing Education Perspectives, 31*(4), 233–236.

11

Selecting Learning Experiences to Achieve Curriculum Outcomes

Martha Scheckel, PhD, RN

The purpose of the curriculum is to present students with a cohesive body of knowledge, attitudes, and skills that are necessary for professional nursing practice. A curriculum provides the means of delivering a course of study designed to support the achievement of intended outcomes (Ellis, 2004). The curriculum is implemented for both faculty and students through teaching strategies and learning activities. This chapter focuses on designing and selecting learning activities for effective implementation of the teaching–learning process. The rationale that guides the design and selection of learning activities is reflected in the understanding that students should be educated for self-development and various nursing roles in society. Selecting experiences that enable meeting curriculum outcomes cannot be accomplished through a casual, hit-or-miss approach; learning activities must be thoughtfully designed to offer students the opportunities necessary to achieve the intended curriculum outcomes.

Defining Learning Activities and Teaching Strategies

In recent years, there has been an increased emphasis on learning and learner-centered instruction, shifting the focus in education away from teacher-centered instruction. Learning activities that are *learner-centered* focus on students becoming empowered to participate in designing learning tasks, which facilitates their responsibility for acquiring the knowledge and abilities specified by curriculum outcomes (Greer, Pokorny, Clay, Brown, & Steele, 2010).

The author acknowledges the work of Pamela R. Jeffries, DNS, RN, FAN, ANEF, and Barbara Norton, RN, MPH, in the previous edition(s) of the chapter.

When faculty design an instructional strategy to provide specific kinds of student learning experiences, the instructional strategy is then referred to as a *learning activity* or a *learning experience*.

Conversely, teaching strategies, teaching methods, and teaching techniques are *teacher-centered* strategies that are used to describe the kinds of activities faculty engage in when teaching. Faculty need to select instructional strategies that match the outcomes, competencies, and objectives of the curriculum (see Chapters 9 and 10) so that students have the opportunity for maximum learning. In contemporary education, for optimal learning, teacher-centered strategies must be counterbalanced with learner-centered strategies.

Student Learning Activities

Faculty are responsible for arranging the learning activities and conditions necessary to ensure that learning occurs. It is essential that faculty understand that learning activities are an integral part of the curriculum and courses and, as such, they must be purposeful, planned, and organized. Learning activities are designed to engage students in listening to and interacting with others, observing, thinking, and doing in a manner that highlights the knowledge, attitudes, competencies, and skills to be acquired. For example, activities situated in narrative pedagogies promote clinical reasoning across time by allowing students to analyze illness trajectories within actual life contexts (Benner, Sutphen, Leonard, & Day, 2010, p. 225).

Other examples of learning activities include participating in simulations, using case studies, doing writing assignments such as journaling, developing care plans and pathways, doing concept mapping, engaging in discussions or debates, and using computer-mediated activities and resources such as computer-assisted instruction and the World Wide Web. Learning activities can be designed for use by individual students, pairs of students, or small groups of students.

Designing Learning Activities

Learning activities should be designed to contribute to the achievement of the major objectives or competencies of a course and the curriculum. Any learning activity should articulate with previous and subsequent activities, providing cohesiveness in such a way that students are able to understand the connections and relationships between facts, concepts, theories, and principles. Activities should provide students with opportunities to acquire knowledge and skills and apply specific areas of content and processes. Faculty need to plan and organize class time so that students become actively involved in the learning process because active involvement can result in increased retention and a deeper understanding of content.

Passive and Active Learning

There are many theories that explain the learning process. Many of these theories are behaviorally, cognitively, or socially based (Jarvis, Holford, & Griffin, 2003) and include, but are not limited to, constructivism, brain-based learning, experiential learning, and adult learning. There are other learning theories that are situated in critical and feminist theory, phenomenology, and postmodernism (Diekelmann & Diekelmann, 2009). Common to each of these theories is the idea that learning may be a passive or an active process. Students typically experience both types of learning throughout their educational career.

Passive Learning

Passive learning, a mode of learning commonly present in many classrooms, occurs when students use their senses to take in information from a lecture, reading assignment, or some form of audiovisual media. Passive learning is commonly used to acquire ideas and information that are subsequently available through recall (Wingfield & Black, 2005).

Advantages

Passive learning provides faculty with the opportunity to present a great deal of information within a short period, and they can select and prepare in advance lecture notes, handouts, and audiovisual media. Faculty usually feel comfortable with these teaching methods because they can present the information that students need to learn in a controlled environment. For a faculty member who is new or one who is teaching new content for the first time, the instructional strategies used in passive learning may enable him or her to feel more comfortable in the teaching situation when presenting the content.

Because many students have been socialized to passive learning, they often prefer this approach to learning. Important concepts and content are identified for students in a concrete manner that helps them organize the material in a meaningful way. With passive learning, students tend to have lower anxiety levels and feel secure in their belief that listening to a lecture, reading the assignments and handouts, taking notes, and copying information from audiovisual media will provide them with all or most of the information they need to be successful in the course.

Disadvantages

Passive learning activities may leave faculty with little opportunity to understand how well students are learning the content. Unless designed otherwise, the time used for presentation of the content may leave little time for questions, clarification, or discussion. Students may not feel comfortable letting faculty know that they do not understand key points or relationships; furthermore, they may be reluctant to ask questions in class or they may not ask enough questions to clarify their misunderstandings. In addition, students may be unable to articulate what it is they do not know or understand.

Listening to a presentation, taking notes, and copying from printed media require little cognitive effort from students and no consistent use of higher-level cognitive skills. Even reading activities, although important, do not provide students with opportunities to apply the concepts about which they are reading. Although many students may prefer passive learning, over time passive learning experiences tend to become tedious.

Active Learning

Active learning involves the student through participation and an investment in exploring content knowledge in all phases of the learning process (Wolf, Bender, Beitz, Wieland, & Vito, 2004). It requires educational activities that provide students with the opportunity to actively engage in courses and respond to the learning situation (Price & Nelson, 2007).

Advantages

The benefits of active learning reported by many authors (Clark, 2007; Price & Nelson, 2007; Snelgrove, 2004) include, but are not limited to:
1. Increased attentiveness to learning
2. Greater interest in learning
3. Desire to use multiple ways of learning
4. Increased retention of information
5. Greater assimilation of learning
6. Deeper understandings of course material
7. Increased critical thinking skills
8. Increased problem-solving skills
9. Enhanced teamwork skills
10. Greater sense of accomplishment in learning

It is not always possible to determine whether students are actively involved in learning because their responses during a learning activity may be reticent. Reticence does not necessarily mean students are not learning. However, there are active learning activities that can make it easier for faculty to assess the degree of active learning. For instance, team-based learning, in which small groups of students work together independently within large classes, allows teachers to observe the extent of student preparation for class, students' use of materials related to the course, and their level of participation in class sessions (Clark, Nguyen, Bray, & Levine, 2008). Peer active learning is an approach in which students make apparent their critical thinking skills through think/pair/share, case-based learning, role playing, interactive presentations, and discussions (Stevens & Brenner, 2009). Virtual learning, while still in its early development, allows teachers to assess deep learning verses surface learning (Sand-Jecklin, 2007). *The Neighborhood* is one example where students experience deep learning through scenarios that unfold over time and that are situated in storytelling, case-based learning, and interpretive pedagogies (Giddens, 2007). Fostering active learning in the classroom is a faculty goal, and some evidence exists to support the view that active learning is preferred by some students (Harton, Richardson, Barreras, Rockloff, & Latané, 2002).

Disadvantages

Faculty need to be aware of content areas and relationships among concepts that usually pose difficulty for students. Organizing learning experiences so that students are engaged in active learning requires faculty to educate themselves about and design teaching strategies that are learner-centered rather than strictly teacher-centered. Examples of such strategies were related above, but can also include activities such as think-write-preview, in which students begin to think about topics by writing everything they know about them in 2 to 3 minutes; board workers, in which students work together to address pertinent questions; and bookends, in which students meet before an oral presentation to share what they know about a particular topic and generate questions to ask during and after the presentation (Price & Nelson, 2007).

Regardless of the active learning strategy employed, the shift to active learning paradigms may be stressful for faculty, particularly when trying these approaches with large groups of students. Furthermore, faculty may have concerns about receiving less favorable evaluations of instruction. Additionally, students are often resistant to changes in the way in which they receive instruction because understanding new ways of learning is stressful. They may be impatient with the process and averse to putting forth the effort needed to alter their learning style. In fact, Sand-Jecklin (2007) suggests that, despite recent evidence supporting active learning and teachers' use of it, nursing students still prefer to learn through memorization and recall. Support from faculty, administration, and peers is important if active learning strategies are to be incorporated into teaching practice.

Matching Learning Activities to Desired Outcomes

To determine the match of learning activities with the desired course outcomes, faculty can create a matrix to examine the relationships between the means (learning activities) and the ends (outcomes). Advance planning for how the learning activities relate to the course objectives facilitates the selection of a variety of activities for the course. Faculty and students enjoy and benefit from a variety of learning experiences. Variety helps prevent faculty and students from becoming bored and makes it more likely that faculty can accommodate different learning style preferences. Faculty should use a systematic approach in designing and selecting the learning activities for a course before actually teaching the course. The learning activity plan shown in Box 11-1 provides a useful approach for planning and evaluating learning activities for each of the course's class sessions.

Principles for Selecting Learning Experiences

Several principles and how to achieve them can guide faculty in planning learning activities (Davis, 2009).
1. Promote intellectual development by:
   a. being sufficiently structured (i.e., use criteria)
   b. encouraging multiple points of view
   c. facilitating thoughtful judgments and decision making

BOX 11-1 Learning Activity Plan

Date: _____
Class content focus:
_____

Learning objective and competency:
_____

Domain and domain level:
_____

Type of activity:
_____

Brief description of activity:
_____

Key concepts to be learned:
_____

Number of students in class:
_____

Types of resources needed:
_____

Time allowed for activity:
_____

Time allowed for debriefing and discussion:
_____

Issues and problems encountered:
_____

Students:
_____

Faculty:
_____

---

2. Help students contextualize information by:
   a. using real-world situations
   b. emphasizing deep learning through manageable work schedules, use of conceptual frameworks, and avoiding recall of meaningless details
   c. accounting for what they already know
3. Help students retain and apply information by:
   a. encouraging repeated review of materials
   b. making activities active rather than passive
   c. encouraging cooperation and group work
   d. giving immediate and specific feedback
4. Facilitate self-regulated learning by:
   a. assisting to manage learning resources
   b. giving students choices
   c. encouraging reflection on progress in learning

Structuring Course Materials

Informing students of the purpose and goals for learning allows teachers and students to use instructional activities to help students understand why they need to know the materials, fosters appreciation for learning, and invites them to learn new content in the future (Blumberg, 2009). It is advantageous to include the learning activities in the materials students receive at the beginning of the course. Placing learning activities in the same logical order as the content, in the sequence in which they will be used, and in proximity to the appropriate objectives or competencies enables students to have a holistic sense of how the learning activities relate to the course objectives and content. Students should be able to determine from the course materials the sequence and patterns of the course.

Structured and Unstructured Learning Activities

Learning activities may be structured or unstructured. Structured learning activities are frequently used and are important in assisting students to address and pose questions, solve problems, create solutions, and consider alternatives (Pascarella & Terenzini, 2005). Although unstructured learning activities may be used at the undergraduate level, they are more likely to be used in honors or honors option courses, independent study courses, and capstone courses. Faculty may also allow students to use unstructured learning activities for bonus credit.

Structured Learning Activities

In structured learning activities, the stimuli for learning are specifically selected. A structured activity consists of a clear, concise description of the purposes, objectives, and competencies related to the activity; the content and processes to be used while engaged in the activity; specific directions presented in a logical sequence indicating each of the steps to be followed; the time for the activity; and the method to be used to report its completion.

A well-structured activity allows students to function with a great deal of independence and creativity while working to achieve the desired outcomes. For example, when assigning students a text, article, or other form of media to study, providing specific questions directly related to the desired objectives and competencies assists students in focusing on the essential concepts. Faculty may choose any one of several methods for students to share the results of their learning experiences. For example, students may be required to do the following:

1. Complete an answer sheet that will be evaluated by peers, faculty, or both.
2. Write a general or specific summary report that addresses the content or processes and submit it to faculty.
3. Present a report to the class.
4. Discuss the experience with another student or small group of students.
5. Initiate a small group or class discussion of the major points, issues, or problems that arise during their work.

These methods can be used separately or in combination with each other. Faculty may also choose to allow the student to select the preferred method of sharing.

Unstructured Learning Activities

Unstructured learning activities are designed to allow students to acquire knowledge and skill with much less specific direction from faculty. This form of activity is derived from Bruner's discovery learning (Bruner, 1977) and, in recent times, has been called *inquiry-based learning* (Levy, Aiyegbayot, & Little, 2009). Discovery learning is believed to do the following:

1. Promote a disposition toward inquiry.
2. Promote independent thinking and enhanced problem solving.

3. Stimulate student motivation and interest.
4. Improve knowledge retention.
5. Facilitate transfer of learning by stimulating the student to seek and find relationships between information and the situation at hand.

A major limitation associated with discovery learning is the need for students to adapt to self-directed learning that is student-centered rather than teacher-centered (Bebb & Pittam, 2004).

In an unstructured learning activity, students may be given an assignment in which they are asked to apply their previous and current knowledge, skills, and experiences either to a specific faculty-designated situation or to a situation of their choice that fits a general profile described by faculty. The situation may be an actual event in the practice setting or an event that is depicted through a simulation, case study, or form of media. For example, in a community health nursing course, a learning outcome for students may be for them to become familiar with the kinds of activities and interactions that occur during a community meeting. Students would be directed to act as a participant–observer at a community-based meeting of their choosing. The meeting could be a support group for a particular health problem, a meeting of constituents with their legislator, a town board meeting, or a neighborhood association meeting. Students could be given the option of describing their experience verbally in class or at a clinical conference or by writing about it in a journal.

Critical Learning Experiences

Critical learning experiences are those that are considered to be essential to the curriculum. They are specific types of experiences that faculty have agreed that all students must achieve before successfully completing the course or program. Critical learning experiences are clearly and directly tied to one or more course objectives or program outcomes. These experiences are carefully selected so that each student engages in an activity that enables him or her to attain the specific essential competencies by the completion of the course or program.

When faculty decide to designate certain learning experiences as "critical" to the curriculum, it becomes necessary for faculty to make sure that all students will have the opportunity to participate in the experience. This does not mean, however, that all students must have exactly the same experience under the same or similar conditions. For example, when teaching about the care of patients with musculoskeletal disorders, faculty may decide that a critical learning experience for all students is to provide care to patients in skin and skeletal traction. The age of the patient, the setting in which the care is provided, and the specific type of skin or skeletal traction would not necessarily be specified in the learning objective. The identification of the concept of care of patients with skin and skeletal traction as a critical learning experience, however, would provide students the opportunity to develop the necessary competencies in caring for a patient in traction but still allow some flexibility and individualization regarding how that experience is designed.

Faculty and students may also collaborate to create different types of experiences that are expected to yield similar results consistent with the course objectives. For example, if a course learning objective states that all students are to develop a family nursing care plan, faculty may decide that this is such an essential part of the course that it will be identified as a critical learning experience. The objective for the critical learning experience would simply state: "The student will be able to develop a family nursing care plan." Faculty may agree on more than one appropriate way in which students may complete this critical learning experience. The following two examples demonstrate how this may be done:

Example 1. Students are required to make a series of visits over a period of weeks to a family in any community setting, such as their home, a day care center, a senior center, an extended care facility, a homeless shelter, or a church function. Over the course of the visits, students use the nursing process to develop a plan of care with the family and provide verbal or written reports to faculty, peers, and agency staff on the visits and the progress they are making. On completion of the visits, students will have completed a family nursing care plan. Faculty may choose to have students share their care plan with others in any one of a variety of ways. For example, students may present their completed care plan either verbally or in writing, either in clinical conference or as a case study, to faculty, peers, and agency staff. When a student develops a case study, faculty may want to obtain the student's permission to use it as a teaching tool with future students.

Example 2. As an alternative to family visits, faculty may offer students the opportunity to use case studies, simulations, or virtual excursions that present a scenario representative of the type of experience in which the students would engage in actual practice. These alternative activities could be used by a small group of clinical students, and care plans could be shared in the manner described in Example 1.

Both of these examples provide students with the opportunity to complete the desired critical learning experience of developing a family care plan, although different learning strategies are used in each example.

Learning Experiences with Technology

There is a growing emphasis on incorporating technology into the nursing curriculum. Technology must be a fixture in today's nursing curriculum; therefore nurse educators and nurses must accept the challenge of incorporating technology into nursing programs. Teaching with technology in the classroom and clinical setting and teaching students to use technology in patient care are both important in preparing nursing students for clinical practice. Teaching with technology currently includes simulation and e-learning modalities. Teaching technology for use in patient care includes developing competencies in informatics.

Simulation

A simulation is an event or situation constructed to reflect clinical practice as closely as possible to teach procedures and critical thinking (Jeffries, 2005). Unlike the traditional classroom setting, a simulation allows the learner to function in an environment that is as close as possible to a real-life situation and provides the opportunity for the learner to think spontaneously and actively rather than passively. Simulations should present realistic situations, require active involvement in problem solving, provide feedback on the process, and require the learner to act on the effects of the harmful actions.

When faculty decide to use simulation in the classroom or in clinical teaching, simulations should be developed at an appropriate level for the beginner or advanced beginner. Simulations should provide opportunities for students to select relevant assessment data, infer patient problems, and take appropriate actions (Jeffries, 2006). Ideally simulations present clinical situations that vary in complexity depending on the number of decisions that must be made, the clarity or ambiguity of the possible choices, and the urgency of the underlying problem. The complexity of each case has to be appropriate for the targeted learners.

When using a simulation, faculty should guide students in understanding why the data are relevant, what the critical issues are, and how the actions relate to the data and the issues. Assistance is also needed in viewing the clinical situation as a whole rather than as isolated segments of information.

Simulations can help enrich an environment by promoting interaction with students' minds, the content, and the equipment. Good educators attempt to make learning meaningful so that students can make connections, problem-solve, and think critically, and simulations are one way of doing that. Faculty should consider both the advantages and the challenges and barriers to simulation when deciding whether to develop and incorporate it into the learning environment (Table 11-1) (Hovancsek, 2007).

E-Learning Modalities

E-learning is the use of electronic learning tools that include, but are not limited to, web-based courses, online programs of study, podcast lectures, personal response systems, blogging, and social networking (Skiba, 2009; Skiba, Connors, & Jeffries, 2008). When using e-learning, the learning experiences must be selected with the same amount of attention to addressing identified competencies or learning outcomes as they are in traditional courses. However, the educator has an opportunity to select experiences that take advantage of e-learning tools. Bonnel and Smith (2010) outline several examples of e-learning tools and note the advantages:

1. Virtual tours that package web-based resources (e.g., use of relevant websites) on concepts learned in class can reinforce learning.
2. Personal response systems allow students to review course information and prepare for examinations.
3. Online courses that include surveys, discussion forums, and shared assignments promote applied learning.
4. Web conferencing software promotes real-time learning opportunities from a distance.
5. Audio-casts allow the creation of podcasts and voice-over PowerPoint to promote engagement in learning.

TABLE 11-1 Advantages and Challenges/Barriers in Using Simulation within the Curriculum

Advantages	Challenges/Barriers
Mistakes can be made without patient harm	More faculty preparation time to develop and conduct simulations
Can provide clinical experiences rarely seen	Only a small number of students per session
Experiences can be repeated to enhance learning	Simulation sessions must be offered repeatedly
Can promote critical reflective analysis of skill sets	Expense (maintaining equipment; fixing equipment; faculty workload; create new positions to maintain labs)
Immediate feedback from peers, teachers, and/or sophisticated equipment	Physical space limitations for equipment, teachers, and students in each simulation
Promotes active learning	Technical support for computer-based simulations
Decreases performance anxiety	Faculty development to ensure computer literacy
Increases critical thinking skills	Is learner-centered, requiring a paradigm shift for students (students need to become active learners)
Increases confidence	Faculty time to validate learning outcomes
Promotes team work	Research needed to ensure is financially and educationally sound

From Hovancsek, M. T. (2007). Using simulations in nursing education. In P. R. Jeffries (Ed.), *Simulation in nursing education: From conceptualization to evaluation* (pp. 5–6). New York, NY: National League for Nursing. (Included with permission.)

Regardless of the e-learning approach used, the role of the educator changes when he or she teaches using e-learning. Whether the electronic interaction occurs either synchronously or asynchronously, the educator becomes a "facilitator of learning." This means that he or she is not necessarily the primary source of information, as in a traditional classroom. Learning experiences are designed to encourage active learning among the students. The instructor assists the students to meet the learning goals and achieve expected outcomes. He or she also guides the students to assume responsibility for identifying their own needs and to be self-directed in the process of achieving expected outcomes. Table 11-2 lists

TABLE 11-2 Traditional Teaching versus E-Learning

Traditional Teaching	E-Learning
Learning is teacher-centered	Learning is student-centered
Classroom environment with a set time for class	Learning can take place anytime, anywhere
Instructor can read verbal and nonverbal cues	Instructor can interact in discussion forums, e-mails, chats, and other online activities
Face-to-face interaction with students	Electronic interactions and communication with students
Typically a fixed academic schedule (e.g., a semester or quarter)	Students may have more freedom in their class session or course start dates and completion times
Student interaction in the classroom	Student interaction can occur within and outside of the physical classroom space
Teaching occurs at a set time (e.g., Tuesdays 9 AM to noon)	Teaching is flexible: synchronous or asynchronous

differences between traditional teaching and e-learning in the curriculum.

Teaching Informatics

Teaching informatics in nursing has traditionally involved students' abilities to locate, evaluate, and use information in ways that support the delivery of nursing care (American Nurses Association, 2001; Graves & Corcoran, 1989). At its more basic level, it has involved developing information literacy. This includes teaching students to search library databases, find information related to a patient care problem, and evaluate the information for such things as authority, credibility, accuracy, objectivity, coverage, and purpose (Flood, Gasiewicz, & Delpier, 2010). At more advanced levels it includes teaching students to use informatics tools (Skiba et al., 2008) to assist them in learning to provide evidence-based practice, make effective clinical decisions, and provide safe, quality patient care. This means that teaching informatics includes more than increasing students' computer skills (Skiba et al., 2008). Rather, it includes assisting students to develop the knowledge, skills, and attitudes needed to use a multitude of health information systems for patient care,

including hardware, software, spreadsheet programs, and databases.

As teachers develop students' informatics competencies, it is important for them to know and integrate the most recent technological advances. Examples include mobile computing devices such as personal digital assistants (PDAs), iPhones, and smart phones (Skiba, 2010), and other technologies available on clinical units such as electronic medical records and data management systems (Bonnel & Smith, 2010). All of these technologies promote immediate access to information. For instance, students may use a PDA to access information on a disease and how to treat it, or to look up a medication. The advantage is the immediate access to information that students can readily apply in clinical practice. Teachers must exercise caution in ensuring that students use appropriate decision-making skills as they apply the information they access to patient situations. Similar to simulation, teachers must develop informatics competencies using beginner to advanced-level frameworks (Flood et al., 2010).

Despite the need to develop students' information literacy, barriers to integrating it into the curriculum include a lack of faculty competencies in information literacy, curricula that are already laden with content, and faculty uncertainty with how to integrate information literacy into the curriculum (McNeil, Elfrink, Beyea, Pierce, & Bickford, 2006). It is important for faculty to access new and emerging resources such as Technology Informatics Guiding Education Reform (www.tigerssummit.com) and Quality and Safety Education for Nurses (Cronenwett et al., 2007) that will allow them to become competent in informatics so that they can effectively contribute to students' competencies in this area of nursing education.

Domains of Learning and Learning Activities

Cognitive, psychomotor, and affective domains of learning provide a framework for learning activities that shape how students learn to provide high-quality care (Duan, 2006). Although the domains address the three aspects of learning (knowledge, skills, and attitudes) separately, they are actually interdependent (Bloom, 1956; Duan, 2006; Krathwohl, Bloom, & Masia, 1964).

After the desired outcomes related to each domain have been clearly delineated, faculty can then think creatively about the types of learning activities that will actively engage students in the process of learning. Learning activities need to be appropriate for the domain and domain level. One learning activity can be designed to meet several outcomes; those with a broad focus are especially helpful.

A sequence of learning activities is designed to provide continuity with previous learning and experiences. Although the same concepts may be used repeatedly, they should be applied to increasingly complex situations. Learning activities are designed to enable students to integrate concepts and recognize relationships. Combining and unifying concepts from the cognitive, psychomotor, and affective domains facilitates integration. For example, an activity focused on a specific skill such as taking a blood pressure requires knowledge, technical skill, communication skills, and valuing the importance of an accurate measurement.

Because nursing is a practice discipline that ultimately requires the application and synthesis of acquired knowledge, skills, and attitudes, faculty must keep in mind that the levels of the domains are sequenced in a hierarchical order progressing from the simple to the complex, thus enabling the learner to move toward these higher levels of learning. The underlying assumption is that each subsequent level builds on and integrates the prior set of knowledge, skills, and attitudes (Anderson & Krathwohl, 2001; Bloom, 1956).

For example, the hierarchical order presented by Bloom's (1956) taxonomy for the cognitive (knowledge) domain consists of six categories: knowledge, comprehension, application, analysis, synthesis, and evaluation. The following reveal the progression from the simple to the most complex cognitive processes:

1. Identifies steps in the epidemiological process (knowledge)
2. Differentiates among the steps in the epidemiological process (comprehension)
3. Applies the epidemiological process to common health conditions (application)
4. Relates the epidemiological process to patients' health conditions (analysis)
5. Proposes interventions based on the epidemiological process for patients' health conditions (synthesis)
6. Determines priorities for patients' health conditions based on the epidemiological process (evaluation)

Krathwohl et al.'s (1964) taxonomy for the affective (attitude) domain consists of five categories: attending, responding, valuing, organization, and characterization by value set. The following reveals the progression from the simple to the most complex affective processes:

1. Listens for patients' concerns about health conditions (attending)
2. Accepts patients' concerns about health conditions (responding)
3. Assumes responsibility for involving patients in decisions about self-care practices (valuing)
4. Develops nursing care plans incorporating patients' belief systems (organization)
5. Revises nursing care plans in accord with patients' preferences (characterizes values)

The separation of the cognitive, psychomotor, and affective domains is intended for classification purposes only, because they are closely interrelated. Behaviors in each domain have dimensions in the others, and one domain may be used as a vehicle to attain the others (Krathwohl et al., 1964). Knowledge must be possessed if it is to be applied, professional nursing values must be internalized if they are to be implemented in practice, and skills must be well practiced if they are to be safely executed in a variety of circumstances. Faculty need to guard against selecting domain levels that are too low on the hierarchy for the outcomes they want students to achieve.

Matching the Learning Activity with the Learning Domain

When choosing instructional materials, faculty need to consider the match between the learning materials, the desired outcomes, the learning domain and domain level, and student attributes. All instructional materials used during the course, such as textbooks, course handouts, articles, and media, including computer-assisted instruction programs, should be selected in accordance with their appropriateness for the learning objective, learning domain, and domain level. Faculty must also take into account the student's academic level, cognitive maturity, learning readiness, motivation, and interests, as well as the complexity of the course content, processes, and skills (Reilly & Oermann, 1990).

Faculty can expect the time required for students to attain the desired learning outcome in each domain to increase according to the complexity of the domain level. A reasonable amount of time for the teaching–learning process to occur needs to be allocated. The learning activity should facilitate learning and also be cost effective in terms of the use of time, effort, and resources for both faculty and students.

The Cognitive Domain

The categories in this domain include knowledge, comprehension, application, analysis, synthesis, and evaluation. Knowledge represents the lowest, or simplest, level of learning in the cognitive domain. At this level the learner focuses primarily on the acquisition and recall of specific facts, concepts, and principles. Ideally learners progress to a higher order of intellectual ability and through the more complex stages of cognitive learning. Higher levels of learning are the ability to understand the meaning of new information (comprehension), the ability to apply this information to a new situation (application), the ability to break down the information into its component parts (analysis), the ability to put together elements to form a new whole (synthesis), and the ability to make judgments about information and ideas (evaluation) (Reilly, 1980).

In recent years Bloom's taxonomy has been revised to reflect progress in contemporary knowledge of how people learn and how teachers teach (Anderson & Krathwohl, 2001). The revised taxonomy includes the six cognitive categories mentioned above, but adds another dimension to the cognitive domain through four kinds of knowledge (Anderson & Krathwohl, 2001, p. 27):

1. Factual: content elements
2. Conceptual: complex organized knowledge
3. Procedural: knowing how to do something
4. Metacognitive: knowledge of cognitive processes

This new dimension to the cognitive domain means that teachers can construct dualistic objectives or objectives that capture both the original cognitive domains and the new kinds of knowledge. Dualistic construction of objectives assists teachers to more effectively plan and diversify instructional strategies and assess the effectiveness of these strategies than using the cognitive domains alone (Ming Su, Osisek, & Starnes, 2005).

The lecture has been perhaps the most commonly used teaching method to instruct learners in the cognitive domain. However, the revised taxonomy encourages the use of not only lecture, but also small group activities, case studies, concept mapping (Ming Su, Osisek, & Starnes, 2004), questioning, and self-reflection activities (Ming Su et al., 2005).

The challenge in this domain is to select an appropriate action verb that clearly describes the desired level of student performance. When designing and selecting learning activities to fit the appropriate domain level, faculty need to consider all aspects of the activities and determine whether they provide students with the opportunities necessary to learn and practice the desired competencies. The following example written for a community health nursing course illustrates how an objective at the application level and learning activity can be matched:

Learning outcome: Students will apply the epidemiological process to common disease conditions.

Learning activity: The following directions are provided to students for the learning activity:

Before class read the assigned text section describing the steps of the epidemiological process. At the beginning of class form into groups of four to discuss your understanding of the reading, then select one disease condition to which you will apply all of the steps in the process. Write a brief summary of your work on a PowerPoint slide and be prepared to report your work to the class. You have 25 minutes to complete your group work and 10 minutes for your presentation. Faculty will be available for consultation.

This activity requires that the group members agree on a single disease condition, share and clarify their knowledge of the content and understanding of the task, and apply the epidemiological process as would be done in actual community health nursing practice. Although designed primarily for the cognitive domain, this activity also focuses students on the affective domain by raising their consciousness (level one) with regard to the importance of and opportunities for disease prevention, which is the primary focus of public health practice.

The Affective Domain

The affective domain of learning encompasses attitudes, beliefs, values, feelings, and emotions. Classification of affective behaviors, like that of the cognitive domain, is hierarchical. The categories are organized along a continuum of stages of internalization that reflect changes in personal growth, moving from an external to an internal locus of control (Krathwohl et al., 1964).

Storytelling, with the use of vivid images, has been recommended as a way of enhancing the development of the affective domain. The story could be an experience, a fantasy, or a combination of both. Learning activities that involve case studies, clinical decision making, group work, practice experiences, and writing also enhance the development of the affective domain.

Competency statements must be clearly written so that faculty can design learning experiences that help students develop the desired competencies and outcomes. It is also important for faculty to develop a systematic manner for assessing and evaluating students' progress (Krathwohl et al., 1964). The following example written for a community health nursing course illustrates how an objective at the valuing level of the affective domain and a learning activity can be matched:

Learning outcome: Students will assume responsibility for involving their patients and families in decisions about disease prevention self-care practices.

Learning activity: The following directions are provided to students for this learning activity:

You are to be prepared to discuss in clinical conference your plan to engage your patient or family in preventive health care decisions. Present your analysis of the patient and family assessment data that led you to identify the existence of an actual or potential problem that could be averted through the use of preventive self-care practices. Describe the approaches you will use to stimulate involvement of your patients in appropriate self-care practices. Be prepared to give a report on your progress in a future clinical conference.

Although this activity is designed to focus primarily on the affective domain, it is clear that students need to possess some in-depth knowledge of the epidemiology of specific health problems and be able to use data collection and communication skills. This activity directs students to integrate disease prevention strategies in the context of promoting self-care practices within the family.

The Psychomotor Domain

For the psychomotor domain, Reilly and Oermann (1990) described three types of skills: fine motor, manual, and gross motor. These are the skills most commonly used in the clinical techniques of nursing practice. Fine motor skills are those needed to implement tasks requiring exactness. Nursing skills such as preparing and administering parenteral medications, manipulating instruments to prepare and apply dressings, and manually adjusting intravenous fluid drip rates are examples of skills that fall into this category. Manual skills are those involving some common coordinated movements of the hand, arm, and eye. Nursing skills involving different types of touch, such as personal hygiene, suctioning, and the physical assessment skills of palpation and percussion, are examples of skills included in this group. Gross motor skills are those that use large muscle masses in body movements. Some nursing skills that require the use of gross motor skills are bed making, transferring and positioning, exercising, and cardiopulmonary resuscitation.

The psychomotor taxonomy suggested by Reilly and Oermann (1990) as the most useful for nursing was the one published in *Psychomotor Levels in Developing and Writing Objectives* (Dave, 1970). Dave's taxonomy is based on neuromuscular movement and coordination; the five levels in the taxonomy are imitation, manipulation, precision, articulation, and naturalization. Reilly and Oermann (1990, p. 84) created criteria for the levels that they believe are consistent with the developmental stages of competency; the criteria may be used to write learner objectives and competencies. Their criteria for each level are as follows:

1. *Imitation level*: The necessary actions are taken with some errors, there are some weaknesses in the smoothness of the gross motor actions, and the time used to complete the actions depends on the learner's needs.
2. *Manipulation level*: Written directives are followed with some degree of accuracy, and variations occur during the coordination of movements and the time taken to execute the actions.
3. *Precision level*: Actions are carried out in a logical sequence with few errors occurring only during some noncritical actions, movements are well coordinated, the time needed to execute the actions continues to be variable.
4. *Articulation level*: Coordinated actions are carried out in a logical sequence with limited errors, and the time used to execute the actions is reasonable.
5. *Naturalization level*: The skill performance demonstrates professional competence in that it is automatic with good coordination.

Within the nursing curriculum, students can learn psychomotor skills in various traditional and nontraditional settings. Different teaching strategies requiring considerable instruction, explanation, support, and facilitation about the process are needed by the educators teaching psychomotor skills. Faculty must orient students to the mechanism of the skill and encourage students to learn and practice the skills in the environment provided. Faculty can use a variety of instructional methods to provide learning, including "hands-on" instruction, even though the content originally may not be delivered in a traditional mode.

The following example created for a physical assessment course in the first semester of a baccalaureate nursing program illustrates how an objective at the articulation level in the psychomotor taxonomy and learning activity can be matched.

Learning outcome: Students will be skillful in using auscultation, palpation, and percussion to assess a person's pulmonary status.

 Learning activity: Students are given the following directions:

Read the assigned text and view the assigned DVDs in preparation for your rehearsal and practice session in assessing pulmonary status. Sign up on the schedule posted for the examining room to rehearse and practice these skills in triads. As a group, first discuss the equipment and manual technique you will use to implement the skills. Describe the sequence, positions, and patterns you will use on the chest during each skill. When you have finished this part of the activity, decide who will be the examiner, the examinee, and the participant-observer for the first round of practice. Begin your examination by describing to the examinee what you will be doing and then perform a complete assessment of your peer's chest in a systematic manner. At the completion of each separate assessment, make a written record of all of your findings. The participant-observer is to provide feedback on the skill and systematic approach used by the examiner. After completing the first examination, reverse roles with the participant-observer and complete the second and third rounds of practice. Compare your techniques and findings and share helpful hints with each examiner. During the rehearsal and practice, feel free to use faculty guidance and validation. At the completion of this activity, be prepared to discuss your experiences with faculty before or during the next class.

Although this learning activity is designed to focus primarily on skill development in the psychomotor domain, it is clear that students need to possess knowledge about how to use and place the stethoscope, how to execute the manual techniques necessary for palpation and percussion, how to find the normal range of results that are obtained from each assessment technique, and how to write a description of the findings with the correct terminology. In addition, students need to demonstrate their willingness to engage in rehearsal and practice, a second-level affective domain response.

Learning Activities to Promote Thinking

The Carnegie Foundation for the Advancement of Teaching's national nursing education study reported that nurse educators must shift from emphasizing critical thinking to emphasizing clinical reasoning and many ways of thinking that include critical thinking (Benner et al., 2010, pp. 84–86). In this study clinical reasoning is defined as the ability to reason when clinical situations change. Other ways of thinking include critical reflection; clinical imagination; and creative, scientific, and formal criterial reasoning (Benner et al., 2010, p. 85). The authors of the study suggest that these ways of thinking promote thinking like a nurse and encourage informed action in clinical practice. They highlight many approaches to teaching these ways of thinking. Some examples include using:

1. Pedagogies of contextualization where the educator teaches students to notice broad contextual concerns that influence how they provide care
2. Integrative teaching and learning in which the educator asks students to integrate multiple pieces of information to ensure quality care
3. Stories and cases whereby the educator teaches students to recognize the salience (relevance) of patient information (e.g., signs and symptoms of illness)
4. Dialogue and questioning in which the educator promotes students' clinical reasoning abilities

In addition to this hallmark study, nursing education has a rich supply of literature on developing students' thinking. For instance, Turner (2005), in completing a concept analysis on critical thinking, emphasized critical thinking as a skill. She related that, in nursing, critical thinking is most consistent with the 1990 American Philosophical Association's

Delphi Report. It is within this context that Turner describes critical thinking in nursing as

> a purposeful, self-regulatory judgment associated in some way with clinical decision making, diagnostic reasoning, the nursing process, clinical judgment, and problem solving. It is characterized by analysis, reasoning, inference, interpretation, knowledge, and open-mindedness. It requires knowledge of the area about which one is thinking and results in safe, competent practice and improved decision making, clinical judgments, and problem solving. (p. 276)

By designing and selecting learning activities that require active learning, faculty can cultivate thinking in students. Over time, approaches in nursing education that have contributed to developing students' thinking include using reading strategies, case studies, and questioning (Hoffman, 2008) and using concept maps, role playing, and "think aloud" strategies (Walsh & Seldomridge, 2006). Others have emphasized the need for educators to use narrative pedagogy to develop students analytic, reflective, embodied (intuitive), and pluralistic ways of knowing and understanding (Scheckel & Ironside, 2006). See Chapter 15 for information about how faculty can use writing and thinking exercises to develop students' critical thinking skills.

Constraints to Choosing and Implementing Learning Activities

Constraints to choosing and implementing learning activities may arise from faculty, students, time, and resources. Although it may not be possible to eliminate all constraints, by making a careful assessment of each source of constraint during the planning phases, faculty will be able to avoid many pitfalls. Faculty gain an appreciation of the benefits and limitations of any learning activity after implementing it, reflecting on how students responded, and assessing how the activity contributed to learning. Taking time to debrief themselves after an activity helps faculty decide whether to repeat, revise, or delete the activity. Table 11-3 presents a summary of the sources of constraint in selecting and implementing learning activities.

Faculty Constraints

Some constraints in choosing and implementing learning activities arise from faculty. A faculty member's lack of experience in teaching in an academic

TABLE 11-3 Sources of Constraint in Choosing and Implementing Learning Activities

Source	Constraint
Faculty	• Faculty–student ratio • Lack of experience • Lack of knowledge of course content • Lack of understanding of students' knowledge and skills • Personal attributes: • Personality • Vocal qualities
Students	• Distractions • Inability to use equipment and technology • Lack of prerequisite knowledge and skills • Resistance to active participation • Stress and anxiety • Student–faculty ratio too large
Time	• Inadequate for activity • Inadequate for debriefing
Resources	• Copyright restrictions • Inadequate clinical or classroom facilities • Inadequate funds • Unavailable audiovisual equipment • Unavailable electronic technology

setting or in teaching students at the course level assigned may present some difficulty when he or she is choosing and implementing learning activities. Faculty are more likely to select appropriate activities when they have a reasonable understanding of the cognitive abilities of their students and some familiarity with the knowledge base and previous school and life experiences that their students bring to the course. Overestimating or underestimating the abilities and experiences of students can undermine the intended value of the learning experience. Another pitfall that faculty may encounter is the failure to adequately appreciate a student's inability to engage in an activity. This inability may be attributed to an activity that is too sophisticated or complex, or perhaps to a learning experience that is not challenging enough for a student.

Novice faculty, and even experienced faculty who are teaching a new course, may not possess a comfortable or adequate command of the content and processes required by the learning activity. In addition, they may not be comfortable in dealing with questions, problems, or issues that may arise during the activity. Even under the best of circumstances it is often difficult for faculty to fully appreciate the various perspectives that students may bring to the activity. Students may raise questions and issues that faculty may not have even remotely considered as being related to the activity. Consulting with senior faculty who have taught the course or who have had experience teaching the same level of students before designing the learning activities can provide valuable input that can help reduce the potential for difficulties. Because learning activities are student centered, faculty must not only be prepared to deal with any ambiguity that may arise but also be willing to be flexible, to go with the flow of the learning experience while taking advantage of the opportunity to learn from students how they process the experience. Feedback from students about the different ways they interpreted the learning activity, or certain elements of it, can be used as points of discussion and thus expand the learning experience.

Demands on students outside the classroom can complicate and put constraints on faculty. Retaining standards and rigor while providing appropriate academic expectations for students with numerous job and family demands makes teaching a challenge and can have major implications for pedagogy. Yoder and Saylor (2002) found that students expected to be challenged, implying a higher level of intellectual effort, yet class preparation was far below the expectations of faculty. Concerns of the educators included whether assignments were reasonable and whether the effort to reduce preparation time simply dilutes course expectations to an unacceptable level. Incorrect assumptions and mismatched expectations, which might be increased if there is cultural diversity in the classroom, between students and teachers can promote an academic challenge and provide a critical focus and direction to establishing better nursing education policy and research with these issues.

Faculty may have personal attributes that interfere with their ability to establish a climate that engages student interest in learning activities. Having a soft or a poor-quality voice, talking too fast or too slow, or speaking in a monotone may make it difficult for students to attend to and follow verbal presentations. Faculty with reserved or shy personalities, or those with a matter-of-fact orientation, may be perceived by students as distant, aloof, or uncaring. Personal habits that faculty may be unaware of may also be distracting for students and interfere with their ability to fully focus on the learning experience. Although students may be reluctant to share some of their perceptions about faculty's personal attributes, inviting a colleague to attend a class can provide helpful input that can be used to improve classroom performance. It may also be helpful for faculty to learn the Concernful Practices of Schooling Learning Teaching, which emphasize practices that are important to fostering positive learning climates (Diekelmann & Diekelmann, 2009).

Student Constraints

Student constraints may be due to the number of students enrolled in a course. There may be too many students to ensure that they all have the same or a comparable experience. The student–faculty ratio may make a particular activity too labor- and time-intensive.

Students may lack some of the prerequisite knowledge and skills required for an activity, knowledge and skills that faculty reasonably assumed the students would possess. There are usually some students, regardless of the clarity of the activity and the directions, who fail to understand the activity or who are unable to connect parts of the activity with previous knowledge and experience. Some students may have difficulties with comprehension and may be unable to adequately follow directions.

Stress or anxiety may interfere with some students' ability to attend to and participate in an activity. Distractions such as mechanical noise in the classroom and noise from outside the building may also interfere with learning activities. Students working in groups may make enough noise to interfere with others working in proximity.

Resistance to participation in learning activities is another constraining force. Students socialized to a passive learning model may be resistant to engaging in some or all types of activities. Students may perceive learning activities as a form of busywork that has little or no meaning for them and not accept the activities as a meaningful experience.

Students may not have the skill or experience in using the resources, equipment, or electronic technology required for a learning activity. Although many types of computer equipment are easily and quickly learned, there are students who lack experience, skill, and comfort in using computers for any purpose.

Time Constraints

Time is an all too common constraint in teaching. Faculty must carefully weigh the trade-off between faculty-centered and student-centered activities when determining how to use class time most effectively. For all learning activities, faculty must prioritize and then select the objectives or competencies and the related content and processes. Faculty must also assess the complexity of the learning activity to ensure that it can be accomplished given the ability of the students and the allotted time.

For an activity to be meaningful and worthwhile, adequate time needs to be allowed for both students and faculty to actively plan and participate in the activity. Time should also be allowed for debriefing following the completion of the activity. Although the need to debrief after the activity depends on the nature of the activity, debriefing is an important part of learning, and it has several benefits for both students and faculty. It extends the learning process because students share what they did with their peers, it enables faculty to gain a more comprehensive perspective of the kinds of thinking processes students use, and it provides a window of opportunity for students to identify issues or problems that came up during the activity. Faculty can use this information as the basis for further discussion of issues and problems relevant to the student's immediate learning situation. Information gleaned from students about their difficulties with the directions, elements, or focus of the activity itself is useful to faculty when deciding whether to retain, revise, or delete the activity.

Resource Constraints

Resources may be another source of constraint. The resources used to support learning activities include clinical facilities; learning resource centers; physical examination rooms; classrooms; supplies and equipment; print materials; audiovisual equipment and programs such as films, DVDs, and audiotapes; computer-assisted instructional programs; and a variety of information technologies. The use of a particular learning activity or type of activity may not be possible because of a lack of the appropriate resources needed to implement the activity. For example, a clinical unit may not be able to accommodate the students; the type of clinical facility desired may not be available; classroom size

or design may not be adequate; audiovisual equipment may be unavailable for the specific class day and time; or films, DVDs, or computer software may not be accessible because of heavy demand or lack of funds to acquire them. In addition, licensing or copyright restrictions may prohibit or limit faculty use of a particular resource.

Information technology, e-mail, and other electronic messaging and conferencing systems are useful tools that can be used as a vehicle for selected learning activities. Although faculty may inform students in advance of the course that skill and experience in using electronic technology are required, students often report that they are too busy to allocate the time to acquire the necessary training on their own time. In addition to time, money may also be a barrier. Some academic institutions charge students to learn how to use electronic messaging systems or computer software programs. Faculty who are committed to using some form of computer or electronic technology as a means of implementing one or more learning activities may find it necessary to schedule training sessions for students during class time.

Evaluation of Learning Activities

Evaluation of teaching and learning is a continuous process for both faculty and students. Faculty need to be aware that in education two types of evaluation are commonly used: formative and summative. Selecting the appropriate type of evaluation for use at the appropriate time is important. Formative and summative evaluations are further discussed in Chapter 25.

Formative Evaluation

Formative evaluation is conducted while the teaching–learning process is unfolding. Faculty use formative evaluation to (1) appraise learning activities while they are developing and using them, (2) assess student learning and ability to apply the content, and (3) identify any difficulties that come up during the implementation.

Students use formative evaluation to appraise (1) the effectiveness of their learning strategies; (2) the extent to which they are grasping the knowledge, skills, and attitudes presented in the course; (3) the need for additional clarification of the material; and (4) the need for further study.

Clearly differentiating between learning and evaluation and allocating specific time for each purpose is essential. However, separating learning from evaluation does not mean that frequent formative assessment of student learning can be neglected. Collecting systematic verbal and written feedback from students is an integral and essential component of the teaching–learning process. These data enable faculty to monitor student progress and design appropriate strategies to improve student achievement.

When most students demonstrate problems in achieving the desired outcomes for a specific content topic, it may be necessary for faculty to select a different activity to present and reinforce the content. Faculty can use a variety of other strategies to facilitate student learning, such as giving supplemental assignments, organizing students with different levels of ability into learning groups, scheduling personal conferences with individuals or groups of students, and referring students to tutors. Students deserve to be informed about when they will be evaluated and the purpose of the evaluation. Because formative evaluation data can provide valuable feedback to students about their performance, faculty should frequently share these data with students in both verbal and written form.

Summative Evaluation

Summative evaluation is conducted by faculty at the completion of the course and program; it is the final outcome. Faculty use summative evaluation to (1) appraise the student's learning outcomes, (2) determine the effectiveness of all instructional strategies and learning activities used during the course, and (3) plan appropriate revisions to the planned learning activities of the course.

Because evaluation of learning should be done in the same manner in which students learned, the same types of learning activities that were used as part of the instructional strategies may also be used for the summative evaluation. Many types of learning activities, such as case studies, simulations, and audiovisual media, can also be included in an examination. Faculty may choose to use these types of learning activities for the complete examination or only part of it. For example, when faculty use case studies or simulations or other approaches designed to promote in-depth thinking and problem solving, they may prefer to test students by using

short-answer essay questions based on the content presented in a case study. Although short-answer essay questions are an excellent testing method, grading them can be a labor-intensive activity, especially if there are a large number of students in the course. In this situation, one strategy that faculty may choose is to create an examination that combines traditional multiple-choice items with a few essay questions.

Another useful strategy for handling the grading of essay examinations is to have students exchange examinations and provide one another feedback, with faculty assigning the final grade. In this model faculty may also choose to grade the students on their ability to critically examine their peers' performance. Students must sign their names on the examination they are reviewing. This helps them focus on the content of the examination rather than on the person who wrote the examination, who may be a friend. If faculty wish to preserve the anonymity of students, identification codes rather than student names may be used. Although this approach requires that more time be allocated for the examination, it provides students with an opportunity to learn from others' work as they critically assess the quality of the responses.

A third strategy that serves to reduce the workload of grading essay examinations is to allow students to work in pairs or small groups. This strategy is sometimes used with a cooperative learning model.

Cooperative learning (Baumberger-Henry, 2005; Khosravani, Manoochehri, & Memarian, 2005) uses instructional strategies that structure the environment to encourage and promote students working actively together in small groups on academic tasks. These strategies are designed to maximize students own and each other's learning. Research evidence indicates that cooperative learning increases students' critical thinking abilities, creates positive relationships among students, and promotes a healthier psychological adjustment than learning in a competitive or individualistic mode.

Maximum benefits of cooperative learning are derived when learning groups are carefully designed and facilitated. Cooperative learning requires that group members (1) develop positive interdependence among themselves, (2) assume responsibility for promoting each other's learning, (3) assume individual responsibility and accountability for doing a fair share of the work, (4) know and use appropriate interpersonal and small group process skills, and (5) actively process how effectively they are working together.

SUMMARY

Selecting learning activities is an intentional, systematically planned effort that is time consuming. It requires attention to several important issues. Faculty must keep in mind that learning activities that require students' active engagement in their own learning have positive benefits for students and faculty. Within this context faculty must consider when to use structured or unstructured activities; whether learning activities are needed for

critical learning experiences; how to appropriately match the objectives and competencies, learning domain, and domain level with the instructional materials and the learning activities; and how to design and incorporate formative and summative evaluation strategies.

In addition, faculty must determine how and where it is appropriate to integrate critical thinking skills, simulations, and technology into the activities. Using a set of principles for selecting learning experiences helps ensure that the learning activities will maximize student learning. Faculty also need to be conscious of the sources of constraints that may interfere with choosing and implementing learning activities.

REFLECTING ON THE EVIDENCE

1. What type of evidence and how much evidence do nursing faculty need to understand learning strategies that are effective and learning strategies that are ineffective?

2. To what extent have teachers become learner-centered in their approaches to teaching?

3. What nursing education research evidence is needed to determine whether faculty decisions about critical

learning experiences actually prepare students for contemporary nursing practice?

4. What evidence is needed in nursing education to address the meaning and efficacy of the domains of learning as a framework for developing learning strategies?

5. How do faculty in schools of nursing who promote and support risk taking and innovation overcome barriers to implementing novel and progressive learning strategies?

REFERENCES

American Nurses Association. (2001). *Scope and standards of nursing informatics practice.* Washington, DC: Author.

Anderson, L. W., & Krathwohl, D. R. (2001). *A taxonomy for learning, teaching, and assessing: A revision of Bloom's taxonomy of educational objectives.* New York, NY: Longman.

Baumberger-Henry, M. (2005). Cooperative learning and case study: Does the combination improve students' perception of problem solving and decision-making skills? *Nursing Education Today,25* (3), 238–246.

Bebb, H., & Pittam, G. (2004). Inquiry-based learning as a "whole curriculum approach": The experiences of first year nursing students. *Learning in Health and Social Care,3* (3), 141–153.

Benner, P., Sutphen, M., Leonard, V., & Day, L. (2010). *Educating nurses: A call for radical transformation.* San Francisco, CA: Jossey-Bass.

Bloom, B. S. (Ed.). (1956). *Taxonomy of educational objectives. Handbook 1: Cognitive domain.* New York, NY: Longman.

Blumberg, P. (2009). *Developing learner-centered teaching: A practical guide for faculty.* San Francisco, CA: Jossey-Bass.

Bonnel, W. E., & Smith, K. V. (2010). *Teaching technologies in nursing and the health professions: Beyond simulation and online courses.* New York, NY: Springer.

Bruner, J. (1977). *The process of education.* Cambridge, MA: Harvard University Press.

Clark, C., Nguyen, H. T., Bray, C., & Levine. R. E. (2008). Team-based learning in an undergraduate nursing course. *Journal of Nursing Education, 47*(3), 111–117.

Clark, M. C. (2007). Using team-based learning as a substitute for lectures in a required undergraduate nursing course. In L. K. Michaelsen, D. X. Parmelee, K. K. McMahon, & R. E. Levine (Eds.), *Team-based learning for health professions education: A guide to using small groups for improving learning* (pp. 151–160). Sterling, VA: Stylus.

Cronenwett, L., Sherwood, G., Barnsteiner, J., Disch, J., Johnson, J., Mitchell, P., & Warren, J. (2007). Quality and safety education for nurses. *Nursing Outlook, 55,* 122–131.

Dave, R. (1970). *Psychomotor levels in developing and writing objectives.* Tucson, AZ: Educational Innovators Press.

Davis, B. G. (2009). *Tools for teaching* (2nd ed.). San Francisco, CA: Jossey-Bass.

Diekelmann, N., & Diekelmann, J. (2009). *Schooling learning teaching: Toward a narrative pedagogy.* New York, NY: iUniverse.

Duan, Y. (2006). Selecting and applying taxonomies for learning outcomes: A nursing example. *International Journal of Nursing Education Scholarship, 3*(1), 1–12.

Ellis, A. (2004). *Exemplars of curriculum theory.* Larchmont, NY: Eye on Education.

Flood, L. S., Gasiewicz, N., & Delpier, T. (2010). Integrating information literacy across a BSN curriculum. *Journal of Nursing Education, 49*(2), 101–104.

Giddens, J. F. (2007). The neighborhood: A web-based platform to support conceptual teaching and learning. *Nursing Education Perspectives, 28*(5), 251–256.

Graves, J. R., & Corcoran, S. (1989). The study of nursing informatics. *Image, 21,* 227–231.

Greer, A. G., Pokorny, M., Clay, M. C., Brown, S., & Steele, L. L. (2010). Learner-centered characteristics of nurse educators. *International Journal of Nursing Education Scholarship, 7*(1), 1–15.

Harton, H. C., Richardson, D. S. Barreras, R. E., Rockloff, M. J., & Latané, B. (2002). Focused interactive learning: A tool for active class discussion. *Teaching of Psychology, 29* (1), 10–15.

Hoffman. J. J. (2008). Teaching strategies to facilitate nursing students' critical thinking. In M. H. Oermann (Ed.), *Annual review of nursing education: Clinical education.* New York, NY: Springer.

Hovancsek, M. T. (2007). Using simulations in nursing education. In P. R. Jeffries (Ed.), *Simulation in nursing education: From conceptualization to evaluation* (pp. 5–6). New York, NY: National League for Nursing.

Jarvis, P., Holford, J., & Griffin, C. (2003). *The theory & practice of learning* (2nd ed.). Sterling, VA: Kogan Page.

Jeffries, P. R. (2005). A framework for designing, implementing, and evaluating simulations used as teaching strategies in nursing. *Nursing Education Perspectives, 26* (2), 96–103.

Jeffries, P. R. (2006). Designing simulations for nursing education. In M. H. Oermann & K. T. Heinrich (Eds.), *Annual review of nursing education* (pp. 161–178). New York, NY: Springer.

Khosravani, S., Manoochehri, H., & Memarian, R. (2005). Developing critical thinking skills in nursing students by group dynamics. *Internet Journal of Advanced Nursing Practice, 7*(2), 1–20.

Krathwohl, D., Bloom, B., & Masia, B. (1964). *Taxonomy of educational objectives. Handbook II: Affective domain.* New York, NY: Longman.

Levy, P., Aiyegbayot, O., & Little, S. (2009). Designing for inquiry-based learning with the learning activity management system. *Journal of Computer Assisted Learning, 25,* 238–251.

McNeil, B. J., Elfrink, V., Beyea, S. C., Pierce, S. T., & Bickford, C. J. (2006). Computer literacy study: Report of qualitative findings. *Journal of Professional Nursing, 22,* 52–59.

Ming Su, W., Osisek, P. J., & Starnes, B. (2004). Applying the revised Bloom's taxonomy to a medical-surgical lesson. *Nurse Educator, 29* (3), 116–120.

Ming Su, W., Osisek, P. J., & Starnes, B. (2005). Using the revised Bloom's taxonomy in the clinical laboratory: Thinking skills involved in diagnostic reasoning. *Nurse Educator, 30*(3), 117–122.

Pascarella, E. T., & Terenzini, P. T. (2005). *How college affects students: A third decade of research* (Vol. 2). San Francisco, CA: Jossey-Bass.

Price, K. M., & Nelson, K. L. (2007). *Planning effective instruction: Diversity responsive methods and management* (3rd ed.). Belmont, CA: Thomson Higher Education.

Reilly, D. E. (1980). *Behavioral objectives: Evaluation in nursing.* New York, NY: Appleton-Century-Crofts.

Reilly, D. E., & Oermann, M. H. (1990). *Behavioral objectives: Evaluation nursing* (3rd ed.). New York, NY: National League for Nursing.

Sand-Jecklin, K. (2007). The impact of active/cooperative learning on beginning nursing students learning strategy preference. *Nurse Education Today, 27,* 474–480.

Scheckel, M. M., & Ironside, P. M. (2006). Cultivating interpretive thinking through enacting narrative pedagogy. *Nursing Outlook, 54* (3), 159–165.

Skiba, D. J. (2009). On the horizon: Dialogues for the nursing academy. *Nursing Education Perspectives, 30,* 330–331.

Skiba, D. J. (2010). On the horizon: Technologies coming to your school soon. *Nursing Education Perspectives, 31,* 114–115.

Skiba, D. J., Connors, H. R., & Jeffries, P. R. (2008). Information technologies and the transformation of nursing education. *Nursing Outlook, 56,* 225–230.

Snelgrove, S. R. (2004). Approaches to learning of student nurses. *Nursing Education Today, 24,* 605–614.

Stevens, J., & Brenner, Z. R. (2009). The peer active learning approach for clinical education: A pilot study. *The Journal of Theory Construction & Testing, 13*(2), 51–56.

Turner, P. (2005). Critical thinking in nursing education and practice as defined in the literature. *Nursing Education Perspectives, 26* (5), 272–277.

Walsh, C. M., & Seldomridge, L. A. (2006). Critical thinking: Back to square two. *Journal of Nursing Education, 45*(6), 212–219.

Wingfield, S. S., & Black, G. S. (2005). Active versus passive course designs: The impact on student outcomes. *Journal of Education for Business, 81*(2), 119–125.

Wolf, Z. R., Bender, P. J., Beitz, J. M., Wieland, D. M., & Vito, K. O. (2004). Strengths and weaknesses of faculty teaching performance reported by undergraduate and graduate nursing students: A descriptive study. *Journal of Professional Nursing, 20,* 118–128.

Yoder, M., & Saylor, C. (2002). Student and teacher roles: Mismatched expectations. *Nurse Educator, 27*(5), 201–203.

Service Learning: Developing Values, Cultural Competence, and Social Responsibility

Carla Mueller, PhD, RN

For two decades, agencies and commissions concerned with higher education and preparation of the professions (American Association of Colleges of Nursing, 2008a; Campus Compact, 2001; National Service-Learning Clearinghouse, 2010; Pew Health Professions Commission, 1998) have recommended that educational programs include experiences that require civic engagement and community involvement. Institutions of higher education and their schools of nursing are therefore seeking opportunities for students to develop moral judgment, civic responsibility, cultural competence, and global awareness, in addition to the basic professional skills set forth in the curriculum. Service learning, a structured component of the curriculum in which students acquire social values through service to individuals, groups, or communities, is one way to provide opportunities for students to develop these values. Service offers opportunities for learning that cannot be obtained any other way. As such, a service experience may be one of the first truly meaningful acts in a student's life. Service learning uses reflective learning to connect learning with students' thoughts and feelings in a deliberate way, creating a context in which students can explore how they feel about what they are thinking, and what they think about how they feel. As it does so, service learning becomes an integral part of students' education. This chapter explains how service learning can contribute to these outcomes in nursing curricula.

The author acknowledges the work of Barbara Norton, RN, MPH, in a previous edition of the chapter.

Service Learning

Service learning evolves from a philosophy of education that emphasizes active learning directed toward a goal of social responsibility and civic engagement. Service learning is not merely volunteerism, nor is it a substitute for a field experience or practicum that is a normal part of a course. Service learning is not the same as a nursing clinical experience because the focus of the learning is on meeting the needs of the host community rather than those of the nursing curriculum. Rather, service learning offers a way in which students can develop cultural competence and a sense of civic responsibility congruent with the tenets of social justice and help create a better world by contributing to national renewal (Amerson, 2010). Both the recipient and the student benefit from the experience.

Service learning is an educational experience in which students participate in a service activity that meets the needs of multiple stakeholders in the professional and community environment within the framework of a specific credit-bearing course. Service learning focuses on developing social values rather than a providing a discrete type of experiential education. Service learning is also defined as a way of connecting academic learning with service; it provides concrete opportunities for students to learn new skills, think critically, and test new roles in situations that encourage risk taking and reward competence.

Service learning is a component of broader educational goals to promote civic engagement (American Psychological Association, 2007; Colby, Ehrlich, Beaumont, & Stephens, 2003). Civic engagement involves individual and collective actions to address areas of societal concern. Civic engagement may include service-learning projects as well as community-focused faculty research. Like service learning, civic engagement involves structured activities that require the student to work with a community to solve a problem, but unlike service learning, the focus of the activity is to promote civic responsibility and development for citizenship.

Often the terms *service learning* and *experiential learning* are used interchangeably; however, they are distinct entities. Experiential learning includes hands-on work and has the learning of work-related skills as its major goal. Traditional nursing clinical experiences are an example of experiential learning. In contrast, service learning involves work that meets actual community needs, has as one of its goals the fostering of "a sense of caring for others," and includes structured time for reflection (Bailey, Carpenter, & Harrington, 2002). Service learning balances the need of the community and the learning objectives of the students. Community agencies are true partners in design, implementation, and evaluation of the experience.

Service learning expands the learning environment for students and faculty. Service learning is population focused and therefore provides opportunities for students to act locally to solve social problems (Eads, 1994). Although a number of similarities are present, key differences exist between traditional learning and service learning (Richardson, Billings, & Martin, 1996). These differences are summarized in Table 12-1.

Colleges and universities may engage in service learning differently because of different institutional missions and traditions (Jacoby, 1996). Some universities embrace service learning as a philosophy, some as part of their spiritual mission. Others embrace service learning as part of a "commitment to citizenship, civic responsibility and participatory democracy, and still others ground their service learning programs in community partnerships" (Jacoby, 1996, p. 17). Regardless of how universities embrace service learning, service learning must do the following (American Psychological Association, 2007; Eyler & Giles, 1999; Jacoby, 1996; Shah & Glascoff, 1998; Worrell-Carlisle, 2005):

1. Be connected to program and course learning outcomes and promote learning
2. Be experiential
3. Allow students to engage in activities that address human and community needs via

TABLE 12-1 Differences between Traditional Learning and Service Learning

	Traditional Learning	Service Learning
Location	Classroom	Classroom, community
Teacher	Professor	Professor, preceptor or facilitator, patients
Learning	Writing	Writing
	Examinations	Examinations
	Passive	Active
	Authoritarian	Shared responsibility
	Structured	Reflective
	Compartmentalized	Expansive, integrative
	Cognitive	Cognitive and affective
	Short term	Short term and long term
Reasoning	Deductive	Inductive
Evaluation	Professor	Professor, preceptor or facilitator, self-assessment by students

structured opportunities for student learning and development
4. Provide time for guided reflection in discussion, writing, or media
5. Develop a sense of caring, social responsibility, global awareness, and civic engagement
6. Involve activities that have real meaning for the participants and promote deeper learning
7. Address problems that are identified by the community and require problem solving
8. Promote collaborative learning and teamwork
9. Embrace the concept of reciprocity between the learner and the person or organization being served

Service learning may be a separate course within the college curriculum or integrated as a thread throughout multiple courses. The trend is toward the latter. Faculty members intentionally and strategically plan to incorporate service-learning experiences as part of a course. When service learning is integrated into existing courses, it is important that it not be added as an "additional" course requirement. Instead it should be a learning activity that replaces one or more learning activities previously used. Credit should be given for the learning and its relation to the course, not for the service alone. The service activity must match course content and enhance learning by allowing application of the theoretical principles taught in the classroom setting. At some colleges and universities, courses with a service-learning component are identified in the course catalogue as having an opportunity for service learning. At the same time, some colleges allow students to select an alternate learning activity if they do not wish to participate in service learning.

Theoretical Foundations of Service Learning

Kolb's (1984) theory of experiential learning has been widely used as a theoretical basis for designing and analyzing service-learning programs. Reflective observation about the experience is essential to the learning process. It links the concrete experience to abstract conceptualizations of that experience. Learning is increased when students are actively engaged in gaining knowledge through experiential problem solving and decision making (Bailey et al., 2002; Dewey, 1933; Kolb, 1984; Miettinen, 2000). Use of reflection is built on the work of Kolb (1984) and Dewey (1916, 1933, 1938). In service learning, reflection is both a cognitive process (Kolb, 1984; Mezirow, 1990; Schön, 1983) and a structured learning activity (Silcox, 1994). Effective reflection fosters moral development and enhances moral decision making. Moral decisions involve an exercise of choice and a corresponding willingness to accept responsibility for that choice (Gilligan, 1981).

Delve, Mintz, and Stewart (1990) developed a service-learning model based on the theories of moral decision making and values clarification (Gilligan, 1982; Kohlberg, 1976). The model includes five phases of development: exploration, clarification, realization, activation, and internalization. It illustrates that service learning is developmental, providing students with an opportunity to move from charity to justice as they become more empathetic. Delve et al. (1990) believe that without that empathy, the student will not come to recognize the members of the patient population as valued individuals in the larger society and as sources for new learning.

The pedagogy of service learning has powerful flexibility. It can be based on subject matter or on learning process; it can connect theory and practice; it integrates several different approaches to knowledge and uses of knowledge; it encourages learning how to learn; and it can focus on a wide range of issues, problems, and interests (Pellietier, 1995). Service learning also lends itself to problem-based learning and case study methodologies.

Outcomes of Service Learning

Service learning in the curriculum provides opportunities for students to attain personal, professional, and curriculum goals. Service learning also contributes to the overall educational experience of the college or university and thus provides benefits to the institution as well. Finally, service learning benefits the community in which it occurs and the clients it serves.

Benefits to Students

A review of the literature on the outcomes of service learning reveals that students benefit from service learning in multiple and integrated ways (Amerson, 2010; Bailey et al., 2002; Batchelder & Root, 1994; Battistoni, 1995; Callister & Hobbins-Garbett, 2000; Carter & Dunn, 2002; Cohen & Kinsey, 1994; Ehrlich, 1995; Fleischauer & Fleischauer, 1994; Giles & Eyler, 1994; Hales, 1997; Herman & Sassatelli, 2002; Macy, 1994; Narsavage, Lindell, Chen, Savrin, & Duffy, 2002; Pellietier, 1995; Redman & Clark, 2002; Reynolds, 2005; Schaffer & Peterson, 2001; Wills, 1992). Benefits can include personal and professional development as well as mastering course outcomes.

Direct participation in the service-learning activity assists with socialization into the profession, introduces new technical or professional skills, increases motivation to learn, and encourages self-directed learning (Bailey et al., 2002; Narsavage et al., 2002; Pellietier, 1995; Reynolds, 2005; Wills, 1992). Several schools of nursing have integrated service-learning components into the freshman experience as a way to introduce nursing students to the role of the nurse (Baumberger, Krouse, & Borucki, 2006; Worrell-Carlisle, 2005). Service learning can also be an opportunity for interprofessional learning and developing collaborative relationships with other professions. Although the majority of service learning occurs in undergraduate programs, graduate programs in nursing are beginning to explore community engagement to further develop students' leadership skills and sense of responsibility, as well as enhancement of their critical thinking skills and learning of academic content (Francis-Baldesari & Williamson, 2008; Narsavage et al., 2002).

Service learning has been found to provide a more thorough understanding of "self" and provides insight into personal strengths and weaknesses (Batchelder & Root, 1994; Ehrlich, 1995). It also has been found to contribute to the development of personal vision, moral sensitivity, clarification of values, and spirituality (Ehrlich, 1995; Eyler, Giles, Stenson, & Gray, 2001; Fleischauer & Fleischauer, 1994; Hales, 1997; Macy, 1994).

Service learning facilitates academic inquiry by connecting theory and practice, enhancing disciplinary understanding and understanding of complex material, bringing greater relevance to course material, and helping students generalize their learning to new situations (Carter & Dunn, 2002; Cohen & Kinsey, 1994; Ehrlich, 1995; Hales, 1997; Jarosinski & Heinrich, 2010; Schaffer & Peterson, 2001; Williams, 1990). Service-learning experiences also develop critical thinking (Battistoni, 1995; Callister & Hobbins-Garbett, 2000; Herman & Sassatelli, 2002), communication (Reynolds, 2005), collaboration, leadership, and professional skills (Anstee, Harris, Pruitt, & Sugar, 2008; Giles & Eyler, 1994; Hales, 1997; Pellietier, 1995; Schaffer & Peterson, 2001; Wills, 1992). Reising, Allen, and Hall (2006a) found that participating in a blood pressure screening service-learning project in the university community provided skills of blood pressure assessment, history taking, and health counseling.

The social impact of service learning includes the development of civic responsibility, increased orientation to volunteerism, increased political and global awareness, development of cultural competence, and improved ethical decision making (Amerson, 2010; Gehrke, 2008; Herman & Sassatelli, 2002; Palmer & Savoie, 2001; Redman & Clark, 2002; Reising, Allen, & Hall, 2006b; Wills, 1992; Worrell-Carlisle, 2005). Students also learn the value of community health promotion (Reising et al., 2006a, 2006b).

Benefits to Faculty

Identifying benefits to faculty are key to obtaining buy-in because of the time commitment involved. "Faculty engagement in service learning energizes teaching and places greater emphasis on student-centered learning" (Hoebeke, McCullough, Cagle, & St. Clair, 2009, p. 634). Even though faculty may not be on-site with students directly supervising the service activities, significant faculty time commitment is required to plan the assignment, obtain community partners, read student journals, and facilitate reflection sessions. Faculty who link service-learning activities in their courses with their research and service interests have increased commitment to continuing its use. Some universities have adopted the Boyer model of scholarship, which enlarged the scholarship perspective to include teaching, service, and practice, in addition to research. By enlarging the scholarship perspective, Boyer (1990) believed that there would be a stronger connection between universities and the communities they served. This scholarship model facilitates integration of service learning into the faculty member's academic role as well as promotion and tenure requirements. The Carnegie Academy for the Scholarship of Teaching and Learning in Higher Education provides an online gallery of interdisciplinary projects, including those that involve service learning that can be used by faculty to transform their teaching. This gallery is available on the Carnegie Foundation for the Advancement of Teaching's website at http://gallery.carnegiefoundation.org/gallery_of_tl/castl_he.html.

Benefits to the Institution

Service learning also has institutional benefits. These include invigoration of the campus educational culture, development of a strong sense of campus community, increased institutional visibility, enhanced appeal to potential donors, and retention of students (Cooper, 1993; Molledahl, 1994; Pellietier, 1995; Rehnke, 1995; Wills, 1992; Worrell-Carlisle, 2005). Service learning invigorates the campus culture by increasing students' engagement in their own learning, revitalizing faculty, and allowing faculty to mesh service projects with research interests (Hoebeke et al., 2009; Pellietier, 1995; Rehnke, 1995; Wills, 1992). The interdisciplinary nature of service learning helps the campus regain a strong ethos of community, keeps students and faculty more engaged in the life of the college, and contributes to student retention (Hamner, Wilder, Avery, & Byrd, 2002; Pellietier, 1995). By placing service-learning experiences early in the program, for example as a freshman-year experience, the student retention rate can be increased

(Worrell-Carlisle, 2005) because students develop self-efficacy and an understanding of the field of study. Increased institutional visibility contributes to increased student recruitment by providing a visible link between the community and the institution and by providing a perception of access to higher education to community members who have not believed higher education to be within their reach (Cooper, 1993; Molledahl, 1994; Pellietier, 1995; Wills, 1992). Service learning enhances the institution's appeal to potential donors by providing a direct link between the college and the community, and it appeals to donors interested in community service educational reform (Pellietier, 1995).

The mentoring environment that is created between students, faculty, staff, administration, and the broader community becomes a "complex ecology of higher education . . . that can provide knowledge, support, and inspiration" (Daloz, Keen, Keen, & Parks, 1996). Service learning also provides a real-world learning environment in the community that facilitates transfer of knowledge and transition to the practice environment. A smooth transition to practice and increased use of community and public health settings were key recommendations for nursing education in the Institute of Medicine (2010) report. The new alliances formed between academic institutions and community service agencies and organizations eliminate or minimize the traditional separation between the "gown and the town." Cotton and Stanton (1990) indicated that the gap between gown and town is bridged by successful service-learning programs that cultivate "a spirit of reciprocity, interdependence, and collaboration" (p. 101).

Benefits to the Community

The community also benefits when colleges and universities include service learning and civic engagement outcomes in their academic programs. For example, Reising et al. (2006b) found that as a result of a service-learning project in which nursing students conducted hypertension screening and health counseling, 1 year later the community recipients had made modifications in their health management behaviors such as diet change and weight loss. In another service-learning course, students in a nursing research course established partnerships with community organizations to develop research proposals, some of which led to submitting for grant funding (Rash, 2005). Benefits to the community may also include students' increasing awareness of community health needs and an interest in working in community settings (Ligeikis-Clayton & Denman, 2005).

Benefits to the Health Care System

While traditional service learning has occurred in community settings, it can also occur within a traditional acute care setting. Hoebeke et al. (2009) noted that service learning within the health care system

> directly benefits the nursing staff because the ideas for projects are initiated by the staff and driven by the needs and priorities identified by nursing . . . Instead of the nursing staff feeling burdened with the additional responsibility of students in the clinical setting, they see students engaging jointly with them in projects that will lead to a positive impact on their daily work . . . , affect health care policy, develop evidence-based patient care protocols and guidelines and improve patient care outcome measures. (p. 634)

Hospitals working toward Magnet status can use these projects to provide support for their application for Magnet recognition.

Integrating Service Learning into the Curriculum

Integrating service-learning experiences into the curriculum requires careful planning. The experience must be developed and resources acquired before the course is offered. Identifying enthusiastic faculty champions and faculty development are keys to success (American Association of Community Colleges [AACC], 2010).

Planning Faculty Development

Planning for a change to service learning begins with faculty development that may be available from the academic institution, workshops, and independent study. These resources will help faculty obtain essential information about how to design and implement service learning. A few of the practical considerations involved in planning service learning include establishing good relationships with community agencies, identifying the types of experiences suitable for the course content, finding agency representative supervisors, structuring the types of activities, and scheduling the activities.

Preparation links the service-learning activities to specific learning outcomes and prepares students to perform the activities. The service needs to be challenging, engaging, and meaningful to the students, and it must focus on meeting an actual community need that students can perceive as important and relevant to their own development.

Preparation also includes finding agencies for student placement. Students involved in service learning typically work in voluntary not-for-profit community or public tax-supported service agencies and organizations that provide services that meet people's actual needs. Agencies and programs are selected on the basis of their congruence with the academic program or course and student goals and objectives. Faculty must also assess the agency's capacity for students and determine that the students' abilities are a match for the agency's needs.

Faculty development provides an explanation of a new pedagogy for many and establishes a common definition and a sound knowledge base. Consultants can be an invaluable aid in this early development process, and many campuses have offices of service learning that can provide or assist with faculty development. It is also helpful for faculty to make contact with faculty in other colleges to identify what others have been doing. The Internet can be a means of making contact with other faculty involved in service learning. Electronic mailing lists are available, and many sources of information that list faculty involved in service learning are available on the Internet. The Internet can also be a source of information about starting service-learning programs, sample course descriptions, syllabi, electronic mailing lists, funding resources, and best practices. Some of the most widely recognized Internet resources are the following:

---

www.compact.org (Campus Compact)
www.cns.gov (Corporation for National
    & Community Service)
www.servicelearning.org (Learn and Serve,
    National Service-Learning Clearinghouse)

Faculty support is also important to cultivating success. Support begins with campus and school administrators who value service learning and will commit resources to its implementation in the curriculum. Although universities have embraced service learning, they have been slow to implement support systems needed for effective implementation (Schmidt & Brown, 2008). Faculty can organize a faculty service-learning committee or advisory board to provide needed support. This group could be an invaluable advocate of service learning as a teaching tool. The committee can establish faculty handbooks and guidelines for service-learning courses, sponsor lunch-and-learn sessions on service learning for particular departments or the entire college, develop webinars, ensure that faculty receive continuing education units for attending service-learning workshops, and organize faculty development opportunities regarding service learning pedagogy (AACC, 2010). This committee also encourages the development of interdisciplinary professional relationships and provides an avenue for sharing ideas, successes, and failures.

The goal of planning and faculty development is to work for sustainability of service learning throughout the curriculum. Funding for service learning can be obtained from the community, from grant funding available locally and nationally, and often from the college or university itself. Although service learning is not expensive, it does require time for planning and course development and the personnel to make the arrangements. A number of colleges and universities have a service-learning office or coordinator. Staff from this office provide assistance in structuring the program, identifying community partners, and placing students according to mutual needs.

Selecting Placement Sites

Anstee et al. (2008) presented a process model for incorporating service learning into an academic class. The six stages of their model were "(a) establishing community collaboration, (b) partnering in the classroom, (c) student training, (d) delivering the service, (e) returning to the classroom, and (f) reporting to the stakeholders" (p. 599). Selecting a placement site and establishing collaboration within the community are important early steps. It is important to match the type of community organization and service with the institutional mission of the college when service-learning experiences are being planned. Before making plans regarding service placements, faculty should conduct a community needs assessment and develop a resource inventory, either informally through personal and telephone contact or formally through surveys or needs assessments. Community agency staff are invaluable in determining where students are needed the most. Allowing community partners to control the identification of the service helps ensure that projects meet agency needs. Involvement of agency staff in the planning process also helps educate community agencies about service learning. Community advisory boards often help ensure continual contact between agencies, students, faculty, and staff and ascertain evolving community needs. Student safety is also an issue, and the agency and school have a responsibility to choose sites that are appropriate for the students' safety needs.

Once placement sites have been determined and service-learning projects are finalized, preceptors must be identified and dates for student orientation and initial meetings must be planned. Written project descriptions, contact information, and a schedule of initial meetings should be available for students on the first day of class. Organization before the start of the semester ensures that students get started on projects promptly and are likely to complete projects within the semester time limit.

Although careful planning prevents many problems, faculty members should be prepared for the unexpected. Occasionally the needs of community agencies change (e.g., because of funding cuts or receiving a grant), there may be conflicts between agencies' needs for services and students' schedules, or there may be dissatisfaction. Sources of dissatisfaction may include students' perception of inequality of time investment between groups, failure of the reality of the situation to match expectations, and problems in communication (Schaffer & Peterson, 2001). Faculty members may need to intervene to prevent the escalation of problems and to renegotiate expectations.

Planning Learning Activities

Service learning can be used as an experientially based pedagogy to bring excitement and vitality to the classroom, to assist community members in need while at the same time learning from them, and to provide students with information and experiences through which they can engage in critical reflection about society's needs and one's responsibility to the community (Palmer & Savoie, 2001). Opportunities for service learning may be discovered from a number of sources. Faculty may identify appropriate situations for service learning from their own service activities in a wide variety of community agencies. Service opportunities may also be suggested by friends, colleagues, agency personnel, or students, or they may be found in the professional or secular literature. When faculty have identified potential service-learning experiences that seem to be appropriate for the course, discussions and negotiations are held with the agency staff.

Legal issues also need to be considered when planning service activities. Any time a student performs service off campus in conjunction with coursework, liability issues can arise. Faculty should seek legal counsel from the college or university regarding activities with potential liability, just as legal counsel is sought when contracts with clinical agencies are established. Institutional Review Board approval should be sought if students are collecting data as a part of their service-learning projects.

Once service-learning experiences have been planned, students must be engaged. Faculty can use groups such as the student nurses association, student government, the student life office, and campus publicity mechanisms (e.g., newspaper, radio station, online learning system bulletin boards) to inform students about service learning. Often courses or service-learning components of courses are open to students from a variety of disciplines, and faculty should distribute the course announcements widely. Service learning's best promoters are its own students, who attract other students by word of mouth.

Student activities are planned so that they relate to the course objectives and content (Kendall, 1990). Types of agencies and programs that could be used for nursing students engaged in service learning include state or county services for persons with different forms of impairment or disability, various types of health and health care facilities, social welfare agencies and day care programs, Meals on Wheels, senior centers, youth services, civic leagues, drug education programs, and groups or committees related to some aspects of government. Community agencies offer many opportunities for students to collaborate with the agency to fulfill unmet needs. Some service experiences will involve assessment, others work in ongoing programs, and still others work on development and implementation of new programs or services. During the final phase of the service experience, students who have developed new programs should work with agency partners to establish plans for sustainability. Students should compile materials to facilitate this continuation. A summary report to the stakeholders should be completed to close the service experience.

Service Learning in the Nursing Curriculum

The Pew Health Professions Commission (1998) identified service learning as a key competency for programs educating health professionals. National organizations such as the American Association of Colleges of Nursing (2008b), the National League for Nursing (2005), and the Institutes of Medicine (IOM) (2010) have noted that nursing curricula should prepare nurses to practice in diverse settings that are global in nature. The IOM report (2010) advocated interdisciplinary learning to facilitate a smooth transition to the workplace, where working as part of an interdisciplinary group is a key skill. Service learning lends itself to interdisciplinary endeavors, and the interdisciplinary nature of the endeavor would enrich and change the experience. Community-based service learning is increasingly being integrated into nursing courses (Callister & Hobbins-Garbett, 2000). Some service-learning endeavors are part of a larger consortium. An example of this is the Community-Campus Partnerships for Health (CCPH), an independent, nonprofit organization that organized the Partners in Caring and Community: Service-Learning in Nursing Education project. The Partners in Caring and Community project works with teams of nursing faculty and students and their community partners to facilitate the integration of service learning into nursing education curricula, increase the understanding and support for service learning in nursing education, and disseminate new knowledge and information about best practices and models of service learning and nursing education (CCPH, n.d.). The CCPH website (http://depts.washington.edu/ccph/index.html) provides links to participatory institutions and a wide variety of information.

The nursing literature provides a variety of examples for ways to integrate service learning into the curriculum. In one program students spend the first half of the semester in the classroom learning background material and the second half of that semester and all of the following semester in a service-learning experience. Past student placements include the Connecticut Women's Health Campaign, where the student coordinated a coalition of organizations and developed fact sheets to educate women and public officials on issues such as breast cancer legislation and access to health insurance, and the Connecticut Department of Health, where the status of the state's safety net providers was analyzed for the Commissioner of Health to assist in planning services and allocating public funds for health care (Cohen & Milone-Nuzzo, 2001).

As one way to promote global awareness, schools of nursing offer international service-learning experiences. In one course, students traveled to Nicaragua to conduct a nutritional needs assessment; provided prenatal education for community health workers and lay midwives, with a special emphasis on nutrition; and supported the relief efforts in refugee camps following Hurricane Mitch (Riner & Becklenburg, 2001). Students were provided with information about the Nicaraguan culture before starting the experience.

Service-learning courses are also designed to provide students an opportunity to work with underserved and vulnerable populations. For example, at one school, course placement sites include a child care center for homeless children, a senior citizens program, a center serving teenage parents, a mission for homeless individuals, Habitat for Humanity, and Head Start (Hales, 1997). Another course provides opportunities for students to work with an underserved sector of society that has a variety of needs and challenges that are often different from their own. Students provide health and developmental screenings, create handouts for parents, assess the social behavior of children, read safety storybooks to the children, and assist with classroom activities (Kulewicz, 2001). Health promotion activities such as education on tobacco use can help to reduce the prevalence of cigarette smoking (Bassi, Cray, & Caldrello, 2008). In another example, working in partnership with a sheriff's department, students conducted health assessments, participated in case findings, and provided health education (Fuller, Alexander, & Hardeman, 2006).

Service learning can also be integrated into faith-based curricula and faith-based nursing practices

(Brown, 2009; Lashley, 2007). In one service-learning project, several Catholic Charities programs were targeted for service experiences, including an emergency shelter for battered women and their children, an addiction recovery treatment center for economically disadvantaged individuals, food pantries, and an inner-city school counseling service. Initially the Department of Nursing focused on students' ability to apply theoretical knowledge during the service experience. However, Herman and Sassatelli (2002) report that as the program evolved, it embraced Brackley's (1988) challenge to have the "courage not to turn away from the eyes of the poor, but to allow them to break our hearts and shatter our world" (p. 38). They also incorporated Dorr's (1993) emphasis on the importance of not only feeling for economically disadvantaged individuals but also discovering what it means to be with them. Faculty and students found that companionship with economically disadvantaged individuals during the service experience encouraged understanding of what it means to be humanly weak and powerless (Herman & Sassetelli, 2002). Brown (2009) reports that a faith-based service-learning experience reduced mental illness stigma in an underserved community and increased students' understanding of mental health problems and substance abuse. Due to the decreased stigma, patients reported greater willingness to seek treatment and use community resources.

Service-learning courses can also take advantage of online learning technologies. For example, faculty at the School of Nursing at the University of Colorado Health Sciences Center extended the reach of their service-learning initiative to include distance education students by reformulating the course in an Internet-based format, with the materials available online (Redman & Clark, 2002). Faculty teaching an online RN to BSN leadership course used service learning to enhance the collaborative teaching–learning relationship and provide a venue for a required change project (Anderson & Miller, 2007). An asynchronous forum allows discussions with opportunities for reflection. Descriptions of agencies and service projects used by on-campus students are posted online to help distance education students find comparable experiences within their own community. Faculty members work collaboratively with students to finalize arrangements with those agencies.

Preparation for Service Learning

Once student placements and focus of the service have been selected, preparation must extend to the classroom setting. Conceiving of service learning as simply a matter of mutually beneficial service ignores the important concept of readiness for the encounter. Radest (1993) introduced the idea of solidarity: "the name of my relationship to the stranger who remains unknown—only a person in an abstract sense—but who is, like me, a human being. Solidarity is then a preparation for the future and at the same time a grounding in the present" (p. 183). Sheffield (2005) notes that "Radest's concept of solidarity develops into a disposition toward democratic interaction and service" (p. 49) and that academic preparation for the encounter is essential. Preparation develops a sense of understanding in the student that gives increased meaning to the service and a realization that the strangers are much like them, further developing the sense of solidarity.

Preparation should include exploration of social issues as well as an introduction to the service environment and the people who will be encountered. It can take the form of reading materials from the agency, reading text-based materials, exploring material available on the Internet, and viewing films, and should be accompanied by discussions to prepare students for the service experience. Preparatory classroom activities should have an overall goal of enhancing understanding and helping the stranger become familiar. Sheffield (2005) notes that "academic preparation not only under girds the particular service activity, but also advances solidarity generally for future encounters with future 'strangers' and develops a habit of readiness to interact open-mindedly with others" (p. 52). Preparation also brings participants a greater understanding of diversity, the ability to embrace and celebrate differences, and a realization of their ethical responsibility to connect with others in the community. Sheffield (2005) notes that "without that understanding, service degenerates into volunteerism where act rather than connection is the focus" (p. 52).

Incorporating Reflection

Reflection is a critical and essential aspect of service learning that further differentiates it from volunteerism, community service activities, and nursing students' clinical experiences (Hatcher & Bringle, 1995; Hoebeke et al., 2009; Kendall, 1990). Reflection is an active, persistent, thoughtful, and intentional consideration of the service activity. Reflection must include the student's behavior, practice, and achievement. Within the reflective process, students must respond to basic questions such as "What am I doing?" "Why am I doing it?" and "What am I learning?" As well, they should critically examine their actions, feelings, and thoughts. During this examination and while responding to the questions posed, students contemplate, think, reason, and speculate about their service experiences (Fertman, 1994).

Reflection is a learning tool that serves to maximize students' highly individualized learning experiences by linking the service experiences with the learning objectives established for the course and curriculum. Reflection combines cognitive and affective activities in a way that bridges the gap between the service experience and the course.

Reflection also provides opportunities for students to improve their self-assessment skills and have insights that help build on their strengths. Because reflection and self-assessment are skills that require development, many students new to service learning find faculty facilitation during reflection activities helpful (Elam, Musick, Sauer, & Skelton, 2002).

Faculty responsibilities include designing reflection activities, coaching students during reflection, monitoring students' reflections, and providing feedback (Rama, 2001). Faculty will also find a wealth of other information on reflection activities available on the Internet.

Reflection is most effective when it is continuous, connected, contextual, and challenging (Eyler, Giles, & Schmiede, 1996; Williams, 1990). Continuous reflection involves reflection before, during, and after the service-learning experience. Connecting service learning with classroom learning assists students to develop a conceptual framework for their service project and to apply concepts and theories learned in class to the experience. Reflection must be appropriate for the context and setting of the experience. Some service-learning experiences lend themselves to formal methods of reflection, such as written papers, whereas others are best suited to informal discussions. Whether formal or informal methods are used, reflection should challenge students to think in new ways, question their

assumptions, and formulate new understandings and new ways of problem solving (Rama, 2001).

Including service partners in the reflective dialogue enhances communication and increases the depth and breadth of learning. Without an emphasis on dialogue between individuals and community partners, reflection becomes one sided, focusing on the isolated views and perceptions of the individual student without coming to an understanding of each person's perspective (Noddings, 1992; Rama, 2001). Keen and Hall's (2009) study noted that this dialogue across boundaries of perceived differences that happened during the service experience and in reflection exercises was the core experience, not the service itself.

One common approach to stimulate reflection is to have students keep a journal or engage in directed writing that faculty read and respond to frequently throughout the course. Journals allow students to record thoughts, observations, feelings, activities, questions, and problems encountered and solved during the service-learning experience. If students are working on a service-learning project as a team, a team journal can be used to promote interaction between team members on project-related issues and to introduce students to different perspectives on the project (Rama, 2001). The team concludes its work with a collective reflection on the service learning.

Portfolios can be developed to organize materials related to the service-learning project and document accomplishments and learning outcomes. Other reflective activities include small group discussions and presentations that relate the service experience to classroom concepts, introduce students to different perspectives, and challenge them to think critically about the service experience. It is helpful for faculty to pose a few questions to guide the discussion, but students should also be allowed to freely discuss and reflect on ideas and issues. In such discussions students often disclose expectations and myths about the service experience. Themes that may emerge during reflections include social analysis of community needs and the importance of civic responsibility (Bailey et al., 2002). A final reflective paper based on the writing done during the semester provides a comprehensive description of students' learning (Hatcher & Bringle, 1995).

Bringle and Hatcher's (1996) guidelines help clarify the nature of effective reflection activities in a service-learning course. Effective reflection activities:

1. Link the service-learning experiences to the learning objectives
2. Are designed, structured, and guided by faculty
3. Are planned so that they occur across the span of service-learning experience
4. Permit faculty feedback and assessment of progress and learning
5. Foster the clarification and exploration of values

Debriefing

Following the experience, debriefing is essential to reinforce classroom theory, allow students to share differing experiences, and reinforce the sense of solidarity that was developed. Debriefing adds to the intentional nature of the service experience and facilitates a dialogue between students who may have been placed in different locations throughout the community. Debriefing can be combined with an evaluation of the service experience. Community partners can also be engaged in the debriefing experience and share their views of outcomes of the experience and what impact the service learning had on the agency in which the students served.

Evaluation

After the completion of service learning, faculty should evaluate student outcomes, the usefulness of the service-learning experience, and the contribution of the experience to overall curriculum goals. Evaluation of students' achievement is based on the students' learning and not merely on their experience or participation in the service activities. Faculty, the agency supervisor, and students' self-assessment provide the evaluation data.

Many faculty administer preservice and postservice surveys that measure students' attitudes toward community service and civic responsibility and toward their coursework. Such instruments not only help faculty evaluate their students and assess the usefulness of service learning but also help students see how much they have learned and how their attitudes may have changed because of their service-learning experience. In addition to the short-term course evaluation, a systematic long-term follow-up of students helps determine any

additional learning that may have occurred after the course is completed.

Challenges

Some of the challenges to implementing service learning result from ordinary budgetary constraints in higher education (Palmer & Savoie, 2001). Multiple departments and programs compete for limited resources. Those beginning a service-learning initiative may need to search for external funding sources and rely on the goodwill of faculty members willing to spend extra time learning about service learning and then incorporating service learning into their courses without extra compensation.

Institutions that lack a dedicated service-learning office may struggle with organization and effective evaluation strategies. When funding issues prevent the establishment of a service-learning office, a service-learning council composed of faculty members from each department on campus can provide direction for faculty development, coordinate student learning activities with community agencies, evaluate service-learning experiences, and facilitate the sharing of information (Palmer & Savoie, 2001).

Convincing faculty members to adopt service learning as an effective pedagogical device can also be a challenge. This resistance is understandable because of the time and effort involved in incorporating service learning into courses. Faculty members involved in service learning often serve as the best change agents as they extol the benefits of service learning, including increased student engagement in the learning process and increased sense of collegiality because of their intradisciplinary and interdisciplinary activities (Palmer & Savoie, 2001).

Challenges encountered by faculty include time constraints; students' commitments to work and family; and students', faculty's, and community partners' heavy workloads. Community partners may struggle with orienting new students each semester and with the lack of students during summer break (Holloway, 2002; Mayne & Glascoff, 2002). Several universities reported designing experiences that lasted more than one semester or encouraging students taking multiple courses with service-learning components to remain at the same community agency to increase continuity (Cohen & Milone-Nuzzo, 2001; Holloway, 2002).

SUMMARY

The ultimate goal of providing opportunities for civic engagement, development of cultural competence, and service learning in institutions of higher education and their schools of nursing is to develop a more caring society and foster social justice. Students, schools, and the community benefit when service learning is a part of the curriculum. Service-learning experiences have the benefits of increasing retention of academic material and fostering global awareness and a sense of social responsibility within participants. Following service-learning experiences, students are often inspired to continue to work for social justice as engaged citizens in their communities. Although integration of service learning into the curriculum requires faculty development and thoughtful planning, service learning is a win–win–win situation for the college, the students, and the community.

REFLECTING ON THE EVIDENCE

1. In what ways is service learning similar to and different from a clinical practicum experience in a nursing program?

2. Plan a service-learning project for a particular curriculum. How does service learning fit within the mission of the college or university and school of nursing? What needs to be considered before initiating service learning? What resources are already available on campus? What will be barriers and facilitators? Where is (are) the most appropriate place(s) for the experience(s)?

3. What are the best practices for service learning in the curriculum? What evidence exists? What additional evidence needs to be established? Pose a research question and design a study.

REFERENCES

American Association of Colleges of Nursing. (2008a). *Cultural competency in baccalaureate nursing education.* Retrieved from http://www.aacn.nche.edu/Education/pdf/competency.pdf

American Association of Colleges of Nursing. (2008b). *The essentials of baccalaureate education for professional nursing practice.* Retrieved from http://www.aacn.nche.edu/Education/pdf/BaccEssentials08.pdf

American Association of Community Colleges. (2010). Creating a climate for service learning success. Retrieved from http://www.aacc.nche.edu/Resources/aaccprograms/horizons/Documents/creatingaclimate_082010.pdf

American Psychological Association. (2007). Retrieved from http://www.apa.org/ed/slce/home.html

Amerson, R. (2010). The impact of service-learning on cultural competence, *Nursing Education Perspectives, 31*(1), 1822.

Anderson, S., & Miller, A. (2007). Implementing transformational leadership as a model for service learning activities in an online RN to BSN leadership course. *Online Journal of Nursing Informatics, 11*(1). Retrieved from http://ojni.org/11_1/Miller.htm

Anstee, J. L. K., Harris, S. G., Pruitt, K. D., & Sugar, J. A. (2008). Service learning projects in an undergraduate gerontology course: A six-stage model and application. *Educational Gerontology, 34*(7), 595–609.

Bailey, P. A., Carpenter, D. R., & Harrington, P. (2002). Theoretical foundations of service-learning in nursing education. *Journal of Nursing Education, 41*(10), 433–436.

Bassi, S., Cray, J., & Caldrello, L. (2008). A tobacco-free service-learning project. *Journal of Nursing Education, 47*(4), 174–178.

Batchelder, T. H., & Root, S. (1994). Effects of an undergraduate program to integrate academic learning and service: Cognitive, prosocial cognitive, and identity outcomes. *Journal of Adolescence, 1*(4), 341–355.

Battistoni, R. (1995). Service learning, diversity, and the liberal arts curriculum. *Liberal Education, 81*(1), 30–35.

Baumberger, M. L., Krouse, A. M., & Borucki, L. C. (2006). Giving and receiving: A case study in service learning. *Nurse Educator, *(6), 249–252.

Boyer, E. L. (1990). *Scholarship reconsidered: Priorities of the professoriate.* New York, NY: The Carnegie Foundation for the Advancement of Teaching.

Brackley, D. S. J. (1988). Downward mobility: Social implications of St. Ignatius's two standards in studies of spirituality of Jesuits. *Studies in Spirituality of Jesuits, 20*(1), 38.

Bringle, R. G., & Hatcher, J. A. (1996). Implementing service learning in higher education. *Journal of Higher Education, 67*(2), 221–239.

Brown, J. F. (2009). Faith-based mental health education: A service learning opportunity for nursing students. *Journal of Psychiatric and Mental Health Nursing, 16*(6), 581–588.

Callister, L. C., & Hobbins-Garbett, D. (2000). Enter to learn, go forth to serve: Service learning in nursing education. *Journal of Professional Nursing, 16*(3), 177–183.

Campus Compact. (2001). Retrieved from http://www.compact.org

Campus Community Partners for Health. Retrieved from http://depts.washington.edu/ccph/index.html

Carter, J., & Dunn, B. (2002). Educational innovations: A service-learning partnership for enhanced diabetes management. *Journal of Nursing Education, 41*(10), 450–452.

Cohen, J., & Kinsey, D. F. (1994). "Doing good" and scholarship: A service-learning study. *Journalism Educator, 48*(4), 4–14.

Cohen, S. S., & Milone-Nuzzo, P. (2001). Advancing health policy in nursing education through service learning. *Advances in Nursing Science, 23*(3), 28–40.

Colby, A., Ehrlich, T., Beaumont, E., & Stephens, J. (2003). *Educating citizens: Preparing America's undergraduates for lives of moral and civic responsibility.* San Francisco, CA: Jossey-Bass.

Cooper, J. (1993). Developing community partnerships through service learning programs. *Campus Activities Programming, 26*(1), 27–31.

Cotton, D., & Stanton, T. K. (1990). Joining campus and community through service learning. In C. I. Delve, S. D. Mintz, & G. M. Stewart (Eds.), *Community service as values education: New directions for student services* (pp. 101–110). San Francisco, CA: Jossey-Bass.

Daloz, L. A., Keen, C. H., Keen, J. P., & Parks, S. D. (1996). Lives of commitment. *Change, 28*(3), 11–15.

Delve, C. I., Mintz, S. D., & Stewart, G. M. (1990). Promoting values development through community service: A design. *New Directions for Student Services, 50*(2), 7–29.

Dewey, J. (1916). *Democracy and education.* New York, NY: Macmillan.

Dewey, J. (1933). *How we think.* Boston, MA: Heath.

Dewey, J. (1938). *Experience and education.* New York, NY: Macmillan.

Dorr, D. (1993). *Options for the poor: A hundred years of Vatican social teaching.* Maryknoll, NY: Orbis Books.

Eads, S. E. (1994). The value of service learning in higher education. In R. J. Kraft & M. Swadner (Eds.), *Building community: Service learning in the academic disciplines* (pp. 35–40). Denver, CO: Colorado Campus Compact.

Ehrlich, T. (1995). Taking service seriously. *AAHE Bulletin, 47*(7), 8–10.

Elam, C. L., Musick, D. W., Sauer, M. J., & Skelton, J. (2002). How we are implementing a service-learning elective. *Medical Teacher, 24*(3), 249–253.

Eyler, J., & Giles, D. (1999). *Where's the service in service learning?* San Francisco, CA: Jossey-Bass.

Eyler, J., Giles, D. E., & Schmiede, A. (1996). *A practitioner's guide to reflection in service learning: Student voices and reflections.* A technical assistance project funded by the Corporation for National Service. Nashville, TN: Vanderbilt University.

Eyler, J., Giles, D. E., Stenson, C., & Gray, C. (2001). *At a glance: What we know about the effects of service learning on college students, faculty, institutions and communities, 1993–2000.* Retrieved from http://www.servicelearning.org/filemanager/download/aag.pdf

Fertman, C. L. (1994). *Service learning for all students.* Bloomington, IN: Phi Delta Kappa Educational Foundation.

Fleischauer, J. P., & Fleischauer, J. F. (1994). College credit for community service: A "win-win" situation. *Journal of Experiential Education, 17*(3), 41–44.

Francis-Baldesari, C., & Williamson, D. C. (2008). Integration of nursing education, practice, and research through community partnerships: A case study. *Advances in Nursing Science, 31*(4), E1–10.

Fuller, S. G., Alexander, J. W., & Hardeman, S. M. (2006). Sheriff's deputies and nursing students service-learning partnership. *Nurse Educator, 31*(1), 31–35.

Gehrke, P. M. (2008). Civic engagement and nursing education. *Advances in Nursing Science, 31*(1), 52–66.

Giles, D. E., & Eyler, J. (1994). The impact of a college community service laboratory on students' personal, social, and cognitive outcomes. *Journal of Adolescence, 17*(4), 327–339.

Gilligan, C. (1981). Moral development in the college years. In A. Chickering (Ed.), *The modern American college* (pp. 139–157). San Francisco, CA: Jossey-Bass.

Gilligan, C. (1982). *In a different voice: Psychological theory and women's development.* Cambridge, MA: Harvard University Press.

Hales, A. (1997). Service-learning within the nursing curriculum. *Nurse Educator, 22*(2), 15–18.

Hamner, J. B., Wilder, B., Avery, G., & Byrd, L. (2002). Community-based service learning in the engaged university. *Nursing Outlook, 50*(2), 67–71.

Hatcher, J. A., & Bringle, R. G. (1995). Reflection: Bridging the gap between service and learning. (Unpublished manuscript). Indiana University–Purdue University, Indianapolis, IN.

Herman, C., & Sassatelli, J, (2002). DARING to reach the heartland: A collaborative faith-based partnership in nursing education. *Journal of Nursing Education, 41*(10), 443–445.

Hoebeke, R., McCullough, J., Cagle, L., & St. Clair, J. (2009). Service learning education and practice partnerships in maternal-infant health. *Journal of Obstetric, Gynecologic, and Neonatal Nursing, 38,* 632–639.

Holloway, A. S. (2002). Educational innovations: Service-learning in community college nursing education. *Journal of Nursing Education, 41*(10), 440–442.

Institute of Medicine. (2010). Transforming education. In Institute of Medicine, *The future of nursing: Leading change, advancing health* (pp. 139–186). Retrieved from http://books.nap.edu/openbook.php?record_id=12956&page=139

Jacoby, B. (1996). *Service-learning in higher education: Concepts and practices.* San Francisco, CA: Jossey-Bass.

Jarosinski, J. M., & Heinrich, C. (2010). Standing in their shoes: Student immersion in the community using service-learning with at-risk teens. *Issues in Mental Health Nursing, 31*(4), 288–297.

Keen, C., & Hall, K. (2009). Engaging with difference matters: Longitudinal student outcomes of co-curricular service learning programs. *Journal of Higher Education, 80*(1), 59–79.

Kendall, J. C. (1990). *Combining service and learning: A resource book for community and public service.* Raleigh, NC: National Society for Internships and Experiential Education.

Kohlberg, L. (1976). Moral stages and moralization: The cognitive-developmental approach. In T. Lickona (Ed.), *Moral development and behavior: Theory, research and social issues* (pp. 31–53). New York, NY: Holt, Rinehart & Winston.

Kolb, D. A. (1984). *Experiential learning: Experience as the source of learning and development.* Englewood Cliffs, NJ: Prentice Hall.

Kulewicz, S. J. (2001). Service learning: Head Start and a baccalaureate nursing curriculum working together. *Pediatric Nursing, 27*(1), 27–43.

Lashley, M. (2007). Nurses on a mission: A professional service-learning experience with the inner-city homeless. *Nursing Education Perspectives, 28*(1), 24–26.

Ligeikis-Clayton, C., & Denman, J. Z. (2005). Service learning across the curriculum. *Nurse Educator, 30*(5), 191–192.

Macy, J. E. (1994). A model for service learning: Values development for higher education. *Campus Activities Programming, 27*(4), 62, 64–69.

Mayne, L., & Glascoff, M. (2002). Service learning: Preparing a health care workforce for the next century. *Nurse Educator, 27*(4), 191–194.

Mezirow, J. (1990). How critical reflection triggers transformative learning. In J. Mezirow (Ed.), *Fostering critical reflection in adulthood: A guide to transformative and emancipatory learning* (pp. 1–20). San Francisco, CA: Jossey-Bass.

Miettinen, R. (2000). The concept of experiential learning and John Dewey's theory of reflective thought and action. *International Journal of Lifelong Education, 19*(1), 54–73.

Molledahl, A. K. (1994). Student volunteers live out Catholic mandate of service. *St. Thomas, 1,* 27–30.

Narsavage, G. L., Lindell, D., Chen, Y., Savrin, C., & Duffy, E. (2002). A community engagement initiative: Service-learning in graduate nursing education. *Journal of Nursing Education, 41*(10), 457–461.

National League for Nursing. (2005). *Transforming nursing education.* Retrieved from http://www.nln.org/aboutnln/PositionStatements/transforming052005.pdf

National Service-Learning Clearinghouse. (2010). Retrieved from http://www.servicelearning.org/

Noddings, N. (1992). *The challenge to care in schools: An alternative approach to education.* New York, NY: Teachers College Press.

Palmer, C. E., & Savoie, E. J. (2001). Service learning: A conceptual overview. In G. P. Poirrier (Ed.), *Service learning: Curricular applications in nursing* (pp. 17–22). Boston, MA: Jones & Bartlett.

Pellietier, S. (1995). The quiet power of service learning: Report from the National Institute on Learning and Service. *The Independent, 95*(4), 7–10.

Pew Health Professions Commission. (1998). *Recreating health professional practice for a new century.* San Francisco, CA: The Center for Health Professions.

Radest, H. (1993). *Community service: Encounter with strangers.* Westport, CT: Praeger.

Rama, D. V. (2001). *Using structured reflection to enhance learning from service.* Retrieved from http://www.compact.org/disciplines/reflection

Rash, E. M. (2005). A service learning research methods course. *Journal of Nursing Education, 44*(10), 477–478.

Redman, R. W., & Clark, L. (2002). Educational innovations: Service learning as a model for integrating social justice in the nursing curriculum. *Journal of Nursing Education, 41*(10), 446–449.

Rehnke, M. A. F. (1995). Teaching and learning: Why should colleges encourage community service learning? *The Independent, 95*(2), 6.

Reising, D. L., Allen, P. N., & Hall, S. G. (2006a). Student and community outcomes in service-learning: Part 1—Student perceptions. *Journal of Nursing Education, 45*(12), 512–515.

Reising, D. L., Allen, P. N., & Hall, S. G. (2006b). Student and community outcomes in service-learning: Part 2—Community outcomes. *Journal of Nursing Education, 45*(12), 516–518.

Reynolds, P. J. (2005). How service-learning experience benefits physical therapist students' professional development: A grounded theory study. *Journal of Physical Therapy Education, 19*(1), 41–51.

Richardson, B., Billings, D. M., & Martin, J. S. (1996, January). *Service learning as a pedagogy for community-based nursing education.* Poster presented at the NLN-CRNE 13th Conference on Research in Nursing Education, San Antonio, TX.

Riner, M E., & Becklenberg, A. (2001). Partnering with a sister city organization for an international service-learning experience. *Journal of Transcultural Nursing, 12*(3), 234–240.

Schaffer, M. A., & Peterson, S. J. (2001). Teaching undergraduate research and group leadership skills through service learning projects. In G. P. Poirrier (Ed.), *Service learning: Curricular applications in nursing* (pp. 41–47). Boston, MA: Jones & Bartlett.

Schmidt, N. A., & Brown, J. M. (2008). Girl Scout badge day as a service learning experience. *International Journal of Nursing Education Scholarship, 5*(1), 1–14.

Schön, D. A. (1983). *The reflective practitioner: How professionals think in action.* New York, NY: Basic Books.

Shah, N., & Glascoff, M. (1998). The community as classroom: Service learning in Tillery, North Carolina. In J. Norbeck, C. Connelly, & J. Koerner (Eds.), *Caring and community: Concepts and models for service-learning in nursing* (pp. 111–118). Washington, DC: American Association for Higher Education.

Sheffield, E. C. (2005). Service in service-learning education: The need for philosophical understanding. *The High School Journal, 89*(1), 46–53.

Silcox, H. C. (1994). *A how to guide to reflection: Adding cognitive learning to community service programs.* Holland, PA: Brighton Press.

Williams, R. (1990). The impact of field education on student development: Research findings. In J. C. Kendall (Ed.), *Combining service and learning: A resource book for community and public service* (pp. 130–147). Raleigh, NC: National Society for Internships and Experiential Education.

Wills, J. (1992). Service: On campus and in the curriculum. *Educational Record, 73*(2), 32–36.

Worrell-Carlisle, P. J. (2005). Service-learning: A tool for developing cultural awareness. *Nurse Educator, 30*(5), 197–202.

13

From Teaching to Learning: Theoretical Foundations

Lori Candela, EdD, MS, RN, FNP-BC, CNE

Teaching and learning are interactive processes. The roots of the paradigm shift away from an emphasis on the teacher and teaching to the learner and learning can be traced back to the works of Carl Rogers (1969), Malcolm Knowles (1980), and Jack Mezirow (1975), among others. This shift places the purpose of the educational enterprise on the outcomes of the learning process and is of particular interest in nursing, which relies on this process for effective practice.

The learning paradigm, as opposed to the instructional paradigm, "frames learning holistically, recognizing that the chief agent in the process is the learner" (Barr & Tagg, 1995, p. 21). Within this process, faculty are responsible for "creating environments and experiences that bring students to discover and construct knowledge for themselves" (Barr & Tagg, 1995, p. 15). In the learning paradigm, the learning environment and learning experiences are learner centered and learner mediated. Learning is a two-way process of teacher as senior learner and student as junior learner (Rogers, 1969), resulting in both being transformed (Diekelmann, 1989). It is viewed as a fundamental social activity by Chan and Pang (2006), who emphasize the co-construction of ideas and development of learning communities. In contrast, the instructional paradigm positions the faculty as knowledge disseminator and student as passive recipient whose primary responsibility is to take in this knowledge and recall it during activities and examinations.

The purposes of this chapter are to (1) differentiate between the processes of teaching and learning,

(2) explore the dimensions of the teaching–learning process, and (3) provide an overview of selected learning theories and pedagogical or educational frameworks that can be used to guide faculty and learners in their quest to discover nursing knowledge. Theoretical frameworks have historical and evolutionary value. The adoption of an innovation or theory is most often a long-term commitment and affected by the creativity of the adopter, thus contributing to change or evolution. Original citations as well as subsequent adaptations and applications that may be judged as dated or old are classics—useful and necessary to contemporary educators interested in theory-based education. Perhaps the adage "things old made new again" is nowhere more applicable than in the use of theory.

Teaching

Teaching is a complex and abstract concept that has several definitions. Teaching is a system of directed and deliberate actions that are intended to induce learning through a series of directed activities (Heidgerken, 1953; Hyman, 1974). Bevis (1989a) defined teaching as an art and science in which the content is structured and the processes used enable student learning. For Bevis (1989a), teaching includes determining the objectives, arranging the instructional materials, creating the learning activities, and evaluating student learning. However, Bevis (1989c) addressed the need for teachers to restructure their perception of teaching from a focus on establishing the climate, structure, and teaching role to a focus on establishing the climate, structure, and dialogues that engage students' intellectual processes. This redirected focus is necessary so that students will be able to find

The author acknowledges the work of Melissa Vandeveer and Barbara Norton in the previous editions of the chapter.

patterns that can eventually be used as their proto-types for clinical practice. Intellectual engagement is promoted through the use of questions that direct students to read, observe, analyze, and reflect on the care of patients. The new pedagogies with a focus on teaching and learning thinking rather than increasing and impossible demands on memorization produce adaptive students with the capacity to solve problems (Ironside, 2005). Within this context, teachers are also involved in nurturing students, ethical ideals, caring, creativity, curiosity, assertiveness, and dialogue. The journey to this restructure requires that the teacher think about how their own thinking changes with the adoption of new paradigms and strategies (Diekelmann & Lampe, 2004).

Davis (1993) also viewed teaching as a science and an art. In nursing education, the science aspect of teaching is based in a body of knowledge derived from the theories and research from natural and social science disciplines, such as microbiology, anatomy, physiology, anthropology, psychology, so-ciology, and speech communication. In addressing the art aspect of teaching, Eisner (1983) used the analogy of an orchestra conductor for the teacher because conductors and teachers must use a wide variety of skills while making judgments about complex issues that arise while conducting or teaching. The teacher and conductor must be pre-pared to deal creatively with unexpected events. For example, although the conductor and teacher are knowledgeable about the musical score and content for a given session, both persons must pro-vide appropriate guidance, attend to the responses from the participating members, maintain and ad-just the desired pace, make every effort to evoke the best responses, and be flexible and creative when the members have problems producing the desired effect.

The concept of teaching has evolved from what and how content is taught and evaluated. Current thinking also includes what Duffa (2005) calls the "who I am" as a teacher. Style significantly influences learners and the learning environment. The person-ality of the teacher is reflected in the style in which he or she teaches. This makes it important for teach-ers to reflect on thoughts and feelings regarding edu-cational philosophy, life biography, and class and clinical practices as a part of the complex concept of teaching (Demetriou, Wilson, & Winterbottom, 2009; Niyozov, 2008).

Learning

In general, learning is considered a change in a per-son that has been caused by experience (Slavin, 1988). Learning is a process of understanding, clari-fying, and applying the meanings of the knowledge acquired. Furthermore, learning is the exploration, discovery, refinement, and extension of the learner's meanings of the knowledge (Heidgerken, 1953). Learning occurs when an individual's behavior or knowledge changes.

Learning has also been defined from the perspec-tives of two major bodies of learning theory: behav-iorism and cognitivism. The behavioristic perspec-tive views learning as a change in observable behavior or performance resulting from some external rein-forcers that stimulate the change. To be considered learning, a change in performance must come about as a result of the learner's interaction with the envi-ronment (Driscoll, 1994). In contrast, the cognitive perspective views learning as occurring when a new experience alters some unobservable mental pro-cesses that may or may not be manifested by a change in behavior or performance.

Bevis (1988) proposed that the distinction between training and education is essential for the development of curriculum and indicated six types of learning (Box 13-1). The first three types of learning are associated with technical aspects and may be observed. The last three are associated with mental processes that may or may not produce an observable change.

Learning is self-active; it can be accomplished only by the learner. The use of multiple theories to guide educational practice is evident in the follow-ing sentence. Learning is influenced by a person's profile of intelligences (Gardner, 1983), background,

---

BOX 13-1 Six Types of Learning

- Directive learning
- Item learning
- Rational learning
- Contextual learning
- Inquiry learning
- Syntactical learning

From Bevis, E. O. (1988). New directions for a new age. In *Curriculum revolution: Mandate for change* (pp. 27–52). New York, NY: National League for Nursing.

and experience; by the type of learning activities and the degrees of participation in the teaching–learning situation (Barr & Tagg, 1995); and by the power structure that dictates what knowledge is valid (Freire, 1993/1971).

Learning is explained by Alexander, Schallert, and Reynolds (2009) as a complex set of principles and dimensions. They set out nine principles, including the process of learning as change, interaction, possible resistance, and process and product. The what, who, where, and when of learning dimensions provide a framework through which the principles can be understood.

Teaching–Learning Process

The teaching–learning process or transaction is a complex cooperative and personal relationship between faculty and students. When viewed from the perspective of the "learning paradigm" rather than the "instructional paradigm," the teaching–learning process is a personal interactive relationship that extends beyond the subject matter. Within the interactive relationship, faculty relate to students with dignity and respect, with the expectation that students will be supported and stimulated to develop intellectual integrity and independent judgment (Hyman, 1974). The roles of the teacher are facilitator, learner, guide, coach, and mentor acting in partnership with students. The student roles become those of learner-inquirer and seeker of knowledge within an active participative student–faculty relationship.

In a humanistic model both the faculty, as senior learner, and the student, as junior learner, are engaged in the teaching–learning process (Rogers, 1969). According to Diekelmann (1989), both teacher and learner engage in a transformed relationship as a result of meaningful dialogue with one another. Shared responsibility and an egalitarian relationship between student and teacher are also key components of feminist pedagogy (Wheeler & Chinn, 1989).

Bevis (1988) identified the purpose of nursing education as twofold: to ensure safety and to provide the climate, structure, and dialogue that promote praxis (the application of a skill as opposed to its theory). The roles associated with these purposes include raising questions; nurturing creative drive, caring, assertiveness, and ethics; designing ways to engage mental processes; and interacting with students as persons of worth, dignity, intelligence, and high scholarly standards.

The four steps of the teaching–learning process are assessment, planning, implementation, and evaluation. The process is circular, with each step interacting with the preceding and subsequent step.

Assessment

Assessment has three major components: the curricular attributes, the faculty attributes, and the student attributes. The program and course objectives, critical learning experiences, and learning outcomes must be thoughtfully examined. These curricular components provide the foundation for identifying and preparing the appropriate content that is to be taught.

Faculty also need to appraise their own attributes, including their level of content knowledge, their philosophy and attitudes about teaching, and the instructional skills they already possess and those they want to develop. Faculty should be well informed about various theories of learning and other theories relevant for teaching and learning. Appropriate theories relevant to learning are used as a framework to design the teaching–learning process.

Students' personal attributes that are particularly relevant are those associated with successful learning. Student attributes having significant bearing on the decisions made for the entire teaching–learning process include the students' entry knowledge and skills, cognitive abilities, learning styles, motivation to achieve, study habits, readiness to learn the content, and preference for instructional methods.

Data about students' personal attributes can be obtained from various sources. Students' entry knowledge and skills can be obtained from a brief review of the course materials and texts used for prerequisite courses; this helps establish reasonable expectations of the students. Informal discussions with faculty and students are another excellent source of entry-level information. During the first or second class meeting, students' interest in the course and content and their perception of the class's relationship with previous and concurrent courses can be elicited through class discussion. Students can also be asked about individual skills, abilities, and personal gifts that have not been directly associated with their formal education in a nursing program. This type of discussion often stimulates a lively interaction and helps students become aware of faculty interest in the student as a whole person. Individual learning styles and preferences can also be elicited. See Chapter 2 for further discussion of assessment of student learning styles.

Planning

Assessment data are used as a foundation for instructional planning. Instructional plans are essential for good teaching; plans serve to help faculty better prepare to meet their teaching responsibilities. Instructional plans can be thought of as maps developed at the course, unit, and lesson level.

Instructional planning includes selecting and organizing the appropriate and essential concepts and content in a logical and meaningful sequence, with attention given to the appropriate delineation of the important relationships between facts, concepts, and principles. Planning also includes selecting the instructional strategies and designing learning activities. Developing a map of all of the lesson plans before the course begins is beneficial because it helps ensure that the content will be adequately addressed and allows faculty to examine the variety of instructional strategies and learning activities to be used throughout the course. See Chapter 10 for further discussion of planning learning experiences and developing instructional plans.

Implementation

To enhance student achievement, faculty should be flexible when adapting and modifying preselected instructional strategies or when implementing the predesigned lesson plan. Students' verbal and nonverbal responses during the lesson usually provide cues that indicate a need for some further explanation, clarification, or additional practice in applying the content. The common saying "There is the lesson you planned to give, the lesson you gave, and the lesson you wished you had given" provides some insight into the need for flexibility and an awareness of recognizing that the practice of teaching is an ever-evolving process.

Evaluation

Evaluation is the final step in an iterative teaching–learning model. Formative and summative evaluations are two common forms of evaluation used during instruction. Formative evaluation is used to determine student progress throughout the course and is often used during a class session. It is helpful to teachers in assessing what students understand and in providing feedback to them that can be used for improvement (Nicol, 2009). Informal strategies such as questions, discussion, and feedback about student participation and success in attaining the objectives of the learning activities provide faculty with valuable information about student comprehension and achievement during the lesson. Having students participate at the end of class in constructing a summary of the key points of the lesson also provides valuable information. Formative evaluation strategies can be considered diagnostic tools in that they help faculty focus on difficulties students are having in attaining the learning outcomes and provide opportunities for corrective interventions designed to further facilitate learning (see Chapter 24).

Summative evaluation is conducted at the end of a course and is used to determine the extent to which students have achieved the desired learning outcomes. Strategies used for summative evaluation include multiple-choice, essay, and short-answer examinations; simulations; case studies; and formal papers. Faculty may choose to use the results of a combination of formative and summative evaluation data as the basis for assigning student grades.

The formative and summative evaluation strategies selected to determine student learning need to be consistent with the approaches used during the instructional strategies and learning activities. For additional information on evaluation and evaluation strategies, see Unit V.

Learning Theories and Educational Frameworks and Philosophies

Learning theories and educational frameworks and philosophies provide the structure that guides the selection of faculty-centered instructional strategies and student-centered learning activities. Faculty's beliefs about learning provide the assumptions that underlie the approaches used in their teaching. Being cognizant of various theories is a prerequisite to effective teaching. Experienced and novice faculty are challenged to select theories that best support the school philosophy and at the same time complement individual teaching preferences.

Learning theories focus on how people learn, whereas educational frameworks and philosophies focus on identifying the methods that will provide students with the conditions that are most likely to facilitate attainment of the learning outcomes (Reigeluth, 1983). As faculty shift the emphasis from teaching to learning, educational frameworks may be used to enhance the faculty-facilitated learning environment (Barr & Tagg, 1995).

Discussion of learning theories and educational frameworks and philosophies is organized in the following manner. After a brief overview of each theory or framework, additional information is presented from the perspectives of the basic premise, the setting or climate in which the theory or framework may be used, the role of the faculty, the role of the student, some of the advantages and disadvantages associated with the theory or framework, and application. Summaries of the premises for the learning theories and educational frameworks and philosophies are presented in Box 13-2 and Table 13-1, respectively.

Learning theories and frameworks are descriptive in that they focus on and describe the processes used to bring about changes in either the way in which students perform or the way in which they understand or organize elements in their environment. Theories of learning include sets of concepts of psychological variables that are presented as laws or principles about learning. Theories of learning

---

TABLE 13-1 Premises of Educational Frameworks and Philosophies

Framework	Premise
Adult education	Adults are self-directed and problem centered and need to learn useful information.
Authentic learning	Focuses on real-world situations as the context for students to develop skills that are important in nursing practice.
Brain-based learning	Emphasizes the maximization of learning by enhancing the conditions under which the brain learns best: relaxed alertness; orchestrated immersion; and active, regular processing of experiences.
Caring	Education consists of an integration of humanistic-existential, phenomenological, feminist, and caring ideologies.
Critical	The liberation of thought occurs through analysis of power and relationships within social structure information.
Deep learning	An intentional, intrinsically motivated strategy that integrates previous knowledge to what is being learned in order to create new meaning and actions.
Feminism	Intellectual growth, activism, and empowerment can change injustice and inequity for all persons.
Humanism	Education motivates the development of human potential.
Narrative pedagogy	A practical discourse using nine themes allows knowledge gained through experiences of teachers, students, and clinicians to direct nursing education.
Patterns of knowing	Patterns of knowing (empiric, aesthetic, personal, and ethics) provide the nursing professional in practice, education, and research with new means to understand meaning within situational contexts.
Phenomenology	Understanding the hows and ways in which humans experience and perceive events that result in learning.
Postmodern discourse	Truth is related to specific context and is constantly being constructed.

BOX 13-2 Premises of Learning Theories

Behavioral: All behavior is learned and can be shaped and rewarded to attain desired ends.

Cognitive: Conditions of learning influence acquisition and retention by modifying existing cognitive structures. Assimilation, accommodation, and construction of knowledge are basic processes in learning.

Cognitive development: Development is sequential and progresses in an uneven and interrupted manner through several identifiable phases.

Cognitive development: sociocultural historical influences: Learning is interactive and occurs in a social, historical context. Knowledge, ideas, attitudes, and values are developed as a result of relationships with people.

Multiple intelligences: Human beings have unique profiles composed of varying degrees of 9 research-based intelligences.

---

can be used as prescriptions that provide a focus for creating an environment and conditions in which the instruction will occur (Driscoll, 1994).

Psychologists have developed two principal types of learning theory—behavioral and cognitive—to explain how people learn. In addition to the cognitive theories, educators and counselors are using cognitive development theories because they focus on the ways in which thought processes develop over time and the influence those processes have on other dimensions of personality development (Widick & Simpson, 1978). Adult education and humanistic theories are also commonly used in educational programs. There is no single behavioral, cognitive, cognitive development, adult education, or humanistic theory; variations exist for each type of theory.

The learning theories discussed are behavioral; cognitive (including information processing, constructivism, and assimilation); cognitive development; sociocultural historical influences; multiple intelligences; and authentic, brain-based, and deep learning.

Behavioral Learning Theories

Ivan Pavlov and Edward Thorndike established the roots for behaviorism in the late nineteenth century with their systematic scientific investigation of how animals and human beings learn (Hilgard & Bower, 1966). This work provided the basis for what became known as behaviorist psychology. Pavlov and Thorndike associated behavior with physical reflexes (Hilgard & Bower, 1966). However, Thorndike believed that the behavior was in response to rewards or reinforcements; he called this the *law of effect*. The focus of their research later became known as *stimulus–response theory*.

Skinner's (1953) principles of operant conditioning focus on arranging consequences for learner behavior (Slavin, 1988). Skinner suggested a different type of behavior associated with learning that he named *operant behaviors*. Operant behaviors are a person's responses that act on the environment as an immediate response to the consequence resulting from the behavior. A behavior is strengthened or weakened in response to positive or negative consequences. Positive consequences are referred to as *reinforcers* because they strengthen or increase the frequency of behaviors, whereas negative consequences weaken the behavior by not reinforcing it (Skinner, 1953; Slavin, 1988).

Complex behaviors are acquired by shaping through providing reinforcement. Reinforcement is an essential condition for learning because reinforced responses are remembered. Skinner defined learning as a process of behavioral change. A learning act consists of discrimination stimulus, learner response, and a consequence.

Although all behaviorists do not have the same framework for their theories, there are some fundamental similarities in that they all look for behavioral change in the learner and define learning as permanent change in behavior. In addition, they all place great importance on the external environment as a main element in controlling what people learn (Dembo, 1988).

Since the 1950s, the principles of behaviorism have been incorporated into the widely promulgated work of several renowned educators. Tyler (1949) addressed the psychology of learning, the learning setting, and learning conditions and presented a model for writing behavioral objectives. Bloom, Englehart, Furst, Hill, and Krawthwhol (1956) compiled a taxonomy of the cognitive domain incorporating the use of action verbs to differentiate levels of cognition. Mager (1962) developed a model for writing highly prescriptive behavioral objectives that consist of three components: specification of the behavior to be acquired, conditions under which the behavior is to be demonstrated, and the criteria for how well the behavior is to be performed.

The prominent nurse educators of the 1970s and 1980s who adopted the behavioristic paradigm into their works include Bevis (1973, 1978, 1982, 1989a), deTornyay (1971, 1982), deTornyay & Thompson (1987), Reilly (1975, 1980), and Reilly and Oermann (1990). As a result of these publications, programs in nursing education once made extensive use of the principles of behaviorism.

Premise

All behavior is learned; it can be shaped and rewarded to achieve appropriate and desired ends. Learning results from a process of attaching one element of learning to another in an environment in which external reinforcement stimulates a change in behavior (Grippin & Peters, 1984).

Setting and Climate

Behavioristic principles are used in classrooms, clinical settings, and learning resource centers in which the faculty design and control highly structured learning environments.

Role of Faculty

Faculty dominate the highly structured learning environment and perform as an authority, dispensing knowledge while exercising control of the learning experiences. Formal control of the learning situation is clearly established by creating all of the favorable conditions required for learning, by providing all of the content and audiovisual media to be used, and by determining the time allowed for instruction and practice as well as for breaks. Stimuli to which students are to respond are carefully selected. Learning occurs in an environment that consists of clearly established learning objectives and highly structured learning experiences in which student behavior is intentionally shaped and managed by faculty's cues, prompts, directions, and redirections.

Faculty establish a positive learning climate by responding to student success with a previously determined system of positive reinforcers (rewards) to shape behavior. The desired learner behavior or correct performance is reinforced by tangible rewards, such as praise or bonuses, whereas an absence of the desired behaviors, lack of achievement, or deviant behavior is ignored. Faculty's focus is on what the student is doing correctly rather than on what is being done incorrectly. Achievement is monitored by looking for behavior patterns demonstrated over a period.

Role of Student

Students follow faculty's directions and use the behavioral objectives as a prescription for what is to be learned. Students work to achieve and demonstrate the desired behavior as determined by faculty and plan the time needed to practice as much as necessary to attain the desired behavior. Student motivation for achievement is obtained from the tangible rewards that reinforce the desired behavior.

Advantages

Faculty find that behaviorist principles are very appropriate for highly structured situations in which the objectives can be clearly established in a step-by-step sequence and the desired behavior can be defined, quickly learned, and observed. Behaviorist principles are particularly useful for skills training in which the steps and sequences can be clearly delineated and observed.

Disadvantages

The organization of instruction is dominated and directed by behavioral objectives and learning outcomes that can be specified, observed, and measured. Common criticisms of the behavioristic model for instruction are that it is mechanistic and decreases or minimizes student involvement in learning. Less visible and unobservable processes involved in complex mental processes, such as concept formation, problem solving, and critical thinking, are not deemed appropriate in the behavioristic paradigm. Romyn (2001) challenges such criticism with the claim that a professional shift in value orientation from one of learning outcomes based on a behaviorist paradigm to social change based on an emancipatory paradigm is the foundation of this criticism. In the emancipatory or interpretive pedagogies, the egalitarian, shared responsibility for learning replaces fixed, directive outcome objectives with meaningful dialogue (Tanner, 1990). Romyn (2001) suggests an inclusive approach in which both emancipatory and behaviorist paradigms are available to nursing education and practice is the solution to this criticism.

Students vary in response to clearly defined steps presented in a highly structured learning situation. Some students prefer to explore and discover their own ideas outside of a highly structured and directive environment.

Application

The instructional focus is on the stimuli that lead to the desired behaviors; the existing classroom climate needs to be analyzed and changed if necessary to develop a positive classroom climate. If the climate is one in which behaviors or attitudes about learning are negative, faculty can change the climate by responding to and emphasizing only student successes rather than pointing out what students are doing incorrectly. Other positive reinforcer approaches include calling the class's attention to and praising students who made correct responses, writing positive comments on written work, and enlisting students with correct responses to serve as peer tutors for students who did not respond correctly. Serving as a peer tutor enhances self-esteem and stimulates students to continue their efforts to perform well.

Determining the type of positive student behaviors to receive reinforcement and appraising the students' responses to the reinforcer help faculty develop other effective tangible reinforcers. In addition to faculty's list of tangible reinforcers, students can provide suggestions for reinforcers they would appreciate and respond to positively.

Cognitive Learning Theories

The initial focus on the cognitive aspects of learning is attributed to the work of the Gestalt psychologists during the early 1900s. *Gestalt,* a German word, means "patterns" or "configurations." Gestalt psychologists emphasized perception, and learning was interpreted in terms of perceptual principles of organization. Gestalt psychologists believe that people respond to whole situations or patterns rather than to parts (Shuell, 1986).

Insight is an important concept in Gestalt psychology. Insight is often referred to as the "a-ha" phenomenon. Insight is primarily a matter of perception that is explained as a procedure of mental trial and error that results in a solution. When a person's perceptual field is disorganized, order is imposed by restructuring problems into a better gestalt (pattern); the restructuring may occur through a process of trial and error (Dembo, 1988). Lewin (1951) believed that because human beings have a basic need to bring order to the situation, the motivation to learn is stimulated by the ambiguity perceived in the situation.

During the 1960s, criticism of the limitations of behaviorism as a system for explaining learning led to the development of other theoretical formulations in cognitive and developmental psychology that focused on how people learn. Cognitive psychology has several perspectives and approaches that try to explain particular aspects of human behavior (Weinstein & Meyer, 1991).

Cognitive theorists focus on and emphasize the mental processes and knowledge structure that can be inferred from behavioral indices. Cognitive learning theorists are concerned with the mental processes and activities that mediate the relationship between stimulus and response; the learner selects from stimuli in the environment according to his or her own internal structures (Grippin & Peters, 1984; Slavin, 1988).

Cognitive theorists seek the factors that explain complex learning; they are concerned with meaning rather than behavior. In cognitive systems of learning, behavior is not automatically strengthened by reinforcers; the reinforcers provide affective and instructional information. The specific focus is on mental processes that include perception, thinking, knowledge representation, and memory, with emphasis on understanding and acquisition of knowledge and not merely on acquiring a new behavior or learning how to perform a task.

Cognitive theories define learning as an active, cumulative, constructive process that is goal oriented and dependent on the learner's mental activities (Shuell, 1986; Wittrock, 1992). Learning is an internal event in which modification of the existing internal representations of knowledge occurs. Learning is processing information; it is experiential and formed by a person's experience of the consequences.

In cognitive models of learning, students have active rather than passive roles in the instruction and a new responsibility for learning. A transfer of information from faculty to student does not automatically result in learning; students must discover meaning by using information processing strategies, memories, and attentional and motivational mechanisms to organize and understand it (Wittrock, 1992).

Some authors associated with cognitive learning theory are Anderson (1980, 1985); Ausubel (1960, 1978); Ausubel, Novak, and Hanesian (1968); Ausubel and Robinson (1969); Piaget (1970a, 1970b, 1973); Rumelhart and Ortony (1977); Shuell (1986); Tulving (1972, 1985); and Wittrock (1977, 1978, 1986).

Information Processing Theories

Information processing theories emerged during the 1970s; they focus on describing the way in which information is tracked, the sequences of mental operations, and the results of the operations (Anderson, 1980). A computer model provides the basis on which the theories were developed. The primary focus of information processing investigations is the various ways in which individuals perceive, organize, and remember large amounts of information.

In the information processing theory, memory is viewed as a complex organized system. Memory selects the sensory data to be processed and transforms the data into meaningful information before storing it for later use. Information is processed through three components of the memory system: the sensory register, short-term memory, and long-term memory. The sensory register receives stimuli from visual and auditory information from the physical environment; only some of these data are retained for further processing. Information that is retained then enters the short-term (working) memory, where it is either forgotten or encoded into some meaningful form. Short-term memory is believed to be brief (a few seconds) and to have a limited capacity of six to seven items (the capacity can be enlarged by chunking related items). Some of the information may be quickly used and not further processed for transfer to the third component, long-term memory. Rehearsal of the information is important for retention in short-term memory and helps it persist long enough to move to long-term memory (Atkinson & Shiffrin, 1968; Norman, 1989; Simon, 1979).

The capacity for long-term memory or for permanent storage of information is believed to be limitless. Information in long-term memory may be moved from short-term memory even while new information is being received from the environment. Information in long-term memory is stored in a complex system of nodes that are interrelated through learning. A node has one information item or a cluster of related items. In the event that some elements in a cluster are activated, all elements are likely to be activated.

Long-term memory has at least three parts—episodic, semantic, and procedural—all of which are organized differently (Tulving, 1972, 1985). Episodic memory contains the memories of personal experiences. Semantic memory is organized into networks that have connected ideas or relationships that are referred to as schemata (Anderson, 1985), which hold meaningful information. Schemata are packages of knowledge that include different concepts that are organized into larger groups in an outline form (Rumelhart, 1981). Procedural memory is where the ability to do a task or skill resides.

Graff (2003) contends that memorization reflects only recall and not how students think about or make sense of the content. This covering of the context to which thinking occurs is a result of confusing memorization with thinking. The problem in nursing education occurs when memorization is

rewarded in the didactic portion of the curriculum and expected knowledge is not applied in the practice setting. Recognizing that these are two different expected outcomes can redirect learning strategy design.

Cognitive load theory was first advanced in the 1980s to better understand the nature of short-term or "working" memory and subsequent instructional design (Ozcelik & Yildirim, 2005; van Merrienboer & Sweller, 2010). Information capacity is limited in terms of amount and duration in the working memory so information is quickly either chunked into an existing long-term memory schema (thereby expanding and transforming the schema) or lost unless reinforced with rehearsal (de Jong, 2010; Merrienboer & Sweller, 2010). In order to promote transfer to long-term memory, teachers need to avoid nonessential content, align new content with previous learning, and promote learning through student engagement (de Jong, 2010).

Constructivism

Constructivism, a psychology of learning theory, is based on the work of Piaget (1970a, 1970b, 1973) and Vygotsky (1986/1962). Constructivism theory holds that learning is development (Fosnot, 1996) and that assimilation, accommodation, and construction are the basic operating processes in learning. A learner constructs new knowledge by building on an internal representation of existing knowledge through a personal interpretation of experience. Constructivists assume that learners build knowledge in an attempt to make sense of their experiences and that those learners are active in seeking meaning. Constructive processes operate in all types of learning; learners form, elaborate, and test their mental structures until they get one that is satisfactory to them. In the constructivist paradigm, knowledge representation is open to change as new knowledge structures are added to the existing foundational structure and connections (Reigeluth, 1983; Walton, 1996). Piaget's (1970a, 1970b, 1973) theory of cognitive development introduced the notion of knowledge construction. Wittrock's (1977, 1986, 1992) generative learning theory and the works of Ausubel and colleagues (Ausubel, 1978; Ausubel & Robinson, 1969; Ausubel et al., 1968) also fit within the constructivist paradigm. The concepts of self-efficacy, self-regulation, and metacognition have underpinnings in constructivism (McInerney, 2005).

Mezirow (1975, 1981), describing learning as transformation, studied women participating in re-entry college programs and discovered 10 elements associated with perspective transformation. This transformation process began with a disorienting dilemma, progressing to self-examination and critical assessment, then connecting the discontent to similar experiences shared by others, resulting in a building process and construction of new knowledge. Components of the building process included acquiring knowledge and skills, planning a course of action, trying new roles, and finally reintegrating into society with a new perspective.

Assimilation Theory

Ausubel and colleagues (Ausubel, 1978; Ausubel & Robinson, 1969; Ausubel et al., 1968) developed assimilation theory to describe meaningful learning processes involved in assimilating old meanings with the new meanings that form a more highly differentiated cognitive structure. Cognitive structure refers to a person's store of information. Cognitive structure provides an overall framework that incorporates new knowledge, and it is a prerequisite to meaningful learning. Ausubel (1978) held that prior knowledge is the most significant factor in determining the occurrence of new learning.

Ausubel and Robinson (1969) and Ausubel (1978) held that a learner may incorporate received information by either a meaningful or a rote approach and that the information can be learned by one of two methods: reception or discovery. In the rote reception method learning is acquired by memorization, whereas in the meaningful reception method learning results from information that is logically organized and presented to the learner in a final form. This information is then integrated into the learner's own existing cognitive structure.

Meaningful learning can be attained only if (1) the learner has a mental set to learn the task in a meaningful way, (2) the task has a logical meaning, and (3) specific and relevant concepts in the learner's cognitive structures can interact with the new material (Ausubel, 1978).

Ausubel (1960) and Ausubel and Robinson (1969) proposed the use of different aids to facilitate students' learning processes. Aids help students fit new material into existing cognitive or affective structures. One aid is prompting learners about what they already know by questioning, giving, and asking for examples and recalling their existing knowledge for them and showing how it relates to points presented in an explicit introductory example. Another aid is the use of advanced organizers. Advanced organizers are process-oriented introductory presentations that emphasize the context for the content; they are developed at a higher level of abstraction and are presented before students engage in the learning task. Advanced organizers provide a broad conceptual framework that students can use to gain clarity about the subsequent material. Advanced organizers may consist of verbal or written prose or a visual presentation (Ausubel & Robinson, 1969; Hartley, 1976; Mayer, 1979).

Premise

In cognitive learning theory, the conditions of learning primarily influence the meaningful acquisition and retention of ideas and information by modifying the existing cognitive structure. Learning involves perceptual reorganization because individuals respond to meaningful wholes. Analysis begins with the situation as a whole, from which the component parts are differentiated.

Setting and Climate

Cognitive theories can be applied in any formal or informal academic setting and in continuing education classes. The climate must allow for time and flexibility so that the learner can experience and make meaning of that which is to be learned. Twomey (2004) suggests constructionist theory as supportive of online education with emphasis on Vygotsky's theory (Learning Theories Knowledgebase, 2011) to add the social element and "scaffolding" as a technique to structure learning activities.

Role of Faculty

Emphasis is on designing an active, constructive, and goal-directed learning environment appropriate for the students' cognitive abilities. Faculty relinquish some control of the learning situation to the students and actively involve students in reflective thinking, examination of assumptions, and assessing what they have learned (King & Kitchener, 2004). Creating a rich, real-world context in the classroom facilitates students' learning constructive processes that can be applied outside the classroom. It is important for students to have the opportunity to construct knowledge for themselves; group discussions of topics that involve a number of different variables enhance knowledge construction.

A primary focus is on changing the learners by modeling and encouraging the use of appropriate teaching strategies. Understanding how students process information helps faculty in selecting and implementing teaching strategies. Using think-aloud protocols, which is the process of having students verbalize their thinking while they are thinking, helps faculty gain some understanding of how students are processing information (Corcoran, Narayan, & Moreland, 1988; Muth, Britton, Glynn, & Graves, 1988).

Using an introduction with an advanced organizer before actually beginning a lesson helps faculty prepare students for the subsequent learning experience (Ausubel, 1960). An advanced organizer includes only broad concepts presented in a hierarchical order; following this presentation with some discussion of the interrelationships between the topics helps students see linkages and patterns. An advanced organizer does not contain specific content material that is to be learned.

Faculty selecting other appropriate instructional strategies and learning activities will assist students in assimilating and accommodating new information. For example, concept mapping, sometimes referred to as mind mapping, is a strategy based on Ausubel's assimilation theory (Ausubel & Robinson, 1969; Ausubel et al., 1968). Concept mapping has been shown to be effective in helping students assimilate and accommodate the concepts (Novak, Gowin, & Johansen, 1983; Rooda, 1994).

McKeachie (1980) recommended that faculty relate new information to students' existing cognitive structure. Faculty often discover that students know more than they think they do; students may need some prompting and cues to recognize that the new information being presented is a variation or extension of something they have previously learned and applied. Auditory and visual cues help students activate and connect what has been previously learned to the new knowledge.

Faculty can create an organizational structure for the content, such as cause and effect, time sequence, parallel organization, phenomenon to theory to evidence, problem to solution, pros versus cons to resolution, familiar to unfamiliar, and concepts to application. Faculty should also present a prototype model and make every effort to ensure that students understand it before progressing to new concepts (Norman, 1989).

Limiting the number of elements presented at one time to the six or seven that can be contained in short-term memory and helping students rehearse the information is beneficial; this tactic facilitates learning and retention. Providing examples of concepts and asking students for additional examples from their own perspective encourage concept development and learning. Presenting a prototype model and making every effort to ensure that students understand it before progressing to new concepts are important. The use of periodic summaries and reiteration of the relationships between the concepts is also beneficial. In addition, faculty can provide some suggestions to students about ways to improve their learning strategies. For example, using mental elaboration, attending to verbal and visual cues, and drawing pictures and diagrams can help stimulate imagery of old and new information (Wittrock, 1992).

Role of Student

Students have the responsibility to embrace more control of the learning situation and their own learning. They become actively engaged in the instruction and the learning process. This engagement occurs when they are cognitively interacting with the subject matter. Concentrating and thinking about the content, making relationships between the concepts and principles, completing assignments, participating in learning activities, asking questions, seeking clarification, giving examples from their own experiences, and interacting in dialogues with faculty and peers are some examples of active engagement in learning.

Passively receiving information from faculty or instructional materials does not automatically result in learning; students must discover the meaning by using information processing strategies, memories, and attentional and motivational mechanisms to organize and understand information (Wittrock, 1992). Students may discover the meaning of information by presenting analogies, using and describing prior knowledge and experiences, and having dialogues with faculty and peers about real-life situations that require application of the content. With faculty and peer support, students can acquire an increased self-awareness about what is known and become aware of how the new knowledge fits into their existing knowledge structure. Reflection, an intentional retrospective process focused on the meaning of the content and the learning experiences, is a process students can use to enhance and extend their learning.

Advantages

Cognitive learning theories provide some specific direction to faculty about instructional approaches. Cognitive instructional approaches are expected to enhance retention of concepts and relationships between concepts and promote improved problem solving and critical thinking. Students' prior knowledge is valued and used as the basis for acquiring new knowledge. Students may sense more ownership of their learning and feel an increase in their self-esteem as a learner while being able to see the real-world relevance of their newly acquired knowledge. Learning may become more effective and efficient when students develop schemata and improve their ability to make more extensive linkages between their schemata. Further research is expected to add to the body of evidence needed to guide faculty in actual practices that involve active learning. The National League for Nursing's position statement titled *Transforming Nursing Education* (May 9, 2005) indicated support of more than 50 research studies specific to nursing education in support of practices that will do more than update, add, and rearrange content.

Disadvantages

Faculty may need to consciously and purposefully let go of control over learners. This, in turn, requires or forces a change in the learner. These changes likely produce tension and the urge by both faculty and students to return to more familiar and comfortable methods of educational styles. While the outcome for both can be positive, acknowledgment may be delayed. Faculty must prepare for possible poor evaluations as students transition into self-direction. Colleagues operating in the more traditional "dominator social system" may judge faculty engaged in a more partnership-based social system as incompetent. The use of cognitive approaches may require some reduction in the amount of content for which learners will be held accountable so that their learning has more meaning

and depth and will be more effective for ongoing contextual application.

Application

The key to learning in the cognitivists' paradigm is the use of cognitive apprenticeship, reflection on the collaboration required in real-life problem solving, and the use of tools available in the problem situation. In the learning paradigm, faculty create the learning environments and experiences that assist students to move toward discovering and constructing knowledge for and of themselves (Barr & Tagg, 1995; Bevis, 1989c).

The use of the perspective transformation theory (Mezirow, 1975, 1981) has direct application in nursing programs seeking to advance from basic to higher degrees or to role change instruction. Such programs (RN to BSN, APN, and ADN to MSN programs) can structure didactic material in consideration of the 10 elements associated with reentry to couple professional advancement with an expected need for psychosocial transformation.

Concept mapping (Rooda, 1994) and problem-based learning (Heliker, 1994; van Niekerk & van Aswegen, 1993) are examples of instructional approaches that incorporate principles derived from cognitive theories. The use of journals for didactic and clinical courses enables students to take time to reflect on and describe their own learning and meaning making; journals also provide faculty with opportunities to communicate with students through writing. Fay, Johnson, and Selz (2006) apply constructionist theory to the online learning environment to develop an action-based model with the acronym ALINE (A = action based, students are actively engaged; L = learner centered, action shifts from teacher to student; I = interactive, students interact to gain competency; N = nursing competency oriented, skill building over time; E = evaluative, students are continuously involved in performance assessment). Azzarello and Wood (2006) suggest an approach to encourage well-developed situational mental models by unfolding case studies. Through selective release of case information the student has the opportunity to actively engage in a problem related to a specific situation. As the case unfolds, the context changes and the mental exercise becomes more complex, offering a series of discoveries.

Cognitive Development Theories

Cognitive development theories provide a practical model of the student and present ways in which the organization and structure of instruction can be designed to accommodate the students' readiness to learn (Widick & Simpson, 1978). Cognitive development occurs in sequential, predictable stages; in each stage aspects of the previous stage are expanded.

Perry's (1970) model of intellectual and ethical development of college students is presented here because it has received increased attention in the nursing education literature. Perry (1970) and his associates developed the model based on the results of a study of undergraduate students who volunteered to report on their college experiences. The study sample included men at Harvard and women at Radcliffe; the students were interviewed at the end of each academic year for a period of four years during the late 1950s and early 1960s (Perry, 1970). Analysis of the interview data revealed dominant themes with regard to students' orientation to authority; the nature of knowledge; and other themes such as simplicity versus complexity, good versus bad, right versus wrong, orientation to responsibility, reasoning, open versus closed mental perspective, rationale for differences of views, and concreteness versus abstractness (Perry, 1970, 1981; Valiga, 1988).

Perry organized the phenomenological themes into nine positions that were further categorized into four broad categories: dualism, multiplicity, relativism, and commitment. Students progress through the positions in each of these categories in a sequential manner, demonstrating specific intellectual skills and values. At any point in time, however, further development may be halted or suspended. Growth is usually not linear and usually occurs in fluctuating surges (Perry, 1970, 1981).

In the two positions of dualism, students view knowledge and values with the assumption that all knowledge can be either right or wrong; learning consists of finding and knowing the right answers. Progress to the category is indicated by students having some ability to accept the legitimacy of diversity and uncertainty with their own explanations that the authority has not yet found the answers. Perry (1970, 1981) referred to this latter stage as *multiplicity*.

The two positions of relativism begin with movement to accept that views of right and wrong and good and bad are not sufficient to deal with real-life situations. Continued progress in development is demonstrated by the recognition that knowledge is contextual, uncertain, and relative. Students develop the ability to abstract and weigh information to problem-solve in specific situations. Perry considered that the progression of cognitive development that occurs between the stages of the legitimacy of uncertainty and the acceptance that knowledge is contextual is a revolutionary change in cognitive restructuring. This stage is necessary for students to fully engage in critical thinking activities (McGovern & Valiga, 1997).

The last category in this model is marked by the students' understanding that making a commitment is necessary to become oriented to a world of relativism. At this stage "commitment is foreseen as the resolution of the problems of relativism, but it has not yet been experienced" (Perry, 1970, p. 137). In commitment, continued cognitive development focuses on the affective domain. Responsibility is the theme in this phase of development. Progression is through phases of initial commitment, orientation in implications of commitment, and developing commitment. Students reveal the ability to take a risk by making an initial commitment in some particular area. Movement to this phase involves realization of the implications of what the experience of commitment means in terms of responsibility. Here students affirm their identity and accept the reality that commitment is a continuing experience that is revealed through a personal lifestyle.

Baxter Magolda (2004) traces the evolution of her qualitative research and development of the epistemological reflection model over 20 years and contributes important concepts leading to the consideration of learning and gender reasoning patterns, development, types of knowing, and managing uncertainty. She traces participants' journeys as well as her own, acknowledging *contextual knowing*, meaning that knowledge exists in a context. In her study, 70% of freshman college students assumed that knowledge was certain and demonstrated this reasoning as absolute knowing. Transitional knowing (assuming knowledge to be more uncertain) was evidenced in 30% of freshman and in 80% of those in the senior year. Contextual knowledge, characterized by the belief that knowledge exists in context, was found in only 2 of the 80 participants in the senior year. She also found that postcollege environments prompted movement toward independent and contextual knowing faster than the college environment. Gender-related reasoning patterns associated with absolute knowing included the receiving pattern, used more often by women, and the mastery pattern, evidenced more in men. In transitional knowing, women were found to use an interpersonal pattern (connecting to others) and men an impersonal pattern (focus on self).

Research findings from studies in which Perry's model (1970) was used have particular relevance for nursing education because of the responsibility that faculty have for preparing graduates who need highly developed critical thinking skills and the ability to deal with uncertainty if they are to provide care in an increasingly complex society and health care system. Baxter Magolda (2004) contributes evidence of an expected developmental sequence during the college years and evidence that use of contextual knowledge is more common in the postgraduate years.

Valiga (1988) summarized several variables identified through research with Perry's (1970) model that relate to cognitive development. Variables that pertain to the student include age, sex, socioeconomic status, verbal fluency, student's hometown population, educational motivation, and learning style preference. Variables related to the development and implementation of the curriculum and courses include the subject matter discipline of the curriculum, the amount of structure and flexibility, the degree of challenge and support given, the types of course assignments, the nature of student–peer interactions, the openness of student–faculty relationships, and the degree of fit between the students' positions in the Perry (1970) model and the learning environment.

Frisch (1990) reported on the results of Collins' (1981) study that revealed that baccalaureate nursing students functioned in the dualistic stage. Frisch's (1987) study of junior baccalaureate nursing students revealed that most students operated at the end of the dualistic stage, whereas only one had attained multiplicity, which occurs at the beginning of the relativism stage. Frisch (1990) noted that these findings are consistent with studies conducted on other college students. Valiga (1988) reported her study results on a sample of 123 nursing students.

At the beginning and at the end of the academic year, most of the students were at the dualistic stage. Although some showed no change, a few gained almost two positions, moving them into the relativism stage. Positive gains in cognitive development were found by Zorn (1995) and Frisch (1990) with some students who had an international learning experience in Mexico.

Premise

Cognitive development progresses in a sequential but fluctuating manner. Growth begins with a narrow, absolute, right versus wrong view of the world; it moves to further development, in which knowledge and values are perceived as contextual and relative, and finally to the stage in which a responsible commitment is made to establish a personal identity in a pluralistic world.

Setting and Climate

Perry's (1970) model of intellectual and ethical development and Baxter Magolda's (2004) model of epistemological reflection are appropriate for generic undergraduate and RN to BSN and RN to MSN mobility students enrolled in undergraduate programs. The climate is one in which the student's cognitive development is considered. Baxter Magolda offers additional assistance in understanding the greater potential for contextual learning in the second degree student who comes to nursing education with postbaccalaureate experience.

Role of Faculty

Implementing a cognitive development model requires that faculty give attention to the cognitive and interpersonal characteristics of the students who will actually be in the classes rather than focus only on increasing the subject matter content. Guardo (1986) contended that faculty design curriculum for imaginary students, with little or no regard for their cognitive and interpersonal characteristics. Information about the students may be collected at the time of entry into the program or at the beginning of a semester or course. Data such as age, sex, socioeconomic status, verbal fluency, the type and composition of a student's hometown, educational motivation, learning style preference, and life experiences can be elicited through informal conversation. These conversations also facilitate development of a closer student–faculty relationship and begin the trust-building process.

Developing an open, honest, and supportive partnership with students within the context of challenging experiences promotes intellectual development. Rewards for thinking should be available according to an appropriate developmental expectation. Open discussions that reveal the faculty's own sense of uncertainty helps to legitimize students' own sense of uncertainty.

Role of Student

Students must be willing to be socialized to the college experience and risk entering into new experiences with others whose backgrounds and views are different than their own. Having an open and receptive attitude and a disposition to become comfortable in revealing aspects of the self is important. Students' being aware of the importance of their active participation in new and challenging experiences that will stretch their cognitive abilities is beneficial for their development. Students can also expect that progression through school will bring increased intellectual demands, challenging faculty expectations, and some disruptions in their sense of certainty about their world.

Advantages

The use of the intellectual development and the epistemological transformation models offers faculty opportunities for further personal and professional development and increased satisfaction in relationships with students, as well as satisfaction about their students' progressing cognitive development. The increased use of a variety of instructional strategies encourages faculty creativity and has the potential to energize teaching.

Students who progress into different developmental positions experience increased sophistication in their view of the world; they can expect to receive rewards for improved cognitive ability and look forward to a more challenging and stimulating life.

Disadvantages

Faculty who are interested in using these models for curriculum, course, and instructional development will need to study the model and related materials to become knowledgeable about the different positions and divisions. Although this study takes time, it is essential before attempting to implement the model in the curriculum, courses, and instructional strategies. Faculty may find it difficult to find time for informal interactions with students outside of the classroom.

Program design and course materials will need significant revision. Frustrations may arise as the demands on faculty time increase when planning and evaluating the new course requirements. Faculty who chose to implement the model in their own courses may find a lack of this type of student consideration in other courses.

Students who developmentally focus on certainty or absolute answers may be stressed to develop answers to contextual situations that exist in nursing practice. These students may adopt a negative attitude about the amount of time and effort required to meet the program and course objectives. Thus the context of their learning becomes a negative experience in and of itself.

Application

Valiga (1988) recommended that faculty design curricula that require students to have organized experiences with other students who have alternative ways of thinking, reasoning, and viewing the world. These experiences should be introduced during the freshman year. In addition, requiring courses in different disciplines that provide gradual degrees of complexity should be part of the curricular design.

Other instructional and evaluation strategies suggested include instructional strategies that minimize the use of lecture and promote faculty–student interactions and student-to-student interactions. Role play, debate, discussion, frequent use of questioning, and use of materials that present opposing opinions and positions are appropriate. Evaluation strategies should include essay examinations, position and reaction papers, projects, and journals, with less frequent use of multiple-choice examinations. Allowing students choices in some content areas and assignments facilitates development (Valiga, 1988).

Hodges (1996) described how she developed a model for journal writing for RN to BSN students. The model incorporated concepts from Knowles' model of adult education, Perry's model of intellectual development, and qualitative research on women's ways of knowing. The model progresses through four levels: dualism, multiplicity, relativism, and commitment. Colucciello (1988) also recommended the use of Perry's model as a way to create a powerful learning environment after she found students operating at the dualistic stage of conceptualization. Colucciello (1988) identified several instructional strategies and learning activities that are consistent with those already described. She concluded that powerful learning environments are essential if faculties are to prepare graduates to achieve a professional career rather than function at the technical level.

McGovern and Valiga (1997), using Perry's model, report the use of developmental instructional strategies to promote cognitive change in freshman nursing students. They used interactive teaching strategies in the classroom to provide diversity in learning experiences, integrate previously learned information, and encourage the use of active learning strategies such as group projects. Although students were at lower levels of cognitive development, they did show cognitive growth.

Lessons about implementing Perry's model can be found in other disciplines. For example, Thoma (1993) has described how he developed instructional strategies in an economics course that specifically focus transitions from dualism through relativism. Ward (1992) used the Perry model as a framework for developing writing exercises in a legal environmental course.

Cognitive Development: Sociocultural Historical Influences

An emphasis on the social nature and thus the cultural influences on the expressions of cognitive development were central to the research and subsequent theories attributed to Lev Vygotsky, a Russian psychologist (Newman & Holzman, 1993; van der Veer & Valsiner, 1994; Wertsch, 1985). While acknowledging a biological base to the human development potential and recognizing cognitive learning theory such as that suggested by Piaget, Vygotsky (1986/1962) contributes as key concepts (1) cognitive self-instruction, (2) assisted learning, and (3) the zone of proximal development.

Vygotsky (1986/1962) recognized a process between word and thought, with the thought being more dynamic and never completely expressed in word. The child and beginning learner may use self-talk to mature the thought, eventually not only mastering the thought but also going beyond the basic understanding to create the new and more complex (Ratner, 1991).

Assisted learning requires that a senior learner (adult, teacher) provide the learner with the necessary support to allow the learner to eventually solve the problem. The senior learner gradually diminishes instruction as the student gains independence. Support includes clues, affirmation, reducing the problem to steps, role modeling, and giving examples.

Real learning occurs in the zone of proximal development (Newman & Holtzman, 1993). This is the point at which the learner cannot solve the problem alone but has the potential to succeed and can do so with assistance. The teacher or facilitator must understand what the learner has mastered and what comes next. Unlike for Piaget, who viewed development from a separatist perspective, for Vygotsky both the mastered and the to-be-mastered are heavily influenced by sociocultural exposure (Newman & Holtzman, 1993).

The sociocultural learning movement has grown from the work of Vgotsky and progressed from constructivist and cognitive theories (Grabinger, Aplin, & Ponnappa-Brenner, 2007; Knapp, 2008). Grabinger et al. (2007) identify enculturation as a major goal of sociocultural learning and argue that it proceeds as students develop communities of practice. Niewolny and Wilson (2009) discussed sociocultural learning through the use of situated cognition.

Premise

Learning is interactive and occurs in a social, historical context. Knowledge, ideas, attitudes, and values are developed as a result of relationships with people. Transformative learning occurs through social interactions that are situated in authentic environments (Knapp, 2008).

Setting and Climate

Interactive learning can be used in the classroom, online, and in the clinical setting. The setting of choice for sociocultural learning is one in which dialogue and sharing between learners is fostered.

Role of Faculty

To facilitate further learning, nursing faculty can recognize learners' zones of proximal development and provide assistance through encouragement, affirmation, role modeling, and the breakdown of steps. As nursing education increasingly addresses the positive aspects of cultural differences, faculty may enjoy the challenge of recognizing student differences in learning as a result of individual sociocultural exposure. The focus is on student development through participation with others. Faculty must be comfortable in letting learning emerge. Some facilitation may encourage interaction. For example, the respectful use of higher-level questions can draw out how each student thinks about topics and why. Faculty do need to take the time to understand individual student differences, including experiences.

Role of Student

Students may benefit from recognizing and honoring their unique matured cognitive attributes and their contributions to the specialized profession of nursing. Self-recognition of the expected need for assistance in a developmental and historical sense can alleviate the stress experienced by the novice learner. Students are responsible for their learning. They need to communicate and collaborate with others. This includes reflection, sharing, and questioning as a way to learn from others. Students participate in the design and evaluation of learning.

Advantages

Faculty can recognize learners as having unique cognitive skills influenced by a social and cultural history. Students can learn to appreciate differences in peers in an environment in which the teacher is sensitive to sociocultural differences. Such differences can translate into a greater understanding of the patient in the nurse–patient relationship. A sociocultural approach to learning fosters a growing knowledge of self and others, which facilitates enculturation.

Disadvantages

Faculty may not have enough time to evaluate the social and cultural context that individual learners bring to advanced learning, and therefore it may be difficult for faculty to provide unique or specific assistance. Faculty may resort to general appreciation and a broad application of theory and not be able to capture individual student contributions. Cultivating student engagement may be initially difficult, particularly for students who have come from more traditional learning experiences.

Application

Faculty can encourage student identification of the sociocultural nature of their previous learning through personal reflection, storytelling, and comparisons between textbook or clinical examples and their own experience. Encouraging students to communicate in their own voice in both written and oral presentations can serve to both illuminate and enrich individual and peer learning. Sanders and Welk (2005) developed strategies to scaffold student leaning, applying Vygotsky's zone of proximal development (1986). Scaffolding techniques to be constructed or gradually diminished based on student needs include modeling, feedback, instruction, questioning, and cognitive structuring. An instructing scaffold example was the initial use of a written form called "Making Connections," which promoted student critical thinking regarding patient care; the next scaffold allowed the progressing student to perform the thinking orally as the student moves to self-assistance in learning. The authors offer concrete yet familiar examples in the context of moving the learning to increased independence.

Group interactions in activities such as examination of issues from an actual clinical day promote sociocultural learning. Debriefings following simulation activities provide rich opportunities for feedback and learning. Authentic case studies can be used to foster questioning, dialogue, and even debate among student groups. This may be enhanced if cases are given that are complex and contain less than all of the information needed.

Multiple Intelligences

Howard Gardner (1983) challenged the classical view of intelligence and posited a plurality of intellects. The idea of multiple intelligences (MI) began with a preliminary list of seven constructs. As a result of ongoing empirical research, the list has expanded to nine. Intelligence is defined by Gardner

(1999) as a biopsychological potential specific to the species. Gardner considers the intelligences to be raw, biological potentials that work together to solve problems and lead individuals to vocations, avocations, and cultural end states. The theory suggests that individuals differ in the intelligence profiles they are born with and that profiles work in harmony, changing as influenced by experience and learning throughout life. Incorporating the multiple intelligences in designing and executing instruction enhances student learning (Holland, 2007).

The original seven intelligences were identified as bodily-kinesthetic, visual-spatial, verbal-linguistic, logical-mathematical, musical-rhythmic, interpersonal, and intrapersonal (Gardner, 1983). Two additional intelligences have been added; naturalist and existential (Bowles, 2008; Moran, Kornhaber & Gardner, 2006).

Bodily-kinesthetic intelligence is the ability to solve problems or create using the body. The person who is agile and especially skilled in bodily movement may become notable as a dancer or a surgeon, exhibiting fine and gross motor control. Visual-spatial intelligence is observed in people who enjoy learning through charts, graphs, maps, and drawings and who draw on their ability to maneuver in a spatial world. Sailors, engineers, sculptors, and painters draw on visual-spatial intelligence. Persons with high-profile verbal-linguistic skill (intelligence) demonstrate strength in the language arts: speaking, writing, reading, and listening. Poetry is a highly skilled product of verbal-linguistic skill. Logical-mathematical intelligence is just what the name implies—logical and mathematical skill—and is probably the skill studied by Jean Piaget (Gardner, 1983, 1993), who thought he was studying all intelligences. Musical-rhythmic intelligence is the gift possessed by those who learn through songs, patterns, rhythms, and musical expression. These people are sensitive to pitch, melody, rhythm, and tone. Two forms of personal intelligence are included in the MI list. The first is interpersonal intelligence, which is the ability to be "people smart." The people-smart person is a good listener and communicator and is likely to be an exceptionally good salesperson, politician, teacher, or clinician. The second is intrapersonal intelligence, which is the ability to turn inward. The person with intrapersonal intelligence has the capacity to access his or her own emotions and is in touch with feelings, ideas, and values as a means to understanding self and others. The eighth intelligence is naturalist. Persons who identify and classify demonstrate naturalist expertise. Although it was initially identified as those skills associated with the recognition of flora and fauna in the environment, other classification patterns (e.g., mechanistic sounds such as car engines and heart sounds, artistic styles and behaviors) are thought to tap the naturalist intelligence. Existential intelligence is the capacity to identify oneself in relation to the infinitesimal, to ponder the meaning of life and death, to experience love, and to immerse oneself in a work of art—in other words, the species' potential to engage in transcendental concerns (Gardner, 1993, 1999, 2003).

Premise

Every human being has a unique intelligence profile and expresses the intelligences in varying degrees. Although in any one person one or more of the intelligences may be demonstrated at a higher operant level than the others, it is in the working together of the intelligences that a person solves problems and interacts with the environment.

Setting and Climate

The setting is basically within each individual student and teacher. Problems and solutions can be addressed and demonstrated in the formal classroom, in the clinical setting, and through the use of technology.

Role of Faculty

The relationship between the constructs identified in the nine intelligences identified by Gardner (1985; 1999) and the profession of nursing is evident. Qualities identified in all of the categories can contribute to an optimal patient encounter in a practice profession such as nursing. Because most intelligence tests tap only the logical-mathematical and verbal-linguistic intelligences, students enter nursing with documentation that only partially identifies preparation for nursing. Faculty has the opportunity, using the MI theory, to focus on each student's unique profile and to use students' strengths to enhance contributions to practice and the profession. The MI theory is not a prescriptive theory. Application in educational settings is left to faculty to develop, test, and refine. In this explanatory theory, nursing faculty may enjoy the discovery of untested, undocumented, yet affirmed abilities in students, as well as in themselves, that contribute to nursing.

Role of Student

The student can use the MI theory for self-evaluation and for the evaluation of others. Because there is no hierarchy in the MI theory, no intelligence is thought to be of higher value than any other. The student may enjoy the recognition of untested, undocumented, yet affirmed abilities that can contribute to his or her success in nursing. Students can find direction for within-nursing vocations, as well as other social choices, by giving attention to their personal profiles.

Advantages

A broader, more comprehensive view of the intelligences that nurses, students, faculty, and other health care professionals bring to the learning encounter can contribute to greater understanding of potential nursing interactions. The complexity of MI and individual profiles mirrors the complexity of holistic nursing. Specific and broadened attention to course and clinical learning goals relative to the constructs in the MI theory may contribute to greater student success and satisfying professional performance.

Disadvantages

The MI theory is not prescriptive. Direct use of the theory may require changes across the curriculum, study of the theory, and identification of a specific application in nursing. Adult students who have developed through a traditional primary and secondary school curriculum followed by a focus on the sciences in their professional education may not have had the opportunity to develop intelligences in which they have great strength and that could be of service in their nursing career. This is not a disadvantage of the theory but of its application at the postsecondary level.

Application

Although not a prescriptive theory, MI provides a framework for understanding intelligence that can benefit both students and teachers. Teachers can empower students to recognize their own unique gifts to the nursing encounter by acknowledging profiles of problem-solving abilities that consider more than the narrow range of verbal-linguistic and logical-mathematical abilities traditionally associated with intelligence quotient (IQ) testing. The development of teaching strategies to complement all MI categories would be of benefit to nursing.

Educational Frameworks and Philosophies

In addition to behavioral and cognitive learning theories and cognitive developmental theories, nursing faculty use other frameworks, such as adult education models and interpretive pedagogies, to guide the development of the curriculum and the teaching–learning process. These educational frameworks tend to assist faculty in adjusting students' attitudes and the environment to facilitate learning. The interpretive pedagogies discussed are critical, feminist, postmodern, and phenomenological. Nursing faculties have advanced concepts inherent in, or applicable to, the interpretive pedagogies that include caring, patterns of knowing, and narrative pedagogy. Table 13-1 indicates the educational frameworks and philosophies and premises discussed in the following sections.

Adult Education Theory

Andragogy is the term used to refer to the education of adults; it is used in contrast to *pedagogy*, the term used for the education of children. Knowles (1980) defined *andragogy* as "the art and science of helping adults learn" (p. 43). From a psychological perspective, adults are persons with a self-concept of being self-directing and being responsible for their own life (Knowles, 1990). Cross (1981) proposed that learners who are adults should be conceptualized from a developmental perspective that includes the physical, psychological, and sociological aspects of the learner.

Knowles (1980) described adult learners as persons who do best when asked to use their experience and apply new knowledge to solve real-life problems. Adult learners' motivation to learn is more pragmatic and problem centered than that of younger learners. Adults are more likely to learn if they view the information as personally relevant and important (Mitchell & Courtney,

2005; Petersson, 2005). The basic assumptions about adult learners are that they are increasingly self-directed and have experiences that serve as a rich resource for their own and others' learning. Their readiness to learn develops from life tasks and problems, and their orientation to learning is task centered or problem centered. Adult learners' motivation is internal; it arises from their curiosity (Knowles, 1990).

The following five additional characteristics of adult learners have been described by Jackson and Caffarella (1994):

1. Adults have more and different types of life experiences that are organized differently from those of children.
2. Adults have preferred differences in personal learning style.
3. Adults are more likely to prefer being actively involved in the learning process.
4. Adults desire to be connected to and supportive of each other in the learning process.
5. Adults have individual responsibilities and life situations that provide a social context that affects their learning.

Adults make a commitment to learning when the learning goals are perceived as immediately useful and realistic and as important and relevant to their personal, professional, and career needs. The learning behaviors of adults are shaped by past experiences; their maturity and life experiences provide them with insights and the ability to see relationships.

Some contemporary authors associated with adult learning are Caffarella and Barnett (1994), Cross (1981), Galbraith (1991a, 1991b), Hiemestra and Sisco (1990), Knowles (1980, 1984, 1986, 1990), Merriam and Caffarella (1991), and Schön (1983).

Premise

Adults are not content centered; adults are self-directed and problem centered, and they need and want to learn useful information that can be readily adapted. Adults need a climate that enables them to assume responsibility for their learning.

Setting and Climate

The learning setting is unique for each individual; it becomes individualized and personalized. Adult education takes place in formal and informal classrooms in which academic courses, continuing education, self-development, and personal enrichment courses are presented. Opportunities to teach based on adult learning methods are increasing in nursing education in traditional classroom settings, in distance learning, and in other settings where staff development and continuing education occur. Learning opportunities are becoming increasingly available in the home and workplace through the use of audiovisual media and computer technology. Social interaction in the learning environment is important, and opportunities for social interaction are available with distance learning through computer technology.

Role of Faculty

Because adults fear failure, faculty must create a relaxed, psychologically safe environment, while developing a climate of trust and mutual respect that will facilitate student empowerment. Faculty facilitate, guide, or coach adult learners. Courses that rely heavily on pedagogical teaching strategies must be modified to meet the needs of adult learners.

Although faculty assume responsibility for being the content expert, a collaborative relationship and use of the democratic process are essential with adult learners. As content experts, faculty need to design learning activities that are as close as possible to the actual practice they represent so that learning transfer becomes a reality. The activities should stimulate and encourage reflection on past and current experiences and be sequenced according to the learners' needs. Faculty attend to adult learners' needs and concerns as legitimate and important components of the learning process; this helps ensure that their learning experiences are maximized.

Course materials are sequenced according to learner readiness. Learning plans are actually learning contracts established with learners. Learning contracts are often used with adult learners in formal academic classrooms and staff development. Contracts are developed collaboratively and should specify the knowledge, skills, and attitudes (KSA) that students will acquire; the means by which students will attain the objectives; the criteria and evidence by which they will be judged; and the date for completion of the work (Knowles, 1980). The development of KSA is central to the Quality and Safety Education for Nurses (QSEN) competencies (QSEN Project Overview, n.d.). Learning contracts allow students some control when they are given the option to select their learning experiences.

Learning activities should include independent study and inquiry projects that focus on inquiry and experiential techniques (Caffarella & Barnett, 1994). Field-based experiences such as internships and practicum assignments provide experiential learning. Reflective journals, critical incidents, and portfolios are other types of activities that allow adult learners to introduce their past and current experiences into the content of the learning events (see Chapters 11 and 15). These activities also help learners make sense of their life experiences, providing added incentive to learn (Caffarella & Barnett, 1994).

The use of adult learning principles is actually a constructivist instructional model because consideration is given to how previously learned knowledge and experience influence new learning. Teaching adult learners is a reflective practice in which faculties stimulate learners to develop, from a single experience, new ideas and ways of thinking through an internal dialogue. In reflective practice the process is to bring forth past events to a conscious level and then determine some appropriate ways to think, feel, and behave in the future (Brookfield, 1995; Schön, 1983). Within the context of the content, faculty help learners use their experience, intuition, and trial-and-error thinking to define, solve, or rethink a particular problem or issue (Schön, 1983).

Evaluation is shared with the students and peers; students should have some options for selecting the tools or approaches. The basis for the judgment of performance is criterion referenced, not norm referenced. Students collect evidence that is validated by peers and facilitators.

Role of Student

Students must be able, with support from faculty and peers, to determine their own learning needs and work collaboratively in negotiating their learning experiences. Self-directedness and the ability to pace learning and monitor progress toward completion of goals are essential attributes of adult learners.

Advantages

Faculties using adult learning principles assume very different roles in using a process structure for the course experiences in which students are provided considerable freedom and responsibility. The use of adult learning principles actively involves students and stimulates the use of a broader variety of resources as students work collaboratively with others to achieve their personal learning objectives. Box 13-3 identifies the teaching and learning principles associated with Knowles' adult learning model (Knowles, Holton, & Swanson, 2005).

Students' ability to be self-directed is increased, their sense of accountability is increased, and their motivation for learning is maximized. Adult learners are able to find their own level of comfort within

---

BOX 13-3 Adult Teaching and Learning Principles Based on Knowles' Model of Adult Learning

1. Faculty
   a. Relate to learners with value and respect for their feelings and ideas
   b. Create a comfortable psychological and physical environment that facilitates learning
   c. Involve learners in assessing and determining their learning needs
   d. Collaborate with learners in planning the course content and the instructional strategies
   e. Help learners to make maximum use of their own experiences within the learning process
   f. Assist learners in developing their learning contracts
   g. Assist learners in developing strategies to meet their learning objectives
   h. Assist learners in identifying the resources to help meet their learning objectives
   i. Assist learners in developing their learning activities
   j. Assist learners in implementing their learning strategies
   k. Encourage participation in cooperative activities with other learners
   l. Introduce learners to new opportunities for self-fulfillment
   m. Assist learners in developing their plan for self, peer, and faculty evaluation
2. Learners
   a. Accept responsibility for collaborating in the planning of their experiences
   b. Adopt goals of learning experiences as their goals
   c. Actively participate in the learning experience
   d. Pace their own learning
   e. Participate in monitoring their own progress

their learning experiences. The means for systematic feedback from faculty is established in collaboration with faculty (Knowles, 1980).

Disadvantages

The roles and responsibilities of faculty as facilitators and mentors in the learning process should be clearly described and explained (Knowles, 1980). Adult learning principles generate more ambiguous learning directives than those experienced in a traditional classroom; therefore participants may not be comfortable with the requirement that they establish their own learning needs and objectives. Students who lack experience in the domains or topics of the course or lesson may not be able or willing to actively participate. The absence of a highly structured experience may be disconcerting and stressful. The demands of an adult learning model may require that students change their attitudes and beliefs about learning. Some of these difficulties may be overcome by the way in which faculty attend and respond to the affective aspects presented by individual students during learning experiences. It may be possible to move dependent learners toward independence by involving them in group learning activities and peer support groups and providing overt praise for their independent activities. In addition, faculty may choose to use class time to discuss adult learning styles and preferences. Giving attention to students' personal concerns in a caring and supportive manner may help improve their comfort level.

Adult learning methods are not necessarily suitable for all adult learning situations; they may be inappropriate for courses in which the content is totally unfamiliar to the learners and for courses that focus on interpersonal skills, group dynamics, or psychomotor skill development.

Application

Opportunities to use adult learning methods are increasing in nursing education in traditional classroom settings. Adult learning methods are also appropriate for courses in nursing mobility programs (e.g., baccalaureate degree completion nursing programs designed for LPN or RN students; RN to MSN students). Hodges (1996) developed a model for journal writing in which she used principles of adult learning. The model was developed for use with RN to BSN students for the purpose of assisting students to develop writing and critical thinking skills and to assist in their "social, cognitive and professional development" (p. 137).

Adult learning theory can also be applied in clinical practice because nurses are becoming more actively involved in teaching adult patients in acute care, long-term care, and various community settings about self-care practices and about interventions for health promotion and disease prevention. Nurses must understand and incorporate principles of adult education when teaching patients.

Humanism

Humanism has been used as an approach to education. Sometimes referred to as the human potential movement, humanism became an important force during the 1970s, although its roots can be traced from pre-Socratic times (Traynor, 2009). Generally, its early beginnings in recent times are attributed to Abraham Maslow's *Motivation and Personality*, published in 1954. Humanistic psychologists, building on Maslow's (1954, 1962) work, refer to themselves as "third force" psychologists. Third force psychologists have been concerned with the study and development of self-actualizing or fully functioning persons. The use of these descriptors is associated with Maslow (1954, 1962) and Rogers (1954, 1961, 1969).

The humanistic approach to education was developed as a strong reaction to the excessive use of drill and practice that had been common in education (Holt, 1964). Humanistic education is considered a successor to John Dewey's (1916, 1938, 1939) progressive movement in the early 1900s. Humanistic psychologists are primarily concerned with motivating students for growth toward becoming self-actualized. Individual behavior is described according to the person rather than the observer.

Humanistic education has been defined as a "commitment to educational practice in which all facets of the teaching–learning process give major emphasis to the freedom, value, worth, dignity and integrity of persons" (Combs, 1981, p. 446). Learn (1990) indicated that humanism in education is both a philosophy and a "practice-oriented program of education for professional nurses" (p. 235). Humanistic education focuses more on the affective outcomes of education, with helping students learn how to learn and promoting creativity and human potential as its primary concerns (Glasser, 1969; Rogers, 1961, 1969). Rogers (1961) conceptualized the notion of student-centered teaching. The humanistic approach supports and promotes the dignity of the individual, values students' feelings, and promotes the development of a humanistic perspective toward others.

Educators adopting this approach use learning experiences that emphasize the affective aspects of development, promoting the students' sense of responsibility, cooperation, and mutual respect. Honesty and caring are considered equally important as the learning goals that focus on the cognitive and psychomotor domains (Slavin, 1988). Traditional forms of evaluation of learning, such as letter grades and standardized examinations, are inconsistent with the philosophy of humanistic education. Learning is defined as a process of developing one's own potential with the goal of becoming a self-actualized person. Proponents of the humanistic movement in education include Combs (1959, 1981, 1994), Glasser (1969), Kohlberg (1984), Learn (1990), Leininger (1978), Maslow (1954, 1962), and Rogers (1961, 1969).

Premise

Education motivates students to develop their human potential so that they can progress toward self-actualization.

Setting and Climate

Humanistic education is appropriate for a formal or informal setting and involves a climate in which there is recognition and valuing of individual freedom and worth. It may be the framework for traditional academic courses, continuing education courses, staff development programs, and personal development seminars and courses.

Role of Faculty

Faculty create an educational environment that fosters and promotes self-development by establishing an informal and relaxed climate. This can be accomplished by taking about 15 minutes at the beginning of the first few classes to use "icebreaker" strategies that invite students to mingle and become acquainted with each other and the teacher. For example, students can be asked to complete a 5- × 8-inch index card with their name and some personal information, such as a list of three things they like most and three things they like least, and wear it as a name tag for several class periods. This allows students to find out about each other and helps students and faculty to remember each other's names.

One way to help students learn the behaviors consistent with the humanistic movement is through modeling. Faculty can consistently model the desired behaviors and attitudes that are integral components of humanistic education; these behaviors include being a caring, empathetic person and demonstrating genuineness while being consistently respectful of self and others. Faculty's recognition of themselves as a co-learner in educational transactions encourages more egalitarian student–teacher relationships.

Faculty help students recognize and develop their own unique potential by facilitating their growth process. This may be facilitated by praising students' positive behaviors, asking students to draw on and share their own experiences, asking questions that enable students to contribute to discussions, and elaborating on students' responses and questions.

Prepared lessons are rarely presented to the whole class; instructional time is spent working with individuals or small groups. Faculty- or student-created case studies promote self-directed experiences. Faculties develop learning contracts with students to allow them to negotiate their own objectives and pace their own learning. A strong focus is on the frequent use of open-ended activities in which students find their own information; make decisions; solve problems; and create their own, rather than required, products (Slavin, 1988). Selective and appropriate field trips allow students to explore and learn from real-life settings.

Role of Student

Students are responsible for their own learning; determine their own needs, goals, and objectives; and conduct self-evaluations. Students become actively engaged in the learning process, assume responsibility, are open to discussion, and are able to use reflection and introspection. In addition, students adopt the respectful and caring behaviors modeled by faculty.

Advantages

Humanistic education focuses on honesty, integrity, manners, respect for the rights of others, caring, and accepting responsibility for self-development; these are important ethical and moral dimensions. Faculty and students are able to draw on prior school and life learning experiences. The environment provides opportunities to maximize use of the "teachable moment." Students are actively engaged in all aspects of the learning experience.

Disadvantages

Direction by faculty is necessary to ensure that all domains of learning (cognitive, affective, and psychomotor) are adequately addressed. Although self-evaluation is key to humanistic growth, teachers must maintain responsibility in verifying clinical competence and content mastery (Learn, 1990).

Application

The humanistic approach to education is appropriate for courses in the social sciences and humanities, as well as for teaching communication skills, interpersonal dynamics, and group dynamics. Duncan, Cribb & Stephenson (2003) described the need for humanistic skills in patient–physician relationships that has relevance to nursing. A humanistic approach is also appropriate for courses in which the goal is to teach approaches to problem solving and different points of view (Slavin, 1988). The general precepts of humanistic education are relevant to all forms of formal and informal educational experiences.

Interpretive Pedagogies: Critical, Feminist, Postmodern, and Phenomenological Theories

The interpretive pedagogies focus on exploring, deconstructing, and critiquing experiences. They embrace multiple epistemologies, ways of knowing, and practices of thinking (Diekelmann, 2001). The interpretive pedagogies are methods to use when the educational emphasis is to understand or appreciate the nature of experience. The interpretive pedagogies empower the student, decenter authority, encourage social action, and construct new knowledge.

Critical Pedagogy

Critical pedagogy guides the learner to discover practices that oppress and silence people (Hartrick, 1998). Wink (2011) has described critical pedagogy as learning, relearning, and unlearning through questioning and reflection. The commitment is to social action, community building, and collective good. Critical pedagogy is based on the critical theory and work of Paulo Freire (1993/1971). Freire, a Brazilian educator and theorist, posited that those in power for the purpose of marginalizing the masses maintain oppressive social reality. For Freire, the purpose of education was to encourage conscious understanding of the oppressive context to eliminate domination. The ultimate goal is social transformation through the liberation of thought.

Education as an act of freedom is first the analysis of one's own experiences within ongoing relationships with power, giving meaning and expression to one's own needs and voice for the purpose of self-empowerment and social empowerment. Naming one's own experience, therefore, is the beginning of understanding the political nature of the limits and possibilities that make up the larger society (Freire & Macedo, 1987). Teachers, nurses, students, and patients all have experiences and relationships with power and can be situated in marginalized positions. These marginalized positions are to be discovered, understood, and analyzed for the purpose of eliminating oppression.

The concept of marginalization was expanded on in nursing and proposed by Hall, Stevens, & Meleis (1994) as a guiding concept for valuing diversity in nursing knowledge. The concept has relevance to all of the interpretive pedagogies, as well as to the strategies related to cultural competence. Marginalized people are vulnerable within the health care system as a result of discrimination, environmental dangers, severe illness, trauma, and restricted access to health care (Hall, 1999). A discussion of marginalization and seven properties with associated risks and resilience can be found in Hall et al. (1994) and Hall (1999). The seven properties are intermediacy, differentiation, power, secrecy, reflectiveness, voice, and liminality.

Premise

Critical pedagogy is the liberation of thought through analysis of power and relationships within social structure. Opportunity exists, through critical social examination, for education to give meaning and expression to self and social empowerment (Freire & Macedo, 1987).

Setting and Climate

Critical pedagogy can be used in any climate in which it is desirable to focus and understand people or groups of people who are marginalized through the formal and informal educational experience. Analysis is appropriate for students, teachers, and patients as individuals or populations.

Role of Faculty

Faculty identify and accept student identification of literature, issues, and clinical examples that relate to the course content and are amenable to critical review. Faculty decenter authority and empower students (Ironside, 2001). Faculty accept the power shift with an examination of values and position of self in the sociopolitical structure. Assignments constructed around the properties of marginalization can guide greater understanding of risks and resilience in vulnerable populations.

In the clinical setting, faculty support student identification of injustices and imbalances in power and guide analysis of issues and support action for change. Learning issues come from the field of faculty, student, and patient experiences.

Role of Student

Students are challenged to understand themselves and others relative to sociopolitical power. Responsibility to accept empowerment requires self-direction and the examination of values and the position of self in the sociopolitical structure.

Advantages

Personal and professional growth are made possible through critical examination of social power structures between and among faculty, students, patients, education, and health care systems. The potential exists for interrupting systems of oppression.

Disadvantages

The nature of critical social examination exposes the individual to the realization of a position of relative power or powerlessness within a system or systems. This realization can be personally meaningful and emancipating or it can produce a painful realization. The educational climate must be appropriate and supportive for all contingent realizations.

Application

Depending on the course content, any or all of the following power structures and relationships may be identified for critical review in nursing curricula: individuals or populations of patients and health care systems; local, state, and federal governments; student–faculty and faculty–administration relationships; and nursing schools in relationship to accrediting agencies. Assignments that address issues can include a deconstruction of the issue relative to the identification of stakeholders and power structures. Support for action for change is possible through written assignments, field trips, and experience with professional lobbyist organizations and organizations that support change. Kellner and Kim (2010) apply critical pedagogy through the use of media activism in assignments that require the use of the Internet in promoting learning potential via communication that may include writing via social networking sites and YouTube (www.youtube.com).

Feminist Pedagogy

Feminist pedagogy is associated with critical pedagogy in that the approach is a commitment to overcoming oppression but with a focus on gender. The challenge is to embrace inclusiveness, cooperation, collaboration, multiple ways of knowing, and collective action in learning.

Feminism is described as an ideology of beliefs and values about women and relationships of gender (Boughn & Wang, 1994; Morse, 1995; Webber, 2006). The life, work, and writings of early leaders in professional nursing, such as Nightingale, Wald, and Sanger, demonstrate feminist perspectives (Chinn & Wheeler, 1985). Nursing and feminist theory are interrelated because they both have central beliefs that reflect a reverence for life and respect for the uniqueness of each individual (Chinn & Wheeler, 1985).

Feminist pedagogy is based on the assumptions that traditional models of education do not meet all of the educational needs of women and that "education must serve as a means for individual development and social change in order to meet those needs" (Hayes, 1989, p. 56). Boughn (1991) indicated that nursing curricula are beginning to incorporate a feminist perspective as a way to focus on gender issues pertinent to the roles of women as consumers of health care services and as providers of that care.

According to Chinn and Wheeler (1985), the feminist approach values all persons regardless of gender and has a goal of bringing an end to the dehumanizing polarizations that have traditionally existed. The long history of oppression in nursing has been revealed through the absence of autonomy in practice, lack of professional power, inadequate social status, and income inequities (Boughn & Wang, 1994). Benefits from using a feminist theory in nursing education are viewed as being consistent with professional nursing values; some of these include heightened self-awareness, independence, and empowerment (Beck, 1995; Boughn, 1991; Boughn & Wang, 1994; Ruffing-Rahal, 1992).

Boughn (1991) believes that feminist theory provides a basis for restructuring nursing education. Chinn (1989b) indicated that a more complete understanding of nursing's patterns of knowing can be achieved through the contributions of feminist thought.

From the feminist perspective, the caring aspect of nursing should focus on care of self and patients. Care of self includes behaving autonomously, having high self-esteem, understanding power and its use, holding a commitment to other nurses, and advocating for patients served (Boughn, 1991). Feminism is considered to be "a personal, philosophical and political means for analyzing the realities of women's lives as lived in patriarchal systems" (Chinn & Wheeler, 1985, p. 77). Ruffing-Rahal (1992) viewed feminism as an ideology that can change nursing's caring ethic into a political agenda that promotes social justice for the people served; feminism also has the potential for changing professional nursing into a worldwide network of competent, caring, and activist healers.

Premise

In feminist pedagogy the commitment is the emancipation of women (Ironside, 2001). It provides a framework that promotes and enables the development of intellectual growth, activism, and empowerment in nursing (Ruffing-Rahal, 1992).

Setting and Climate

Feminist theory may be used in any setting that provides formal and informal learning experiences for nurses. The theory has relevance for nursing

education in all courses. Many of the concepts and principles may be used when emphasizing group dynamics, interpersonal relationships, power and authority, and the understanding of personal meaning. The application of feminist theory may be useful for continuing education, staff development, and personal growth programs.

Role of Faculty

Faculty strive to foster partnerships with and among students, reducing traditional barriers between faculty and students. The feminist teacher exposes gender bias and oppression in education and health care. Instructional strategies and learning activities that encourage, facilitate, and support students' development in terms of personal autonomy, independence, assertiveness, and sense of achievement should be selected. Insofar as is possible, a course should be structured to allow students to select some of the content and to propose topics or issues that they will address, as well as to revise or omit topics.

Formative and summative evaluations are a collection of information obtained from students' self-evaluations combined with evaluations from faculty and peers (Boughn & Wang, 1994). A desired outcome of students' learning experiences is that they develop positive attitudes and behaviors for all women and nurses. Another desired outcome is that students understand and endorse professional nursing organizations to advance professional nursing (Boughn, 1991).

Role of Students

Students become actively engaged in the course and willing to accept responsibility for contributing to discussions and participating in consensus building. Students listen and talk while sharing life experiences, engage in introspection, support their peers, and become comfortable in relating to the faculty as colleagues rather than as authority figures.

Advantages

The use of feminist theory and methods is described as promoting positive benefits for both male and female nursing students. The potential exists for significant change in the sociopolitical arena with the empowerment of professional nursing. Empowerment of professional nursing has the potential to revolutionize the way in which men and women live their lives and to initiate and sustain major changes in the practice of nursing within the health care delivery system.

Disadvantages

Feminism is perceived by many as an emotional issue because it challenges the basic structure of a worldwide societal view (Chinn & Wheeler, 1985). Despite the feminist position that both male and female students can benefit from learning nursing from the feminist perspective, some male and female faculty and students may struggle with the ideology because it is not in accord with their own beliefs or construct of reality.

Application

Feminism upholds personal lived experience as the content for analysis in research investigations (Belenky, Clinchy, Goldberger, & Tarule, 1986). Chinn (1989a) presented a detailed description of a prototype course with the pedagogical strategies and feminist philosophy she developed as a way of assisting others who are interested in integrating a feminist philosophy into their teaching. The research method or the findings of lived experiences can be used as part of a course's content. Feminist theory and methods have been used in some undergraduate and graduate courses (Ruffing-Rahal, 1992; Walton, 1996). Boughn (1991) described using the feminist perspective in an elective course on women's health for junior- and senior-level baccalaureate nursing and nonnursing students. Teaching women's health can be influenced by feminist values and beliefs (Morse, 1995). A feminist perspective also has been used in conjunction with a model for cooperative learning in a baccalaureate course on professional nursing for male and female RN students (Beck, 1995). Hodges (1996) used feminist theory as a partial framework for developing a model for journal writing for RN to BSN students.

Postmodern Discourse

The postmodern position is that of multiple meanings of reality. It rejects the metanarrative in favor of recognizing what is "real" as that which is socially constructed within specific contexts (Hall, 1999). The postmodernist will keep everything in process, avoiding the power and domination of one central truth (Traynor, 1997).

The deconstruction of the rules and principles of education and practice clarifies who is served by the rules and principles, drawing attention to the changing, fragmented, and political nature of difference, of knowledge, and of the uses of knowledge. Thus the historic, social, cultural, and fluid construction of knowledge is exposed (Ironside, 2001). Deconstruction allows the student and teacher to review how knowledge is both possible and problematic (Escolano, 1996; Traynor, 1997).

Premise

The specific context is essential in understanding what is real (true). Truth is constantly being constructed and is in process.

Setting and Climate

The application of postmodern thinking is appropriate in climates in which ambiguity is possible and concrete application of knowledge is not required. It is useful for beginning students to understand context-specific reality and essential for advanced students to evaluate and prepare for changing perceptions in themselves, patients, and the profession.

Role of Faculty

Faculty work with students to develop an appreciation of the multiple ways of understanding socially constructed systems in health care and education. While in the deconstruction mode, faculty must resist jumping to conclusions and instead support the idea of multiple realities, yet they must work in a system or systems in which rules, regulations, and single truths are clearly established.

Role of Student

Students learn a method of analysis that exposes a stated position, rule, policy, or truth and become familiar and comfortable working with the notion of multiple changing truths. In a learning environment with rules and expectations, motives and rationales are examined.

Advantages

Postmodern approaches serve to expose multiple truths in socially structured educational and health care climates, with the expectation of a single or better truth and the requirements for actions based on set principles. Personal and professional growth is enhanced through academic examination of changing truths.

Disadvantages

Postmodernism has been critiqued for its lack of practical application (Ironside, 2001; Kaufmann, 2000). There is scant documentation on how to apply the theory in concrete terms. Postmodern theory, including deconstruction, provides no results, no conclusion, and no final decision on which to base a nursing action. The application of postmodern thought is theoretical.

Application

A postmodern approach is desirable in an academic situation in which faculty wish to deconstruct a situation to illustrate how subjects, individuals, ideologies, and relationships all hold different and multiple positions in society (Giroux & McLaren, 1992). Deconstruction exercises may be used to encourage pluralistic appreciation. Examples can be found in any clinical and educational setting or situation.

Phenomenology

Phenomenology is a philosophy and a qualitative research method nurse scholars use to study the lived human experience. It is an inductive, descriptive approach used to explain the phenomenon of the human experience (Omery, 1983). Van Manen (1990) wrote that "phenomenology is, on the one hand, a description of the lived-through quality of lived experience, and on the other hand, description of meaning of the expressions of lived experience" (p. 25). Phenomenology has been used by philosophers such as Heidegger (1962/1927) and Merleau-Ponty (1962/1945).

Phenomenology is a research method that "acknowledges and values the meanings people ascribe to their own existence" (Taylor, 1993, p. 173). Phenomenology is concerned with communicating understandings of meanings of phenomena and offers multiple approaches to examine problems at any system level. It involves reflection and discourse through a dialogue of language and experience of caring about phenomena from which meanings are transformed into themes that capture the phenomenon that one is trying to understand (Van Manen, 1990). When applied in nursing education and clinical practice, phenomenology can be used to gain some understanding of the phenomena that are the focus of nursing in clinical practice. The phenomenon of concern of nursing includes nurses themselves as students and practitioners and, of course, their patients. The concerns include, but are not limited to, human experiences such as pain, suffering, loss, grief, and hope (Taylor, 1993).

Phenomenology offers a way to describe the nature of nursing practice in actual practice settings; it is a flexible and fluid pedagogy that is situated in the entire universe of professional nursing as viewed through a holistic lens. This view enables perception of the gestalt of the lived experience of nurses and patients. The physical and social environments merge into a personal, intimate, and holistic experience. A phenomenological approach establishes a view that shifts the focus from a technical skills orientation to one that is concerned with the whole human being.

Phenomenology restructures the relationship between knowledge and skill because of the holistic view of the phenomena of interest in the human being. The themes elicited in the phenomenological approach become the pedagogy (Van Manen, 1990). Faculty can integrate themes elicited through phenomenology into the appropriate content portion taught in the classroom. Students can be shown how to expand their databases to include aspects of the lived experiences of patients with specific health problems or concerns and integrate this type of knowledge into case studies. Case studies are a useful instructional strategy and learning activity through which various layers of the meaning of the phenomena pertaining to patients' experiences may be extracted (Boyd, 1988).

Phenomenology has been used by nurse scholars such as Benner (1983, 1984, 1985); Benner and Tanner (1987); Benner and Wrubel (1989); Bevis (1989b); Diekelmann (1988, 1989); Kondora (1993); Paterson and Zderad (1976); Tanner (1987); and Tanner, Benner, Chesla, and Gordon (1993).

Premise

The goal of phenomenology is to understand human experience—the hows and ways in which events are experienced. Phenomenology informs "the discipline of nursing about phenomena of concern to it" (Taylor, 1993).

Setting and Climate

Phenomenology can be used in the classroom; in clinical practice; and in any other situation in which patients, nurses, and nursing students are the phenomena of interest. Both the beginning and the more advanced student can learn from this inductive approach to what is relevant. The beginning student will have an opportunity to be impressed with the power of the theory and the more advanced student will have the option of assimilating new information into existing constructs.

Role of Faculty

Faculty select phenomena from professional literature that is relevant to the course content and explore them in the classroom. Faculty can also demonstrate ways in which aspects of a patient's or nurse's lived experience can be elicited through the use of open-ended and probing questions. Guest speakers may enhance classroom learning experience by sharing their own personal knowledge of the lived experience of patients or themselves.

In clinical practice settings, expert nurse clinicians assume the primary instructional role; if the expert clinician is other than the faculty member, the faculty member assumes a secondary role. Control of the agenda and learning experiences is left to students and to the expert clinicians. Faculty guide and show students how to learn from the expert clinician. Faculty assume responsibility for identifying, negotiating, and collaborating with the expert clinicians who guide and mentor students' learning experiences in clinical practice. In addition, faculty initiate discussion and debate, offer critiques without judgments, and guide the agenda without controlling it. Faculty become listeners and responders and enter into dialogues with students. The climate provides opportunities for students to become empowered.

Role of Student

The role of students varies according to the level of exposure to the issue or subject of interest. Students assume an active role in making meaning out of information. Students must be self-directive in seeking out what they want and need to learn from the expert clinician or faculty.

Advantages

Faculty and students have unique opportunities to gain knowledge and learn new skills from all subjects. Patients, expert clinicians, students, and faculty all have a story to unfold. Phenomenology clearly acknowledges the value of the students in making meaning out of stories while promoting trust, creativity, and inquiry. These learning experiences have the potential to promote a more in-depth understanding and enhance the caring aspects of students' clinical practice.

Disadvantages

Faculty must have an understanding of phenomenology and some knowledge of the phenomenological themes that have been elicited through clinical practice and research. When serving in a secondary role in the teaching–learning process, faculty must be willing to relinquish considerable control and power in the classroom to the students and in the clinical setting to the clinician.

Students must assume the primary responsibility for their own learning and seek understanding of the lived experience of others along with the tasks of nursing that often are the focus of the beginner.

Application

The anecdotal phenomena from which faculty and student may draw are unlimited. Bevis (1988) suggests the following: the nurse–patient relationship, the patient and his or her circumstance as object, the nurse (self) as object, the vicarious experience, the patient's description of his or her experience, and the nurse's and patient's indirect expressions. Bevis (1988) also suggests expanded database formats, clarified nursing perspectives, nursing prose, logs, case studies, anecdotal recordings, dialogue, fictional and autobiographical accounts of experience, responses to art, and artistic expression.

Patterns of Knowing in Nursing

Carper (1978) proposed four patterns of knowing in nursing as a typology of knowledge forms: empirics, aesthetics, personal knowledge, and moral knowledge. Empirics is the science of nursing: the systematic collection of facts, laws, and theories for the purpose of describing, explaining, and predicting phenomena of concern to nursing. Since 1950 the increasing emphasis on establishing a science of nursing has been generally associated with empirical knowledge as discovered through logical positivistic methods. In contrast, the aesthetic pattern of knowing involves creation and subjective expression of imagined possibilities. The knowledge gained by subjective means is specific and unique and associated, by Carper, with the experience of helping and the concept of nursing the whole patient. Personal knowledge is an interpersonal process and involves interactions, relationships, and transactions between the nurse and patient. The resulting nurse–patient relationship is authentic and personal within a process of becoming. The fourth and final pattern of knowing is the moral component, which focuses on matters of obligation or what ought to be done. It goes beyond knowing the norms or ethical codes of the discipline and is based on specific, concrete situations. Carper suggested that the application of the fundamental patterns of knowing addresses new, developing, and unsolved problems that reference the structure of the discipline and its changing, developing nature. Jacobs-Kramer and Chinn (1988) expanded on Carper's typology with descriptions of developmental processes and product outcomes, expressions of the patterns and process context for assessing knowledge associated with the pattern. They assert that all knowledge patterns must be integrated into the "art-act" of nursing to facilitate clinical choices and dynamic meaning.

Premise

Nursing knowledge is more than that which is discovered through the scientific method. Patterns of knowing provide the nursing professional in practice, education, and research with new means to understand meaning in context to a specific situation.

Setting and Climate

An emphasis on all or select patterns is possible in any nursing clinical or academic setting.

Role of Faculty

Emphasis is on the development of student consciousness of the four patterns through study and application. Faculty focus on the development of the individual patterns, with a goal of total patient consideration. The nature of the aesthetic, personal knowledge and moral patterns necessitates that faculty seek to understand their own personal understanding and experience for the purpose of role modeling the theory.

Role of Student

Students must broaden their understanding of their own personal beliefs to engage in total patient care based on all four patterns of knowing. Some students will be stronger in some areas than in others (similar to Gardner's [1999] MI theory) and will need to seek assistance to apply the theory completely.

Advantages

Carper (1978) provided leadership in articulating the art of nursing and therefore nursing as much more than a profession based on knowledge discovered through the scientific method. By introducing empirics, aesthetics, personal knowledge, and moral patterns of knowledge, she effectively legitimized the art of holistic nursing.

Disadvantages

In today's nursing education climate, faculty desiring to embrace the patterns of knowing in a curriculum may find it difficult to balance learning opportunities in the art of nursing patterns with those in empirical knowledge, which is the focus of licensure and accreditation.

Application

The use of the patterns of knowing will require that faculty embrace the concepts as central to a school or program philosophy. The curriculum framework must be designed to include the patterns of knowing and ensure learning opportunities. Seminars, postconferences, and care plan discussions may be designed around the four patterns as a means of valuing each pattern contribution. Opportunities to discuss all patterns relative to clinical experiences can be afforded in clinical, postconference, and classroom environments. Specific assignments can be designed to focus on each of the patterns.

Narrative Pedagogy

Narrative pedagogy is a research-based alternative for reforming nursing education and uses conventional, phenomenological, critical, and feminist pedagogies. Narrative pedagogy is the application of these pedagogies, along with postmodern discourses in nursing education. A 12-year study produced 9 themes from interview texts obtained from teachers, students, and clinicians (Diekelmann, 2001). The experience of learning and teaching is articulated in the common and shared experiences of what is really important in nursing education. The concernful practices of schooling learning teaching outlined by Diekelmann (2001, p. 57) are as follows:

- *Gathering*: Bringing in and calling forth
- *Creating places*: Keeping open a future of possibilities
- *Assembling*: Constructing and cultivating

- *Staying*: Knowing and connecting
- *Caring*: Engendering community
- *Interpreting*: Unlearning and becoming
- *Presencing*: Attending and being open
- *Preserving*: Reading, writing, thinking, and dialoguing
- *Questioning*: Meaning and making visible

Narrative pedagogy is a commitment to practical discourse in which knowledge gained through the experiences of teachers, students, and clinicians can be used to reform nursing education. It is the collective interpretation of common experience that encourages shared learning.

Premise

Narrative pedagogy is the dialogue and debate among and between teachers, students, and clinicians that questions both what is concealed and what is revealed. We come to know one another through our narratives (Brown, Kirkpatrick, Mangum, & Avery, 2008). The nine themes listed earlier exemplify concernful practices of schooling learning teaching.

Setting and Climate

The concernful practices are applicable in any setting and offer a climate of productive dialogue among and between clinicians, teachers, and students.

Role of Faculty

Faculty must develop an understanding and skill in using the nine themes of concernful practices to expose the hidden understandings and provoke new possibilities in nursing education. Faculty must also understand the nature of the interpretive pedagogies in contrast to and along with conventional pedagogy. Faculty will likely engage in personal and professional introspection because the nine concernful practices will illuminate both positive and negative attributes.

Role of Student

Students share the responsibility for discourse and deconstruction with clinicians and faculty.

Advantages

Narrative pedagogy gathers and explores contemporary successes and failures in nursing education. It uses all pedagogies and creates new possibilities for schooling, teaching, and learning that not only meld the conventional and interpretive pedagogies but also move beyond the issues of power, critique, and deconstruction (Diekelmann, 2001).

Disadvantages

Narrative pedagogy represents a new frontier in nursing education and currently relies on the theoretical understanding of the concepts and theories leading up to the discovery of the nine themes.

Application

Faculty construct activities for content and skills acquisition through encouraging meaning making in students relative to stories about experience. This can be done through the narratives of others—for example, viewing and discussing a movie, presentation, or a book (McAllister et al., 2009). Gazarian (2010) describes how students can use digital media to tell their stories. This strategy makes use of the visual and musical aspects of computers. Through listening and responding to stories and personal perceptions, knowledge is developed in context. Scheckel and Ironside (2006) conducted a phenomenological study on how student thinking is affected by use of narrative pedagogy. A subtheme of cultivating interpretive thinking emerged, exemplified by students' discussion of what it meant to be able to make their own clinical assignments. The authors noted that the use of self-assignment was not as novel as was the use of postconference to describe what it meant to be able to do so. Questions and discussion around stories enact narrative pedagogy as a means for shifting thinking from what is known to what is important and needs to be known.

Caring

Watson (1989) indicated that "the ethic of caring provides an expanded context for nursing education by calling upon the highest ethical self in the process of an evolving consciousness" (p. 53). The caring curriculum movement refers to a reconceptualization of nursing education that has been presented as a "curriculum revolution." The movement has been extensively described by Bevis (1988, 1989a, 1989b, 1990, 1993), Bevis and Murray (1990), Diekelmann (1988, 1989), Munhall (1988), Tanner

(1988), and Watson (1988). The caring curriculum model integrates the pioneering work of Bevis (1989a), Leininger (1981), Murray (1989), Watson (1988), and others who believe that caring represents the moral ideal and central essential core of nursing (Bevis, 1989b).

The model integrates, within a human science orientation, concepts and principles drawn from the humanistic-existentialist perspective and feminist philosophy, as well as from phenomenology (Bevis, 1990). Benner's work (1983, 1984, 1985), presented in several publications (Benner & Tanner, 1987; Benner, Tanner, & Chesla, 1992; Benner & Wrubel, 1989), about novice to expert clinical practice is considered an important model for educative experiences. Although no specific component focuses on cognitive learning theories, the concept of constructivism is an integral part of the caring curriculum model. Symonds (1990) advocated that a feminist philosophy and principles become an integral part of a new model for nursing education. Diekelmann (1989) suggested that faculty engage in hermeneutic inquiry as a way of assisting students to gain new meanings for their clinical practice.

The caring movement mandates significant changes in the design and implementation of nursing curriculum; this directive is based, in part, on the rationale that nursing education thus far has not been successful in advancing nursing as a professional discipline (Bevis, 1988, 1989c). Advocates for the movement assert that the behavioristic learning model used in nursing education since the 1950s is more suitable for industrial training than for a professional educative experience (Bevis, 1988, 1993; Diekelmann, 1988).

Valiga (1988) indicated that evidence supports a lack of progress in nursing education and a lack of any significant change in the cognitive development of students. In addition, social forces associated with the increasingly complex and multifaceted nursing roles needed to meet the health care needs of a diverse multicultural society require well-educated and well-trained nurses who are highly skilled scholar-clinicians.

The goal of the caring curriculum is to create an educational experience in nursing that is more in accord with true education and consistent with the professional nursing philosophy and values that are an integral part of contemporary nursing practice, research, and education. Bevis (1988, 1990) and Bevis and Murray (1990) described the caring curriculum model as providing education for professional nursing that emphasizes analytical, problem-solving, and critical thinking skills.

Content and student learning experiences must be based on the science of human caring and grounded in and derived from the actual reality of lived experience as ascertained from phenomenology rather than merely the content that nurse educators have traditionally taught or the content as they believe it should be. Although theory traditionally has been taught to inform practice, in the new models, theory and practice are viewed as informing each other. A restructured focus of learning is based in clinical practice and uses content as the substance to actively involve students in scholarly endeavors (Bevis, 1988).

Caring theory is also well described in practice. Mitchell (2005) lays out the assumptions underlying caring theory as used to develop a model of clinical practice that considers patient and staff perspectives. It can also be used as a framework for nursing leadership (Britt Pipe, 2008). Incorporation of caring concepts in the curriculum can lay a solid foundation for how future practice is perceived and realized.

Premise

Curriculum is based on the integration of humanistic-existential, phenomenological, feminist, and caring ideologies (Bevis, 1990). The educative experience requires caring faculty–student relationships.

Setting and Climate

The caring curriculum model can be implemented in any setting that encourages an interactive relationship between faculty and students.

Role of Faculty

Faculty implementing a caring curriculum work to discover ways to eliminate adversarial relationships with students (Diekelmann, 1989); faculty also strive to maintain open, honest, caring, and supportive relationships. It is within this context that faculty create a climate and structure that promotes the desired learning environment. Faculty develop and model the spirit of inquiry that helps students to develop maturity in their learning and cognitive abilities. Students are guided as they examine information, concepts, and principles and struggle with uncertainty (Bevis, 1989d). The content selected is basic to what is needed in accord with the program's philosophy and desired graduate outcomes. Although the primary content may be presented as information, faculty focus their efforts on helping students see beyond the information to discern the underlying assumptions (Bevis, 1989c).

To provide students with an in-depth educative learning experience, faculty function in different roles and become experts in learning and in the subject matter. Frequent use of instructional strategies that facilitate active learning, such as the use of questioning and dialogue, is important. Faculty-initiated dialogues with students focus on developing the attributes of intellectual curiosity, caring, caring roles, ethical ideals, and assertiveness (Bevis, 1988). Dialogues occur within the context of a spirit of inquiry and should stimulate and enhance faculty and student learning as meanings of the content are explored.

The use of lecture as an instructional strategy is minimized; instead, faculty use instructional strategies such as role play, debate, discussion, questioning, and case studies (see Chapter 15). Exploration of the cases of actual lived experiences of patients cared for by expert nurses rather than constructed case studies allows examination of the real-life complexities encountered in nursing practice. This approach enables faculty to find out how students develop meanings for their practice (Bevis, 1989c). In addition, instructional materials that present opposing or different points of view and different ways of doing things expand students' cognitive development (Bevis, 1989d).

Tools for evaluating learning, such as essay examinations, position and reaction papers, reflective journals, and projects that involve active student participation, are used because they are consistent with the teaching and learning strategies (Bevis, 1989d). (See Chapter 24 for further information about the evaluation of learning outcomes.)

Role of Student

Students adopt different learning styles that include assuming responsibility for active learning and seeking support and guidance from faculty. It is important that students shift their conception of faculty as authority figures to that of colleagues in the learning enterprise because students are expected to function as active participants in the decision-making structure. Flexibility, tolerance for ambiguity, the ability to manage diversity and conflicts, and the ability to organize their own knowledge and experiences are additional student characteristics considered to be essential for learning within the caring curriculum paradigm (Valiga, 1988).

Advantages

Faculty gain new and challenging opportunities to engage in the scholarship of teaching as they become knowledgeable about and able to apply new theoretical models in curriculum development and instructional strategies. They also have increased opportunities to use creativity and problem solving to deal with instructional issues and improve the way in which students are taught.

Changes in the faculty's relationship with students promote an energized climate in which faculty become allies with students. Students' active engagement in the teaching–learning process allows more opportunities for faculty to observe increases in students' self-esteem, self-confidence, and competence. Students experience an increase in their internal motivation and sense of responsibility. Opportunities to observe students' increased intellectual growth and commitment to professional nursing should provide more personal satisfaction to faculty. Furthermore, the status of professional nursing is enhanced as nurses in clinical practice demonstrate higher levels of competence.

Disadvantages

Implementation of the caring curriculum model is a labor-intensive and time-consuming process that includes advanced long-term planning for curriculum redesign, creation of new instructional strategies, and development of faculty. The model may not be feasible for courses or programs with large enrollments because of the demands placed on faculty and students for new teaching–learning behaviors. Development of these new behaviors involves trust and socialization to instructional approaches that are different from the traditional behavioristic model. The shift to a student-centered and learning-centered focus from a teacher-centered focus is challenging for both faculty and students. Faculty should expect and be prepared to provide more support to students as they adapt to this new approach to learning. Students need to have attained a level of cognitive development that enables them to shift from the behavioral model.

Application

Heliker (1994) suggested that problem-based learning has many features that are consistent with the goals and elements presented in caring curriculum models. Content should be substantive and based on the reality of actual clinical practice so that practice and theory inform each other. Small groups of students can dialogue cooperatively about real cases of the lived experience of patients, and questions designed to initiate and stimulate inquiry for each paradigm case can guide the dialogues.

Authentic, Brain-Based, and Deep Learning Concepts

Authentic Learning

Authentic learning is concerned with bringing the "real" world into the academic setting so that students are better equipped to navigate the complex and often ill-defined environments that make up life beyond school. Typically, the emphasis is on constructing solutions to situations that exist or may exist in practice. Rule (2006) notes that these situations are typically open ended and require investigation through multiple sources, collaboration with others, and individual and group reflection. Authentic learning has been likened to the knowledge construction fundamental to experiential learning. Knobach (2003) compared three tenets associated with authentic learning (construction of knowledge, discipline of inquiry, and value beyond school) to those of experiential learning and found similarity between both. An important concept in authentic learning is situated cognition. This is "thinking that is embedded in the context in which it occurs" (Elsbach, Barr, & Hargadon, 2005, p. 423).

Premise

Focusing on real-world situations provides opportunities for students to develop skills important in practice, including problem solving, collaboration, communication, and creativity.

Setting and Climate

Authentic learning naturally occurs in clinical settings and can be facilitated in classroom and laboratory settings.

Role of Faculty

Faculty need to consider current and projected practice realities, including the multiple influences of interdisciplinary teams and patient families. This can then be used to align course objectives to authentic learning experiences and assessments. In addition to current knowledge of practice, faculty need to resist the tendency to supply answers and encourage student exploration and innovation in finding answers.

Role of Student

Students need to be inquisitive and able to "think outside the box." Active participation in groups and the ability to weigh different alternatives are important for authentic learning students. Also, students need to be able to articulate their reasoning.

Advantages

Authentic learning can motivate and engage learners who see the relevance to actual practice. It promotes a broader, inquiry-based view to finding innovative ways to solve or manage situations. Authentic learning also develops collaboration and communication skills.

Disadvantages

If not carefully thought out prior to use, authentic learning can be frustrating for students and teachers. If objectives, learning experiences, and assessments are not well aligned and articulated, students may not see the relevance to practice and may not be fully engaged.

Application

Authentic learning may consist of realistic case studies, simulation, and performance in class or lab, for instance. Examples include demonstration of history taking or role playing, or group projects culminating in a final product, such as the creation of a teaching program for adolescent diabetics. Portfolios can serve to demonstrate learning and promote student reflection on areas of strength and weakness.

Brain-Based Learning

The concept of brain-based learning arose through research in neuroscience, psychology, and biology over the last 30 years and focuses on optimal conditions for the brain to learn (Jensen, 2008). Early work in the area was noted with Gardner's (1993) multiple intelligences and right–left hemisphere brain function. Complex and interconnected functions in the brain work to process incoming information from memory or outside senses and route for immediate action, elimination, or further processing and storage. The way the brain learns is affected by multiple factors, including time of day, nutrition, and stress (Jensen, 2008). Twelve principles of brain learning have been advanced by Caine and Caine (1991). Among these are the emotional aspect of learning and enhancing learning through non-threatening challenges.

Premise

Learning may be maximized by enhancing the conditions under which the brain learns best:
- Relaxed alertness: a learning environment of high challenge and low threat
- Orchestrated immersion of learners in authentic, complex, multiple experiences
- Active, regular processing of experiences to develop meaning (Caine & Caine, 1991)

Setting and Climate

Any setting can foster brain-based learning that encourages interaction, authentic experiences, and learning challenges balanced in a low-threat environment.

Role of Faculty

It is important for faculty to create and maintain a learning environment that engages learners and encourages expression of the "how and why" of thinking. As the "orchestrator," faculty need to design learning experiences that help learners to make connections. Faculty need to understand that each learner is unique; learners attend to and process information in different ways. It is up to the faculty to set the learning environment tone by demonstrating caring, valuing, and trust (Jensen, 2000). Enthusiasm and organization can be helpful in stimulating student motivation to learn.

Role of Student

Having positive feelings (emotions) and motivation to learn will increase a student's capacity to take in and process information. Coming to class or clinical prepared and well rested can positively influence both emotion and motivation.

Advantages

Brain-based learning is effective in further developing learning pathways and deeper learning. It encourages a more holistic view of how the brain, body, and environment affect learning.

Disadvantages

The major disadvantage to brain-based learning is the commitment on the part of both teacher and learner. For the teacher, nonessential content needs to be reviewed and eliminated to allow for more time to "dwell" in essential concepts. More time is needed to create authentic learning experiences that connect prior to new learning. Thoughtful time is also necessary to reflect on the environment and how to make it learner friendly. For students, more time will need to be allocated to being prepared to learn. Some students may initially feel uncomfortable expressing themselves.

Application

Brain-based learning is fostered through activities that require knowledge construction and connection to previous knowledge. Examples include authentic case studies that adapt based on new content and initial responses; simulation exercises; group projects; in-depth, multifaceted exploration of a patient; and reflection on how and why decisions are made.

Deep Learning

Deep versus surface learning distinctions have been made for decades. Deep learning is learning to understand and create meaning (Smith & Colby, 2007). Learners become more persistent and able to contend with more challenging learning situations (Majeski & Stover, 2007). Wittmann-Price and Godshall (2009) discussed deep, strategic, and surface learning. Surface learning is usually extrinsically motivated and involves memorizing information, often for tests. Deep learning, in contrast, is intrinsically motivated and involves a desire to learn in order to understand. Strategic learning is a combination of deep and surface learning, with students being goal oriented and doing what is necessary to achieve their goals.

Premise

Deep learning is an intentional, intrinsically motivated strategy to understand and connect knowledge to create new meaning and actions.

Setting and Climate

Deep learning can be fostered in classroom or clinical settings that offer the time and space for interactive discourse.

Role of Faculty

Faculty may need to fundamentally reconceptualize a course from "covering" content via one-way lectures to exploring topics with students. It is important to hone questioning skills that draw out student understanding.

Role of Student

Students need to regularly assess their learning and be actively engaged in the learning process with peers and teachers. It is also important to value learning for new insights versus just a good grade.

Advantages

The advantages of deep learning are real and far reaching. Learners benefit through a more conceptual understanding that fosters meaning and relevance (Clare, 2007). Intrinsically motivated learners are likely to value lifelong learning as a way to learn and grow.

Disadvantages

Deep learning is time consuming for teachers due to advance planning of learning experiences and detailed feedback. Additionally, students who typically are extrinsically motivated to learn are at a real disadvantage.

Application

Student concept mapping to explain topics can be used as activities to promote deep learning and for faculty to assess it (Hay, 2007). Dialogue between students and teachers aimed at deconstructing a complex issue in order to construct new meaning and ways to make an impact, such as access to health care, can be carried out in face-to-face or online environments. Semester-long or two-stage projects that allow for specific, formative assessment and feedback can facilitate deep learning (Rushton, 2005).

SUMMARY

The main focus of the educational experience is the learner as active participant in transaction with the teacher, peers, and the larger environment. Students are given considerable control over the development of learning experiences, and they construct and create knowledge. Faculty assume a primary role as designers of the learning environment and learning experiences in a shared governance approach with students and others contributing to the learning climate.

The learning theories and frameworks presented in this chapter provide a guide for faculty to use within the four steps of the teaching–learning process. Each theory or framework has varying degrees of usefulness depending on the faculty's philosophy about teaching; the philosophy that guides the curriculum; the setting and climate in which the teaching is to occur; student characteristics; and the purpose, nature, and content of the course. Within these contextual variables, faculty need to weigh the advantages and disadvantages of each theory or framework and select those that are most appropriate.

Recent literature in education and nursing education indicate that the current and future emphasis in the learning paradigm is and will be on having learners construct and create knowledge while faculty serve as designers, facilitators, coaches, guides, and mentors. For most learning experiences in higher education and for nursing in particular, behavioristic principles have limited relevance. Current and emerging concepts and principles in cognitive, humanistic, and adult learning theories and Perry's model for intellectual and cognitive development, as well as those included in the interpretive pedagogies, patterns of knowing, narrative pedagogies, and caring, are consistent with the thrust of a learning paradigm to guide nursing education. Faculty create the environment and contextual learning experiences and the student assumes control over learning through active engagement.

REFLECTING ON THE EVIDENCE

1. Baxter Magolda (2004) found that contextual knowledge is not well established during the college years for the traditional student and the understanding that knowledge exists in context occurs at a greater rate after graduation. What strategies could the clinical teacher use to meet student nurses' development from absolute knowing to transitional knowing to contextual knowing?

2. The National League for Nursing's position statement titled *Transforming Nursing Education* (May 9, 2005)

calls for nursing education to do more than update, rearrange, and add content. What theoretical supports provide direction to reform nursing education?

3. The Institute of Medicine points to the increased complexity and diversity of patients and the health care system as the driving force for nurses to be able to adapt, learn, and function effectively within health care teams. How can clinical and classroom faculty promote collaboration and knowledge construction in interdisciplinary learning environments?

REFERENCES

Alexander, P. A., Schallert, D. L., & Reynolds, R. E. (2009). What is learning anyway? A topographical perspective considered. *Educational Psychologist, 44*(93), 176–192.

Anderson, J. R. (1980). *Cognitive psychology and its implications.* San Francisco, CA: W. H. Freeman.

Anderson, J. R. (1985). *Cognitive psychology and its implications* (2nd ed.). San Francisco, CA: W. H. Freeman.

Atkinson, J. R., & Shiffrin, R. M. (1968). Human memory: A proposed system and its control processes. In K. W. Spence & J. T. Spence (Eds.), *The psychology of learning and motivation: Advances in research and theory* (pp. 89–115). New York, NY: Academic Press.

Ausubel, D. P. (1960). The use of advance organizers in the learning and retention of meaningful verbal material. *Journal of Educational Psychology, 51*(5), 267–272.

Ausubel, D. P. (1978). *Educational psychology: A cognitive view* (2nd ed.). New York, NY: Holt, Rinehart & Winston.

Ausubel, D. P., Novak, J. D., & Hanesian, H. (1968). *Educational psychology: A cognitive view.* New York, NY: Holt, Rinehart & Winston.

Ausubel, D. P., & Robinson, F. G. (1969). *School learning: An introduction to educational psychology.* New York, NY: Holt, Rinehart & Winston.

Azzarello, J., & Wood, E. (2006). Assessing dynamic mental models: Unfolding case studies. *Nurse Educator, 31*(1), 10–14.

Barr, R., & Tagg, J. (1995). From teaching to learning. *Change, 27*(6), 13–25.

Baxter Magolda, M. B. (2004). Evolution of a constructivist conceptualization of epistemological reflection. *Educational Psychologist, 39*(1), 31–42.

Beck, S. E. (1995). Cooperative learning and feminist pedagogy: A model for classroom instruction in nursing education. *Journal of Nursing Education, 34*(5), 222–227.

Belenky, M. F., Clinchy, B. M., Goldberger, N. R., & Tarule, J. M. (1986). *Women's ways of knowing.* New York, NY: Basic Books.

Benner, P. (1983). Uncovering the knowledge embedded in clinical practice. *Image, 15*(2), 36–41.

Benner, P. (1984). *From novice to expert.* Menlo Park, CA: Addison-Wesley.

Benner, P. (1985). Quality of life: A phenomenological perspective on explanation, prediction, and understanding in nursing science. *Advances in Nursing Science, 8*(1), 1–14.

Benner, P., &. Tanner, C. (1987). Clinical judgment: How expert nurse uses intuition. *American Journal of Nursing, 87*(1), 23–31.

Benner, P., Tanner, C., & Chesla, C. (1992). From beginner to expert: Gaining a differentiated world in critical care nursing. *Advances in Nursing Science, 14*(3), 13–28.

Benner, P., & Wrubel, J. (1989). *The primacy of caring: Stress and coping in health and illness.* Menlo Park, CA: Addison-Wesley.

Bevis, E. O. (1973). *Curriculum building in nursing: A process.* St. Louis, MO: Mosby.

Bevis, E. O. (1978). *Curriculum building in nursing: A process* (2nd ed.). St. Louis, MO: Mosby.

Bevis, E. O. (1982). *Curriculum building in nursing: A process* (3rd ed.). St. Louis, MO: Mosby.

Bevis, E. O. (1988). New directions for a new age. In *Curriculum revolution: Mandate for change* (pp. 27–52). New York, NY: National League for Nursing.

Bevis, E. O. (1989a). *Curriculum building in nursing: A process* (3rd ed.). New York, NY: National League for Nursing.

Bevis, E. O. (1989b). The curriculum consequences. In *Curriculum revolution: Re-conceptualizing nursing education* (pp. 115–134). New York, NY: National League for Nursing.

Bevis, E. O. (1989c). Teaching and learning: The key to education and professionalism. In E. O. Bevis & J. Watson (Eds.), *Toward a caring curriculum* (pp. 153–188). New York, NY: National League for Nursing.

Bevis, E. O. (1989d). Teaching and learning: A practical commentary. In E. O. Bevis & J. Watson (Eds.), *Toward a caring curriculum* (pp. 217–259). New York, NY: National League for Nursing.

Bevis, E. O. (1990). Has the curriculum become the new religion? In *Curriculum revolution: Redefining the student-teacher relationship* (pp. 57–66). New York, NY: National League for Nursing.

Bevis, E. O. (1993). All in all it was a pretty good funeral. *Journal of Nursing Education, 32*(2), 101–105.

Bevis, E. O., & Murray, J. P. (1990). The essence of the curriculum revolution: Emancipatory teaching. *Journal of Nursing Education, 29*(7), 326–331.

Bloom, B. S., Englehart, M. D., Furst, E. J., Hill, W. H., & Krawthwhol, D. R. (1956). *Taxonomy of educational objectives: Handbook 1, Cognitive domain.* New York, NY: David McKay.

Boughn, S. (1991). A women's health course with a feminist perspective: Learning to care for and empower ourselves. *Nursing & Health Care, 12*(2), 76–80.

Boughn, S., & Wang, H. (1994). Introducing a feminist perspective to nursing curricula: A quantitative study. *Journal of Nursing Education, 33*(3), 112–117.

Bowles, T. (2008). Self-rated estimates of multiple intelligences based on approaches to learning. *Australian Journal of Educational & Developmental Psychology, 8,* 15–26.

Boyd, C. O. (1988). Phenomenology: A foundation for nursing curriculum. In *Curriculum revolution: Mandate for change* (pp. 65–87). New York, NY: National League for Nursing.

Britt Pipe, T. (2008). Illuminating the inner leadership journey by engaging mindfulness as guided by caring theory. *Nursing Administration Quarterly, 32*(2), 117–125.

Brookfield, S. D. (1995). *Becoming a critically reflective teacher.* San Francisco, CA: Jossey-Bass.

Brown, S. T., Kirkpatrick, M. K., Mangum, D., & Avery, J. (2008). A review of narrative pedagogy strategies to transform traditional nursing education. *Journal of Nursing Education, 47*(6), 283–286.

Caffarella, R. S., & Barnett, B. G. (1994).Characteristics of adult learners and foundations of experiential learning. *New Directions for Adult and Continuing Education, 62,* 29–42.

Caine, R. N., & Caine, G. (1991). *Making connections: Teaching and the human brain.* Retrieved from http://www.eric.ed.gov/PDFS/ED335141.pdf

Carper, B. (1978). Fundamental patterns of knowing. *Advances in Nursing Science,1* (1), 13–23.

Chan, C. K. K., & Pang, M. P. (2006). Teacher collaboration in learning communities. *Teaching Education, 17*(1), 1–5.

Chinn, P. L. (1989a). Feminist pedagogy in nursing education. In *Curriculum revolution: Re-conceptualizing nursing education* (pp. 9–24). New York, NY: National League for Nursing.

Chinn, P. L. (1989b). Nursing patterns of knowing and feminist thought. *Nursing & Health Care, 10*(2), 71–75.

Chinn, P. L., & Wheeler, C. E. (1985). Feminism and nursing. *Nursing Outlook, 33*(2), 74–77.

Clare, B. (2007). Promoting deep learning: A teaching learning and assessment endeavour. *Social Work Education, 26*(5), 433–446.

Collins, M. S. (1981). *An investigation of the development of professional commitment in baccalaureate nursing students.* (Unpublished doctoral dissertation). Syracuse University, NY.

Colucciello, M. L. (1988). Creating powerful learning environments. *Nursing Connections,1* (2), 23–33.

Combs, A. W. (1959). *Individual behavior: A perceptual approach to behavior* (Rev. ed.). New York, NY: Harper.

Combs, A. W. (1981). Humanistic education: Too tender for a tough world? *Phi Delta Kappa, 62*(6), 446–449.

Combs, A. W. (1994). *Helping relationships: Basic concepts for helping professions* (4th ed.). Boston, MA: Allyn & Bacon.

Corcoran, S., Narayan, S., & Moreland, H. (1988). Thinking aloud: A strategy to improve clinical decision making. *Heart & Lung, 77*(5), 463–468.

Cross, K. P. (1981). *Adults as learners: Increasing participation and facilitating learning.* New York, NY: Jossey-Bass.

Davis, J. R. (1993). *Better teaching, more learning: Strategies for success in postsecondary settings.* Phoenix, AZ: Oryx Press.

De Jong, T. (2010). Cognitive load theory, educational research, and instructional design: Some food for thought. *Industrial Science, 38*(2), 105–134.

Dembo, M. H. (1988). *Teaching for learning: Applying educational psychology in the classroom* (3rd ed.). Santa Monica, CA: Goodyear.

Demetriou, H., Wilson, E., & Winterbottom, M. (2009). The role of emotion in teaching: Are there differences between male and female newly qualified teachers' approaches to teaching? *Educational Studies, 35*(4), 449–473.

deTornyay, R. (1971). *Strategies for teaching nursing.* New York, NY: Wiley.

deTornyay, R. (1982). *Strategies for teaching nursing* (2nd ed.). New York, NY: Wiley.

deTornyay, R., & Thompson, M. (1987). *Strategies for teaching nursing* (3rd ed.). New York, NY: Wiley.

Dewey, J. (1916). *Democracy and education.* New York, NY: Macmillan.

Dewey, J. (1938). *Education and experience.* New York, NY: Macmillan.

Dewey, J. (1939). *Freedom and culture.* New York, NY: G. P. Putnam Sons.

Diekelmann, N. L. (1988). Curriculum revolution: A theoretical and philosophical mandate for change. In E. Bevis (Ed.), *Curriculum revolution: Mandate for change* (pp. 137–157). New York, NY: National League for Nursing.

Diekelmann, N. L. (1989). The nursing curriculum: Lived experiences of students. In V. Waters (Ed.), *Curriculum revolution: Re-conceptualizing nursing education* (pp. 25–41). New York, NY: National League for Nursing.

Diekelmann, N. (2001). Narrative pedagogy: Heideggerian hermeneutical analysis of lived experiences of students, teachers, and clinicians. *Advances in Nursing Science, 23*(3), 53–71.

Diekelmann, N., & Lampe, S. (2004). Student-centered pedagogies: Co-creating compelling experiences using the new pedagogies. *Journal of Nursing Education, 43*(6), 245–247.

Driscoll, M. P. (1994). *Psychology of learning for instruction.* Boston, MA: Allyn & Bacon.

Duffa, D. (2005). Nurturing an education: Acknowledging what we do. *College Quarterly,8* (2), 1–9.

Duncan, P., Cribb, A. & Stephenson, A. (2003). Developing 'the good healthcare practitioner': clues from a study in medical education. *Learning in health and Social Care, 2*(4), 181–190.

Eisner, E. (1983, January). The art and craft of teaching. *Educational Leadership, 40*(4), 4–13.

Elsbach, K. D., Barr, P. S., & Hargadon, A. B. (2005). Identifying situated cognition in organizations. *Organization Science, 16*(4), 422–433.

Escolano, A. (1996). Postmodernity or high modernity? Emerging approaches in the new history of education. *Paedagogica Historica (International Journal of the History of Education), 32*(2), 325–331.

Fay, V. P., Johnson, J., & Selz, N. (2006). Active Learning in Nursing Education (ALINE). *Nurse Educator, 31*(2), 65–68.

Fosnot, C. T. (1996). *Constructivism: Theory, perspectives and practice*. New York, NY: Teachers College Press.

Freire, P. (1993/1971). *Pedagogy of the oppressed*. (M. B. Ramos, Trans.). New York, NY: Continuum.

Freire, P., & Macedo, D. (1987). *Learning: Reading the word and the world*. Westport, CT: Greenwood.

Frisch, N. C. (1987). Value analysis: A method for teaching nursing ethics and promoting the moral development of students. *Journal of Nursing Education, 26*(8), 328–332.

Frisch, N. C. (1990). An international nursing student exchange program: An educational experience that enhanced student cognitive development. *Journal of Nursing Education, 29*(1), 10–12.

Galbraith, M. W. (1991a). *Adult learning methods*. Malabar, FL: Krieger.

Galbraith, M. W. (1991b). *Facilitating adult learning: A transactional process*. Malabar, FL: Krieger.

Gardner, H. (1983). *Frames of mind*. New York, NY: Basic Books.

Gardner, H. (1985). *The minds' new science*. New York, NY: Basic Books.

Gardner, H. (1993). *Multiple intelligences: The theory in practice*. New York, NY: Basic Books.

Gardner, H. (1999). *Intelligence reframed: Multiple intelligences for the 21st century*. New York, NY: Basic Books.

Gardner, H. (2003, April). *Multiple intelligences after twenty years*. Paper presented at the American Educational Research Association, Chicago, IL.

Gazarian, P. K. (2010). Digital stories: Incorporating narrative pedagogy. *Journal of nursing Education, 49*(5), 287–290.

Giroux, H., & McLaren, P. (1992). Writing from the margins: Geographies of identity, pedagogy, and power. *Journal of Education,174* (1), 7–30.

Glasser, W. L. (1969). *Schools without failure*. New York, NY: Harper & Row.

Grabinger, S., Aplin, C., & Ponnappa-Brenner, G. (2007, October). Instructional design for sociocultural learning environments. *e-Journal of Instructional Science and Technology, 10*(1). Retrieved from http://www.ascilite.org.au/

Graff, G. (2003). *Beyond the classroom walls: Ethnographic inquiry as pedagogy*. New York, NY: Routledge Falmer.

Grippin, P., & Peters, S. (1984). *Learning theory and learning outcomes*. Lanham, MS: University Press of America.

Guardo, C. J. (1986). Designing curricula for imaginary students. *Liberal Education, 72*(3), 213–219.

Hall, J. M. (1999). Marginalization revisited: Critical, postmodern, and liberation perspectives. *Advances in Nursing Science, 22*(1), 88–102.

Hall, J. M., Stevens, P. E., & Meleis, A. I. (1994). Marginalization: A guiding concept for valuing diversity in nursing knowledge development. *Advances in Nursing Science, 16*(4), 23–41.

Hartley, J. (1976, Spring). Preinstructional strategies: The role of pretests, behavioral objectives, overviews and advanced organizers. *Review of Educational Research, 46*(2), 239–265.

Hartrick, G. (1998). A critical pedagogy for family nursing. *Journal of Nursing Education, 37*(2), 80–84.

Hay, D. B. (2007). Using concept maps to measure deep, surface, and non-learning outcomes. *Studies in Higher Education, 32*(1), 39–57.

Hayes, E. R. (1989). Insights from women's experience for teaching and learning. In E. Hayes (Ed.), *Effective teaching styles: New directions for adult and continuing education* (p. 43). San Francisco, CA: Jossey-Bass.

Heidegger, M. (1962/1927). *Being and time*. (J. Macquarrie & E. Robinson, Trans.). New York, NY: Harper & Row.

Heidgerken, J. E. (1953). *Teaching in schools of nursing* (2nd ed.). Philadelphia, PA: J. B. Lippincott.

Heliker, D. (1994). Meeting the challenge of the curriculum revolution: Problem-based learning in nursing education. *Journal of Nursing Education, 33*(1), 45–47.

Hiemestra, R., & Sisco, B. (1990). *Individualizing instruction*. San Francisco, CA: Jossey-Bass.

Hilgard, E. R., & Bower, G. H. (1966). *Theories of learning*. New York, NY: Appleton-Century-Crofts.

Hodges, H. F. (1996). Journal writing as a mode of thinking for RN-BSN students: A leveled approach to learning to listen to self and others. *Journal of Nursing Education, 35*(3), 137–141.

Holland, F. (2007). Bringing the body to life: Using multiple intelligence theory in the classroom. *SportEx Dynamics, 14*(Oct), 6–8.

Holt, J. (1964). *How children fail*. New York, NY: Pitman.

Hyman, R. T. (1974). *Ways of teaching* (2nd ed.). Philadelphia, PA: J. B. Lippincott.

Ironside, P. M. (2001). Creating a research base for nursing education: An interpretive review of conventional, critical, feminist, postmodern, and phenomenologic pedagogies. *Advances in Nursing Science, 23*(3), 72–87.

Ironside, P. M. (2005). Teaching thinking and reaching the limits of memorization: Enacting new pedagogies. *Journal of Nursing Education, 44*(10), 441–449.

Jackson, L., & Caffarella, R. S. (1994). *Experiential learning: A new approach*. San Francisco, CA: Jossey-Bass.

Jacobs-Kramer, M., & Chinn, P. (1988). Perspectives on knowing: A model of nursing knowledge. *Scholarly Inquiry for Nursing Practice: An International Journal, 2*(2), 129–139.

Jensen, E. (2000). *Brain-based learning: The new science of teaching and training* (Rev. ed.). San Diego, CA: The Brain Store.

Jensen, E. (2008). *Brain-based learning: The new paradigm of teaching* (2nd ed.). Thousand Oaks, CA: Corwin Press.

Kaufmann, J. (2000). Reading counter-hegemonic practices through a postmodern lens. *International Journal of Lifelong Education, 19*(5), 430–447.

Kellner, D., & Kim, G. (2010). YouTube, critical pedagogy, and media activism. *The Review of Education, Pedagogy, and Cultural Studies, 32*(1), 3–36.

King, P., & Kitchener, K. (2004). Reflective judgment: Theory and research on the development of epistemic assumptions through adulthood. *Educational Psychologist, 39*(1), 5–18.

Knapp, M. S. (2008, August). How can organizational and sociocultural learning theories shed light on district instructional reform? *American Journal of Education, 114*(4), 521–539.

Knobach, N. A. (2003). Is experiential learning authentic? *Journal of Agricultural Education, 39*(4), 22–34.

Knowles, M. S. (1980). *The modern practice of adult education*. Chicago, IL: Follett.

Knowles, M. S. (1984). *The adult learner: A neglected species* (3rd ed.). Houston, TX: Gulf.

Knowles, M. S. (1986). *Using learning contracts*. San Francisco, CA: Jossey-Bass.

Knowles, M. S. (1990). *The adult learner: A neglected species* (4th ed.). Houston, TX: Gulf.

Knowles, M. S., Holton, E. F., & Swanson, R. A. (2005). *The adult learner: The definitive classic in adult education and human resource development*. Burlington, MA: Elsevier.

Kohlberg, L. (1984). *The psychology of moral development: The nature and validity of moral stages*. San Francisco, CA: Harper & Row.

Kondora, L. L. (1993). A Heideggerian hermeneutical analysis of survivors of incest. *Image, 25*(1), 11–16.

Learn, C. D. (1990). The moral dimension: Humanism in education. In M. Leininger &. J. Watson (Eds.), *The caring imperative in education* (pp. 235–245). New York, NY: National League for Nursing.

Learning Theories Knowledgebase. (2011, February). Social development theory (Vygotsky). Retrieved from http://www.learning-theories.com/vygotskys-social-learning-theory.html

Leininger, M. (1978). *Transcultural nursing: Concepts, theories and practice*. New York, NY: Wiley.

Leininger, M. (1981). Some philosophical, historical, and taxonomic aspects of nursing and caring in American culture. In M. Leininger (Ed.), *Caring: An essential human need* (pp. 133–144). Detroit, MI: Wayne State University Press.

Lewin, K. (1951). *Field theory in social science*. New York, NY: Harper & Row.

Mager, R. F. (1962). *Preparing instructional objectives*. Palo Alto, CA: Fearon.

Majeski, R., & Stover, M. (2007). Theoretically based pedagogical strategies leading to deep learning in asynchronous online gerontology courses. *Educational Gerontology, 33*(3), 171–185.

Maslow, A. (1954). *Motivation and personality*. New York, NY: Harper & Row.

Maslow, A. (1962). *Toward a psychology of being*. Princeton, NJ: D. Van Nostrand.

Mayer, R. E. (1979). Twenty years of research on advanced organizer: Assimilation theory is still the best predictor of results. *Instructional Science, 8*(2), 133–167.

McAllister, M., John, T., Gray, M., Williams, L., Barnes, M., Allan, J., & Rowe, J. (2009). Adopting a narrative pedagogy to improve the student learning experience in a regional Australian university. *Contemporary Nurse, 32*(1–2), 156–165.

McGovern, M., & Valiga, T. M. (1997). Promoting the cognitive development of freshman nursing students. *Journal of Nursing Education, 36*(1), 29–35.

McInerney, D. M. (2005). Educational psychology—Theory, research, and teaching: A 25 year retrospective. *Educational Psychology, 25*(6), 585–599.

McKeachie, W. J. (Ed.). (1980). Improving lectures by understanding students' information processing. In W. J. McKeachie (Ed.), *Learning, cognition and college teaching*,(pp. 25-35). San Francisco, CA: Jossey-Bass.

Merleau-Ponty, M. (1962/1945). *Phenomenology of perception*. (C. Smith, Trans.). New York, NY: Humanities Press.

Merriam, S. B., &. Caffarella, R. S. (1991). *Learning in adulthood: A comprehensive guide*. San Francisco, CA: Jossey-Bass.

Mezirow, J. (1975). *Education for perspective transformation: Women's re-entry programs in community colleges*. New York, NY: Columbia University, Teachers College, Center for Adult Education.

Mezirow, J. (1981). A critical theory of adult learning and education. *Adult Education, 32*(2), 3–24.

Mitchell, G. (2005). Advancing the practice of nursing theory: Evaluating nursing as caring. *Nursing Administration Quarterly, 18*(4), 313–319.

Mitchell, M. L., & Courtney, M. (2005). Improving transfer from the intensive care unit: The development, implementation, and evaluation of a brochure based on Knowles' adult learning theory. *International Journal of Nursing Practice, 11*(6), 257–268.

Moran, S., Kornhaber, M. & Gardner, H. (2006). orchestrating multiple intelligences. *Educational Leadership, 64*, 23–27.

Morse, G. G. (1995). Reframing women's health in nursing education: A feminist approach. *Nursing Outlook, 43*(6), 273–277.

Munhall, P. L. (1988). Curriculum revolution: A social mandate for change. In E. Bevis (Ed.), *Curriculum revolution: Mandate for change* (pp. 217–230). New York, NY: National League for Nursing.

Murray, J. (1989). *Developing criteria to support new curriculum models for doctoral education in nursing*. (Unpublished doctoral dissertation). University of Georgia, Athens, GA.

Muth, K. D., Britton, B. K., Glynn, S. M., & Graves, M. F. (1988). Thinking aloud while studying text: Rehearsing key ideas. *Journal of Educational Psychology, 80*(3), 315–318.

Newman, F., & Holzman, L. (1993). *Lev Vygotsky: Revolutionary scientist*. London, UK: Routledge.

Nicol, D. (2009). Assessment of learner self-regulation: Enhancing achievement in the first year using learning techniques. *Assessment & Evaluation in Higher Education, 34*(3), 335–352.

Niewolny, K. L., & Wilson, A. L. (2009). What happened to the promise? A critical (re)orientation of two sociocultural learning traditions. *Adult Education Quarterly, 60*(1), 26–45.

Niyozov, S. (2008). Understanding teaching beyond content and method. *European Education, 40*(4), 46–69.

Norman, D. A. (1989). What goes on in the mind of the learner. In W. J. McKeachie (Ed.), *Learning, cognition and college teaching*, (pp. 37-49). San Francisco, CA: Jossey-Bass.

Novak, J. D., Gowin, D. B., & Johansen, G. T. (1983). The use of concept mapping and knowledge vis-à-vis mapping with junior high school science students. *Science Education, 67*(5), 625–645.

Omery, A. (1983). Phenomenology: A method for nursing research. *Advances in Nursing Science, 5*(2), 49–63.

Ozcelik, E., & Yildirim, S. (2005). Factors influencing the use of cognitive tools in web-based learning environments. *The Quarterly Review of Distance Education, 6*(4), 295–308.

Paterson, J., & Zderad, L. (1976). *Humanistic nursing*. New York, NY: Wiley.

Perry, W. G. (1970). *Forms of intellectual and ethical development in the college years: A scheme*. New York, NY: Rinehart & Winston.

Perry, W. G. (1981). Forms of cognitive and ethical growth: The making of meaning. In A. W. Chickering (Ed.), *The modern American college: Responding to the new realities of diverse students and a changing society* (pp. 76–116). San Francisco, CA: Jossey-Bass.

Petersson, G. (2005). Medical and nursing students' development of conceptions of science during three years of studies in higher education. *Scandinavian Journal of Educational Research, 49*(3), 281–296.

Piaget, J. (1970a). Piaget's theory. In P. H. Musen (Ed.), *Carmichael's manual of psychology* (pp. 703–752). New York, NY: Wiley.

Piaget, J. (1970b). *Structuralism*. New York, NY: Basic Books.

Piaget, J. (1973). *To understand is to invent: The future of education*. New York, NY: Grossman.

QSEN Project Overview. (n.d.). Retrieved from http://www.qsen.org/overview.php

Ratner, C. (1991). *Vygotsky's sociohistorical psychology and its contemporary applications*. New York, NY: Plenum.

Reigeluth, C. M. (1983). Instructional design: What is it and why is it? In C. M. Reigeluth (Ed.), *Instructional-design theories and models: An overview of their current status*. Hillsdale, NJ: Erlbaum.

Reilly, D. E. (1975). *Behavioral objectives in nursing evaluation of learner attainment*. New York, NY: Appleton-Century-Crofts.

Reilly, D. E. (1980). *Behavioral objectives: Evaluation in nursing* (2nd ed.). New York, NY: Appleton-Century-Crofts.

Reilly, D. E., & Oermann, M. H. (1990). *Behavioral objectives: Evaluation in nursing* (3rd ed.). New York, NY: National League for Nursing.

Rogers, C. R. (1954). *Client-centered therapy*. Boston, MA: Houghton Mifflin.

Rogers, C. R. (1961). *On becoming a person*. Boston, MA: Houghton Mifflin.

Rogers, C. R. (1969). *Freedom to learn*. Columbus, OH: Charles E. Merrill.

Romyn, D. R. (2001). Disavowal of the behaviorist paradigm in nursing education: What makes it so difficult to unseat? *Advances in Nursing Science, 23*(3), 1–10.

Rooda, L. A. (1994). Effects of mind mapping on student achievement in a nursing research course. *Nurse Educator, 19*(6), 25–27.

Ruffing-Rahal, M. A. (1992). Incorporating feminism into the graduate curriculum. *Journal of Nursing Education, 31*(6), 247–252.

Rule, A. C. (2006). Editorial: the components of authentic learning. *Journal of Authentic Learning, 3*(1), 1–10.

Rumelhart, D. E. (1981). *Understanding understanding*. La Jolla, CA: University of California, San Diego, Center for Human Information Process.

Rumelhart, D. E., & Ortony, A. (1977). The representation of knowledge in memory. In R. C. Anderson, R. J., Spiro, & W. E. Montague (Eds.), *Schooling and the acquisition of knowledge* (pp. 99–135). Hillsdale, NJ: Erlbaum.

Rushton, A. (2005). Formative assessment: A key to deep learning? *Medical Teacher, 27*(6), 509–513.

Sanders, D., & Welk, D. S. (2005). Strategies to scaffold student learning: Applying Vygotsky's zone of proximal development. *Nurse Educator, 30*(5), 203–207.

Scheckel, M. M., & Ironside, P. M. (2006). Cultivating interpretive thinking through enacting narrative pedagogy. *Nursing Outlook, 54*(3), 159–165.

Schön, D. (1983). *The reflective practitioner: How professionals think in action*. New York, NY: Basic Books.

Shuell, T. J. (1986). Cognitive conceptions of learning. *Review of Educational Research, 56*(4), 411–436.

Simon, H. A. (1979). Information processing models of cognition. *Annual Review of Psychology, 30*, 363–396.

Skinner, B. F. (1953). *Science and human behavior*. New York, NY: Macmillan.

Slavin, R. E. (1988). *Educational psychology: Theory into practice* (2nd ed.). Englewood Cliffs, NJ: Prentice Hall.

Smith, T. W., & Colby, S. A. (2007). Teaching for deep learning. *The Clearing House, 80*(5), 205–210.

Symonds, J. M. (1990). Revolutionizing the student–teacher relationship. *Curriculum revolution: Redefining the student–teacher relationship*. New York, NY: National League for Nursing.

Tanner, C. (1987). Teaching clinical judgment. *Annual Review of Nursing Research, 5*, 153–173.

Tanner, C. (1988). Curriculum revolution: The practice mandate. *Nursing & Health Care, 9*(8), 427–430.

Tanner, C., Benner, P., Chesla, C., & Gordon, D. R. (1993). The phenomenology of knowing the patient. *Image, 25*(4), 273–280.

Tanner, C. A. (1990). Reflections on the curriculum revolution. *Journal of Nursing Education, 29*(7), 295–299.

Taylor, B. (1993). Phenomenology: A way to understanding nursing practice. *International Journal of Nursing Studies, 30*(2), 171–179.

Thoma, G. A. (1993). The Perry framework and tactics for teaching critical thinking in economics. *Journal of Economic Education, 24*(2), 128–136.

Traynor, M. (1997). Postmodern research: No grounding or privilege, just free floating trouble making. *Nursing Inquiry, 4*(2), 99–107.

Traynor, M. (2009). Humanism and its critiques in nursing research literature. *Journal of Advanced Nursing, 65*(7), 1560–1567.

Tulving, E. (1972). Episodic and semantic memory. In E. Tulving & W. Donaldson (Eds.), *Organization of memory* (pp. 381–403). New York, NY: Academic Press.

Tulving, E. (1985). How many memory systems are there? *American Psychologist, 40*(4), 385–398.

Twomey, A. (2004). Web-based teaching in nursing: Lessons from the literature. *Nurse Education Today, 24*(6), 425–458.

Tyler, R. W. (1949). *Basic principles of curriculum and instruction*. Chicago, IL: University of Chicago Press.

Valiga, T. M. (1988). Curriculum outcomes and cognitive development: New perspectives for nursing education. In E. Bevis (Ed.), *Curriculum revolution: Mandate for change* (pp. 177–200). New York, NY: National League for Nursing.

Van der Veer, R. & Valsiner, J. (1994). The Vygotsky Reader. Cambridge, MA: Blackwell Publishing.

Van Manen, M. (1990). *Researching lived experience: Human science for an action sensitive pedagogy*. Albany, NY: State University of New York Press.

van Merrienboer, J. J., & Sweller, J. (2010). Cognitive load theory in health professional education: Design principles and strategies. *Medical Education, 44*(1), 85–93.

van Niekerk, K., & van Aswegen, E. (1993). Implementing problem-based learning in nursing. *Nursing RSA Verpleging, 8*(5), 37–41.

Vygotsky, L. (1986/1962). *Thought and language*. Cambridge, MA: MIT Press.

Walton, J. C. (1996). The changing environment: New challenges for nursing education. *Journal of Nursing Education, 35*(9), 400–405.

Ward, P. C. (1992). Two legal environment writing exercises following the Perry scheme of cognitive development. *The Journal of Legal Studies Education, 10*(1), 87.

Watson, J. (1988). Human caring as moral context for nursing education. *Nursing & Health Care, 9*(8), 423–425.

Watson, J. (1989). Transformative thinking and a caring curriculum. In E. O. Bevis & J. Watson (Eds.), *Toward a caring curriculum: A new pedagogy for nursing* (pp. 51–60). New York, NY: National League for Nursing.

Webber, M. (2006). Transgressive pedagogies? Exploring the difficult realities of enacting feminist pedagogies in undergraduate classrooms in a Canadian university. *Studies in Higher Education, 31*(4), 453–467.

Weinstein, C. E., & Meyer, D. K. (1991). Spring cognitive learning strategies and college teaching. In R. J. Menges & M. D. Svinicki (Eds.), *New directions for teaching and learning: College teaching: From theory to practice* (pp. 15–25). San Francisco, CA: Jossey-Bass.

Wertsch, J. V. (1985). *Vygotsky and the social formation of mind.* Cambridge, MA: Harvard University.

Wheeler, C., & Chinn, P. (1989). *Peace and power: A handbook of feminist process* (2nd ed.). New York, NY: National League for Nursing.

Widick, C., & Simpson, D. (1978). Developmental concepts in college instruction. In C. A. Parker (Ed.), *Encouraging development in college student* (pp. 227–259). Minneapolis, MN: University of Minnesota Press.

Wink, J. (2011). *Critical pedagogy: Notes from the real world.* Boston, MA: Pearson.

Wittmann-Price, R. A., & Godshall, M. (2009). Strategies to promote deep learning in clinical nursing courses. *Nurse Educator, 34*(5), 214–216.

Wittrock, M. C. (1977). Learning as a generative process. In M. C. Wittrock (Ed.), *Learning and instruction* (pp. 621–631). Berkeley, CA: McCrutchan.

Wittrock, M. C. (1992). Generative learning processes of the brain. *Educational Psychologist, 27*(4), 531-541.

Wittrock, M. C. (1986). Students' thought processes. In M. C. Wittrock (Ed.), *Handbook of research on teaching* (pp. 297–314). New York, NY: Macmillan.

Zorn, C. R. (1995). An analysis of the impact of participation in an international study program on the cognitive development of senior nursing students. *Journal of Nursing Education, 34*(2), 67–70.

14

Managing Student Incivility and Misconduct in the Learning Environment

Karen M. Whitney, PhD

Susan Luparell, PhD, ANCS-BC, CNE

On today's campuses of higher education, there appears to be increasing incidence of incivility among students (Clark & Springer, 2007). When preparing a learning environment for students and faculty, how can faculty ensure that it is one that is safe and productive for all, one in which a quality teaching and learning experience can be provided? This chapter introduces developmental, legal, and risk management issues related to classroom learning environments and methods to minimize student conduct that disrupts learning. Instructional strategies are discussed to assist faculty in achieving a robust and engaging learning environment through management of the students' actions.

Management of actions includes student in-class behaviors and extends to out-of-class course-related activities, both on- and off-campus internship, clinical, and practicum experiences. Specifically, this chapter explores methods to nurture and support learning and describes effective responses for situations in which student behavior could disrupt your learning objectives for the students with an emphasis on (1) a continuum of student misconduct, (2) proactive response strategies, and (3) effective use of campus resources.

The learning outcomes of this chapter include gaining an understanding of problem or disruptive student behavior and an understanding of specific steps faculty can take to minimize disruptions to your learning environments. The content of this chapter is based on case law, statutory law, research, and more than 20 years of experience working with college students and college student misconduct. As a cautionary note, it is strongly recommended that faculty consult with the administrators responsible for student conduct at their institution, their immediate supervisor, campus police, and campus legal counsel regarding issues specific to their institution.

Incivility in the Higher Education Environment

Most experienced faculty will tell you that they get much pleasure from working with students much of the time. However, on occasion, interactions between students and faculty may be somewhat uncomfortable, slightly challenging, or even distressing. Despite the "ivory tower" moniker, the academy, as a microcosm of society, is not immune to the problems of society. Thus incivilities of various types and among various individuals can and do occur in higher education. However, this is an aspect of the teaching role that tends to surprise novice faculty.

Both faculty and students have reported that incivility is a moderate problem in nursing education (Clark, 2007, 2008a). More specifically, Lashley and deMeneses (2001) found that all faculty who responded to a survey of student misconduct in nursing had experienced students being late, inattentive, or absent from class, and more than 90% reported student cheating as a problem. In some more rare instances, faculty experience more serious episodes of misconduct, including verbal or physical abuse (Lashley & deMeneses, 2001; Luparell, 2004). Stress in both faculty and students has been identified as contributing significantly to uncivil behavior in nursing education (Clark, 2008b).

While the majority of this chapter will address how student misbehavior can be managed, it is important that faculty have an appreciation for the overall context in which misconduct and incivility occur. Student misconduct and incivility rarely occur in a vacuum. In both the general workplace and in nursing education, experts suggest that incivility is reciprocal in nature (Andersson & Pearson, 1999; Clark, 2008b). If student misbehavior is viewed as a form of communication, it necessitates that we view it in a broader context that includes student interactions with faculty and the learning environment.

There is evidence to suggest that faculty play a pivotal role in establishing classroom behavioral norms and also may contribute to the problem in a variety of ways. In a landmark study, Boice (1996) concluded that faculty are the most crucial initiators of incivility in the classroom. Poor teaching skills may lead to student frustration and misbehavior. Additionally, lack of instructor willingness to address classroom incivility sends a message that such behavior is acceptable.

Additionally, Clark (2008a) found that students sometimes experience incivility at the hands of faculty. Students perceive condescending remarks or putdowns by faculty as uncivil. A long list of additional behaviors that students identify as uncivil on the part of faculty include exerting superiority, being unavailable outside of class, refusing or being reluctant to answer questions, canceling scheduled classes and activities without warning, ignoring disruptive behaviors, not allowing open discussion, and using ineffective teaching styles or methods.

Thus, although it is tempting to focus on student misconduct and incivility from a narrow perspective, it is prudent to avoid this. Poor student behavior and incivility, although never appropriate, may be influenced by a broad spectrum of variables, including stress levels and lack of general civility within the environment. Additionally, lack of teaching acumen by faculty may serve to increase student stress and frustration. Although this chapter provides a starting point for managing misbehavior and incivility when it occurs in the classroom, the thoughtful practitioner should consider multiple variables when considering how to best prevent and manage conduct problems in the classroom environment.

A Continuum of Misconduct

In considering student conduct, one size does not fit all. It is important to examine each incident in terms of the behaviors observed and reported. It is also vital to use a framework from which to evaluate student behavior. With few exceptions, every institution of higher education has a policy that informs the student of behaviors that are or are not expected of the student. These policies can be described in many ways, such as a Student Code of Conduct, an Honor Code, Student Rights and Responsibilities, or some other variation. These policies provide the filter through which one takes a set of observed and reported behaviors and considers the extent to which a specific situation may or may not violate a code of conduct.

For purposes of analyzing student behaviors, all behaviors will fall within one or more of the following three categories: (1) annoying acts, (2) administrative violations, and (3) criminal conduct (Fig. 14-1). It is possible that a single behavior, such as stealing a test, can be both an administrative violation and criminal conduct. It is also possible that a behavior repeated over time, such as interrupting a lecture repeatedly, can be considered both an annoying act and an administrative violation. Occasionally a lecture disruption might be annoying, but the behavior moves from annoying to a violation of campus policy if the disruptions persist after the student has been counseled that the behavior exceeds reasonable limits. Regardless of where the behavior may lie on the continuum, it is critically important to create a teaching approach wherein faculty are in a position to observe student behaviors objectively. The focus should be on actions and not on emotion, rumor, or innuendo. Furthermore, it is important that faculty remain cognizant of student behaviors and their potential impact on learning in order to, at the earliest opportunity, consider the extent to which student actions fall within this framework. Awareness is the first step in managing the learning environment. Box 14-1 lists examples of student misconduct that fall within the categories of annoying acts, administrative violations, and criminal conduct.

Annoying Acts

Annoying acts are behaviors that may not be desired but do not violate an administrative code of conduct. Annoying acts are usually behaviors that

A Continuum of Student Behaviors

| Annoying acts | Administrative violations | Criminal conduct |

Figure 14-1 A continuum of student behaviors.

BOX 14-1 Examples of Student Misconduct in the Classroom

ANNOYING ACTS

- Sleeping in class
- Talking in class
- Discourteous
- Uncooperative
- Late to class
- Poor hygiene
- Eating, drinking
- Pagers, cell phones
- Early exits

ADMINISTRATIVE VIOLATIONS

- Dishonesty; false accusations or information; forgery; alteration or misuse of any university document, record, or identification
- Disorderly conduct
- Actions that disrupt the academic process
- Failure to comply with directions of authorized university officials
- Cheating, plagiarism, fabrication

CRIMINAL CONDUCT (ALSO CAN BE CONSIDERED ADMINISTRATIVE VIOLATIONS)

- Threats of violence against self or others
- Actions that endanger one's self or others in the university community
- Physical or verbal abuse
- Possession of firearms
- Conduct that is lewd, indecent, or obscene
- Intimidation, harassment, stalking
- Alcohol or drug possession or sale
- Theft

these types of behaviors can escalate. Although these behaviors are at the more benign end of the continuum, it is best to document any observed behaviors and interactions with students regarding their conduct.

The key in responding to annoying behaviors is to keep grounded in the learning experience, even though the behavior is annoying to you. When talking with students about annoying behaviors, focus on the importance of the learning environment and on the goal of meeting or exceeding the course learning objectives. You are not simply asking the student to be polite or thoughtful; rather you are exploring with the student how his or her behavior is not serving him or her, you, or the rest of the learning community. Based on these authors' experience, most likely once faculty have met with a student who displays annoying behavior, brought these behaviors to the attention of the student, and suggested new behaviors, no further misconduct will occur. In fact, coaching sessions can often lay the foundation for a productive teaching–learning–mentoring relationship.

From a professional educational standpoint, it is important to note that these annoying acts, left unchecked, can later manifest themselves in the student's professional workplace. Bartholomew (2006) summarizes a relatively recent body of literature that describes this set of behaviors as "horizontal hostility" or "lateral violence." Examples of "horizontal hostility" include peers (e.g., students to students or nurses to nurses) acting uncivilly, acting abruptly, undermining individual and group efforts, withholding work-related information, and demonstrating a general lack of collegiality. As a result, clearly and consistently holding students accountable for their actions has an immediate impact on the individual as a learner and a future impact on the individual in his or her professional life.

Administrative Violations

Administrative violations are behaviors that violate an administrative code of conduct. Administrative violations can be a variety of behaviors that significantly disrupt the learning process, such as acts of intimidation or harassment. These behaviors can be motivated by a desire to gain an academic advantage through scholastic misconduct, such as cheating, plagiarism, or fabricating results. Because

include poor interpersonal communication skills, such as monopolizing class discussion, or discourteous, abrasive, aggressive, or hard-to-get-along-with behaviors. Annoying acts may also include poor time or life management skills, such as entering class late or leaving class early, or repeated excuses for poor performance. From a developmental perspective, there is a tremendous opportunity to assist the student toward improvement.

It is important to communicate with a student regarding annoying behaviors. In confronting students regarding annoying behaviors, faculty are keeping small problems small and possibly avoiding an escalation of behaviors along the continuum. The risk management level is low, but over time codes or policies of student conduct are unique to each institution, it is strongly recommended that faculty acquaint themselves with the code in order to know when a student may have violated institutional policy. Chapter 3 further discusses the ethical issues related to academic dishonesty.

From a developmental perspective, there may be an opportunity to assist the student, but this will depend on the incident and the student's disposition and attitude for change. For instance, an incident involving an alcohol-impaired student coming to an on-campus class that has a zero tolerance for such behavior would limit faculty's ability to work with the student in a coaching capacity. If faculty have reason to believe that a student has violated the campus student code, the best approach is to document the faculty's observations, when reasonably possible talk with the student, and engage the student in order to fully understand the situation. If after talking with the student it continues to appear that a violation has occurred, then documentation of the student's behavior should be referred to the appropriate administrative officer as prescribed by campus policy.

It is important to communicate with a student regarding any allegations of misconduct. In confronting students regarding possible violations, the sooner you confront the student the better, and it might be advisable to contact your department chair to assist you in talking with the student. In confronting the student immediately, you avoid an escalation of behaviors along the continuum. The risk management level is moderate but over time these types of behaviors can escalate and increase the administrative severity and the possibility of the behavior violating local, state, or federal law. These behaviors should be documented, as should interactions with students regarding their conduct. Faculty should expect that the incident will be referred to the appropriate administrative office for disciplinary review.

Criminal Conduct

Criminal conduct can be characterized as behaviors that violate local, state, or federal criminal law. Criminal conduct can be a variety of behaviors that significantly disrupt the learning process, such as threats or acts of violence, stalking, intimidation, harassment, possession of firearms, drugs, alcohol, or theft. Because local and state laws can vary and

the application of the law to college populations can vary as well, it is strongly recommended that faculty acquaint themselves with the practices at their institution. It is also recommended that faculty discuss these legal issues with their department chair and fellow colleagues so that they become familiar with the historical context and institutional practice.

From a developmental perspective, acts that are determined to be criminal allow very little opportunity to assist the student but quickly are relegated to campus and local law enforcement personnel for investigation and disposition. For instance, an incident involving a student threatening to injure a fellow student limits faculty's ability to work with the student in a coaching capacity. If faculty have reason to believe that a student has acted criminally, the best approach is to document their observations and immediately report the observations to the appropriate campus law enforcement personnel.

When criminal conduct is suspected, it is important for faculty to inform their immediate supervisor (e.g., department chair) of the incident and contact campus law enforcement. Each situation will dictate the faculty's role regarding any further engagement with the student regarding her or his behavior. In many cases, as the student's instructors, faculty may know the student best and could become a vital resource as to the most constructive approach to take with the student to minimize any threat of violence or disruption to the student and to the greater learning community. The risk management level is high and all exchanges with the student should be carefully coordinated with campus law enforcement and the campus office responsible for student conduct in order to limit an escalation of criminal conduct.

The campus administration may further hold the student accountable for an administrative violation of the student code of conduct following an investigation of the alleged behavior. It is important to understand that a university or college cannot and should not insulate the student from being held accountable for criminal actions. These behaviors should be well documented. Faculty should expect that the incident will be referred to the appropriate administrative unit for disciplinary review. Pursuing a single incident through multiple levels of the university as well as pursuing both criminal and administrative action is not considered double jeopardy; rather it is a result of multiple jurisdictions properly responding to a single behavior.

Proactive Response Strategies

Under the philosophy of keeping small things small, this section provides a series of actions that faculty can implement when managing a learning environment. These strategies can be applied to learning in a conventional classroom, in off-campus settings, and in online learning environments. It is also recommend that faculty within a department discuss these strategies and adopt common practices. Students will notice common practices from class to class, which helps to reinforce these strategies.

Forewarning in the Course Syllabus

An important first step in managing the learning environment is taking early action to prevent problematic behavior. This can be done in a variety of ways, including being attentive to creating a climate of civility from day one of class. Novice faculty tend to assume that college students intrinsically understand professional behavioral expectations of them. This may be a false assumption. Therefore it is imperative that appropriate behavior be explicitly described, both in the syllabus and on the first day of class.

In the course syllabus, faculty should express their expectations for the learning environment. The program or institution may also have specific expectations or policies that faculty are required to insert into syllabi. The syllabus is a performance agreement between faculty and students. As such, it is an opportunity to express the ground rules and guidelines for engagement. This is the time that faculty should outline what student behaviors matter most to them as educators. Faculty should keep the discussion positive and indicate the behaviors they wish to see demonstrated by students. Faculty should also connect these behaviors to the achievement of the learning outcomes established for the course.

For example, if students arriving to class on time and remaining through the entire class period is an important component of the learning environment, then express this expectation in the syllabus and also indicate the rationale for this expectation. For all expectations, it is also recommended that faculty provide students with a way to manage these expectations. If a student knows that he or she will not be able to arrive at a class on time, what should the student do? Should the student not attend at all? Should the student call faculty in advance of the class and discuss the need to arrive late? Is there a place (e.g., the back row of the class) that has been designated as an area where students who arrive late or must leave early should sit so as not to inconvenience the learning of others?

Expressing expectations in writing to students from the first day together helps students understand the behaviors faculty expect from the outset. This approach also provides faculty with a guide in case a student acts in a manner that has been indicated as unacceptable. As the instructor, faculty are in a position to set standards that students must meet. These standards may be both academic and behavioral. The key is that they are clearly expressed and consistently expected of all students.

The syllabus is historically the document that articulates the basic relationship between student and instructor. While a syllabus cannot present text for every concern, including text that expresses "the ground rules" or the rules of engagement between the instructor and students is often one way to create an environment designed to minimize conflict. Three types of suggested text are offered for your consideration in Box 14-2. The examples offered are suggestions and should be customized to support the established culture and values of your particular program and university or college.

Reviewing the Institutional Code of Conduct

With expectations clearly outlined in the syllabus, the first class meeting of the semester is a time to outline expectations for the course. In addition to sharing individualized faculty expectations, it is also appropriate to inform students about any policies that the institution has established to guide student conduct. It is recommended that faculty briefly address the sections of the institutional student conduct policy that have meaning for the specific learning objectives of the course. This is the time for faculty to review their expectations and interpretations of the code. It is also appropriate for faculty to provide positive examples of the behavior they wish to see exhibited by the students and engage the students in a discussion about these expectations. One exercise is to ask the students to

---

BOX 14-2 Examples of Text for the Syllabus

TEACHING–LEARNING PHILOSOPHY

My expectation is that you are a self-motivated learner. By the end of the semester you will have invested your time, energy, and resources to complete this course and I want you to be successful. My responsibility as your instructor is to provide a context and environment that supports your learning through mindful, intentional curriculum that guides your investigations and learning. I expect you to be an involved, active member of this learning community who will contribute with thorough preparation, active discussion participation, and timely participation in course activities. I further expect that you will treat everyone, including the instructor, with respect and civility. Learning in this course takes place through lectures, readings, written analysis, reflective discussions, critical reflection, and written assignments.

CLASS EXPECTATIONS

This course will be most successful when all participants commit to developing a learning community in which the beliefs of all may be discussed in an open, civil, and understanding environment. Everyone will be expected to consider multiple perspectives, engage in critical reflection, and take intellectual risks built on one's confidence in the course content. Class activities will focus on critical analysis of (1) course readings, (2) video cases, (3) group work, and (4) research findings. Your personal experiences are important but require critical reflection and analysis. Hence the ability to interact with the material in a personal and self-reflective manner is essential.

PROFESSIONAL EXPECTATIONS

Becoming a professional is not simply a matter of possessing a degree. Becoming a professional is agreeing to a set of standards of behavior now, as a student, that models the behavior that will be expected of you once you complete your professional program.

1. Be on time. Arrive 10 minutes prior to your expected time and be prepared to begin class or lab. Leave with plenty of time in case you encounter delays.
2. Be present every day! Your instructor has created specific lesson plans with the expectation that you will be present every class day. On what should be a rare occasion, it is imperative that if you are unable to keep your commitment, you contact your instructor as soon as possible. Ask the instructor what is the best way for you to communicate with them. Write down his or her e-mail or phone number and have it with you at all times.
3. Be professional! Maintain a professional attitude and be positive! You never get a second chance to make a first impression.
4. Know what is expected of you every day. Read your syllabus. Note all course obligations on your calendar and check your calendar daily.
5. Leave your cell phone off and out of site. Focus on being present in the class and with your work.
6. Collegiality. Now, as a student, and in the future, as a professional, you will interact with and work extensively with your peers and colleagues. Work to be a positive influence and a productive colleague to your peers.
7. Ethics. As a student, learn and reflect on the ethical expectations of the profession and begin reflecting on your current daily decisions within an ethical context. Realize that the decisions and choices you make every day build on your ability to make decisions and actions on behalf of others you will be responsible for in the future.
8. Collaboration. As a professional you will collaborate with patients, family members, and other professional colleagues in providing care. As a student today you will be expected to collaborate in a positive, civil, and mutually beneficial way that will build your skills and understanding of working with groups of people to achieve a common goal.

---

describe annoying or disruptive behaviors they have seen from their fellow classmates in other classes and to talk about how each person will agree to not act in a manner that disrupts learning in the classroom.

Being Transparent

Another way in which faculty can minimize problematic behavior is to be as transparent as possible with students regarding development of assignments and rationale for decision making and grading. Open communication about how the course has been developed and how decisions have been made serve to decrease student perceptions that an instructor's actions are arbitrary or even malicious. Evidence suggests that students may potentially respond disruptively when they disagree with grading decisions, when they receive an unsatisfactory clinical grade, or when they receive a failing grade for a course (Luparell, 2004). Perceptions that an instructor acts in an arbitrary manner, especially where grades are concerned, may result in a student misbehaving out of frustration.

Establishing a Trusting Environment

A trusting relationship between student and faculty is essential to creating an environment in which students can mature professionally. As faculty, we frequently need to deliver critical feedback that is constructive in nature. It is false to assume that students understand the benevolent motives behind providing such feedback; they are often unprepared to receive feedback that is not wholly positive. Consequently, it is beneficial to elucidate the purpose of constructive feedback in students' professional development. A sample script for initiating this discussion can be found in Box 14-3. Once the underlying basis of trust has been established, a more conducive environment for the give and take of constructive feedback is created.

Providing Effective Behavioral Feedback

Students often are unaware of how their behaviors are perceived. In a trusting environment in which the student's professional development is a priority, faculty have a responsibility to provide concrete and specific feedback regarding behaviors that may impede a student's progress. A template for crafting such a discussion has been shared elsewhere (Luparell, 2007a) and may be found in Box 14-4. It is important to note that the script provides students with the choice to continue the behavior or not, based on whether they are concerned with the outcomes of their behavior. Students almost always

---

BOX 14-4 Sample Script for Giving Feedback Related to Problematic Behavior

Hi _____,

Thank you for coming in to see me. Remember the first day of class when we talked about the role of trust in giving feedback? I have some feedback to share with you now that may be a bit difficult to hear. Please remember that I'm sharing it with you so you can successfully meet your goal of becoming a competent nurse.

When you do _____, it leaves me with the impression that _____. If I have that impression, it's likely that others may have it as well. If you are okay with people drawing this conclusion about you, then keep on doing what you are doing. If you are not comfortable with people potentially drawing this conclusion, you may want to consider a change.

An example of the script put to use with a student who does not put good effort into completing postclinical paperwork:

Hi Mary,

Thank you for coming in to see me. Remember the first day of class when we talked about the role of trust in giving feedback? I have some feedback to share with you now that may be a bit difficult to hear. Please remember that I'm sharing it with you so you can successfully meet your goal of becoming a competent nurse.

When you turn in your clinical packet so insufficiently completed, it leaves me with the impression either that you really don't understand what is going on with your patient or that you are a bit of a slacker. If I have that impression, it's likely that others may have it as well. If you are okay with people drawing the conclusion that you really don't understand what you are doing or that you are a slacker, then keep on doing what you are doing. If you are not comfortable with people potentially drawing this conclusion, you may want to consider a change.

BOX 14-3 Elucidating the Role of Trust in Giving Constructive Feedback

Providing you with feedback on your performance and progress is a crucial component of this course. While often that feedback will be positive and address your strengths, at times I may need to share constructive feedback that focuses on areas that are not as well developed. I am willing to trust that you want this feedback in order to meet your educational goals. I ask that you trust that my sole motivation for giving you this feedback is to help you be successful in your development.

---

choose to discontinue the annoying behavior. However, if the behavior continues you will need to address it more assertively by requesting unequivocally that it stop.

Know Who to Contact for Consultation

Sooner or later faculty will need to consult with someone regarding a student's behavior. Students are coming to college more stressed, more financially challenged, more distracted, and more overcommitted than previous generations (Levine & Cureton, 1998). Every college or university has designated individuals who respond to issues regarding student behavior. There are no consistent titles or standardized credentials, and every institution through its history, context, mission, vision, values, and goals has constructed individualized approaches to how student behavior is managed.

It is best if faculty reacquaint themselves annually with the key people on campus who should be consulted regarding student behavior concerns. Consultants can include staff from such offices as the dean of students, counseling, advising, student health services, student ombudsman, student advocate, faculty professional development, student affairs, student life, or the campus police. Faculty can inquire of other faculty and administrators as to which offices and which staff have provided helpful counsel in the past, depending on the student situation. Faculty should also know who is responsible for administering the institutional student code of conduct. It is helpful to have established a working relationship with these individuals in advance of contacting them with a particular student concern. The key point is that, as instructors, faculty are not unsupported in responding to student conduct in the classroom, but instead should have the institutional support of other professionals with expertise in handling student issues.

Know When to Call for Consultation

Just as important as knowing who to call for consultation is knowing when to call for consultation and knowing when to refer an unresolved matter to others. Quite often faculty dwell on an unresolved matter with a student much longer than necessary, which is distracting to the teaching and learning experience for the entire class. Let us assume that a faculty member has outlined the behaviors that are expected from her or his students to facilitate learning. Let us further assume that the faculty member has had a discussion with the students during the first class regarding these expectations and has indicated that there is a set of institutional policies (a student code of conduct) that supports expecting these behaviors of students. If the faculty member has outlined student behavior expectations in the syllabus, met with the student, and made the student aware that his or her behavior is not meeting the standard that has been set for the class, and if the student either refuses or is unable to change the behavior to meet the expected standard, then the

faculty member should immediately consult with others, such as the department chair, to identify other ways to work with the student or to request a referral to another office on campus. As mentioned earlier, the timing of a referral will also depend on the unique circumstances and the continuum of behaviors observed. If at any time faculty feel their safety or the safety of others is at risk, then campus law enforcement should immediately be contacted. If, on the other hand, faculty are responding to an annoying act, then they may wish to meet with the student on repeated occasions to address a variety of issues that are adversely affecting the student's academic success.

Documentation and Communication

"When in doubt write it out" is one of the first things one of these authors learned as a young administrator. It is important for faculty to keep notes of student behaviors that have been observed. Faculty may observe behaviors that are not desired but that do not violate the classroom standard that has been set or the campus student code. One reason to note these "below the radar" behaviors is that they can escalate to a level that would ultimately violate the classroom standard or the campus standard. At that time it will be helpful when faculty meet with a student to be able to note that specific patterns of behaviors have been observed. Students are often surprised that faculty have taken note of them and want to talk with them about their conduct.

Keeping personal notes may also be helpful if faculty need to refer an incident to others. The information to document includes time, day, and place where the behavior was observed. It is also important to use descriptive and not evaluative statements. To say that the student was "rude" is not helpful; however, to document that "the student has arrived late to four of the last six classes, which disrupted the class lecture when the student attempted to locate a seat in class" is helpful, because it is specific and allows the faculty to talk with the student in a way that focuses on student behaviors and not on how the faculty may feel about those behaviors.

There is often a misunderstanding among faculty and staff throughout colleges and universities regarding documentation and communication of students' behaviors and students' privacy rights. These misunderstandings center around an interpretation of federal legislation called the Family Educational Rights and Privacy Act (FERPA). Pursuant to FERPA (United States Department of Education, 2007), faculty and staff may and in fact should share information about a student when a "legitimate educational interest" exists. Matters of classroom management, student conduct or misconduct, and behaviors of concern fall within a legitimate educational interest. The Department of Education acknowledges that there is a balance between students' rights to privacy and the university's responsibility to ensure stability and public safety. As such,

> The University [may] disclose education[al] records without a student's prior written consent under the FERPA exception for disclosure to school officials with legitimate educational interests. A school official is a person employed by the University in an administrative, supervisory, academic or research, or support staff position (including law enforcement unit personnel and health staff); a person or company with whom the University has contracted as its agent to provide a service instead of using University employees or officials (such as an attorney, auditor, or collection agent); a person serving on the Board of Trustees; or a student serving on an official committee, such as a disciplinary or grievance committee, or assisting another school official in performing his or her tasks.

Therefore you should communicate with your department chair when you become aware of possible student behavioral concerns. It is good practice to keep the department chair updated as to any documentation, meetings, or other actions regarding student behavior issues.

Discipline as an Educational Experience

Faculty may want to simply eject a student from a class, because the faculty is offended, annoyed, or feels that the student has acted in a disrespectful manner; however, it is vitally important for faculty to frame their interactions with the student within an educational framework. Setting standards of conduct within a learning environment is part of the educational and professional preparatory experience. Students learn that there are standards of conduct and consequences to not meeting these standards, which contributes to their preparation for their postdegree work. Developing the discipline and focus to arrive to class on time will contribute

to students' ability to effectively complete work-related duties and helps increase their understanding of the importance of collegiality, connectedness, and teamwork as a means toward achieving a quality working environment. The integrity required to ethically complete laboratory work by submitting only the results that they have personally calculated and not use the work of other students is the same integrity that will be required of graduates when they are in the workforce completing work-related reports.

Responding to Student Misconduct

When faculty have reason to believe that a student may be acting inappropriately, there are six steps to use when responding to allegations of misconduct:

1. *Gather and document information.* The information should objectively describe the student's actions and note the date, time, and others who were present.
2. *Engage and confront the student about behaviors observed.* At the earliest time possible, meet with the student privately to discuss the behaviors that have been observed. This meeting will inform the student of faculty concerns, allow the student to express his or her perspective on the situation, and provide an opportunity for the student to understand how the behavior affects others and is disrupting the learning outcomes of the course.
3. *Focus on the behavior.* Faculty should always focus on what the student did and not be swayed by ancillary aspects, such as the extent to which one knows or likes the student or the student's academic record. For instance, high-achieving students are just as likely to plagiarize as average students. It is important to be consistent in what is expected from students.
4. *Outline required new behaviors.* The purpose of meeting with the student is to first explore with the student concerns about her or his behavior. If after talking with the student the concerns remain valid, then the second goal of the meeting is to discuss with the student how the behavior should change in the future. Working with the student to change any annoying acts provides the greatest opportunity for a collaborative discussion between the student and the faculty. Any administrative

violations of the code of conduct should be documented and forwarded to the appropriate administrative office and, depending on campus policy, may be followed up administratively in addition to what the faculty has discussed with the student. All criminal conduct should be immediately forwarded to the appropriate campus office and may limit faculty's ability to outline new behaviors.

5. *Outline consequences of compliance and noncompliance.* Faculty interactions with the student should conclude with the hope that the student will choose to make different choices and will choose to comply with the standards that faculty and the campus have set. However, it is also important to be clear with the student that, should he or she fail to comply and continue to disrupt the learning environment, there will be additional follow-up that may include further sanctions.

6. *Refer unresolved or risky cases to other campus resources.* If at any time faculty are working with a student and it comes to their attention that the student's misconduct is not being resolved as planned, or if there is evidence that the incident may escalate in terms of level of disruption or safety to either the faculty or other students, the situation should automatically be referred to other campus resources.

Campus Resources

As stated previously, it is recommended that faculty become familiar with the services, programs, and personnel who staff their institution's campus support resources before they actually need their assistance. Campus resources can include counseling services, student health services, police, department chair, dean of students, and services for students with disabilities. Depending on the history and context of the institution, there may be other support services, including campus ministries and specialized centers for specific populations of students such as women, people of color, or gay and lesbian students. Regarding behaviors of concern that rise to the level of safety for individuals or groups, universities have increasingly established formal committees that convene to conduct a broad review of a student's behavior in order to coordinate a comprehensive and organized response. Working with a team of professionals who can

work together to assess threats and identify problems is preferred to individual faculty working alone. It is best to have multiple offices come together on a case-by-case basis and form a team to assess the situation and achieve the desired results. One easy way to develop relationships with these support services is to invite personnel from one or two of these offices to present introductory information about their offices to faculty within the nursing program and explore how and when students should be referred as a part of the program's faculty professional development activities.

Implications for Practice

Novice faculty are frequently unprepared for the diverse challenges that arise in classroom management. It is important to recognize early that you are likely to experience some degree of student misconduct in your teaching career. *Thus it is wise to consider in advance how you might respond in specific situations.* Working with students effectively and managing the classroom learning environment in a manner that meets or exceeds the learning objectives of the course requires instructors to consider how they will approach the management of the learning environments for which they have accepted responsibility. Faculty may find it helpful to consider their emotional assets as discussed in Goleman's (2005) work on emotional intelligence. His book *Emotional Intelligence* is a helpful guide for developing the faculty's role as a learning facilitator and developing strategies for engaging students in interventions regarding their conduct.

Additionally, because it is tempting to ignore inappropriate behavior, it may be helpful for faculty to consider various ethical imperatives that serve as a compelling rationale for action. For example, most nursing education programs have established objectives or standards related to professional behavior. The American Association of Colleges of Nursing (2008) has gone so far as to stipulate that "in order to demonstrate professionalism, civility must be present" (p. 26). Additionally, we are reminded in the Code of Ethics for Nurses (American Nurses Association, 2001) that educators are responsible for assuring that our students demonstrate "commitment to professional practice prior to entry" (p. 13) into practice. When students consistently behave inappropriately, there is an argument to be made that they do not meet the standard of professionalism.

When managing the learning environment, faculty are setting both learning and behavioral expectations. In setting these expectations, faculty must also monitor and evaluate how these expectations are fulfilled. As such, faculty's own self-awareness becomes important when considering the extent to which students meet the standards that have been set. It is important that faculty observe themselves and recognize their feelings as they engage with students. As the instructor, faculty have administrative power over the student and the responsibility to act civilly, objectively, and consistently.

To effectively manage the learning environment, faculty need to appropriately and effectively manage their own emotions. Nursing faculty have reported experiencing negative emotions when subjected to student incivility, including feelings of decreased self-esteem, a loss in their confidence as teachers, resentment related to the time involved in documenting student misconduct incidents, and a loss of motivation to teach (Luparell, 2007b). It is paramount that faculty be cognizant of their own feelings about students and what is behind these personal responses to student behavior. Of course, the ultimate responsibility of faculty is to find ways to manage their emotions so that they do not interfere with the learning environment. Feelings such as fear, anxiety, anger, and sadness can cause faculty to avoid engaging students. Failing to engage or confront students limits faculty ability to manage the learning environment. These feelings can also skew faculty observations of student behavior. If a faculty member believes that a student is acting inappropriately, and remains reluctant to engage the student in a discussion about these behaviors, the faculty's feelings may be an underlying issue that needs to be addressed as well. Campus faculty teaching and professional development services can be a valuable resource in assisting faculty to develop strategies for effective student conferences.

As faculty engage with their students in learning experiences, a key to effective management is maintaining sensitivity to others' feelings and concerns and the ability to consider others' perspectives. Clark and Springer (2007) conducted a study of nursing faculty and students that indicated that students and faculty had different perceptions of what constituted uncivil behavior on the part of students *and* faculty. Baxter and Boblin (2007)

also stated that nursing faculty and students may disagree on what constitutes dishonest behavior, especially in the classroom. When confronting a student about behavior and how it appears that the behavior is disrupting the learning environment, appreciating the differences in how people perceive and respond to situations will be helpful when talking with students about what constitutes appropriate behavior in the learning environment. These differences in perceptions between faculty and students also further illustrate the importance of faculty being explicit about the behaviors that are expected of students at the very initiation of the learning experience.

The Faculty–Student Learning Relationship

Faculty often ask what their rights and responsibilities as instructors are and what rights and responsibilities students have as learners. Rights and responsibilities are guided by constitutional law, state law, and institutional policy. Private and public colleges and universities have been treated differently by the courts in that private institutions are seen more as private corporate entities and public institutions are considered to be agents of the government (Kaplin & Lee, 2006). Regardless of the type of institution, see Box 14-5 for an example of the rights and responsibilities that are generally held as good practice when working with students in a learning setting.

If an institution or program does not have clearly established expectations for the behaviors of students and faculty, these policies should be developed (Clark & Springer, 2007). In addition to faculty development activities, student development activities should also be provided by the institution to assist students in coping with the multiple stressors many are facing in their lives and to help students identify appropriate and inappropriate behaviors.

SUMMARY

Faculty have more contact time with students than anyone else in the educational setting. Faculty are the key to developing quality learning environments that allow for the civil exchange of information and ideas. Faculty and administrators must be able to recognize the early warning signs of student misconduct such

---

BOX 14-5 Code of Student Rights, Responsibilities, and Conduct

STUDENTS HAVE THE RIGHT TO:

- Exercise their rights as a citizen
- Exercise constitutional freedoms and responsibilities without university interference or fear of university disciplinary action for such activity
- Be present at all aspects of any disciplinary proceedings (as complainant or accused) in which witnesses provide evidence
- Not be falsely accused of violating the code

STUDENTS HAVE THE RIGHT TO EXPECT FACULTY TO:

- Clearly state the course goals and inform students of testing and grading systems; moreover, these systems should be intellectually justifiable and consistent with the rules and regulations of the academic division
- Plan and regulate class time with an awareness of its value for every student and meet classes regularly
- Remain available to students and announce and keep liberal office hours at hours convenient to students
- Strive to develop among students respect for others and their opinions by demonstrating faculty's own respect for each student as an individual
- Strive to generate a proper respect for an understanding of academic freedom by students
- Allow students to raise relevant issues pertaining to classroom discussion, to offer reasonable doubts about data presented, and to express alternative opinions to those being discussed without concern for any academic penalty

FACULTY HAVE THE RESPONSIBILITY TO:

- Be sensitive to the student's personal or political beliefs expressed in a private manner in connection with coursework
- Not publicly disclose student's grades or class standing without the student's permission
- Obtain a clear statement of student basic rights, obligations, and responsibilities concerning both academic and personal conduct

STUDENTS HAVE THE RESPONSIBILITY TO:

- Uphold and comply with the student code
- Not make false statements
- Respect each other's personal rights and dignity
- Select a major field of study, choose an appropriate degree program within the discipline, plan class schedules, and meet the requirements for the chosen degree
- Take appropriate advantage of the educational opportunities presented by the university, participate in the learning process in a serious and conscientious manner, and respect the rights of other members of the university community with regard to academic affairs

Adapted from the *Indiana University code of student rights, responsibilities, and conduct*. Available at www.iupui.edu/code.

---

as unhealthy obsessions and specific verbal clues—expressions of hopelessness, direct or indirect threats, or suicidal language—and then report them. Working with a team of campus professionals and faculty to effectively engage troubled students is a critical aspect to classroom management. When a student is struggling in a class or is affected by drugs or alcohol, or financial or relationship problems, faculty are often the key to successfully assisting students. When a student's behavior interferes with the educational process or campus safety, the institution can consider a range of options in response. This chapter provided some insight into those options.

This chapter provided a brief summary of developmental, legal, and risk managing aspects of student misconduct and learning, in addition to specific actions that can be used to reduce in-class disruptions and maintain a well-managed learning environment that allows both the instructor and students to meet their learning objectives in a civil manner. The goal of this chapter is to help future faculty gain an understanding of problem or disruptive student behavior, in addition to an understanding of specific steps one can take and available professional resources one can use to minimize disruptions in a learning environment.

CASE STUDIES FOR FUTURE DISCUSSION

The following are three case studies that illustrate the continuum of student misconduct behaviors, the developmental opportunities, and the instructional management risks that faculty may experience when managing the learning environment.

Annoying Acts

The Situation: Alexandra

Alexandra is a first semester student who wants to talk with you before, during, and after class, often about personal noncourse-related items. Alexandra appears emotionally needy and does not appear to have any friends in class. Lately she has started interrupting others during in-class discussion. The other students don't listen to her and have asked not to be in her lab group.

At the point that Alexandra's behavior begins to disrupt your ability to lecture in class and the students' ability to learn, you need to meet with her. At the end of one class session you ask her to come to your office. During your meeting with Alexandra, you let her know that you value her as a student and that you have enjoyed getting to know her but that recently you have noticed that she has begun interrupting students during class discussion. You ask her about her studies and how she feels the class is progressing. She mentions that she is having a tough time making friends in her program and does not know what to do, and that at times she feels very alone and isolated. You let her know that her comments are valuable, but that she also needs to allow other students to be heard. You point out that listening is a part of learning and that you would like her to wait and allow her fellow students time to make their points in class. You also let Alexandra know that making friends is important and studying in groups is helpful to learning. You suggest that Alexandra talk with a counselor at the campus counseling center to gain some ideas on how to develop these friendships on campus. As a follow-up to your meeting, you set a time to meet in three weeks to talk about her work in class and her overall progress in the program.

Administrative Violations

The Situation: Adam

It is the middle of the semester and it has become common for Adam to dominate the conversation in class. He has often become angry and visibly agitated and he uses incendiary language when interacting with other students. He is constantly challenging the material you present. When he is not present, the class is more productive and more relaxed. You realize that you have put off talking with Adam. You talk with him, describe his behaviors in class, and talk about how you would like him to participate in class discussion in the future and the importance of working cooperatively with his fellow students. Adam begins to argue with you and refuses to consider that he should reflect on his own conduct. He blames other students who have "disrespected" him. During the next class, Adam's behavior escalates and is disruptive to the point that you are not able to cover the material planned for that day. You decide to forward a referral to your department chair for review and advice as to next steps.

The department chair receives your documentation and informs you that two other faculty have sent him similar reports about Adam over the last year. The department chair contacts the dean of students' office and forwards all three referrals for review and action. Adam's lack of cooperation makes it difficult to approach him developmentally and his response pushes the situation to a level that violates administrative policies. The risks to manage are increasing as well, which makes it important to involve other campus offices.

The department chair, associate dean, and you meet with Adam. A behavioral contract is drawn up between the department chair and Adam. Adam agrees to adhere to the standards set in your class, and his conduct is being referred to the dean of students for administrative review as a violation of the student code of conduct.

Criminal Cases

The Situation: Cathy

Cathy is a senior in her last year of the program. You have taught Cathy before in a previous class and you are surprised that she has almost completed the program, because she has been a chronically weak student and has difficulty working with others in a clinical setting. About three weeks into the semester a student reports to you that Cathy is very angry with a fellow student in class and has vandalized the student's car in order to "get even." You contact your department chair, who contacts the campus police and the dean of students' office. The police investigate the allegations and criminal charges are brought against Cathy by the police. The dean of students initiates administrative disciplinary proceedings and Cathy is placed on disciplinary probation until she completes her degree. Cathy is moved to another class and is told to have no contact with the student whose car she vandalized. A condition of Cathy's probation is to attend counseling.

REFLECTING ON THE EVIDENCE

1. From a student perspective, faculty are central to the learning experience. Many of our students spend the greatest amount of time in class interacting with faculty. As such, faculty have the opportunity to cultivate relationships with students and are often in the best position to become aware of inappropriate conduct. How can faculty cultivate an environment that positively contributes to learning and proactively responds to student misconduct?

2. As faculty, you have became aware that during the ninth week of the semester, one of your students went from performing quite well with good attendance, submitting all assignments on time and well done, and displaying a generally collegial demeanor to suddenly missing class, not turning in weekly assignments, and not returning e-mails. What is the best way to respond to this student?

3. While grading a lab assignment you notice that four students appear to have submitted identical work to the extent that you have become concerned that the students may have presented other people's work as their own. What is the best way to approach this situation? What could you have done to avoid or minimize this type of incident?

4. Under what circumstances do you ask for help in responding to possible student misconduct?

REFERENCES

American Association of Colleges of Nursing. (2008). *The essentials of baccalaureate education for professional nursing practice.* Washington, DC: Author.

American Nurses Association. (2001). *Code of ethics for nurses with interpretive statements.* Washington, DC: American Nurses Publishing.

Andersson, L. M., & Pearson, C. M. (1999). Tit for tat? The spiraling effect of incivility in the workplace. *Academy of Management Review, 24*(3), 452-471.

Bartholomew, K. (2006). *Ending nurse-to-nurse hostility: Why nurses eat their young and each other.* Marblehead, MA: HCPro.

Baxter, P., & Boblin, S. (2007). The moral development of baccalaureate nursing students: Understanding unethical behavior in the classroom and clinical settings. *Journal of Nursing Education, 46*(1), 20–27.

Boice, B. (1996). Classroom incivilities. *Research in Higher Education, 37*(4), 453-486.

Clark, C., & Springer, P. (2007). Incivility in nursing education: A descriptive study of definitions and prevalence. *Journal of Nursing Education, 46*(1), 7–14.

Clark, C. M. (2008a). Faculty and student assessment of and experience with incivility in nursing education. *Journal of Nursing Education, 47*(10), 458.

Clark, C. (2008b). The dance of incivility in nursing education as described by nursing faculty and students. *Advances in Nursing Science, 31*(4), E37.Goleman, D. (2005). *Emotional intelligence.* New York, NY: Bantam Books.

Kaplin, W. A., & Lee, B. A. (2006). *The law of higher education* (4th ed.). San Francisco, CA: Jossey-Bass.

Lashley, F. R., & de Meneses, M. (2001). Student civility in nursing programs: A national survey. *Journal of Professional Nursing, 17*(2), 81–86.

Levine, A., & Cureton, J. S. (1998). *When hope and fear collide: A portrait of today's college student.* New York, NY: Wiley.

Luparell, S. (2004). Faculty encounters with uncivil nursing students: An overview. *Journal of Professional Nursing, 20*(1), 59–67.

Luparell, S. (2007a). Dealing with challenging student situations: Lessons learned. In M. H. Oermann & K. T. Heinrich (Eds.), *Annual review of nursing education: Vol. 5. Challenges and new directions in nursing education* (pp. 101–110). New York, NY: Springer.

Luparell, S. (2007b). The effects of student incivility on nursing faculty. *Journal of Nursing Education, 46*(1), 15–19.

United States Department of Education. (2007, October). *Balancing student privacy and school safety: A guide to the family educational rights and privacy act for colleges and universities.* Retrieved from http://www2.ed.gov/policy/gen/guid/fpco/brochures/postsec.html

15 Strategies to Promote Critical Thinking and Active Learning

Connie J. Rowles, DSN, RN

Nursing faculty spend a considerable amount of their time planning experiences to facilitate student learning. The selection of teaching strategies and learning experiences traditionally has been governed by behavioral objectives. However, nursing education has been undergoing a major revolution, with attention focused on how to teach students to think critically. Therefore nurse educators are continually reexamining the "best" way to teach and to empower students for learning. The purpose of this chapter is to identify strategies that students and faculty can use to promote learning. The chapter begins with a discussion of critical thinking as the basis for any teaching strategy. Developing effective learning experiences comes next. A variety of teaching strategies are then presented with a discussion of their use, advantages, disadvantages, and tips for making the learning experience interactive and meaningful.

Critical Thinking and Active Learning

Thinking, reflective thinking, and critical thinking have been topics of discussion among educators for many years (Bandman & Bandman, 1995; Brookfield, 1987, 1995; Dewey, 1933; Facione, 1990; Halpern et al., 1994; Hunkins, 1985; Kurfiss, 1988; McPeck, 1981; Norris & Ennis, 1989; Paul, 1995; Perry, 1970; Siegel, 1980; Watson & Glaser, 1984). A recent search in the Cumulative Index to Nursing and Allied Health (CINAHL) located 58 articles about critical thinking even when the search was limited to full-length articles in English in the time frame of July 2009

through July 2010. One excellent source from the search is Romeo (2010). She reviewed the critical thinking literature and found issues related to the definition of critical thinking as well as issues in the use of instruments to measure critical thinking. She also cited the lack of findings that show a clear-cut correlation with factors that interest nurse educators, such as licensing exam pass rates and changes in critical thinking over time in the program. So, while there is still a lot in the literature about critical thinking, there are some who recommend a change in the dialogue about thinking in nursing. A brief discussion of some of the newer terms found in the literature follows. A common thread with the newer ideas is that they all build on a foundation of critical thinking.

Clinical Reasoning

Clinical reasoning is the ability of the nurse to use critical thinking skills in the ever-changing clinical environment. It should include the ". . . context and concerns of the patient and family" (Benner, Sutphen, Leonard, & Day, 2010, p. 85). Clinical imagination and reflection are also part of clinical reasoning (Benner et al., 2010). The thought is that critical thinking is more a snapshot in time while clinical reasoning can accommodate the changing nature in clinical settings.

Clinical Judgment

Clinical judgment can be defined as "an interpretation or conclusion about a patient's needs, concerns, or health problems, and/or the decision to take action (or not), use or modify standard approaches, or improvise new ones as deemed appropriate by the patient's response" (Tanner, 2006, p. 204).

The author acknowledges the work of Carole Brigham, EdD, RN, and Barbara L. Russo, MSN, RN, in the previous edition(s) of the chapter.

Tanner acknowledges that problem solving, critical thinking, decision making, and clinical judgment are often used in the literature to mean the same thing.

Metacognition

Metacognition is the "self-communication process in which a person engages before, during and after performing a task" (Beitz, 1996, p. 23) and more commonly thought of as thinking about thinking. It is an active process of monitoring your own thinking. Kuiper and Pesut (2004) contend that it is the combination of metacognition (reflective thinking) and critical thinking that better describes the thinking necessary in nursing.

Clinical reasoning, clinical judgment, and metacognition are all important in nursing. However, the basis of all of these is critical thinking. This chapter focuses on critical thinking, the ideal critical thinker, and the related cognitive skills.

The Ideal Critical Thinker Defined

Most experts agree that if an individual is a critical thinker, he or she not only has well-developed critical thinking skills but also exhibits what are variously described as the disposition, attitude, or traits of a critical thinker (Baron & Sternberg, 1986; Facione, Facione, & Sanchez, 1994; Ford & Profetto-McGrath, 1994; Kataoka-Yahiro & Saylor, 1994; Paul, 1995; Pless & Clayton, 1993; Turner, 2005; Watson & Glaser, 1984).

This chapter uses Facione's (1990) definition of an ideal critical thinker. This description was derived by a consensus of experts in critical thinking who participated in a Delphi study. The panel of experts included "46 scholars, educators and leading figures in critical thinking theory and critical thinking assessment research" (p. 34). The experts essentially agreed that

> The ideal critical thinker is habitually inquisitive, well-informed, trustful of reason, open-minded, flexible, fair-minded in evaluation, honest in facing personal biases, prudent in making judgments, willing to reconsider, clear about issues, orderly in complex matters, diligent in seeking relevant information, reasonable in the selection of criteria, focused in inquiry, and persistent in seeking results which are as precise as the subject and the circumstances of inquiry permit. (p. 3)

Facione et al. (1994) suggest that the Delphi study description of an ideal critical thinker describes a nurse with ideal clinical judgment.

Cognitive skills (subskills) of critical thinking were also delineated in Facione's (1990) Delphi study. These include the cognitive skills and subskills of analysis (examining ideas, identifying arguments, analyzing arguments), evaluation (assessing claims, assessing arguments), inference (querying evidence, conjecturing alternatives, drawing conclusions), interpretation (categorizing, decoding significance, clarifying meaning), explanation (stating results, justifying procedures, presenting arguments), and self-regulation (self-examination and self-correction) (Facione, 1990).

Critical Thinking in Nursing and Nursing Education

Nurses need a high level of critical thinking skills and a critical thinking disposition because nurses encounter multiple patients with the same health care needs. However, each patient responds to those needs differently. Therefore nurses are required to use their holistic nursing knowledge base to think through each situation to provide individualized, effective (evidence-based) care rather than simply to follow routine procedures.

Jones and Brown (1993) believe that nursing is practiced in complex environments with humans, who are complex beings. Technological advances and a knowledge explosion have also changed the face of health care. Thinking skills of the nurse become more important than the ability to perform the associated psychomotor skills. Case (1994) discussed the changing arenas for decision making as being not only at the bedside but also in quality assurance processes, delegation activities, shared governance, and management and executive roles. As health care reform extends patient care from the predominantly structured inpatient arena to the more unstructured outpatient or community arenas, critical thinking skills and empowerment become even more important.

Carlson-Catalano (1992), in discussing empowering nurses, believed that traditional curricula encourage students to be obedient, dependent, and fearful in caring for patients. She suggests that nurses in professional practice should be empowered and that students need to be treated as valued members of the profession. She offers analytic nursing, change activities, collegiality, and sponsorship as strategies for empowering nurses. These strategies would be addressed if nursing faculty adopted the principles of critical thinking as the foundation for practice.

Students must develop higher-order thinking skills. Brigham (1993) contends that faculty need to assist students to recognize how systems respond to specific health problems. Students need to know what nursing measures will be needed when they read laboratory reports with abnormal results; they do not need to memorize normal laboratory values. Jones and Brown (1991) argue that nurse educators can no longer convey facts to nursing students. "There are far too many facts, but there are far too many facts that become erroneous over time" (Jones & Brown, 1991, p. 533). Miller (1992) concurs:

> More emphasis should be given to the mental processes students engage in as they solve nursing problems and less given to simply identifying the correct answer. Focusing on making clinical inferences from given data, recognizing unstated assumptions, deductive reasoning, weighing of evidence and distinguishing between weak and strong arguments emphasizes the importance of the processes of thinking. (p. 1406)

Scheffer and Rubenfeld (2000) conducted a Delphi study to develop a consensus statement about critical thinking in nursing education. A panel of 55 experts from 9 countries determined that

> Critical thinking in nursing is an essential component of professional accountability and quality nursing care. Critical thinkers in nursing exhibit these habits of the mind: confidence, contextual perspective, creativity, flexibility, inquisitiveness, intellectual integrity, intuition, open-mindedness, perseverance, and reflection. Critical thinkers in nursing practice [possess] the cognitive skills of analyzing, applying standards, discriminating, information seeking, logical reasoning, predicting and transforming knowledge. (p. 357)

In summary, Jackson (1995) states, "Every patient deserves caregivers who think critically . . . . The ability to think critically can be empowering. Practitioners must commit to a struggle of balancing an explosion of objective and intuitive information in an explosive health care environment" (p. 187). Therefore nurse educators are challenged to help students develop necessary critical thinking skills as the students progress through the curriculum.

Roles of Faculty and Students in Developing Critical Thinking Skills

The development of students' critical thinking skills and dispositions requires faculty to reconsider their philosophy of teaching. The faculty-dominated classroom is not conducive to development of critical thinking. It is the responsibility of faculty to think about the roles of the teacher and student, as well as to create an environment that empowers students. Transmitting information through rote lecture to students does not guarantee learning. Students must be actively engaged with the information for it to be transformed into knowledge. Lesson plans must be designed to foster the development of critical thinking skills (cognitive) and a critical thinking disposition (affective) as students engage with the theoretical, affective, and psychomotor content that is nursing. Students must become empathetic, empowered, and able to critically think about every situation if they are to succeed in nursing (Bevis, 1993; Ford & Profetto-McGrath, 1994).

Faculty Roles

Faculty must become facilitators of learning rather than teachers of content (Bevis, 1993; Brigham, 1993; Brookfield, 1995; Creedy, Horsfall, & Hand, 1992; Jones & Brown, 1993). Ford and Profetto-McGrath (1994) believe that the teacher–student relationship must become a "working with" relationship—an egalitarian relationship. Burns and Egan (1994) suggest that faculty should demonstrate critical thinking as content is presented. For example, when teaching content such as medical acidosis and alkalosis, faculty could demonstrate their own problem-solving skills by thinking aloud as they discuss a relevant case study. Students should think aloud while interacting with the content so that faculty can identify inappropriate thinking processes and provide immediate constructive feedback.

Creedy et al. (1992) propose that faculty can empower students by valuing their contributions, encouraging expression of their opinions, exploring mistakes objectively without demeaning the students, and promoting risk taking. Brookfield (1987) cites the following principles that will facilitate students to think critically:

- Affirm the critical thinkers' self-worth (p. 72).
- Listen attentively to critical thinkers (p. 73).
- Show that you support critical thinkers' efforts (p. 74).

- Reflect and mirror critical thinkers' ideas and actions (p. 75).
- Motivate people to think critically (p. 76).
- Regularly evaluate progress (p. 78).
- Help critical thinkers create networks (p. 79).
- Be critical teachers (p. 80).
- Model critical thinking (p. 85).

Thus according to Brookfield (1987), the facilitator of learning must enter into an egalitarian relationship to support the learners' attempts to engage in critical thinking. Faculty can only provide learning experiences for students; faculty cannot teach (impart knowledge); they can only share their knowledge. Students must transform the content into their own knowledge.

Student Roles

Learning to think critically requires active student participation (Meyers, 1986); students must become active creators of their own knowledge (Creedy et al., 1992). At this time, it can be assumed most students have come from faculty-dominated classrooms in which the students have been the recipients of endless amounts of facts to be memorized and recalled for examinations (Valiga, 1983). Students have probably not been asked to apply those facts to real-life situations. Therefore students will have to be assisted with the transition from the passive to active learner role. Faculty need to create a risk-free environment that is conducive to active student participation. The discussion later in this chapter related to creation of an anticipatory set serves as an example of helping students to make the transition from passive to active learners. Repeated encounters with active learning situations are needed before students can become comfortable with the active learner role.

Active learners must come to class prepared. They cannot rely on the faculty to tell them what they need to know. "Preclass written assignments, study guides, quizzes and short in-class writings" (Brigham, 1993, p. 52) are effective in stimulating students to come to class prepared to engage with the content while interacting with faculty and fellow students in planned learning activities.

Classroom Environment for the Development of Critical Thinking Skills

The classroom environment changes when the principles of critical thinking are adopted. Active learning can be a very threatening situation. Faculty must create a risk-free environment that allows students to explore the content, make mistakes, reflect on the content, associate the content with experience, and transform the content into knowledge (McCabe, 1992).

Brigham (1993) suggests that faculty set the stage by sharing that their philosophy of teaching is to enhance critical thinking. This should be done when students are being introduced to the course. Students need to know that learning experiences have been designed for them to actively engage with the information and with each other while faculty facilitate the activities and learning process. Students must understand that, through the interactions, information will be converted into knowledge (Bevis, 1993).

Classroom environments should establish a sense of connection between faculty and students and among students themselves. Students should understand that neither faculty nor students have all of the answers and that no one answer is correct in all situations. Open discussion and student willingness to take risks should be supported while faculty guide the group toward the preestablished learning outcome.

Students need to be aware that there are conflicting ideas about some concepts. Faculty at some schools of nursing do not adopt a specific textbook for their courses; rather, the bookstore stocks appropriate textbooks by different authors and students select the textbook they would like to use. This particular idea is intriguing because it certainly provides a basis for discussion of information from multiple points of view. When contradictions are found, it helps students recognize that the written word should be questioned.

The physical component of the classroom is important; however, any classroom can be conducive to active student learning. Students should be able to make eye contact with each other and with faculty. MacIntosh (1995) suggests rearranging chairs into small or large circles. Faculty can be creative in modifying the physical characteristics of the classroom. For example, in classrooms where desks are bolted down, students could sit on the tops of the desks to be able to face others in the group.

Student Responses to Active Learning

Beck (1995) conducted a study using a cooperative learning model based on feminist pedagogy that resulted in positive teacher–student and student–student interactions and satisfactory learning.

Hezekiah (1993) cites the five basic feminist goals for the classroom—"atmosphere of mutual respect, trust and community, shared leadership, cooperative structure, integration of cognitive and affective learning, and action oriented field work" (pp. 55–56)—that would establish an environment for the development of critical thinking skills as the learner transforms information to knowledge. Wake, Coleman, and Kneeland (1992) discuss shared governance in the classroom. They note that shared governance in nursing education produces professional nurses who will be prepared to practice in an ever-changing health care environment.

Price (1991) found that "interaction between the student and teacher ranked high as a positive contributor to learning" (p. 170). Price cited the following student responses to the benefits of an interactive classroom:

> What's good is your understanding of conflicts we may be facing as new students, your continual encouragement, and the fact that you're always available to answer questions . . . I don't function well, never have, when the question is memorizing. . . . I tend to learn very abstractly and not sequentially; my learning is not textbook learning. . . . I really find that I learn the most when I can apply it to myself and to someone else; that's the thing I can underline and say, "Yes, I learned that very well." . . . It's practical application, where it's applied to life, where your pattern of behavior is changed, something you can apply in your relationship with another human being. (pp. 170–171)

Summary

Nurses must possess a high level of critical thinking skills and a critical thinking disposition. Faculty must create opportunities for students to develop critical thinking as they progress through the curriculum. Faculty must become facilitators of learning and students must become active learners.

Critical thinking should be at the forefront of planning learning experiences for nursing students. If educators believe that "students can and should think their way through the content of their courses, . . . gain some grasp of the logic of what they study, . . . develop explicit intellectual standards, then they can find many ways to move instruction in this direction" (Barnes, 1992, p. 22). Faculty must create an environment that develops the traits of an ideal critical thinker and plan learning experiences that include strategies to develop the cognitive skills and subskills of critical thinking.

Planning Learning Experiences

Planning challenging encounters that will entice students to learn and develop critical thinking skills is a major task for any faculty member. Effective planning of any kind requires much time and effort; planning learning experiences is no exception. Careful planning of each learning experience gives teachers more self-confidence and aids in formative and summative evaluation of teaching. At least six steps are used in designing learning experiences:

1. Determine the learning outcomes for the specific class period.
2. Create an anticipatory set.
3. Select teaching and learning strategies.
4. Consider implementation issues.
5. Design closure to the learning experience.
6. Design formative and summative evaluation strategies.

Each of the stages is discussed in detail. All steps can be planned by both students and faculty. Novice faculty may find it helpful to design learning experiences in great detail (Table 15-1), whereas more experienced faculty may use only a more general outline form.

Determining the Learning Outcomes

The first step is to determine the learning outcomes of the class. Several activities must be carried out before specific outcomes for any class period are developed. The first activity is assessment of the overall curriculum outcomes and the placement of the specific course in meeting these outcomes. Typically, general curriculum outcomes are stated in very broad terms and will likely not give the teacher any information about what to include in a specific class period. However, a thorough understanding of the broad curriculum goals is necessary so teachers can "connect" the specifics for the day to the broad curriculum outcomes. Course objectives and outcomes need to be reviewed to ascertain how the particular course "fits" within the curriculum (Ayer, 1986; Torres & Stanton, 1982). See Chapters 8 to 11 for additional information.

Teachers tend to design learning experiences within their own belief and value systems. Their

TABLE 15-1 Sample Plan for a Learning Experience: Ethics in Leadership

1. Outcomes: Identify ethical theory used for own decision making. Discuss implications of use of ethical theories in the workplace.

Activity	Content	Time	Strategies
2. Anticipatory set a. Preclass assignment b. In-class exercise	a. Ethical theories b. Ethical case examples c. Ethical situations	a. 2 hr b. 10 min	a. Text reading b. Ethical survey c. Individual reflection to identify the most difficult question on the survey and write how and why answered
3. Implementation tools a. Projector b. PowerPoint slides	a. Three ethical theories from text b. Application (1) Identify own theory used. (2) Apply to familiar situation. (3) Apply to new situation. (4) Apply to workplace decision making.	a. 40 min b. 30 min	a. Large group discussion (1) Slides of the theories' main points (2) At each main point ask, "What does this mean to you?" and "Give an example of how the point would be seen in practice." b. Small group discussion (1) "Which theory do you use?" (2) "Give example of how you used the theory." (3) "How would a nurse administrator use the theory to make ethical decisions?" (4) "How could use of the theories lead to conflict in the workplace?"
4. Closure	Emphasize class outcomes.	20 min	a. Small group reports b. Overall summary

own philosophies about teaching, learning, the curriculum, the ability of students, and how and what a nurse educator "should" do all influence the development of activities for a specific class period. Teachers need to be aware of these value systems and recognize the influence of them on their teaching and selection of teaching strategies (Creedy et al., 1992).

With these activities in mind, outcomes for a given experience can be established. There are several ways to identify outcomes. One way is to use behavioral objectives (see Chapters 9 and 10). For many, however, behavioral objectives imply rigid lists of specific content, faculty-dominated classrooms, and only one right answer to each examination question. Some believe that specific behavioral objectives need to be abandoned, given the important issue of development of critical thinking abilities in students (Bevis, 1993). In another approach, general outcomes or competencies are identified, and the path to achieving them is left open. How they are written depends on individual school requirements, the overall curriculum design, the content of the course, and the beliefs or values of the individual faculty member.

Creating an Anticipatory Set

The second major step in planning a learning experience is to create an environment that invites all students to become interested in the content and to participate in the learning process. This activity is referred to as *creating an anticipatory set* (Ayer, 1986; deTornyay & Thompson, 1982; Maas, 1990). The activity typically takes little in-class time and merely sets the stage for active involvement in the learning process. Maas (1990) includes three elements in an anticipatory set: active participation, relevance to the students, and relevance to the class period. Preclass readings; active, thought-provoking questions; and a class exercise that emphasizes students' prior knowledge are examples of activities that can be used as an anticipatory set. The anticipatory set prepares students for the main activity or content of the class period.

Selecting a Teaching Strategy

Selecting the particular teaching strategy is the third step in lesson planning. Faculty must consider multiple factors as they select a particular strategy.

The first factor is the content itself. For example, teaching abstract concepts is probably better accomplished through mind mapping (Rooda, 1994), whereas psychomotor skills are better taught through demonstration (Kelly, 1992). The philosophy underlying the broad curriculum outcomes also influences the selection of teaching strategies. In a school that has adopted the principles of critical thinking, the traditional lecture would seldom be used as a strategy. Last, faculty must consider teaching strategies that are feasible. Questions to consider may include the amount of time available, room size, distance learning delivery system being used, the availability of equipment, the number of students, time and money costs for both the teacher and the student, and learning styles of the students.

With these factors in mind, many different teaching strategies would be appropriate for any student group and class content. Throughout the course it is important to vary the strategies. Using the same type of anticipatory set followed by lecture and then the same closure can be very boring for students. For example, faculty may create interest for the students by using lecture some of the time and role play, demonstration, and reflection at other times.

Varying the strategies also has the advantage of appealing to all types of learners (see Chapter 2). Few of the teaching strategies are equally stimulating to all types of learners. It is not particularly important that teachers use strategies that appeal to all learners in every class, but it is important for them to use strategies that appeal to all types of learners throughout the course. Questioning is a teaching strategy that should be used consistently; it can even be used in every class (Paul, 1995). "Helping students to ask their own questions should perfect their ability to think critically about information and how to process it" (Hunkins, 1985, p. 296). Strategies that appeal to one type of learner can also be used for the preclass assignments or activities, and strategies for other types of learners can be used for the classroom experience.

Teaching Strategies and Critical Thinking

The actual steps in designing learning experiences do not change when critical thinking concepts are applied to the curriculum. Teaching strategies should be selected for the development of critical thinking skills. Development of these skills in students should be a planned activity throughout all stages of the curriculum. Any strategy selected should be selected for a particular reason, and all strategies should lead to the development of advancing levels of critical thinking.

Cognitive Levels

Cognitive levels must be considered during lesson planning. Several theorists have written about the various cognitive levels of students. Perry (1970) identifies four levels including nine stages of intellectual development. Belenky, Clinchy, Goldberger, and Tarule (1986) have demonstrated that women and men differ in intellectual development in several major areas. One example is that women typically have a silent stage of cognitive development, which is the first level. This stage is characterized by a powerless, dependent fear of authority figures. Men typically do not go through the silent stage.

Hickman (1993) examined the theories of Perry (1970), Belenky et al. (1986), and others and integrated their thinking on cognitive levels with Benner's (1984) levels of skill acquisition. Hickman's (1993) thoughts are related directly to the licensed nurse, but her ideas can also be applied to the undergraduate nursing student. The beginning nursing student is a novice in critical thinking. Thinking is characterized as dualistic (everything is black or white). Little or no critical thinking is used. The novice depends on authority for knowledge and is usually silent. The next cognitive level is the advanced beginner. In this stage, thinking at the multiplicity level occurs. Students use subjective knowledge to begin seeing recurring themes, but they fail to differentiate important cues. Students at this level require assistance in establishing priorities. The next stage is the competent student nurse. At this stage, students continue to use subjective knowledge, but they do so consciously and they use the subjective knowledge in deliberate planning activities. The last cognitive level is the proficient student nurse, who is at the relativistic level of intellectual development. Relativism is the recognition that opinions differ in quality and require supporting evidence to be valid. Relativism is equated with procedural knowledge, connected knowledge, or both. Students no longer see information as only black and white; they begin to see how things "fit" together and notice where information is missing. They begin to think critically.

It would be hoped that students completing a basic nursing education program would have attained the relativism level of cognitive development. Most undergraduate students will not have attained the final level, which is commitment in relativism. Commitment in relativism describes the expert nurse who integrates knowledge with experience and uses personal reflection to derive constructed knowledge (Hickman, 1993). Many graduate students will have already moved to this level. Undergraduate nursing students will likely move to the final level of cognitive development after they are licensed and have many more real-life nursing experiences and the time to reflect on and integrate those experiences.

The cognitive level of students must be addressed when learning experiences are designed. Moving students from the cognitive level of dualism to the level of relativism should be a major goal of nursing education. The level of cognitive development also influences the selection of teaching strategies. Bowers and McCarthy (1993) suggest that students who exhibit thinking at the informed commitment (relativistic) level would probably feel frustrated if they were expected to think at a dualistic level. For example, proficient student nurses would rather discuss implications of abnormal blood gas values (relativistic thinking) than respond to questions about normal findings (dualistic thinking).

Implementation Issues

The fourth stage of lesson planning is implementation of the learning experience. In this stage, two major activities are considered. The first is the timing. How much time will be spent on the strategies selected to develop the anticipatory set? What backup plans are made to account for a lesson that takes much less or more time than anticipated? What can be cut or what can be added? What are the most crucial concepts to be covered if time is short? The sample plan (see Table 15-1) contains estimated times, with more detail included in a more extensive version of the plan.

The second activity in this stage is to plan for the tools needed to implement the class. In this case, tools can refer to many things. Tools can be instructional media and equipment such as a projector, computer, or video information system (see Table 15-1). Tools can also refer to the information technology tools used to establish the learning community, such as computer conferencing or

video conferencing. Plan to check the equipment for correct working order. Nothing can ruin a well-planned learning experience quite as effectively as instructional media that do not work! Tools could also be the classroom itself. How should the chairs be arranged? Do you want to use a podium? Does the screen for the projector or computer work? The last set of tools is the paper products. What handouts does the faculty member need? How much lead time is needed for typing and copying the handouts? Are the computer slides or transparencies ready? Are there items that need to have copyrights cleared? Who does that and how much time does it take? Assessing and planning for the amount of time and the tools necessary for implementation of the teaching strategy are activities that should not be left to the last minute.

Designing Closure

The last step in designing the learning experience is planning for closure. Closure may be as simple as a few sentences that summarize the major concepts. In this case, the time allowed for closure would be very short. However, closure can take a large amount of class time, especially when dealing with sensitive or emotional content. Applying major concepts to similar or new areas of interest is another example of a closure technique (deTornyay & Thompson, 1987). This time may also be used to create the anticipatory set for the next class period by discussing how the content of the class relates to the content of the next class period.

Designing Formative and Summative Evaluation Strategies

During the lesson planning phase, both formative and summative evaluation need to be considered (Ayer, 1986). Chapter 16 contains information about classroom assessment, and Chapters 24 to 26 contain information about assessment of learning outcomes. These chapters should assist in this stage of planning.

Evaluation activities should occur throughout the learning experience. Many formative evaluation techniques are available (see Chapter 16). Frequent formative evaluation is important for assessment of students' understanding of content. Varying the types of formative evaluation used is important. For example, sometimes the objectives can be evaluated and at other times the teaching strategy used can be evaluated. Frequent self-evaluation is critical. Faculty should ask whether the time, tools, strategy, and content were organized and planned effectively and what could have been done differently to enhance student learning.

Summary

Designing effective learning experiences involves at least six distinct stages. A well-designed experience that enhances student learning cannot be done in a haphazard manner or at the last minute. Enhanced student learning and the development of critical thinking skills are the outcomes of well-planned learning experiences.

Teaching Strategies

There are many different teaching strategies. Those with the most application to nursing education are presented throughout the rest of the chapter. Each strategy is described with its advantages and disadvantages, teaching tips, and additional references where the reader may find a more detailed description of the strategy.

Simulation is a teaching strategy that is growing in use in nursing education; it is discussed in detail in Chapter 20. Other teaching strategies may be more appropriate for the online learning environment. A detailed discussion can be found in Chapter 23. Any discussion about teaching strategies would be incomplete without a review of learning resources, including instructional media or distance education delivery systems. These are discussed in Chapters 19 to 23.

The lecture is presented first, because this teaching strategy is frequently used by many teachers. Many other strategies can be used in nursing education. These strategies are alphabetized for ease of location. Each strategy discussed may have its place in a course, but its use depends on the content, the teacher, and the learners.

Most of the strategies described after the lecture involve active learner participation in the learning process and emphasize adult learning and critical thinking concepts. Both teachers and students may resist this type of learning because the strategies are more flexible and less teacher centered than those typically used in the traditional college classroom. However, if one accepts that the learner must actively engage with the content or information to transform it into knowledge, the classroom should become student centered. Thus the traditional lecture may not always be the most appropriate strategy.

Lecture

Definition. Teacher presentation of content to students, usually accompanied by some type of visual aid or handout.

Use. Clarify complex, confusing, or conflicting concepts; provide background information not available to students; change of pace from more experiential learning strategies; cover background information from scattered sources.

Teaching Tips.

1. Increased student participation can be achieved if the format of the feedback lecture is used (Fuszard, 1995). For example, in a feedback lecture of 1 hour, a 6- to 10-minute group discussion period is inserted between two 20-minute lecture times.
2. Use visual aids, handouts, and study guides so students can follow the sequence of the lecture.
3. Students learn in various ways so add activities to the lecture that stimulate all learners.
4. Read the article "What Is the Most Difficult Step We Must Take to Become Great Teachers?" by Nelson (2001) for some ideas on how to decrease the amount of class time devoted to lecture.

Advantages. Time efficient for covering complex material; should raise further student questions that lend themselves to other teaching strategies.

Disadvantages. Decreases student involvement in learning when content is readily available and easy to understand in a text or other reading assignment; lengthy preparation time for faculty; little involvement in the topic for students other than sitting through the lecture; may have a high cost in preparation and development of handouts and visual aids.

Additional Reading. Amerson, 2006; Beers & Bowden, 2005; deTornyay & Thompson, 1982; Fuszard, 1995; Hoover, 1980; Johnson & Mighten, 2005; McKeachie, 1986; Nelson, 2001.

Algorithms

Definition. Step-by-step procedure for solving a complex procedure; breaks tasks into yes or no steps.

Use. Any course in which frequent practice is required for student mastery of content, in which rules aid in problem solving, or in which the content can be broken into yes or no stages.

Teaching Tips.
1. Assess content for appropriate use of algorithm as a teaching strategy.
2. Develop algorithm and accompanying student explanations of how to use.
3. Allow 6 to 8 hours for the development of the first algorithms.
4. Additional algorithms on similar content typically take less time to develop.

Advantages. Shows students how to "spot" the most relevant information for problem solving; develops reliable, complex problem-solving abilities even in novice students; decreases the amount of one-on-one instruction often required when teaching problem-solving techniques; effective in teaching complex procedures that involve many steps; when used with case studies, may enhance learning; saves faculty teaching time over lecture type of presentations; saves student time in trying to remember and understand complex phenomena.

Disadvantages. Teacher must clearly define the steps or students will not be able to complete the task accurately; students may need to be taught how to use algorithms in problem solving; development of algorithms can be time consuming for faculty.

Additional Reading. Connor & Tillman, 1990; Rathbun & Ruth-Sahd, 2009.

Argumentation, Debate, Structured Controversy, and Dilemmas

Definition. The process of inquiry or reasoned judgment on a proposition aimed at demonstrating the truth or falsehood of something; involves the construction of logical arguments and oral defense of a proposition; requires the recognition of assumptions and evidence and use of inductive and deductive reasoning skills; allows identification of relationships.

Teaching Tips.
1. Strategy works best in an issues or topics course for students at a higher level of cognitive thinking.
2. For the purpose of forming productive debate teams, it is helpful for students to know each other.
3. Faculty should introduce the basic topics and structure the debate format early in the course to allow students adequate preparation time.
4. Debate teams usually consist of five students: two students debate for the topic, two debate against the topic, and the fifth acts as the moderator.
5. Debates follow a specified format, including opening comments, presentation of affirmative and negative viewpoints, rebuttal, and summary (Fuszard, 1995).
6. Encouraging students to debate the opposite of their personal opinion will increase student learning.

Advantages. Develops analytical skills; develops ability to recognize complexities in many health care issues; broadens views of controversial topics; develops communication skills; increases student abilities to work in groups.

Disadvantages. Requires a fairly high level of knowledge about the subject on the parts of both those presenting the debate and the audience; may require teaching students the art of debate; requires increased student preparation time; can create anxiety and conflict for students because of the confrontational nature of debate; students without adequate public speaking skills may also have increased anxiety; high time cost for students to work in groups.

Additional Reading. Brookfield, 1992; Candela, Michael, & Mitchell, 2003; Fuszard, 1995; Garity, 2008; Garrett, Schoener, & Hood, 1996; Metcalf & Yankou, 2003; Mottola & Murphy, 2001; Pederson, 1993.

Case Study, Case Problem, Case Report, Research Case, Case Scenario, and Sociodrama

Definition. In-depth analysis of a real-life situation as a way to illustrate class content; applies didactic content and theory to real life, simulated life, or both. Sociodrama combines the attributes of a case study and role play through the theatrical presentation of the case.

Teaching Tips.

1. A well-designed case that illustrates the most important class concepts is critical to the success of learning with this method.
2. Before the class period, analyze the case with the intent of determining the potential ways in which students could analyze the case but be prepared for student questions and comments that previously have not been considered (be able to say, "I don't know" or "I haven't considered that before" if necessary).
3. A safe, open, nonthreatening classroom environment is crucial for active student participation.
4. During the class period, ask pertinent questions, draw out quieter students, correct misconceptions, and support students in their efforts.
5. At the conclusion of the class, provide a summary of the most important points and sources for more in-depth study.
6. Assist in students' comprehension of critical concepts with the use of tools such as concept maps, chalkboards, and slides.

Advantages. Stimulates critical thinking, retention, and recall; associating the practical with the theoretical helps many students recall important information; typical lecture material can be presented in more practical context; problem solving can be practiced in a safe environment without the threat of endangering a patient; especially good for adult learners who desire peer interaction, support for prior experience, and validation of thinking; an experienced nurse can readily devise a case study example from actual patient encounters.

Disadvantages. More effective when used with complex situations that require problem solving; not appropriate when concrete facts are the only content; developing cases is a difficult and time-consuming skill for many and the option of published cases should be considered; requires the use of good questioning skills by the faculty; poor student preparation for class may result in less learning; may frustrate students who desire content to be presented through more traditional strategies such as lecture.

Additional Reading. Cascio, Campbell, Sandor, Rains, & Clark, 1995; Casebeer, 1991; Delpier, 2006; Fuszard, 1995; Pond, Bradshaw, & Turner, 1991; Sprang, 2010; Taylor, Barrick, & Harrell, 1994; Tomey, 2003.

Cooperative Learning, Collaborative Learning, and Group Assignments

Definition. Teams of learners work on assignments and assume responsibility for group learning outcomes.

Teaching Tips.

1. Design meaningful assignments that can be accomplished by small groups (a group of three to five heterogeneous [in ability, gender, ethnic status, experience, and so on] students is ideal).
2. Teach or verify groups' understanding of team roles and group process; assign or ask group to designate "leader," "recorder," "reflector," "reporter," and other roles as necessary.
3. Structuring the group with students who are not homogenous increases the potential for greater student learning (Kinchin & Hay, 2005).
4. Allow adequate time for reporting and processing of group work.

Advantages. Promotes active and reflective learning; encourages teamwork; provides opportunity for students to become accountable for own and others' work; group dynamics skills can be used; large learning assignments and projects can be accomplished efficiently; can be implemented in discussion groups and forums by using the Internet and group conferencing software.

Disadvantages. Students may resist frequent use of group assignments; possibility that not all students will participate equally; student scheduling issues may complicate group assignments; increases student stress if group conflict occurs.

Additional Reading. Dansereau, 1983; Glendon & Ulrich, 1992; Henry, 2006; Kinchin & Hay, 2005; Matthews, Copper, Davidson, & Hawkes, 1995; McAlister & Osborne, 1997; *The Team Memory Jogger*, 1995.

Demonstration

Definition. Show how to do something.

Use. Complex mental or psychomotor skill acquisition.

Teaching Tips.

1. Show the steps of the process clearly, from start to finish.

2. Go through the process a second time, showing the rationale and allowing time for questions.
3. May help to demonstrate the process again.
4. Provide for immediate, individual, supervised practice sessions.

Advantages. Visibly showing a process often aids in retention; complex skills become more understandable as a result of the demonstration; demonstration allows an expert to model the skill; targeted feedback enhances retention (Day, Iles, & Griffiths, 2009).

Disadvantages. Students have differing levels of skill acquisition abilities; students who quickly master skills may become bored while the others are practicing; mastering psychomotor skills is usually very stressful for students; requires adequate faculty supervision, space, supplies, and equipment to provide realistic practice sessions; high faculty workload involved in supervision of student practice times; high cost of supplies and equipment may limit amount of practice time available to students.

Additional Reading. Day et al., 2009; Jeffries, Rew, & Cramer, 2003; Kelly, 1992.

Dialogue, Peer Sharing, Storytelling, and Narrative Pedagogy

Definition. Dialogue involves a conversation between two or more people.

Teaching Tips.
1. A clear connection must be made between the objectives and the strategy or students will think the activity is a waste of time.
2. Create a possible list of topics and allow students to choose what they are interested in to promote active student learning.
3. Creating relevance in the stories or peer sharing will also increase student learning.
4. Informal meetings between faculty and students may help clarify and structure questions used to promote in-class discussion.
5. These strategies probably work best with small groups.

Advantages. Provides a point of reference from which to explore concepts from multiple points of view, including theoretical and practical; promotes reflection and critical analysis; truth seeking is activated; enhances affective learning and caring; increases contextual learning.

Disadvantages. Requires that faculty continually focus on the realistic; faculty may need to assist learners to focus or refocus on concepts being discussed throughout class period.

Additional Reading. Brown, Kirkpatrick, Mangum, & Avery, 2008; Bunkers, 2006; Koenig & Zorn, 2002; MacLeod, 1995; Nehls, 1995; Porter, 1995; Symonds, 1995; Yoder-Wise & Kowalski, 2003.

Films, Film Clips, DVDs, and Online Videos (YouTube)

Definition. Films or film clips are used in the classroom to enrich the classroom learning experience.

Teaching Tips.
1. Consult Chapter 21 for information on using media in the classroom.
2. Strategy should be used with large or small group discussions and include time for debriefing.
3. Specific questions should be used to guide the discussion groups. See Questioning and Socratic Questioning strategy below for hints on question construction.
4. Choose the film or film clip carefully so the use directly relates to class or course objectives.
5. Film clips can emphasize key points and provide visual memory cues for students (Herman, 2006).
6. Consider copyright issues prior to using the film or film clip.
7. Feature films or film clips as well as educational films or film clips may be used.

Advantages. Will probably appeal to younger learners who are used to including video in their learning environment; can expose students to different ideas in a safe environment; discussions can deal with emotional content in a classroom rather than in the clinical setting where it may be more inappropriate; team building can happen if the experience is shaped to support it; better when used once or twice in a semester rather than in every class period; can give students a way to see patients with clinical issues or symptoms before encountering them in a clinical setting; discussions after the film or film clip can stimulate critical thinking.

Disadvantages. Can be time consuming for faculty to find the appropriate film or film clip; may be costly to purchase the film or film clip; some learners may find it difficult to connect the film or film clip to class content; requires extra equipment in the classroom and the ability to run the equipment; equipment may be expensive to acquire; little evidence exists that connects this teaching strategy to improved student outcomes; watching an entire film may consume valuable class time.

Additional Reading. Brown et al., 2008; Herman, 2006; J. C. Masters, 2005.

Games

Definition.
- "Game: An activity governed by precise rules that involves varying degrees of chance or luck and one or more players who compete (with self, the game, one another, or a computer) through the use of knowledge or skill in an attempt to reach a specified goal (gain an intrinsic or extrinsic reward)" (deTornyay & Thompson, 1987, p. 27).
- "Simulation Game: An activity that incorporates the characteristics of both a simulation and a game; a contest that also replicates some real-life situation or process" (deTornyay & Thompson, 1987, p. 27).

Teaching Tips.
1. Use this method for reinforcement of knowledge rather than introduction of new knowledge.
2. An open learning environment is crucial to learning with gaming—faculty must back out—the learning is student to student in this method.
3. Several distinct steps are involved in development of a game. (See Fuszard, 1995.)
4. Debriefing after the game is critical so students clearly connect the game with the important concepts.
5. If faculty do not value gaming as a teaching strategy, they may unconsciously sabotage the game.

Advantages. Increases cognitive and affective learning; improves retention; fun and exciting; increases learner involvement; motivates learner; can help connect practice experiences to theory; students can learn from each other through the experience of the game; good for adult learners who take more responsibility for their own learning; adult learners can receive immediate feedback in learning situation and can also see the immediate application of theory to practice; learning from gaming lasts longer when compared with learning from traditional lecture.

Disadvantages. May be threatening to some learners; may be time consuming; may be costly to purchase or develop; may be difficult to evaluate level of learning if several players are involved; may require greater amount of space; should have introductory and summary sessions; takes longer than traditional lecture; faculty must set guidelines so the game does not get out of control; little evidence exists that connects this teaching strategy to improved student outcomes.

Additional Reading. Batscha, 2002; Bender & Randall, 2005; Blakely, Skirton, Cooper, Allum, & Nelmes, 2009; deTornyay & Thompson, 1987; Flanagan & McCausland, 2007; Fuszard, 1995; Haupt, 2006; Kuhn, 1995; K. Masters, 2005; Metcalf & Yankou, 2003; Royse & Newton, 2007; Sealover & Henderson, 2005.

Humor

Definition. The ability to perceive, enjoy, or express what is comical or funny; the quality of being laughable or comical; funniness.

Use. Provides break in content students may perceive as boring; emphasizes important points.

Teaching Tips.
1. The use of cartoons with relevant content can provide a break in tense class sessions.
2. Content-related quotes work as well as cartoons in many instances.
3. Humor should be used sparingly to be most effective.
4. Assessing the background of students before using humor can help avoid embarrassing moments.
5. Students should not be the target of the humor.
6. Develop your own sense of humor first before implementing humor in a classroom (Ulloth, 2003a).

Advantages. Increased attention and interest, student/teacher rapport, comprehension and retention of material, motivation toward learning, satisfaction with learning, playfulness, positive attitudes and classroom environment, productivity, class discussions, creativity, generation of ideas, quality and quantity of student reading, and divergent thinking, decreased academic stress and anxiety, dogmatism, boredom and class monotony" (Parrott, 1994, p. 37); decreases anxiety and tension; can help with retention of course material; may improve teacher–student relationship.

Disadvantages. Can be seen as "ridicule, sarcasm, racist or ethnic jokes? The wrong kind of humor can be demeaning and destroy self-esteem and confidence, interfere with communication and sever relationships" (Parrott, 1994, p. 37); faculty time spent finding appropriate cartoons, anecdotes, and so on can be extensive; some students may find humor distracting from the topic at hand.

Additional Reading. Englert, 2010; Parrott, 1994; Robbins, 1994; Ulloth, 2002, 2003a, 2003b.

Imagery

Definition. Mental picturing, diagramming, or rehearsal before the actual use of the information in practice.

Use. Best use is in combination with other strategies (e.g., with physical practice in psychomotor skill acquisition).

Teaching Tips.
1. Create a scenario that would mimic a real-life situation.
2. Use the scenario to demonstrate effective use of imagery.
3. Relaxation techniques provide a good example of how to use imagery techniques.
4. A supportive classroom environment is needed for the effective use of this strategy.

Advantage. Superior learning of psychomotor skills when imagery is combined with physical practice.

Disadvantages. Individuals have varying levels of innate imagery skills, so some students may need to be taught how to do imagery; does not provide a substitute for physical practice of a skill; using imagery and physical practice of the skill will require more student study time than if only physical practice is used; stress and performance fears may interfere with the productive use of imagery; may

require teacher education to implement imagery strategy.

Additional Reading. Bucher, 1993; Doheny, 1993.

Learning Contracts

Definition. Individualized written contract between teacher and student.

Teaching Tips.
1. Specific elements need to be included in the learning contract. (See deTornyay and Thompson, 1982.)
2. Learning contracts can be either teacher initiated or student initiated.
3. A high level of trust must be established between the student and the teacher for the successful implementation of learning contracts.

Advantages. Maximizes adult students' needs to direct their own learning; may also provide the structure needed by some adult students; builds on prior knowledge and life experiences of adult students; allows students to work at their own pace (i.e., some may need remediation and others may need more advanced or complex learning objectives); teacher-initiated contracts may be very motivating for some students.

Disadvantages. Students may not be familiar with the process of developing a learning contract and may become frustrated when the "normal" educational classroom is absent; students must be independent thinkers to be able to construct productive learning contracts; students must be self-disciplined to complete the contract; faculty and administrators may need in-service programs in the development, management, and acceptance of learning contracts when they are used as the only form of student summative evaluation for a class; little preparation time but potentially a larger workload for faculty, especially if an entire class has individualized contracts; additional student time will be required for a self-assessment of learning needs and development of the learning contract.

Additional Reading. deTornyay & Thompson, 1982, 1987; Swansburg, 1995.

Literature Analogies, Newspaper Analysis, and Metaphor Examination

Definition. Conceptual clarification with the use of literature to identify similarities and differences of concepts in the literature with those in nursing practice.

Use. Relating unfamiliar to familiar; clarifying abstractions.

Teaching Tips.
1. Requires clear identification of the concepts that would be appropriate to clarify with this strategy.
2. Finding "just the right" piece of literature to use may be difficult. Probably the best way to locate a usable source is to come across it while reading the newspaper for pleasure rather than for work-related reasons.
3. It is important to clarify and summarize the exercise at the conclusion of the class.

Advantages. Allows students to relate foreign concepts to familiar concepts; establishes framework for introducing new materials; raises awareness of multiple meanings associated with human-related concepts.

Disadvantages. Time consuming for faculty to identify appropriate literature related to concepts being studied; learners may have difficulty seeing relationships; reading nonnursing-specific content may be costly in terms of time for students.

Additional Reading. Faulk & Morris, 2010; Halloran, 2009; Kirkpatrick, 1994; Young-Mason, 1988, 1991.

Mind Mapping, Concept Mapping, Pattern Recognition, Chunking, and Argument Mapping

Definition. Learning complex phenomenon by diagramming the concepts and subconcepts. Mind mapping puts the central concept in the center of the page with related concepts surrounding the main concept. Concept maps tend to be a more hierarchical structure (Kern, Bush, & McCleish, 2006).

Teaching Tips.
1. Organizing the course in like subjects can provide an example of mind mapping for the students.
2. This teaching method is frequently used in clinical teaching but is also effective in the classroom.
3. Students can organize patient data prior to entering an actual patient encounter and then add to the map correlating new and existing data to better understand the clinical presentation of the patient.
4. Grouping specific class content can also provide students with examples of mind mapping.
5. Concept map software is helpful when using this technique (Martin, 2009).
6. Concept mapping can be an effective strategy for students with all types of learning styles.
7. Argument mapping techniques are slightly different than other concept mapping techniques and involve depicting the structure of an argument, logic, debate, or clinical reasoning. See Billings (2008) for more information.

Advantages. Better understanding and recall of complex phenomena; especially effective in stimulating long-term recall of like concepts; active involvement by the students in designing the maps will enhance analytic thinking processes; helps students recognize similarities and differences among concepts; helps clarify relationships between concepts; helps link new information with information previously learned; helps students organize information and relate theories to practice; method appeals to the visual learner.

Disadvantages. May take longer initially until both faculty and students understand how to organize the concepts; may not appeal to concrete or auditory learners; both faculty and students will need to learn how to learn before this method can be used effectively.

Additional Reading. All & Huycke, 2007; All, Huycke, & Fisher, 2003; Antonacci, 1991; Beitz, 1998; Billings, 2008; Clayton, 2006; Daley, Shaw, Balistrieri, Glasenapp, & Piacentine, 1999; Hill, 2006; Kern et al., 2006; Kostovich, Poradzisz, Wood, & O'Brien, 2007; Martin, 2009; Reynolds, 1994; Rooda, 1994; Taylor & Wros, 2007; Tschikota, 1993.

Portfolio

Definition. "A portfolio is a collection of evidence, usually in written form, of both the products and processes of learning. It attests to achievement and personal and professional development, by providing critical analysis of its contents" (McMullan et al., 2003, p. 288).

Use. Documentation of student skills from prior courses or life experiences.

Teaching Tips.
1. Students may need an orientation about how to construct a portfolio.
2. A content outline should provide the framework for the portfolio but not limit student creativity.
3. Assessment of portfolios can be complex and difficult. The novice may want to seek consultation from experts for assistance. Consult Jasper and Fulton (2005) and Karlowicz (2010) for ideas on portfolio assessment.
4. Guidelines for the portfolio must be clear.

Advantages. Typically high student motivation because of control over learning; motivated students typically learn more; helps teachers understand individual student goals and aspirations; encourages student reflection of learning; independent, self-confident, and self-directed students will excel with this method; a small, qualitative study reported increased learning with the use of the portfolio (Tiwari & Tang, 2003).

Disadvantages. Must be combined with reflective strategies to encourage student ownership of learning; requires new ways of thinking about the learning process by both teachers and students; portfolios may become bulky unless specific inclusion guidelines are established; students with low self-confidence will need much faculty assistance; time involvement may be high for students in development of portfolios and for faculty in evaluation of portfolios; extra costs may be involved in duplication, construction, and storage of portfolios; unless students clearly see the objective of a portfolio, the work involved may be viewed as busywork.

Additional Reading. Jasper & Fulton, 2005; Jones, 1994; Karlowicz, 2010; Ramey & Hay, 2003; Robertson, Elster, & Kruse, 2004; Tiwari & Tang, 2003.

Poster

Definition. Visual representation of class concepts.
Teaching Tips.
1. Students need instructions about how to construct a poster.
2. Clear guidelines of the expected poster contents, as well as evaluation techniques, need to be developed and presented to students.

3. Poster quality is enhanced when artistic concepts are incorporated in the poster design (Ellerbee, 2006).

Advantages. Students can convey complex ideas through posters; posters can facilitate student creativity; assessment of students' critical thinking abilities can be done through the use of posters; posters provide students with feedback from peers as well as faculty; students can learn from each other; students get a sense of achievement from producing posters; skills developed in the production of a poster will be valuable for students after graduation; evaluation of posters can be done quickly.

Disadvantages. Involves faculty time to develop poster assignment and evaluation techniques; can be frustrating to students who are not visual learners; some students may not be able to financially afford supplies needed to produce a poster.

Additional Reading. Conyers, 2003; Duchin & Sherwood, 1990; Ellerbee, 2006;; Moule, Judd, & Girot, 1998; Russell, Gregory, & Gates, 1996.

Problem-Based Learning and Unfolding Case Studies

Definition. Learning is that "which results from the process of working towards the understanding or resolution of a problem" (Barrows & Tamblyn, 1980). The problem is a clinical situation presented as a stimulus for students to acquire specific skills, knowledge, and abilities in the solution of the problem. Problem-based learning (PBL) is usually used as an approach to the entire curriculum; rather than focusing on separate disciplines or nursing specialties, in PBL clinical problems and professional issues are used as the focus for integrating all of the content necessary for clinical practice. The goals of PBL are to "(1) construct an extensive and flexible knowledge base; (2) develop effective problem-solving skills; (3) develop self-directed, lifelong learning skills; (4) become effective collaborators; and (5) become intrinsically motivated to learn" (Hmelo-Silver, 2004, p. 240). Unfolding case studies follow a patient through a sequence of events that prompts the student to collect data, reflect, integrate knowledge, and make decisions about clinical practice (Azzarello & Wood, 2006). This strategy is appropriately integrated into individual lesson plans and courses as opposed to an approach to the entire curriculum.

Teaching Tips.
1. Develop realistic, comprehensive clinical problems that will prompt and develop intended learning outcomes.
2. The case problem presented is typically accomplished through several scenes containing complex, ill-structured, but realistic information that requires the students to process the available information into the categories of facts, need to know, hypothesis, and learning issues.
3. Faculty workload can increase significantly, particularly during the development stages; requires close collaboration between various disciplines if the case or curriculum is interdisciplinary. See Niemer, Pfendt, and Gers (2010) for help in developing the case scenario.
4. Orient students to PBL approach; allow sufficient time for students to research the problem and discuss answers.
5. Groups of six to nine students are most effective for PBL.
6. More effective in classroom teaching; less effective in clinical teaching (Williams & Beattie, 2008).

Advantages. Fosters active and cooperative learning, the ability to think critically, and clinical reasoning; students use skills of inquiry and critical thinking, as well as peer teaching and peer evaluation; the problem can be developed in paper and pencil formats, videotape and interactive videodisc, computer-assisted instruction, CD-ROMs, or the Internet; students often work in teams or groups; can be used in interdisciplinary learning environments to develop roles and competencies of each discipline; contextual learning motivates students and increases ability to apply knowledge in clinical situations; increases student responsibility for self-directed and peer learning; develops flexible knowledge that can be applied to different contexts; learning method develops lifelong learning skills.

Disadvantages. Involves faculty time in developing the problem situation; requires shifts of roles of faculty and student; extensive time needed for faculty to learn to use PBL; students require orientation to role of learner in PBL setting and must work through potential discrepancies in expectations and goals for learning; student learning seems to be connected to the effectiveness of the case as well as the functioning of the group; difficult and expensive to use as a teaching technique when the class size is large; the evidence about the level of knowledge acquisition using this method is mixed (see, for example, Chaves, Baker, Chaves, & Fisher, 2006, or Hwang & Kim, 2006).

Additional Reading. Alexander, McDaniel, Baldwin, & Money, 2002; Azzarello & Wood, 2006; Baker, 2000a, 2000b; Barrows & Tamblyn, 1980; Chaves et al., 2006; Choi, 2003; Creedy & Hand, 1994; Creedy et al., 1992; Frost, 1996; Hwang & Kim, 2006; McAlister & Osborne, 1997; Niemer et al., 2010; Nieminen, Sauri, & Lonka, 2006; Williams & Beattie, 2008.

Questioning and Socratic Questioning

Definitions.
- *Questioning*: An expression of inquiry that invites or calls for a reply; an interrogative sentence, phrase, or gesture.
- *Socratic questioning*: Probing questioning to analyze an individual's thinking.

Teaching Tips.
1. Allow sufficient time to construct thought-provoking questions.
2. Faculty need to be prepared to facilitate the discussion that should follow a good questioning period.
3. Student learning is enhanced if a preclass assignment that will lead to adequate student preparation is designed.
4. Questioning can be used spontaneously, as an exploratory strategy, or with issue-specific content.
5. An open, trusting classroom environment is needed.
6. Design questions to assess the various cognitive skills and subskills associated with critical thinking (Paul & Elder, 2006).
7. Appropriate phrasing of questions is required so that students do not feel belittled by the questioning experience.

Advantages. Promotes active thinking about conclusions to be drawn; increases interaction between students and faculty; promotes discussion from multiple points of view; allows students to discuss concepts from their own experiences; discloses underlying assumptions;

increases the articulation of evidence; stimulates students to ask higher-level questions; promotes higher level of problem-solving skills; learning is transferred from classroom to clinical environment; promotes thinking skills to enhance test taking abilities.

Disadvantages. Presumes a thorough knowledge of content; preclass preparation by student and faculty must be thorough; student cannot rely on simple recitation of facts; implies there may be no right answer.

Additional Reading. Browne & Keeley, 1990; Ellermann, Kataoka-Yahiro, & Wong, 2006;, 1985; Meyers, 1986; Paul, 1995; Paul & Elder, 2006; Sellappah, Hussey, Blackmore, & McMurray, 1998; Wink, 1993.

Reflection, Clinical Log, Journal, and Critical Incident Analysis

Definition. Students detail personal experiences and connect them to classroom concepts. Critical incident analysis is a specific technique in reflection that asks the students to describe and analyze a particularly meaningful incident they have experienced or observed in the clinical setting.

Teaching Tips.
1. Clear objectives and expectations for the journal may decrease student perception of the exercise as busywork.
2. Using different approaches to journal writing (e.g., writing learning objectives, summary of the experience, a diary, focused argument) may increase student interest in the assignment.
3. Thoughtful feedback (not necessarily lengthy feedback) from the teacher is very important to student learning.
4. Group discussions about the journals and what students are saying may increase learning for all students.
5. Using specific questions in the journal enhances critical thinking.
6. Students may need to be taught how to do reflection.
7. Reflective journals are most often graded pass or fail.
8. Most frequent use is connecting classroom theories and curriculum objectives to actual practice situations.
9. Oral and written reflections are equally effective.

Advantages. Promotes learning from experiences; helps students learn how to transfer facts from one context to another; links the realities of nursing practice to the more ideal classroom model of nursing; encourages students to think about clinical experiences in relation to classroom models; student-centered learning is especially valuable to adult learners; helpful in demonstrating how to become a lifelong learner; stimulates critical thinking; situation provides a feedback loop between teacher and student so teaching emphasis can be modified to enhance student learning; can be used for all levels of nursing education.

Disadvantages. Teachers may want to revert to the expert role rather than concentrating on the students' experiences; student-directed learning may frustrate some teachers; faculty must be ready to support the student if the reflection stimulates unresolved conflict within student; faculty need to direct student learning through questioning and discussion that may cover topics in which they are not prepared; students may see it as only a required exercise and not take the time to make appropriate use of the learning opportunity; high time cost for faculty to construct reflection guidelines, read student reflections, and help individual students process their reflections; high time cost for students to complete reflections.

Additional Reading. Brown et al., 2008; Brown & Sorrell, 1993; Craft, 2005; Fuszard, 1995; Heinrich, 1992; McCaugherty, 1991; Powell, 1989; Rich & Parker, 1995; Rosenal, 1995; Ruland & Ahern, 2007; Schaefer & Curley, 2005; Van Horn & Freed, 2008.

Role Play

Definition. A dramatic approach in which individuals assume the roles of others; usually unscripted, spontaneous interactions (may be semistructured) that are observed by others for analysis and interpretation.

Teaching Tips.
1. Faculty need to plan thoroughly for the role play, but they also need to be prepared to monitor and modify student actions and reactions if necessary.
2. Situations that involve conflicting emotions provide good scenarios for role playing.

3. Typical organization of the role play involves three stages:
   a. Briefing—setting the stage and explaining the objectives, which is usually the shortest stage
   b. Running—acting out the role play, which may take from 5 to 20 minutes
   c. Debriefing—discussion, analysis, and evaluation of the role-playing experience, which may last 30 to 40 minutes or more
4. The debriefing is probably the most important stage of the role play, so students can clarify actions and so decisions and alternative decisions can be explained, observation skills can be enhanced, and other interpersonal reactions can be anticipated.
5. Videotaping or audiotaping of the role play may aid in the debriefing stage.
6. The technique works best with small groups of students so all those not involved in the role play can become active observers.
7. Students should be encouraged to respond naturally to the role play and avoid phony acting.
8. Criticism should be directed to the behaviors exhibited in the role play and not to specific students.

Advantages. Increases observational skills; improves decision-making skills; increases comprehension of complex human behaviors; provides immediate feedback about the interpersonal and problem-solving skills used in the role play; provides a nonthreatening environment in which to try out unfamiliar communication and decision-making techniques; good for adult learners because of the connection to real-life situations and active participation; does not generate extra costs because props, handouts, and so on are typically not used.

Disadvantages. Students may be reluctant to participate; high time cost for faculty to develop scenarios; faculty who like control of the learning environment may be frustrated by this method; stereotypical behavior can be reinforced; role play can be a costly use of class time if it is not planned appropriately.

Additional Reading. deTornyay & Thompson, 1982; Fuszard, 1995; Shearer & Davidhizar, 2003.

Self-Learning Packet, Individualized Learning Packet, Minicourse, and Self-Learning Module

Definition. Information on one concept presented according to a few specific objectives in a format that allows skipping of a section if the student has previously mastered the content; typically includes self-checks (pretests, posttests) of student learning throughout the self-contained packet.

Teaching Tips.
1. A self-learning packet has many distinct sections (deTornyay & Thompson, 1987).
2. Can be used for a single class period, an entire course, enrichment, or remedial learning.

Advantages. Good for adult learners who have busy lives and limited traditional study times; gives students control of when and where learning will occur; learning can occur without the presence of the teacher; flexible according to learner needs; good for teaching psychomotor skills; has been found to enhance learning over combined lecture and discussion methods.

Disadvantages. Students may procrastinate and not complete work in a timely manner; costly in time and money to prepare and update; printing costs may be high; students used to in-class learning may feel abandoned.

Additional Reading. deTornyay & Thompson, 1982, 1987; Kelly, 1992; Schmidt & Fisher, 1992; Swansburg, 1995.

Seminar and Small or Large Group Discussions

Definition. A meeting for an exchange of ideas in some area; guided discussion of concepts.

Teaching Tips.
1. Student preparation time may be reduced by having students rotate as discussion facilitators so the individual student is responsible for in-depth preparation of only a few topics.
2. The teacher is a part of the group, sometimes acting as a participant or a consultant or the leader.
3. Energy, creativity, and planning by the teacher and the students are required for effective use of this strategy.
4. A clear connection of the seminar discussions to the course objectives is necessary or students will be bored and perceive the seminar as a waste of time.

5. Some control is needed so a vocal person (either student or teacher) does not dominate the discussion.

Advantages. Active student engagement with content; collaborative, cooperative learning, peer sharing, and dialogue facilitate comprehension and practical application of concepts; allows teachers to act as role models for concept clarification and expert problem solving; improves articulation in discussion; improves thinking skills; limited development time for teachers, but planning is still necessary to ensure effectiveness; does not typically require additional supplies such as handouts or audiovisuals; students can learn group problem-solving techniques.

Disadvantages. Requires that students possess adequate knowledge for active discussion and comprehension; may require great amount of student preparation time; may allow a student to "slip through" without sufficient knowledge or thinking skills; students may require instruction in how to participate in seminars.

Additional Reading. Alters & Nelson, 2002; Callahan, 1992; Cohen, 1994; Dansereau, 1983; Davidson, 1994; deTornyay & Thompson, 1987; Glendon & Ulrich, 1992; Johnson & Johnson, 1991, 1993; Johnson, Johnson, & Smith, 1991; Johnson, Maruyama, Johnson, Nelson, & Skon, 1981; Kramer, 1993; Nelson, 2000; Rather, 1994; Udvari-Solner, 1994; White, Beardslee, Peters, & Supples, 1990; Wilen, 1990.

Standardized Patient

Definition. "Structured educational simulations using live actors/educators to portray patient in real-life clinical scenarios" (Carter, Wesley, & Larson, 2006, p. 262).

Teaching Tips.
1. A sound lesson plan must be developed so that the content is addressed adequately.
2. Relevance of the standardized patient to real-life situations enhances retention.
3. Training is required for the actor who will portray the standardized patient.
4. Training should include methods to assure portrayal of the standardized patient in a consistent, unvarying manner (Becker, Rose, Berg, Park & Shatzer, 2006).

5. Students need brief information prior to the encounter with the standardized patient.
6. Debriefing after the encounter with the standardized patient is crucial.

Advantages. Students can experience "real" situations without risk to patients; all students can receive the same experience without having to depend on the availability of the experience in the clinical agency; students increase their feelings of self-confidence and competence; can provide immediate feedback, corrective actions, or both; used most often in nursing education with undergraduate and nurse practitioner students to acquire communication or physical assessment skills; cost savings can be seen over use of faculty-led interactions; promotes long-term retention of course content; may be used in the classroom or in the laboratory.

Disadvantages. Must be structured so that all learners will become involved in the situation and problem-solving process; must be realistic enough for transfer of learning to real situations; requires teacher–student summarization of the content to be learned; can be time consuming to develop scenarios and to train the actors.

Additional Reading. Amano et al., 2004; Becker et al., 2006; Carter et al., 2006; Fletcher et al., 2004; Richardson, Resick, Leonardo, & Pearsall, 2009; Yoo & Yoo, 2003.

Team-Based Learning

Definition. Teams of students are created to enhance learning in the course.

Teaching Tips.
1. The four specific principles associated with team-based learning are:
   a. Groups must be properly formed and managed.
   b. Students are accountable for the quality of their individual and group work.
   c. Students must receive frequent and timely feedback.
   d. Team assignments must promote both learning and team development (Michaelsen, Parmelee, McMahon, & Levine, 2008, pp. 10–16).
2. Keep group sizes at 5 to 7 participants.
3. Students stay in the same team for the duration of the course.

4. Students are expected to read class assignments before the start of class and join their team at the beginning of the class time.

Advantages. Strategy can be used in large classes with student to faculty ratio of 200 to 1 (Clark, Nguyen, Bray, & Levine, 2008); gives the students the actual experience of working in a team; the group becomes accountable for learning; increases student involvement in course content.

Disadvantages. Has been used in medical schools but is a strategy little used in nursing education; requires shifts of roles of faculty and student; requires faculty time to learn the new technique; students require orientation to a different way of learning; student scheduling issues may complicate group assignments; increases student stress if group conflict occurs.

Additional Reading. Clark et al., 2008; Michaelsen et al., 2008.

Writing

Definition. Learning through documentation of ideas in, for example, scholarly papers, informal journals, poems, and letters.

Teaching Tips.

1. Teaching the students how to write will increase the quality of student papers (Roberts & Goss, 2009).
2. Structure the writing assignment with final grading in mind.
3. Assess the paper in its entirety rather than concentrating on grammar and style issues.
4. Peer review of drafts may decrease time in grading and stimulate thinking and critiquing skills.
5. Specific grading criteria decrease the amount of subjective grading.
6. Time spent on grading can be decreased with a grading rubric.
7. Increasing complexity in writing experiences through the curriculum increases the effect on stimulating critical thinking abilities.
8. Providing flexibility in topic selection for written assignments recognizes individual student learning needs and empowers students.
9. Teacher review of student drafts allows early assessment of student thinking and processing of the material and allows for early intervention if problems are detected.
10. Writing manuscripts for publication involves different writing skills than the typical course paper. Additional, more specific instruction may be necessary. Mentoring, reflection, and time to learn the different skills are suggested.
11. Many forms of writing can be used, such as journals, formal papers, creative writing assignments (e.g., poems or book reports), summaries of class content, letters to legislators and nurse administrators, and research critiques.

Advantages. Stimulates critical thinking through active involvement with the literature, learning to judge the quality of the literature, organizing interpretation of the literature into logical sequences, and learning to make judgments based on what was learned; students can discover their own beliefs and values when writing, nurses write in many formats, and writing projects in an educational setting allows for learning different mediums and styles; knowledge gained from the writing assignments can give confidence and helps to empower students in their own ideas; improves communication skills.

Disadvantages. Grading writing assignments can be subjective; many students may feel unprepared to complete writing assignments, which may lead to increased frustration and stress; students must understand the importance of learning through writing, or writing assignments will be viewed as just another thing to get completed; may be high time cost for students to complete the writing assignments depending on how the assignment is structured; typically high time cost for teachers to grade; may be almost impossible to implement in large classes; writing to learn concepts may be new to some teachers, and faculty development may be needed before all can fully participate in this type of teaching strategy.

Additional Reading. Bowers & McCarthy, 1993; Bradley-Springer, 1993; Daggett, 2008; Gehrke, 1994; Griffiths, Coppard, & Lohman, 2005; Lashley & Wittstadt, 1993; Pinch, 1995; Roberts & Goss, 2009; White et al., 1990.

SUMMARY

A large part of any faculty member's time is spent in planning learning experiences. Over the past several years, critical thinking and the shift from teaching to learning have assumed greater emphasis in the design of learning experiences in nursing education. Licensed nurses need to be able to think critically in the ever-changing health care environment, and faculty must integrate opportunities to think critically into learning activities so that students will attain appropriate outcomes for critical thinking.

Planning learning experiences involves at least six distinct steps. The steps are determining the outcomes for the specific class period, creating an anticipatory set, selecting a teaching strategy, considering implementation issues, designing closure to the class period, and designing formative and summative evaluation strategies. Careful planning is crucial to the enhancement of student learning.

Many teaching strategies are described in this chapter. Each has been defined along with its advantages, disadvantages, and related teaching tips. It is important to use different teaching strategies throughout the course because different strategies will engage students with varying learning styles, create interest for the students, assist in the development of critical thinking abilities, and enhance retention of the critical body of knowledge needed by licensed nurses.

REFLECTING ON THE EVIDENCE

1. Compare and contrast two different teaching strategies. Which strategy has the "best" evidence to support its use?

2. Which commonly used teaching technique lacks evidence to support its use? How would you design a research study that would provide evidence for its continued use?

3. What is the latest evidence about critical thinking in nursing education?

4. How could you use critical thinking tools that are evidence-based to measure your student's progress with critical thinking?

REFERENCES

Alexander, J. G., McDaniel, G. S., Baldwin, M. S., & Money, B. J. (2002). Promoting, applying, and evaluating problem-based learning in the undergraduate nursing curriculum. *Nursing Education Perspectives, 23*(5), 248–253.

All, A. C., & Huycke, L. I. (2007). Serial concept maps: Tools for concept analysis. *Journal of Nursing Education, 46*(5), 217–224.

All, A. C., Huycke, L. I., & Fisher, M. J. (2003). Instructional tools for nursing education: Concept maps. *Nursing Education Perspectives, 24*(6), 311–317.

Alters, B. J., & Nelson, C. E. (2002). Perspective: Teaching evolution in higher education. *Evolution: International Journal of Organic Evolution, 56*(10), 1891–1901.

Amano, H., Sano, T., Kinuko, G., Kakuta, S., Suganuma, T., Kimura, Y., . . . Saeki, H. (2004). Strategies for training standardized patient instructors for a competency exam. *Journal of Dental Education, 68*(10), 1104–1111.

Amerson, R. (2006). Energizing the nursing lecture: Application of the theory of multiple intelligence learning. *Nursing Education Perspectives, 27*(4), 194–196.

Antonacci, P. A. (1991). Students search for meaning in the text through semantic mapping. *Social Education, 55*(3), 174–181.

Ayer, S. J. (1986). Teaching practice experience: Linking theory to practice. *Journal of Advanced Nursing, 11*(5), 513–519.

Azzarello, J., & Wood, D. E. (2006). Assessing dynamic mental models: Unfolding case studies. *Nurse Educator, 31*(1), 10–14.

Baker, C. M. (2000a). Problem-based learning for nursing: Integrating lessons from other disciplines with nursing experiences. *Journal of Professional Nursing, 16*(5), 258–266.

Baker, C. M. (2000b). Using problem-based learning to redesign nursing administration masters programs. *Journal of Nursing Administration, 30*(1), 41–47.

Bandman, E. L., & Bandman, B. (1995). *Critical thinking in nursing* (2nd ed.). Norwalk, CT: Appleton & Lange.

Barnes, C. A. (1992). *Critical thinking: Educational imperatives.* San Francisco, CA: Jossey-Bass.

Baron, J. B., & Sternberg, R. J. (1986). *Teaching thinking skills: Theory and practice.* New York, NY: W. H. Freeman.

Barrows, H., & Tamblyn, R. (1980). *Problem-based learning: An approach to medical education.* New York, NY: Springer.

Batscha, C. (2002). The pharmacology game. *CIN Plus, 5*(3), 1, 3–6.

Beck, S. E. (1995). Cooperative learning and feminist pedagogy: A model for classroom instruction in nursing education. *Journal of Nursing Education, 34*(5), 222–227.

Becker, K., Rose, L. E., Berg, J. B., Park, H., & Shatzer, J. H. (2006). The teaching effectiveness of standardized patients. *Journal of Nursing Education, 45*(4), 103–111.

Beers, G. W., & Bowden, S. (2005). The effect of teaching method on long-term knowledge retention. *Journal of Nursing Education, 44*(11), 511–514.

Beitz, J. M. (1996). Metacognition: State-of-the-art learning theory application for clinical nursing education. *Holistic Nursing Practice ,10*(3), 23–32.

Beitz, J. M. (1998). Concept mapping: Navigating the learning process. *Nurse Educator, 23*(5), 35–41.

Belenky, M. F., Clinchy, B. M., Goldberger, N. R., & Tarule, J. M. (1986). *Women's ways of knowing: The development of self, voice and mind*. New York, NY: Basic Books.

Bender, D., & Randall, K. E. (2005). Description and evaluation of an interactive jeopardy game designed to foster self-assessment. *Internet Journal of Allied Health Sciences & Practice, 3*(4). Retrieved from http://ijahsp.nova.edu/articles/vol3num4/bender.htm

Benner, P. (1984). *From novice to expert: Excellence and power in clinical nursing practice*. Menlo Park, CA: Addison-Wesley.

Benner, P. B., Sutphen, M., Leonard, V., & Day, L. (2010). *Educating nurses: A call for radical transformation*. San Francisco, CA: Jossey-Bass.

Bevis, E. O. (1993). All in all it was a pretty good funeral. *Journal of Nursing Education, 32*(3), 101–105.

Billings, D. M. (2008). Argument mapping. *The Journal of Continuing Education in Nursing, 39*(6), 246–247.

Blakely, G., Skirton, J., Cooper, S., Allum, P., & Nelmes, P. (2009). Educational gaming in the health sciences: Systematic review. *Journal of Advanced Nursing, 65*(2), 259–269.

Bowers, B., & McCarthy, D. (1993). Developing analytic thinking skills in early undergraduate education. *Journal of Nursing Education, 32*(3), 107–114.

Bradley-Springer, L. (1993). Discovery of meaning through imagined experience, writing, and evaluation. *Nurse Educator, 18*(5), 5–10.

Brigham, C. (1993). Nursing education and critical thinking: Interplay of content and thinking. *Holistic Nursing Practice, 7*(3), 48–54.

Brookfield, S. (1992). Uncovering assumptions: The key to reflective practice. *Adult Learning, 3*(4), 13–14, 18.

Brookfield, S. D. (1987). *Developing critical thinkers: Challenging adults to explore alternative ways of thinking and acting*. San Francisco, CA: Jossey-Bass.

Brookfield, S. D. (1995). *Becoming a critically reflective teacher*. San Francisco, CA: Jossey-Bass.

Brown, H. N., & Sorrell, J. M. (1993). Use of clinical journals to enhance critical thinking. *Nurse Educator, 18*(5), 16–19.

Brown, S. T., Kirkpatrick, M. K., Mangum, D., & Avery, J. (2008). A review of narrative pedagogy strategies to transform traditional nursing education. *Journal of Nursing Education, 47*, 283–286.

Browne, M. N., & Keeley, S. M. (1990). *Asking the right questions: A guide to critical thinking* (3rd ed.). Saddle River, NJ: Prentice-Hall.

Bucher, L. (1993). The effects of imagery abilities and mental rehearsal on learning a nursing skill. *Journal of Nursing Education, 32*(7), 318–324.

Bunkers, S. S. (2006). What stories and fables can teach us. *Nursing Science Quarterly, 19*(2), 104–107.

Burns, K. R., & Egan, E. C. (1994). Description of a stressful encounter: Appraisal, threat and challenge. *Journal of Nursing Education, 33*(1), 21–28.

Callahan, M. (1992). Thinking skills: An assessment model for ADN in the '90s. *Journal of Nursing Education, 31*(2), 85–87.

Candela, L., Michael, S. R., & Mitchell, S. (2003). Ethical debates: Enhancing critical thinking in nursing students. *Nurse Educator, 28*(1), 37–39.

Carlson-Catalano, J. (1992). Empowering nurses for professional practice. *Nursing Outlook, 40*(3), 139–142.

Carter, M. B., Wesley, G., & Larson, G. M. (2006). Lecture versus standardized patient interaction in the surgical clerkship: A randomized prospective cross-over study. *American Journal of Surgery, 191*(2), 262–267.

Cascio, R. S., Campbell, D., Sandor, M. K., Rains, A. P., & Clark, M. C. (1995). Enhancing critical-thinking skills: Faculty-student partnerships in community health nursing. *Nurse Educator, 20*(2), 38–43.

Case, B. (1994). Walking around the elephant: A critical-thinking strategy for decision making. *Journal of Continuing Education in Nursing, 25*(3), 101–109.

Casebeer, L. (1991). Fostering decision making in nursing. *Journal of Nursing Staff Development, 7*(6), 271–274.

Chaves, J. F., Baker, C. M., Chaves, J. A., & Fisher, M. L. (2006). Self, peer, and tutor assessments of MSN competencies using the PBL Evaluator. *Journal of Nursing Education, 45*(1), 25–31.

Choi, H. (2003). A problem-based learning trial on the Internet involving undergraduate nursing students. *Journal of Nursing Education, 42*(8), 359–363.

Clark, M. C., Nguyen, H. T., Bray, C., & Levine, R. E. (2008). Team-based learning in an undergraduate nursing course. *Journal of Nursing Education, 47*(3), 111–117.

Clayton, L. H. (2006). Concept mapping: An effective, active teaching-learning method. *Nursing Education Perspectives, 27*(4), 197–203.

Cohen, E. G. (1994). *Designing groupwork: Strategies for the heterogeneous classroom* (2nd ed.). New York, NY: Teachers College Press.

Connor, S. E., & Tillman, M. H. (1990). A comparison of algorithmic and teacher-directed instruction in dosage calculation presented via whole and part methods for associate degree nursing students. *Journal of Nursing Education, 29*(1), 31–36.

Conyers, V. (2003). Posters: An assessment strategy to foster learning in nursing education. *Journal of Nursing Education, 42*(1), 38–40.

Craft, M. (2005). Reflective writing and nursing education. *Journal of Nursing Education, 44*(2), 53–57.

Creedy, D., & Hand, B. (1994). The implementation of problem-based learning: Changing pedagogy in nurse education. *Journal of Advanced Nursing, 20*(4), 696–702.

Creedy, D., Horsfall, J., & Hand, B. (1992). Problem-based learning in nurse education: An Australian view. *Journal of Advanced Nursing, 17*(6), 727–733.

Daggett, L. M. (2008). A rubric for grading or editing student papers. *Nurse Educator, 33*(2), 55–56.

Daley, B. J., Shaw, C. R., Balistrieri, T., Glasenapp, K., & Piacentine, L. (1999). Concept maps: A strategy to teach and evaluate critical thinking. *Journal of Nursing Education, 38*(1), 42–47.

Dansereau, D. F. (1983). *Cooperative learning: Impact on acquisition of knowledge and skills* (Report No. 341). Abilene, TX: U.S. Army Research for the Behavioral and Social Sciences.

Davidson, N. (1994). Cooperative and collaborative learning: An integrative perspective. In J. S. Thousand, R. A. Villa, & A. I. Nevin (Eds.), *Creativity and collaborative learning: A practical guide to empowering students and teachers* (pp. 13–30). Baltimore, MA: Paul H. Brookes.

Day, T., Iles, N., & Griffiths, P. (2009). Effect of performance feedback on tracheal suctioning knowledge and skills: Randomized controlled trial. *Journal of Advanced Nursing, 65*(7), 1423–1431.

Delpier, T. (2006). Cases 101: Learning to teach with cases. *Nursing Education Perspectives, 27*(4), 204–209.

deTornyay, R., & Thompson, M. A. (1982). *Strategies for teaching nursing* (3rd ed.). New York, NY: John Wiley.

deTornyay, R., & Thompson, M. A. (1987). *Strategies for teaching nursing* (4th ed.). New York, NY: John Wiley.

Dewey, J. (1933). *How we think: A restatement of the relation of reflective thinking to the educative process.* Boston, MA: Heath.

Doheny, M. O. (1993). Mental practice: An alternative approach to teaching motor skills. *Journal of Nursing Education, 32*(6), 260–264.

Duchin, S., & Sherwood, G. (1990). Posters as an educational strategy. *Journal of Continuing Education in Nursing, 21*(5), 205–208.

Ellerbee, S. M. (2006). Posters with an artistic flair. *Nurse Educator, 31*(4), 166–169.

Ellermann, C. R., Kataoka-Yahiro, M. R., & Wong, L. (2006). Logic models used to enhance critical thinking. *Journal of Nursing Education, 45*(5), 220–227.

Englert, L. M. (2010). Learning with laughter: Using humor in the nursing classroom. *Nursing Education Perspective, 31*(1), 48–49.

Facione, N. C., Facione, P. A., & Sanchez, C. A. (1994). Critical thinking disposition as a measure of competent clinical judgment: The development of the California critical thinking disposition inventory. *Journal of Nursing Education, 33*(8), 345–350.

Facione, P. A. (1990). Critical thinking: A statement of expert consensus for purposes of educational assessment and instruction. In *The Delphi report: Research findings and recommendations prepared for the committee on precollege philosophy.* Newark, DE: American Philosophical Association. Retrieved from ERIC Document Reproduction Service (No. ED 315–423).

Faulk, D., & Morris, A. (2010). The perspective transformation journey: Using a metaphor to stimulate student engagement and self-reflection. *Nurse Educator, 35*(3), 103–104.

Flanagan, N. A., & McCausland, L. (2007). Teaching around the cycle: Strategies for teaching theory to undergraduate nursing students. *Nursing Education Perspectives, 28*(6), 310–314.

Fletcher, K. E., Stern, D. T., White, C., Gruppen, L. D., Oh, M. S., & Cimmino, V. M. (2004). The physical examination of patients with abdominal pain: The long-term effect of adding standardized patients and small-group feedback to a lecture presentation. *Teaching & Learning in Medicine, 16*(2), 171–175.

Ford, J. S., & Profetto-McGrath, J. (1994). A model for critical thinking within the context of curriculum as praxis. *Journal of Nursing Education, 33*(8), 341–344.

Frost, M. (1996). An analysis of the scope and value of problem-based learning in the education of health care professionals. *Journal of Advanced Nursing, 24*(5), 1047–1053.

Fuszard, B. (1995). *Innovative teaching strategies in nursing* (2nd ed.). Gaithersburg, MD: Aspen.

Garity, J. (2008). Resolving ethical dilemmas using debates. *Nurse Educator, 33*(3), 101–102.

Garrett, M., Schoener, L., & Hood, L. (1996). Debate: A teaching strategy to improve verbal communications and critical thinking skills. *Nurse Educator, 21*(4), 37–40.

Gehrke, P. (1994). Finding voices through writing. *Nurse Educator,19*(2), 28–30.

Glendon, K., & Ulrich, D. (1992). Using cooperative learning strategies. *Nurse Educator, 17*(4), 37–40.

Griffiths, Y., Coppard, B., & Lohman, H. (2005). From pedestal to possibility: Learning scholarly writing using a unique course assignment. *Journal of Allied Health, 34*(2), 97–100.

Halloran, L. (2009). Teaching transcultural nursing through literature. *Journal of Nursing Education, 48*, 523–528.

Halpern, D. F., et al. (1994). *Changing college classrooms: New teaching and learning strategies for an increasingly complex world.* San Francisco, CA: Jossey-Bass.

Haupt, B. (2006). Diversity BINGO: A strategy to increase awareness of diversity in the classroom. *Nurse Educator, 31*(6), 242–243.

Heinrich, K. T. (1992). The intimate dialogue: Journal writing by students. *Nurse Educator, 17*(6), 17–21.

Henry, P. R. (2006). Making groups work in the classroom. *Nurse Educator, 31*(1), 26–30.

Herman, J. D. (2006). Using film clips in nursing education. *Nurse Educator, 31*(6), 264–269.

Hezekiah, J. (1993). Feminist pedagogy: A framework for nursing education? *Journal of Nursing Education, 32*(2), 53–57.

Hickman, J. S. (1993). A critical assessment of critical thinking in nursing education. *Holistic Nurse Practice, 7*(3), 36–47.

Hill, C. M. (2006). Integrating clinical experiences into the concept of mapping process. *Nurse Educator, 31*(1), 36–39.

Hmelo-Silver, C. E. (2004). Problem-based learning: What and how do students learn? *Educational Psychology Review, 16*(3), 235–266.

Hoover, K. H. (1980). *College teaching today: A handbook for postsecondary instruction.* Boston, MS: Allyn & Bacon.

Hunkins, F. P. (1985). Helping students ask their own questions. *Social Education, 49*(4), 293–296.

Hwang, S. Y., & Kim, M. J. (2006). A comparison of problem-based learning and lecture-based learning in an adult health nursing course. *Nurse Education Today, 26*(4), 315–321.

Jackson, B. S. (1995). Critical thinking. *Capsules & Comments in Critical Care Nursing, 3*, 183–187.

Jasper, M. A., & Fulton, J. (2005). Marking criteria for assessing practice-based portfolios at masters' level. *Nurse Education Today, 25*(5), 377–389.

Jeffries, P. R., Rew, S., & Cramer, J. M. (2003). A comparison of student-centered versus traditional methods of teaching basic nursing skills in a learning laboratory. *Nursing Education Perspectives, 23*(1), 14–19.

Johnson, D. W., & Johnson, R. T. (1991). Cooperative learning and classroom school climate. In B. Fraser & H. Walberg (Eds.), *Educational environments: Evaluation and antecedents and consequences* (pp. 90–104). Oxford, UK: Pergamon Press.

Johnson, D. W., & Johnson, R. T. (1993). Creative and critical thinking through academic controversy. *American Behavioral Scientist, 37*(1), 40–53.

Johnson, D. W., Johnson, R. T., & Smith, K. (1991). *Active learning: Cooperation in the college classroom.* Edina, MN: Interaction Books.

Johnson, D. W., Maruyama, G., Johnson, R. T., Nelson, D., & Skon, L. (1981). Effects of cooperative, competitive, and individualistic goal structures on achievement: A meta-analysis. *Psychological Bulletin, 89*(1), 47–62.

Johnson, J. P., & Mighten, A. (2005). A comparison of teaching strategies: Lecture notes combined with structured group discussion versus lecture only. *Journal of Nursing Education, 44*(7), 319–322.

Jones, J. E. (1994). Portfolio assessment as a strategy for self-direction in learning. In R. G. Brockett & A. B. Knox (Series Eds.), *New directions for adult and continuing education: No. 64. Overcoming resistance to self-direction in adult learning* (pp. 23–29). San Francisco, CA: Jossey-Bass.

Jones, S. A., & Brown, L. N. (1991). Critical thinking: Impact on nursing education. *Journal of Advanced Nursing, 16*(5), 529–533.

Jones, S. A., & Brown, L. N. (1993). Alternative views on defining critical thinking through the nursing process. *Holistic Nursing Practice, 7*(3), 71–76.

Karlowicz, K. A. (2010). Development and testing of a portfolio evaluation scoring tool. *Journal of Nursing Education, 49*(2), 78–86.

Kataoka-Yahiro, M., & Saylor, C. (1994). A critical thinking model for nursing judgment. *Journal of Nursing Education, 33*(8), 351–356.

Kelly, K. J. (1992). *Nursing staff development: Current competence, future focus.* Philadelphia, PA: J. B. Lippincott.

Kern, C. S., Bush, K. L., & McCleish, J. M. (2006). Mind-mapped care plans: Integrating an innovative educational tool as an alternative to traditional care plans. *Journal of Nursing Education, 45*(4), 112–119.

Kinchin, I., & Hay, D. (2005). Using concept maps to optimize the composition of collaborative student groups: A pilot study. *Journal of Advanced Nursing, 51*(2), 182–187.

Kirkpatrick, M. K. (1994). NINE: Newspaper in nursing education. *Nurse Educator, 19*(6), 21–23.

Koenig, J. M., & Zorn, C. R. (2002). Using storytelling as an approach to teaching and learning with diverse students. *Journal of Nursing Education, 41*(9), 393–399.

Kostovich, C. T., Poradzisz, M., Wood, K., & O'Brien, K. L. (2007). Learning style preference and student aptitude for concept maps. *Journal of Nursing Education, 46*(5), 225–231.

Kramer, M. K. (1993). Concept clarification and critical thinking: Integrated processes. *Journal of Nursing Education, 32*(9), 406–414.

Kuhn, M. A. (1995). Gaming: A technique that adds spice to learning? *Journal of Continuing Education, 26*(1), 35–39.

Kuiper, R. A., & Pesut, D. J. (2004). Promoting cognitive and metacognitive reflective reasoning skills in nursing practice: A self-regulated learning theory. *Journal of Advanced Nursing, 45*(4), 381–391.

Kurfiss, J. G. (1988). *Critical thinking: Theory, research, practice and possibilities* (Report No. 2). Washington, DC: Association for the Study of Higher Education.

Lashley, M., & Wittstadt, R. (1993). Writing across the curriculum: An integrated curricular approach to developing critical thinking through writing. *Journal of Nursing Education, 32*(9), 422–424.

Maas, D. (1990). *Maintaining teacher effectiveness.* Available from Phi Delta Kappa International, P.O. Box 789, Bloomington, IN 47402–0789.

MacIntosh, J. (1995). Fashioning facilitators: Nursing education for primary healthcare. *Nurse Educator, 20*(3), 25–27.

MacLeod, M. L. P. (1995). What does it mean to be well taught? A hermeneutic course evaluation. *Journal of Nursing Education, 34*(5), 197–203.

Martin, K. (2009). Computer-generated concept maps: An innovative group didactic activity. *Nurse Educator, 34*(6), 238–240.

Masters, J. C. (2005). Hollywood in the classroom: Using feature films to teach. *Nurse Educator, 30*(3), 113–116.

Masters, K. (2005). Development and use of an educator-developed community assessment board game. *Nurse Educator, 30*(5), 189–190.

Matthews, R. S., Copper, J. L., Davidson, N., & Hawkes, P. (1995). Building bridges between cooperative and collaborative learning. *Change, 27*(4), 35–40.

McAlister, M., & Osborne, Y. (1997). Peer review: A strategy to enhance cooperative student learning. *Nurse Educator, 22*(1), 40–44.

McCabe, P. P. (1992). Getting past learner apprehension: Enhancing learning for the beginning reader. *Adult Learning, 3*(1), 19–20.

McCaugherty, D. (1991). The use of a teaching model to promote reflection and the experiential integration of theory and practice in first-year student nurses: An action research study. *Journal of Advanced Nursing, 16*(5), 534–543.

McKeachie, W. J. (1986). *Teaching tips: A guidebook for the beginning teacher.* Lexington, MA: D. C. Heath.

McMullan, M., Endacott, R., Gray, M. A., Jasper, M., Miller, C., Scholes, J., & Webb, C. (2003). Portfolios and assessment of competence: A review of the literature. *Journal of Advanced Nursing, 41*(3), 283–294.

McPeck, J. (1981). *Critical thinking and education.* New York, NY: St. Martin's Press.

Metcalf, B. L., & Yankou, D. (2003). Educational innovations: Using gaming to help nursing students understand ethics. *Journal of Nursing Education, 42*(5), 212–215.

Meyers, C. (1986). *Teaching students to think critically.* San Francisco, CA: Jossey-Bass.

Michaelsen, L. K., Parmelee, D. X., McMahon, K. K., & Levine, R. E. (2008). *Team-based learning for health professions education.* Sterling, VA: Stylus.

Miller, M. A. (1992). Outcomes evaluation: Measuring critical thinking. *Journal of Advanced Nursing, 17*(12), 1401–1407.

Mottola, C. A., & Murphy, P. (2001). Antidote dilemma: An activity to promote critical thinking. *Journal of Continuing Education in Nursing, 32*(4), 161–164.

Moule, P., Judd, M., & Girot, E. (1998). The poster presentation: What value to teaching and assessment of research in pre- and post-registration nursing courses? *Nurse Education Today, 18*(3), 237–242.

Nehls, N. (1995). Narrative pedagogy: Rethinking nursing education. *Journal of Nursing Education, 34*(5), 204–210.

Nelson, C. (2000). What is the first step we should take to become great teachers? *The National Teaching & Learning Forum, 10*(1), 7–8.

Nelson, C. (2001). What is the most difficult step we must take to become great teachers? *The National Teaching & Learning Forum, 10*(4), 10.

Niemer, L., Pfendt, K., & Gers, M. (2010). Problem-based learning in nursing education: A process for scenario development. *Nurse Educator, 35*(2), 69–73.

Nieminen, J., Sauri, P., & Lonka, K. (2006). On the relationship between group functioning and study success in problem-based learning. *Medical Education, 40*(1), 64–71.

Norris, S. P., & Ennis, R. H. (1989). *Evaluating critical thinking.* Pacific Grove, CA: Midwest.

Parrott, T. E. (1994). Humor as a teaching strategy. *Nurse Educator, 19*(3), 36–38.

Paul, R., & Elder, L. (2006). *The miniature guide to critical thinking concepts and tools.* Dillon Beach, CA: The Foundation for Critical Thinking.

Paul, R. W. (1995). *Critical thinking: How to prepare students for a rapidly changing world.* Rohner Park, CA: Sonoma State University Center for Critical Thinking and Moral Critique.

Pederson, C. (1993). Structured controversy versus lecture on nursing students' beliefs about and attitude toward providing care for persons with AIDS. *Journal of Continuing Education in Nursing, 24*(2), 74–81.

Perry, W. G. (1970). *Forms of intellectual and ethical development in the college years: A scheme.* New York, NY: Rinehart.

Pinch, W. J. (1995). Synthesis: Implementing a complex process. *Nurse Educator, 20*(1), 34–40.

Pless, B. S., & Clayton, G. M. (1993). Clarifying the concept of critical thinking in nursing. *Journal of Nursing Education, 32*(9), 425–428.

Pond, E. F., Bradshaw, M. J., & Turner, S. L. (1991). Teaching strategies for critical thinking. *Nurse Educator, 16*(6), 18–22.

Porter, E. J. (1995). Fostering dialogical community through a learning experience. *Journal of Nursing Education, 34*(5), 228–234.

Powell, J. H. (1989). The reflective practitioner in nursing. *Journal of Advanced Nursing, 14*(10), 824–832.

Price, J. G. (1991). Great expectations: Hallmark of the midlife woman learner. *Educational Gerontology, 17*(2), 167–174.

Ramey, S. L., & Hay, M. L. (2003). Using electronic portfolios to measure student achievement and assess curricular integrity. *Nurse Educator, 28*(1), 31–36.

Rathbun, M. C., & Ruth-Sahd, L. A. (2009). Educational innovations: Algorithmic tools for interpreting vital signs. *Journal of Nursing Education, 48*(7), 395–400.

Rather, M. L. (1994). Schooling for oppression: A critical hermeneutical analysis of the lived experience of the returning RN student. *Journal of Nursing Education, 33*(6), 263–271.

Reynolds, A. (1994). Patho-flow diagramming: A strategy for critical thinking and clinical decision making. *Journal of Nursing Education, 33*(7), 333–336.

Rich, A., & Parker, D. L. (1995). Reflection and critical incident analysis: Ethical and moral implications of their use within nursing and midwifery education. *Journal of Advanced Nursing, 22*(6), 1050–1057.

Richardson, L., Resick, L., Leonardo, M., & Pearsall, C. (2009). Undergraduate students as standardized patients to assess advanced practice nursing student competencies. *Nurse Educator, 34*(1), 12–16.

Robbins, J. (1994). Using humor to enhance learning in the skills laboratory. *Nurse Educator, 19*(3), 39–41.

Roberts, S. T., & Goss, G. (2009). Use of an online writing tutorial to improve writing skills in nursing courses. *Nurse Educator, 34*(6), 262–265.

Robertson, J. F., Elster, S., & Kruse, G. (2004). Portfolio outcome assessment: Lessons learned. *Nurse Educator, 29*(2), 52–53.

Romeo, E. M. (2010). Quantative research on critical thinking and predicting nursing students' NCLEX-RN performance. *Journal of Nursing Education, 49*(7), 378–386.

Rooda, L. A. (1994). Effects of mind mapping on student achievement in a nursing research course. *Nurse Educator, 19*(6), 25–27.

Rosenal, L. (1995). Exploring the learner's world: Critical incident methodology. *Journal of Continuing Education in Nursing, 26*(3), 115–118.

Royse, M. A., & Newton, S. E. (2007). How gaming is used as an innovative strategy for nursing education. *Nursing Education Perspective, 28*(5), 263–267.

Ruland, J. P., & Ahern, N. R. (2007). Transforming student perspectives through reflective writing. *Nurse Educator, 32*(2), 81–88.

Russell, C. K., Gregory, D. M., & Gates, M. F. (1996). Aesthetics and substance in qualitative research posters. *Qualitative Health Research, 6*(4), 542–552.

Schaefer, K. M., & Curley, C. (2005). Use of focus groups and reflective journaling in a hospice experience. *Nurse Educator, 30*(3), 93–94.

Scheffer, B. K., & Rubenfeld, M. G. (2000). A consensus statement on critical thinking in nursing. *Journal of Nursing Education, 39*(8), 352–359.

Schmidt, K. L., & Fisher, J. C. (1992). Effective development and utilization of self-learning modules. *Journal of Continuing Education in Nursing, 23*(2), 54–59.

Sealover, P., & Henderson, D. (2005). Scoring rewards in nursing education with games. *Nurse Educator, 30*(6), 247–250.

Sellappah, S., Hussey, T., Blackmore, A. M., & McMurray, A. (1998). The use of questioning strategies by clinical teachers. *Journal of Advanced Nursing, 28*(1), 142–148.

Shearer, R., & Davidhizar, R. (2003). Using role play to develop cultural competence. *Journal of Nursing Education, 42*(6), 273–276.

Siegel, H. (1980). Critical thinking as an educational ideal. *The Educational Forum, 45*(1), 7–23.

Sprang, S. M. (2010). Making the case: Using case studies for staff development. *Journal for Nurses in Staff Development, 26*(2), E6–E10.

Swansburg, R. C. (1995). *Nursing staff development: A component of human resource development.* Boston, MS: Jones & Bartlett.

Symonds, J. M. (1995). *RN students finding their voices: Narrative in nursing.* Paper presented at the First Annual RN-BSN meeting, Baltimore, MD.

Tanner, C. A. (2006). Thinking like a nurse: A research-based model of clinical judgment in nursing. *Journal of Nursing Education, 45*(6), 204–211.

Taylor, D. E., Barrick, C. B., & Harrell, F. H. (1994). Preparing students for health care reform: An innovative approach for teaching leadership/management. *Journal of Nursing Education, 33*(5), 230–232.

Taylor, J., & Wros, P. (2007). Concept mapping: A nursing model for care planning. *Journal of Nursing Education, 46*(5), 211–216.

The Team Memory Jogger. (1995). Methuen, MA: GOAL/QPC.

Tiwari, A., & Tang, C. (2003). From process to outcome: The effect of portfolio assessment on student learning. *Nurse Education Today, 23*(4), 269–277.

Tomey, A. M. (2003). Learning with cases. *Journal of Continuing Education in Nursing, 34*(1), 34–38.

Torres, G., & Stanton, M. (1982). *Curriculum process in nursing: A guide to curriculum development.* Englewood Cliffs, NJ: Prentice-Hall.

Tschikota, S. (1993). The clinical decision-making processes of student nurses. *Journal of Nursing Education, 32*(9), 389–398.

Turner, P. (2005). Critical thinking in nursing education and practice as defined in the literature. *Nursing Education Perspectives, 26*(5), 272–277.

Ulloth, J. K. (2002). The benefits of humor in nursing education. *Journal of Nursing Education, 41*(11), 476–481.

Ulloth, J. K. (2003a). Guidelines for developing and implementing humor in nursing classrooms. *Journal of Nursing Education, 42*(1), 35–37.

Ulloth, J. K. (2003b). A qualitative view of humor in nursing classrooms. *Journal of Nursing Education, 42*(3), 125–130.

Valiga, T. M. (1983). Cognitive development: A critical component of baccalaureate nursing education. *Image: The Journal of Nursing Scholarship, 15*(4), 115–119.

Van Horn, R., & Freed, S. (2008). Journaling and dialogue pairs to promote reflection in clinical nursing education. *Nursing Education Perspectives, 29*, 220–225.

Wake, M. M., Coleman, R. S., & Kneeland, T. (1992). Classroom shared governance. *Nurse Educator, 17*(4), 19–22.

Watson, G., & Glaser, E. M. (1984). *Watson-Glaser critical thinking appraisal manual.* New York, NY: Harcourt Brace & Jovanovich.

White, N. E., Beardslee, N. Q., Peters, D., & Supples, J. M. (1990). Promoting critical thinking skills. *Nurse Educator, 15*(5), 16–19.

Williams, S. M., & Beattie, H. J. (2008). Problem based learning in the clinical setting—A systematic review. *Nurse Education Today, 28*(2), 146–154.

Wink, D. M. (1993). Effect of a program to increase the cognitive level of questions asked in clinical postconferences. *Journal of Nursing Education, 32*, 257–263.

Yoder-Wise, P. S., & Kowalski, K. (2003). The power of storytelling. *Nursing Outlook, 51*, 37–42.

Yoo, M. S., & Yoo, I. L. (2003). The effectiveness of standardized patients as a teaching method for nursing fundamentals. *Journal of Nursing Education, 42*, 444–448.

Young-Mason, J. (1988). Tolstoi's *The Death of Ivan Ilych*: A source for understanding compassion. *Clinical Nurse Specialist, 2*, 180–183.

Young-Mason, J. (1991). The Secret Sharer as a guide to compassion. *Nursing Outlook, 39*, 62–63.

Improving Teaching and Learning: Classroom Assessment Techniques

16

Connie J. Rowles, DSN, RN

Since the early 1980s, postsecondary education has been carefully scrutinized by political, economic, consumer, and educational forces to ensure appropriate student performance. As a result, institutions of higher education—faculty and students—are being held more accountable for student learning in the classroom (Angelo & Cross, 1993; Curtis, 1985). To improve learning, educators are attempting to reform classroom instruction. One way of doing this is to use classroom techniques that allow assessment of learning (Cross, 1990). These techniques help the teacher gather data that will help to improve teaching and learning (McKeachie, 1994). The purpose of this chapter is to explain these techniques and how nursing faculty can use them to improve teaching and learning.

Classroom Assessment

Formative evaluation is the foundation of classroom assessment. Bloom, Madaus, and Hastings (1981) describe formative evaluation as a tool useful in the process of evaluation to guide revisions and facilitate improvement of classroom instruction and student learning. By the late 1980s, Cross (1990) was advocating the use of teaching activities—classroom research—to ascertain whether students are learning and to discover the best methods for teaching. At present, these activities are called *classroom assessment techniques* (CATs) (Angelo & Cross, 1993; Halpern, 1994).

Classroom assessment "consists of small scale assessments conducted continuously in the college classroom by discipline-based teachers to determine

The author acknowledges the work of Pamela J. Cole, MA, RN, CS, in the previous edition(s) of the chapter.

what students are learning in that class" (Angelo, 1994, p. 5). Classroom assessment is (Angelo, 1994; Angelo & Cross, 1993):

1. *Learner centered*: Students actively learn, become responsible for their own learning, and critically evaluate their own learning.
2. *Teacher directed*: Teachers decide why, when, and how to include CATs in their classes.
3. *Mutually beneficial:* Teachers improve their teaching and students improve their learning with the use of CATs.
4. *Formative*: CATs help with learning, not with the evaluation or grading of student efforts.
5. *Context-specific*: Classes within different disciplines, courses, and even sections of a course develop their own personalities, and the techniques of classroom assessment may need to vary to "fit" the situation.
6. *Ongoing*: Frequent, current feedback to both the student and the teacher is an important feature in improving student learning.
7. *Rooted in good teaching practice*: Classroom assessment puts already established good teaching practices into a more systematic framework.

Thus classroom assessment provides for an assessment of learning in progress for both teachers and students in a nonthreatening environment. In addition, classroom assessment incorporates active learning strategies that facilitate learning (Astin, 1985; Halpern, 1994; McKeachie, 1994).

The term *classroom assessment* represents conceptual thinking. Techniques used for classroom assessment are called CATs. Many sources provide examples of CATs. The most comprehensive is the collection of 50 different techniques presented by Angelo and Cross (1993).

CAT Outcomes

There is an emerging body of evidence about the impact that CATs have on both faculty and students. The evidence seems to support the thinking of Angelo and Cross (Angelo, 1994; Angelo & Cross, 1993). CATs can be a valuable tool for improving student learning. However, the evidence that CATs improve student learning outcomes is mixed. Boles (1999) found that using an e-mail–designed CAT improved student learning in a data communications class. However, Cottell and Harwood (1998) did not find the same results in an accounting class. Their conclusion was that many variables affect student learning outcomes and more study of CATs is needed.

Advantages of CATs

CATs can give immediate feedback to faculty about the learning that is happening in their classrooms. As a result, midcourse classroom improvements can be made. CATs also give students feedback about their own learning. Students have a chance to make midcourse changes in their study habits.

Steadman (1998) studied the effects of using CATs in a community college setting. When using CATS, faculty found the following advantages: "ability to tune into students' voices, opportunity to engage in reflection on and systematic change of their teaching, student improvement and involvement in learning and the opportunity to join a community of other faculty committed to teaching" (Steadman, 1998, pp. 26–27). Student advantages include "increased control and voice in the classroom, students are more involved in their own learning and students benefit from improved teaching because faculty use feedback from CATs to improve instruction" (Steadman, 1998, p. 30).

Disadvantages of CATs

CATs also have disadvantages for students and faculty. They take up classroom time that is typically used for other activities, but the major disadvantage for faculty is the difficulty "in dealing with negative feedback" (Steadman, 1998, p. 27). Students also reported the use of class time as a disadvantage associated with CATs. Use of CATs means that students must be active participants in the classroom. Students who prefer to be passive participants in the classroom do not like the experience of CATs (Steadman, 1998).

Classroom Assessment Techniques

CATs are informal, formative evaluation tools and procedures used to monitor student learning. They involve immediate, continuous interaction between the student and teacher to validate, clarify, and facilitate learning. CATs can be used to assess students' attitudes, knowledge about course concepts, study habits, or even reactions to the teaching strategies used in a particular course. The three phases of developing and using CATs are planning, implementing, and responding (Angelo & Cross, 1993).

Planning CATs

During the planning phase, the teacher chooses a particular class in which to implement the CAT. The decision that formative evaluation could improve teaching and learning is based on information the instructor may have about the students' progress such as examination scores, student inability to verbalize or implement major course concepts, or frequent questions during class time.

During the second activity of the planning phase, the teacher clearly identifies the desired information to be gained by using a CAT. Most teachers have multiple goals for any one class period. These goals may come from a variety of sources, such as the overall curriculum plan, level objectives, course objectives, unit objectives, and so on. Because all of these goals cannot possibly be measured with any one CAT in a single session, the teacher should focus on one specific goal. The activity in this part of the planning phase forces the teacher to reflect on and prioritize what specifically should be assessed (Fox, 2000).

The last activity in the planning phase is identification of the specific CAT to be used. Obviously, the most important feature in the selection of a CAT is a close match between what the CAT will measure and what the teacher has previously identified as the priority goal for use of the CAT. The selected CAT should be adjusted to fit the purpose of administration or the personality of the class. For example, Angelo and Cross (1993) describe an exercise called "everyday ethical dilemmas" (p. 271). They present the exercise as a brief ethical dilemma after which the students respond to two questions. The teacher then analyzes the student answers and presents the responses to the class, which generates further discussion about the ethical situation.

In one application of this CAT, the teacher modified the exercise and used it to frame an entire class period for a graduate class in nursing administration. The reading assignment for the class period described three different theories about ethical decision making. The goal for the class period was for the students to develop a better understanding of the ethical decision-making theories. Several typical situations involving ethical decision making by nurse administrators set the stage for the analysis of the ethical decision-making theories. The situations were discussed from the perspective of each of the theories. At the conclusion of the class, students reported a better understanding of the theories and a better understanding of how they, as individuals, made their own ethical decisions.

Implementing CATs

The second phase is the actual implementation of the CAT. A CAT can be used before, during, or after a class period. The class content can be taught, with administration of the CAT following, or the CAT can be administered first to set the stage for the rest of the class period. The timing of the administration of the CAT depends on the purpose of the classroom assessment and the particular content of the class session. Examining and organizing the results of the CAT into some sort of meaningful framework is the last activity in this phase.

Responding to the CAT

Reporting the results of the CAT to the students represents the final phase of CAT administration. First, the results of the CAT that have been organized in the prior phase need to be interpreted and arranged for presentation to the students. The feedback is presented in a manner that will enhance student learning. The teacher should present results of the CAT to the students during the next scheduled class period. Some CATs involve very time-intensive interpretation and analysis. In such cases, the results of the CAT should be presented as soon as they are available. The less time it takes students to receive results, the greater will be the impact on improvement of student learning as a result of using the CAT.

The last activity in the responding phase is reflection (Angelo & Cross, 1993). The teacher evaluates the use of the CAT. Did use of the CAT accomplish the goal established during the first phase? Did implementation of the CAT occur as it was planned?

Was the outcome of use of the CAT enhanced student learning? What did the students think about the use of the CAT? What did the teacher think about the use of the CAT? Answering these questions and others posed by the teacher completes the three phases of implementing a CAT. However, this phase usually stimulates further action. Use of another CAT, repeated use of the same CAT at a later date, and even course revision are some of the future actions that may result from the evaluation.

Examples of CATs

In examples 1 and 2, formal descriptions of two CATs are given (Angelo & Cross, 1993) and implementation is described. A teacher implemented these CATs in a nursing classroom. Both of the CATs were adjusted by the teacher to best fit the personality of the class. Other examples of the use of CATs can be found in Ruland and Ahern (2007) (free write exercise and 1-minute paper) and in Davidson (2009) (clinical application of CATs).

Example 1: Implementation of the 1-Minute Paper

Implemented When. Before, during, or at the end of class

Purpose or Goal. To assess comprehension of major course concepts

Activities. On a maximum of half a page, the students answer one question, such as:
- What was the most important thing learned in class today?
- What point was most confusing for you today?

Time Involved.
- 5 minutes for administration
- 30 to 45 minutes to evaluate answers
- Variable time in the next class to clarify problem areas

Advantages.
- Little class time is used.
- Minimal time to analyze results.
- Students will think about the class and evaluate what they did or did not learn.

Disadvantage. The desired results depend heavily on asking questions in the correct way.

A variation of this 1-minute paper was used in a first-year associate degree nursing course. The goal for use of the CAT was to help students prioritize which aspects of nursing care were the most important in a variety of case scenarios.

Midsemester, at the end of a class, student groups were given scenarios to complete. Each group presented its scenario in class the following week. Immediately after each of the presentations, 2 to 3 minutes were allowed for students to write the most important point made by the presenters. Because there were 11 scenarios, there were 11 most important points selected by each student. At the conclusion of class, the sheets of most important points were collected. Students stated that they were satisfied with the class format for the day and asked to see how their most important points compared with the responses from the teacher.

During a later class session, each student was given a tally sheet that listed the most important points selected by the students and the most important points identified by the teacher. When students selected different most important points, frequencies were given. Students reported that the results sheet proved to be a good study tool.

Students performed well on the part of the examination regarding the unit taught that day. A drawback of the CAT was the time required to tally 11 most important points for 30 students. This task took approximately 6 hours to complete! Another disadvantage was that students sometimes had difficulty identifying just one most important point. Overall, however, the teacher thought the established goal was met.

Example 2: Implementation of the Self-Confidence Survey

Implemented When. Before, during, or at the end of class

Purpose or Goal. To identify areas of high and low self-confidence

Activity. Answer survey items.

Time Involved.
- 1 to 10 minutes for administration
- 5 to 30 minutes to evaluate answers
- Variable time in the next class to discuss low- and high-confidence areas

Advantages.
- Little time used to administer and analyze results
- Helps identify low- and high-confidence items
- Helps teacher prioritize what to emphasize

- Acknowledging low self-confidence may facilitate remedy of the problem.

Disadvantage. When many areas of low self-confidence are found, both students and faculty may feel depressed.

This self-confidence survey was implemented in a beginning nursing skills classroom course. The survey given to the students is provided in the box. The purpose of administering this CAT was to identify areas in which students did not feel confident and to guide the need for further instruction. Additionally, the teacher hoped students would be able to identify areas they should pursue for learning and boost their self-esteem by noting areas in which they felt confident.

This CAT was quickly prepared, students completed the form in approximately 3 minutes, and student responses were tallied in approximately 30 minutes. Results were shared with the students by using an overhead projector. Discussion ensued regarding areas of low self-confidence. For example, a clear pattern of low self-confidence was noted in the student responses to the following items: knowledge of medication action, side effects and adverse effects, and nursing considerations regarding medications. Through the resulting discussion, both the teacher and the students discovered ways to improve teaching and learning.

SUMMARY

This chapter described classroom assessment and discussed implementation of the techniques associated with classroom assessment. Classroom assessment involves frequent, ongoing assessment learning. The major purpose of classroom assessment is to enhance the processes of teaching and learning. The three phases of classroom assessment are planning, implementing, and responding.

Although the term *classroom assessment* provides the conceptual background, the term *classroom assessment techniques* describes the "how to" of implementing classroom assessment. A description of the actual implementation of two CATs is provided. CATs can be an important aid in helping both students and teachers improve student learning in the classroom.

Nursing Skills Self-Confidence Survey

This survey is to help both of us understand your level of confidence in your nursing skills. Please indicate how confident you feel about your ability to do the various items listed below. (Circle the most accurate response for each.)

Items	Self-Confidence in Your Ability			
Subcutaneous injections	None	Low	Medium	High
Intramuscular injections	None	Low	Medium	High
Hanging intravenous solutions	None	Low	Medium	High
Spiking an intravenous tubing	None	Low	Medium	High
Teaching a client breast self-examination	None	Low	Medium	High
Teaching a client testicular self-examination	None	Low	Medium	High
Administering oral medications	None	Low	Medium	High
Knowledge of medication actions	None	Low	Medium	High
Knowledge of medication side/adverse effects	None	Low	Medium	High
Knowledge of medical and nursing considerations	None	Low	Medium	High
Caring for a client postoperatively	None	Low	Medium	High
Caring for an orthopedic client	None	Low	Medium	High
Caring for a pediatric client	None	Low	Medium	High
Performing a dressing change	None	Low	Medium	High
Discharge planning/teaching	None	Low	Medium	High
Communicating with clients	None	Low	Medium	High
Communicating with staff	None	Low	Medium	High
Communicating with faculty	None	Low	Medium	High

Courtesy P. Cole, RN, MA, Ball State University College of Applied Sciences and Technology, Associate School of Nursing.

REFLECTING ON THE EVIDENCE

1. Explore the Internet for other CATs and design one for your class. Analyze the strengths and weaknesses of the technique you selected.

2. What is the current evidence about CATs? Does the evidence support the assertion that CATs improve learning outcomes?

3. What is the nature of your learners and your content? How can CATs be used to promote learning given your learners and content?

4. Focus on one course objective and design a CAT to assess achievement of that objective.

5. The following are commonly used CATS: 1-Minute Paper and Muddiest Point. Design one version of each that could be used in your classroom.

REFERENCES

Angelo, T. A. (1994). Classroom assessment: Involving faculty and students where it matters most. *Assessment Update: Progress, Trends, and Practices in Higher Education, 6*(4), 1–2, 5, 10.

Angelo, T. A., & Cross, K. A. (1993). *Classroom assessment techniques: A handbook for college teachers.* San Francisco, CA: Jossey-Bass.

Astin, A. W. (1985). Student involvement: The key to effective education. In A. W. Astin (Ed.), *Achieving educational excellence* (pp. 133–157). San Francisco, CA: Jossey-Bass.

Bloom, B. S., Madaus, G. F., & Hastings, J. T. (1981). Formative evaluation. In B. S. Bloom, G. F. Madaus, & J. T. Hastings (Eds.), *Evaluation to improve learning* (pp. 154–178). New York, NY: McGraw-Hill.

Boles, W. (1999). Classroom assessment for improved learning: A case study in using e-mail and involving students in preparing assignments. *Higher Education Research & Development, 18*(1), 145–159.

Cottell, P., & Harwood, E. (1998). Do classroom assessment techniques (CATs) improve student learning? *New Directions for Teaching and Learning, 75,* 37–46.

Cross, K. P. (1990). Teaching to improve learning. *Journal on Excellence in College Teaching, 17,* 9–22.

Curtis, M. H. (Ed.). (1985). *Integrity in the college curriculum: A report to the academic community. (Project on redefining the meaning and purpose of baccalaureate degrees).* Washington, DC: Association of American Colleges.

Davidson, J. E. (2009). Preceptor use of classroom assessment techniques to stimulate higher-order thinking in the clinical setting. *Journal of Continuing Education in Nursing, 40*(3), 139–143.

Fox, D. (2000). Classroom assessment data: Asking the right questions. *Leadership, 30*(2), 22–23.

McKeachie, W. J. (1994). Learning and cognition in the college classroom. In W. J. McKeachie (Ed.), *Teaching tips: Strategies, research, and theory for college and university teachers* (pp. 279–295). Lexington, MA: DC Heath.

Ruland, J. P., & Ahern, N. R. (2007). Transforming student perspectives through reflective writing. *Nurse Educator, 32*(2), 81–88.

Steadman, M. (1998). Using classroom assessment to change both teaching and learning. *New Directions for Teaching and Learning, 75,* 23–35.

Multicultural Education in Nursing

17

Lillian Gatlin Stokes, PhD, RN, FAAN

Natasha Flowers, PhD

Significant changes are occurring in the population demographics in the United States, with shifts occurring in both ethnic and minority groups. In 2008, the Pew Research Center (http://pewsocialtrends. org/2008/02/11/us-population-projections-2005-2050/) projected that by 2050 about 20 per cent of the population will be immigrants or their U.S.-born decedents, and that the Latino population will comprise 29% of the populations. These changes are reflected in nursing schools as they attempt to recruit, enroll, and retain a student body reflective of the community in which the graduates will practice. Although the demographics of minority populations (white, non-Hispanic) fluctuates with periods of growth and decline (National League for Nursing, 2006), the numbers remain significant. Furthermore, diversity is noted in gender, age, culture, learning styles, and sexual orientation.

The number of students whose second language is English is also increasing in nursing programs. In 2005 Asian nursing students were the largest group of English Language Learners (ELL) students enrolled in all combined basic registered nurse programs (5.6%) and highest in all baccalaureate programs (6%) (National League for Nursing, 2006). Increasingly, the literature is reporting the need to increase enrollment of students with disabilities because of the potential of enriching the profession (Marks, 2007). The nature of a global environment has implications for multicultural education as well. These increases in the diversity of the population and of nursing students have implications for teaching and learning in nursing. Faculty must develop curricula to accommodate diversity by choosing appropriate instructional materials, applying principles of multicultural education, and using teaching strategies to accommodate inclusivity in the classroom. Faculty must

also acquire the necessary knowledge, skills, and attitudes that will help to facilitate inclusive teaching as well as help students' development of those skills needed for cultural competence so that patients will receive appropriate care. This chapter provides information about the theoretical foundations of multicultural education, recommends changes in course and curriculum development, offers suggestions for multicultural teaching and learning, and gives examples of instructional strategies and approaches essential to addressing diversity in the classroom. This chapter also includes information about useful strategies to facilitate the development of cultural competence in students.

Multicultural Teaching and Learning

Components of Multicultural Education

Multicultural education shares the same premise of addressing student learning outcomes and success as cultural competence does in addressing health disparities. Table 17-1 describes the differences between these two concepts. Multicultural education has challenged educators and educational administrators to consider equality and inclusion for the benefit of all students. The father of multicultural education, James A. Banks, defines it as "an idea, an educational reform movement, and a process whose major goal is to change the structure of educational institutions so that male and female students, exceptional students, and students who are members of diverse racial, ethnic, language, and cultural groups will have an equal chance to achieve academically in school" (Banks & Banks, 2004, p. 32). With this three-pronged notion of multicultural education, Banks and Banks (2004) provide a wide lens for

TABLE 17-1 Multicultural Teaching and Teaching for Cultural Competence

	Multicultural Teaching	Teaching for Cultural Competence
Focus	Creating curriculum and using instructional strategies and materials to support diverse students (e.g., equity)	Assisting students to learn about their own values, beliefs, and attitudes and those of individuals from other cultural backgrounds
Process	Developmental, a continuum	Developmental, a continuum
Knowledge Assessment	Takes cultural background and attitudes, learning styles, biases, prejudices, and needs into account in planning for teaching and learning	Takes cultural background, attitudes, values, and beliefs into account to promote cultural understanding
Learning Environment	Promotes respect for and among all students	Promotes understanding and respect for all human variations
	Acknowledges alternative, non-Western perspectives to engaging diverse students	Acknowledges alternative approaches; heterogeneity within and between cultural groups
Curriculum	Focuses on learning for diverse students; equity pedagogy	Focuses on varied aspects of culture in relation to patient care
	Ensures instructional materials are free of bias; facilitates use of extracurricular activities to assist student learning	Ensures inclusion of content about various cultures
Instruction	Allows student more responsibility and choices for learning	Promotes understanding, appreciation, and respect among groups
	Uses multiple ways of conveying information to facilitate student understanding	Uses multiple strategies and approaches to facilitate knowledge acquisition
Teaching Strategies	Groups, instructional media, games, journals, ethnographies, guest speakers, panels, role play, textbooks, simulations, articles, discussion, reflection	Role play, games, vignettes, case studies and groups, media, popular books, visits to museums and other community settings, panels, interviews, storytelling, experiential immersion, exchange experiences, service learning, ethnographies, workshops, educational programming, engagement
Assessing Progress	Observe student engagement Curriculum and program review Course evaluation Student evaluation of course and instruction	Measurement of knowledge of cultural concepts (e.g., cultural awareness and cultural sensitivity, cultural competence), course evaluation, student evaluation of extent of perceived cultural competence
Evaluation	Faculty and student self-evaluation Peer evaluation of faculty; evidence of inclusive teaching External review of curriculum for multicultural education Student and alumni review of curriculum and instruction	Testing (multiple choice), writing, role playing discussions, simulation, abilities to provide appropriate cultural care

any educator or educational administrator to understand the critical need to situate the student at the core of any inclusive, engaging learning situation.

In an effort to bring critical attention and solutions to "ideological resistance, lack of teacher knowledge of ethnic groups, and the heavy reliance of teachers on textbooks" (Banks & Banks, 1993, p. 212), Banks outlined and widely shared his Levels of Integration of Multicultural Content. Although Banks accepted that the levels could be mixed and blended in varied teaching situations, his model clearly serves as a four-level developmental approach: (1) contributions, (2) additive, (3) transformative, and (4) social action. These levels range from the initial integration of cultural artifacts and mainstream heroes of particular ethnic groups in the contributions level to the social action level where "students make decisions on important social issues and take actions to help solve them" (Banks & Banks, 1993, p. 199). Banks' Levels of Integration represent one approach to content transformation and echoes the historic battle for ethnic studies that began in the late 1960s and early 1970s when higher education began questioning and embracing the need for diverse cultural content in colleges and universities (Duarte & Smith, 2000).

In addition to his developmental model, Banks (2007) outlined what he called the five dimensions of multicultural education. These dimensions include content integration, knowledge construction, equity pedagogy, prejudice reduction, and empowering school culture and social structure. While not developmental, these five critical components of multicultural education emphasize planning and action steps in empowering cultural groups in the classroom setting.

Theoretical Frameworks

Higher education has benefited from theorists such as Banks as they began to familiarize prospective and current teachers in the K through 12 educational system and slowly hold them accountable for the retention of the growing diversity among college students. Beyond the teacher education programs, notions of multicultural education can be cited in other professional programs such as business, social work, and (not surprisingly) medicine and health sciences. Marchesani and Adams (1992) designed the framework Four Dynamics of Multicultural Teaching to shape faculty development in this area. Current faculty development scholars such as Stanley, Saunders, and Hart (2005) highlight this four-dimensional framework as a step toward faculty reflection and attention to the needs of students from diverse backgrounds. More specifically, Stanley and other colleagues suggest examining the implicit messages embedded within classroom norms and the explicit messages that are found in the curriculum (Stanley et al., 2005). Along with reflection on curriculum and instruction, the Four Dynamics of Multicultural Teaching (Marchesani & Adams, 1992) emphasize faculty understanding of their own biases as well as their students' beliefs and biases. By doing this, faculty

begin to transform their courses to better support the diversity that exists within the classroom and the course content.

To reach multiple disciplines with the same goal to support all learners, special education scholars Margie Kitano and Ann Morey created a resource for academics in higher education (Morey & Kitano, 1997). In addition to gathering the practice and wisdom of professors in areas such as nursing, economics, biology, English as a new language, and mathematics, Kitano developed the Paradigm for Multicultural Course Transformation (Morey & Kitano, 1997). Seemingly untested by the scholars in the faculty development field, this theory effectively charts the benefits of understanding the principles of learning and multicultural education as the first step to multicultural course transformation. Among the three levels Kitano proposes, the third and final transformed level is ideally where students are learning from the nondominant or non-Western perspectives, which are treated as part of the content of the course, and students reflect on their own learning (and not just the letter grade or point). Also, in a transformed curriculum the culture of the classroom is open to dialogue where there is a "challenging of biased views and sharing of diverse perspectives while respecting rules established for group process" (Morey & Kitano, 1997, p. 24). It is important to note that Kitano structures a paradigm that includes more than just a snapshot of what happens in the exclusive, inclusive, and transformed levels. Faculty must consider the four major course components: content, instructional strategies, assessment of student knowledge, and classroom dynamics. Therefore a thorough course analysis is assumed to be a significant component of multicultural course transformation.

Within a thorough course analysis, Morey and Kitano (1997) propose that the multicultural goals help determine the level of course change and the course elements requiring modification. The modification itself can present in various ways. A first step is to identify the expected outcomes, such as what is expected to be achieved. For example, after articulating that one goal for a course is to increase knowledge of bias and ethnocentrism as it relates to the study of various cultural groups, a faculty member may determine that the course's content includes various examples of cultural groups. However, the course may not facilitate opportunities for open and equitable exchanges of ideas and values. Therefore the transformative work may begin in the area of instruction for classroom as well as clinical practice.

Research on Multicultural Education

The ongoing dialogue about multicultural education in higher education does include outcomes from curricular reform and instructional practices. Major studies from 2000 to the present significantly outline the benefits of diversity. In 2000 three research studies on diversity in college classrooms by the American Council on Education and American Association of University Professors rejuvenated this dialogue and pointed to particular challenges and benefits to diversifying the curriculum. The findings are based on (1) the analyses of data from more than 570 faculty members using the Faculty Classroom Diversity Questionnaire, (2) analyses of data from a similar survey of 81 faculty members at one college in the Midwest, and (3) an in-depth, qualitative multiple case study of three interactive multiracial and multiethnic classrooms at a university in the eastern United States. The use of case studies by both faculty members and students revealed that the perspectives of racially and ethnically diverse students generated more complex thinking among all students. In addition, students also shared that classroom diversity is important in subjects such as math, science, and accounting because "biases can be challenged and exposed" (American Council on Education and American Association of University Professors, 2000, p. 7). When asked to rate their comfort level in teaching racially and ethnically diverse classes, 86% of faculty members responded with 4 or 5 on a scale of 1 (not comfortable) to 5 (very comfortable). Although 71% indicated that they felt well prepared to teach in such a setting, only a small portion of this group admitted to initiating discussions of race in class (36%) or assigning students to diverse groups (33%). Even with a sense of preparedness, faculty did not report innovative, interactive strategies to make the most of their diverse classes. These data beg the question of faculty involvement in diversifying the curriculum, which was carefully investigated in Helton's (2000) quantitative research study and "involved" faculty who had participated in the Association of American Colleges and Universities' initiative, American Commitments: Diversity,

Democracy, and Liberal Learning. Among the 63% who responded to the questionnaire, 92% of the faculty identified the following items as "somewhat" or "extensive" in motivating their participation in diversity initiatives:

- Students who represent racial, gender, or sexual diversity need to see themselves in the curriculum.
- Pursuit of the whole truth requires expansion and inclusion of other points of view.
- The desire to add new research findings and knowledge to courses and programs.
- Participating in diversity initiatives is the morally or ethically compelling thing to do.
- I feel a bond with students of marginalized groups.
- Students who represent racial, gender, or sexual diversity need to see themselves in the curriculum.
- Wanting to meet the learning needs of all of my students.
- I want to add new research findings and knowledge to my courses and programs.
- Diversity is an intellectually stimulating, new, and challenging arena for me.

The five perceived benefits from faculty involvement in this study were intellectual challenge (95%), teaching satisfaction (89%), opportunity to influence social change (88%), teaching effectiveness (85%), and student interaction (84%) (Helton, 2000).

Studies that focused on students shared positive findings. In Chang's (2002) study, 112 undergraduates who were completing a diversity course reported less prejudice in comparison to 85 students who had just started taking the course. Smith, Parr, Woods, Bauer, and Abraham (2010) found that roughly three courses that dealt with globalization, inequities, race, class, and gender issues affected 156 graduates' perceptions of multicultural competence and volunteer service. Increased levels of self-reported multicultural competence positively correlated with undergraduate courses with diversity-related content. Findings such as these point to the benefits of diversity courses and the inclusion of multicultural content in the curriculum.

The Curriculum and Multicultural Education

One of the first ways to initiate a multicultural education is to review the curriculum for its responsiveness to student diversity. Different approaches have been identified. For example, Morey and Kitano (1997) identified three levels of change in transforming any course: (1) exclusive, (2) inclusive, and (3) transformed. The *exclusive* level encompasses traditional and mainstream experiences and perspectives. When information is presented in a didactic manner, there is limited discussion and knowledge acquisition is assessed through written examinations. An *inclusive* level involves the addition of alternative perspectives to traditional views. There is support for the use of a variety of methods of teaching to facilitate active learning. To provide rich experiences for students, the emphasis should be placed on the transformed curriculum. In a *transformed* curriculum, the structure is changed to facilitate students to view concepts, issues, and content from a variety of ethnic cultural perspectives (Byrne, Weddle, Davis, & McGinnis, 2003). The desired outcome is significant change—not so much in what is taught, but in how it is taught (Morey & Kitano, 1997).

A comparative review of the two models, Morey and Kitano (1997) and Banks (2006), reveals components that are useful for multicultural education. Emphasis in the former model is on transformation and overall structural changes. The usefulness of the latter model is its distinct identification of dimensions that can serve as a template for changes in curriculum. The intention of the dimensions in the framework affords opportunities to build on previous dimensions as students progress through the nursing program (Bagnardi, Bryant, & Colin, 2009). These are but two examples. Faculty can explore additional frameworks with the goal of an ultimate outcome of inclusion and integration of multicultural content into the curriculum, thus facilitating multicultural education.

Integrating Multicultural Content into the Curriculum

Diverse cultural content must be integrated throughout the curriculum. The multicultural model designed by Banks (2004, 2006) is described as a model that can be adapted to all levels of the curriculum. Bagnardi et al. (2009) describe an experience of integrating Banks' model throughout an undergraduate curriculum. Students should learn to apply various nondominant perspectives (Morey & Kitano, 1997). As Banks suggested, instructors must move beyond the initial level of integrating cultural artifacts such

as names and holidays to an integrative level where students obtain more substantive information about cultural groups (Banks & Banks, 1993, 2004). Educators should make concerted efforts to exhibit attitudes of positive portrayal of diversity and indicate that diversity is valued. Exposing students to various cultural norms, health beliefs, and practices is a feasible first step in diversifying the curriculum. Underwood (2006) used an inquiry approach to facilitate enhanced knowledge and sensitivity related to culture and health. A student assignment was to write three questions about an ethnic group of the student's choice. The themes that emerged from these questions were used to structure the course. Also, students should have assignments that provide opportunities for them to reflect on all aspects of culture: language, communication patterns, family relationships, religion, spirituality, and ethnicities (e.g., Native Americans, Hispanics, Asian Americans, African Americans, Arab Americans). Students should specifically have access to information about groups that are dominant within the areas in which they learn and practice their clinical skills. The content should excite and motivate students to actively facilitate change in communities. The latter represents applications of the social action element previously described.

Because of the diversity of nursing curricula and the variation in levels in course offerings within programs of nursing, no attempt will be made to specifically foster one particular model. Rather, the approach taken will be to share a variety of strategies and approaches that can be helpful as faculty work to infuse multicultural content into teaching and learning. Attention should be drawn to multiple approaches and resources that can facilitate movement beyond basic levels of integration. Immersion experiences have been reported to be beneficial and an approach that can be used to integrate content.

Immersion experiences can occur in several ways. One is through the use of ethnographies. *Ethnography* refers to a written presentation of qualitative descriptions of human social information based on fieldwork. Brennan and Schulze (2004) engaged students in reading an ethnography. The activity was followed by a written assignment of an analysis of the reading. Presentations and discussions of the analysis were made in groups. Results of the ethnographic analyses indicated that students were immersed in the culture.

Group discussion of the analyses was beneficial in providing a multicultural experience for all participants. Experiences can also occur through spending time and engaging with specific cultural groups within the United States (e.g., special populations) and abroad. Immersion is useful not only for teaching and learning, but to facilitate the development of cultural competence as well.

Caffrey, Neander, Markle, and Stewart (2005) conducted a study to evaluate the effect of integrating cultural content in an undergraduate curriculum on students' self-perceived cultural competence and to determine whether a 5-week clinical immersion in international nursing had additional effects on students' self-perceived cultural competence. The results of the study revealed a larger gain of self-perceived cultural competence for students who engaged in the immersion experience.

Inclusive Teaching: Strategies and Approaches

To facilitate inclusivity, faculty should consult resources that are focused on teaching and learning in classroom environments. In *Multicultural Teaching in the University*, Schoem, Frankel, Zuniga, and Lewis (1995) provide specific information related to a variety of teaching–learning strategies. There are excellent texts that provide tips and a variety of ways in which the strategies can be implemented. From these, faculty can acquire information about how to teach students about different cultures. Ukoha (2004) calls for the acquisition of theoretical bases for these. Morrison, Sullivan, Murray, and Jolly (1999) designed an instrument to address the

evidence base of instructional strategies. Faculty could use these or similar designs to evaluate their instructional effectiveness. Refer to Table 17-2 for a list of online resources for multicultural education (and cultural competence).

As attention is given to making curricular and content changes, opportunities must also be provided for clinical practice and engagement so that knowledge is reinforced, skills are developed, and changes occur in attitudes. In designing instruction for multicultural teaching and learning, a variety of instructional methods and materials must be used to support active teaching and learning. In other words, in the classroom faculty must move from *lectures* to *activity* and *variety*, such as the use of case studies, role play, games, drama, films, movies, panels; students' engagement in interviews, assigned readings, writing specific papers, discussions questions; and involvement in real-life experiences. One experience can be service learning with agencies that service culturally diverse patients (O'Grady, 2000) or those that have a specific patient population (see also Chapter 12). The benefits of such experiences are multifaceted (Hunt, 2007). Immersion experiences in specific areas can also serve to engage students. Closely aligned with engagement experiences, attention must also be given to instructional strategies that are used in the classroom, in clinical practice, and online.

Classroom

In the classroom, learning activities should be planned to facilitate knowledge acquisition and interaction and collaboration of diverse groups of students, including age, race, ethnicity, and gender,

TABLE 17-2 Online Resources for Multicultural Education and Cultural Competence	
http://www.diversityweb.org	Association of American Colleges and Universities provides research, classroom practice, and university diversity reform information
http://edchange.org	Resources for diversity assessment, professional development, and research
http://www.tcns.org	Transcultural Nursing Society website with access to TCN certification, professional journal, and membership
http://www.hrsa.gov/culturalcompetence/	U.S. Department of Health and Human Services provides assessment tools, research, and toolkits for the cultural competence of health care providers
http://ctl.iupui.edu/TSSS_modules/inclusive/introduction/1.htm	The Center for Teaching and Learning at Indiana University–Purdue University Indianapolis offers modules to support multicultural teaching and learning in higher education
http://www1.umn.edu/ohr/teachlearn/	The Center for Teaching and Learning at University of Minnesota offers resources for classroom teaching and for supporting non-native speakers of English

depending on the makeup of the class. Each of these variations brings different experiences and perspectives. Systems can be developed to ensure that students have opportunities to engage in learning activities with peers from different racial and ethnic groups, peers with age variations, and peers who are both male and female. In addition to student interaction, a diverse mix of experts from the community can be used for classroom activities as appropriate. These individuals, experts in their own right, are often willing to be involved in the education of students. Faculty should take advantage of the willingness of these individuals and use them to enhance inclusivity.

Morey and Kitano (1997) suggest that faculty create learning activities to promote reflection among students. The opportunities are many. Faculty can engage students by designing written assignments, such as journaling logs or learning diaries (Anderson, 2004; Billings, 2006; Craft, 2005) and personal letters written by and for the student, which can be a precursor to reflection papers. Letters can have a dual purpose of initially addressing personal fears, feelings, assumptions, and expectations about a planned experience or about different racial and ethnic or age groups, and later reflecting on the identified written content in preparation for writing a major paper. The connecting link between the initial letter and the reflection could be an experience such as service learning. Students can read the letters after the experience and reflect on the initial letter in terms of similarities to and differences from their previous thoughts, feelings, and assumptions, thus providing an avenue for deeper reflection, meanings, and considerable learning. The letter strategy, used for 5 years in a course for beginning students, resulted in noted improvement in the quality and specificity of papers and enhanced learning as identified by students (Stokes, Linde, & Zimmerman, 2008). Immersion and service-learning experiences (see Chapter 12) afford opportunities for reflection as well. Activities relating to cultural diversity can also be resources for framing instructional strategies (Eliason & Macy, 1992).

Clinical Practice

Not only should emphasis be placed on inclusive teaching (and learning) in classroom settings but in *clinical practice settings* as well (Millon-Underwood, 1992). Millon-Underwood (1992) suggests that

experiences are planned to align with the nature of the community and that faculty make efforts to ensure that one in every five patients selected for student clinical learning experiences is from a diverse cultural group. To assure the reality of this, systems such as clinical experience checklists or databases can be established for students and faculty to monitor and track the gender, age, racial and ethnic makeup, and socioeconomic status of patients assigned for care. This system and the rationale for its use should be shared with students.

Preparation for clinical practice is also changing. Learning labs have long been the primary method used for students to acquire the necessary skills to facilitate safe practice. Mannequins continue to be used, but have become more sophisticated and technology driven. Gender-specific mannequins have not been uncommon, but the color of these has reflected the majority population. Mannequins and specific attachments now depict people of color to complement ethnic and racial diversity. Faculty should continue to support these items for use in practice learning environments.

With or without challenges being faced with the use of conventional clinical sites, faculty can be creative in exposing students to and engaging students with other cultural heritages. There are benefits that can be acquired from doing so. By visiting urban areas or specific cultural districts, opportunities can be provided for students to view areas of the community that are different from their own. For example, grocery stores, storefronts, houses of worship, health clinics, and businesses are among the destinations. Often manufacturing plants and waste sites may be close to housing communities of the underserved. Students can be directed to books, movies, and stage plays that depict an image of life as experienced by varied cultures. To make these worthwhile experiences, faculty can assist students in developing focus points that can direct their observations, conversations, and discussions before and following the experience.

Online Courses

The use of the online technology can be an avenue for promoting multicultural education. Merryfield (2001) reported results of an online interaction experience indicating that teachers were open, frank, expansive, curious, and confessional in their willingness to share and discuss certain issues and that interaction patterns were more equitable and cross-cultural than the campus-based course. This methodology also has the potential for linking classrooms for the purpose of cultural exchanges, for example, through the use of virtual experiences. Additionally, faculty teaching online courses can facilitate students' awareness of their own beliefs and those of others by posing questions that require students to reflect on their values, beliefs, or culture and contrast them with those of other members in the class (Flowers, 2002). Online surveys and journals are two strategies for prompting these discussions.

Educators must be sensitive to inclusive teaching in online courses as well. An initial challenge is that, with online courses, visual cues as to gender and race of the student and faculty are absent. Faculty can seek to overcome this by establishing a practice of requesting that students post their photos and of faculty doing likewise. Clear norms and netiquette (network etiquette) must be established at the outset of the course to indicate key principles, such as respect for diversity.

Assessing Instructional Resources

As educators choose instructional resources to support teaching and learning, they must make concerted efforts to eliminate bias in their selections. This includes biases in relation to gender, age, race, ethnicity, language, sexual orientation, socio-economics, and abilities. Sadker and Sadker (1994) identified six categories of bias in instructional materials: invisibility or omission, stereotyping, imbalance and selectivity, unreality, fragmentation and isolation, and linguistic bias. Faculty should be cognizant of these categories and direct actions to select material with limited and ideally no bias. For short-term benefits, it may also mean that a variety of materials, articles, and media be used to make up for deficits of limited information and examples in textbooks. Instructors should examine their course materials in terms of the identified deficits and direct efforts to diminish them. For example, Byrne (2001) found that fundamental nursing textbooks omitted the common health problems faced by African Americans. When this is the case, educators must use supplemental content to fill the gaps. Additionally, special documentation such as books and web resources that include photos or illustrations may not include adequate racial,

ethnic, or gender representation. To facilitate the availability of more unbiased instructional materials, evaluation and feedback should be provided to authors, with suggestions to include content that supports a transformed curriculum. The use of a guide similar to the one developed by Byrne et al. (2003) can be useful in the assessment of instructional materials as well as in helping faculty evaluate and create new products.

Faculty should also examine teacher-made course materials for inclusion, exclusion, and bias. For example, course syllabi, handouts, worksheets, and clinical evaluation tools may inadvertently be written with culture or gender bias. Teacher-made tests are also a source of multicultural bias and the faculty should review these tests to eliminate references to the nurse as "she," to remove any cultural stereotyping, to avoid the use of American slang, and to use language that would be understood by all students in order to test fairly (Ukoha, 2004). Teacher-made tests should also be designed to evaluate students' ability to apply concepts of cultural competence.

Classroom Dynamics and Creating Inclusive Learning Environments

Learners within nursing classrooms are becoming more diverse. The composition may include Euro-Americans (the majority), nontraditional students (e.g., older adults), underrepresented students (e.g., African Americans, Asian Americans, Latinos, Native Americans, Arab Americans), males, international students, and students with differences in sexual orientation, abilities, and life experiences. Such a mixture can provide a rich learning environment. Educators must capitalize on this richness by making concerted efforts toward equity in the learning environments. For example, by listening to the voices of diverse and nontraditional students as they share varied perspectives about their culture, and by engaging other students in dialogue, the worth of these shared messages can be realized.

Exemplars of Equity in Teaching

Three prerequisites have been identified to equity in teaching students: attitude, personal perspective, and knowledge (Lou, 1994). The *attitudinal perspective* relates to an openness to make improvement in classroom practices. Inherent in such openness is to divorce one's teaching from traditional modes to more innovative and engaging modes of instruction. A common example is to move from lecture or one mode of teaching to multiple modes of teaching. Nelson (1996) contends that traditionally taught college courses are biased against nontraditional students and that "neutral teaching practices function to keep courses less accessible to students from nontraditional backgrounds" (p. 165). If the goal is for all students to excel, then it is imperative that strategies be used that are favorable for all.

Another essential prerequisite to teaching students equally is for the teacher to gain an understanding of his or her own *cultural perspective* that might be brought into the classroom. This perspective may include biases, stereotypes, and prejudices. Concerted efforts must be made to assess and reflect on these in order to gain understanding of how they may affect the teaching of diverse students.

A third requirement is for educators to be *knowledgeable* about learning styles or modes of learning of students (see Chapter 2). The implication here is to provide a variety of learning activities that appeal to varying styles of learning, and for students to understand how their own learning style preferences affect their learning. In addition, teachers should have working knowledge of students' cultures and, for some students, their marginalizing experiences and the impact of these on engagement and classroom interactions.

Subconscious Biases

Promoting equity in teaching also means that teachers are aware of subconscious biases and differential treatment (Lou, 1994). Two common examples are gender bias and reactions to students for whom English is not their first language.

Research on *gender bias* in classrooms has supported tendencies for teachers to interact with one gender more than another (Salter, 2004). Specifically in classrooms with predominantly majority students, the reported tendency is for teachers to interact with white male students more than they interact with women and men of color. For example, the latter groups are less likely to be called on. With nursing being a predominately female profession, a valid

assumption could be that nurse educators call more frequently on female students than on the male students in the class. With this awareness, teachers should make concerted efforts to provide equal treatment by engaging all students. This includes the quiet student who speaks up infrequently. Deliberate efforts can be taken to accomplish this by devising a system for engaging students regardless of gender or ethnicity. Such efforts will facilitate inclusion of every student in the classroom at some point.

With increasing numbers of male students in nursing programs, it is essential to refrain from using gender-oriented language. One key is to use gender-neutral statements and to avoid words that would exclude male students, for example, the use of gender-specific terms such as *her* and *she*. Depending on the context of the point, rather than "he or she experienced" it is more appropriate to say "the student experienced." Faculty must be cognizant of gender dynamics as well, for example, those students (male or female) who tend to dominate discussions. Create ways to involve all students. In a class with diverse students, faculty should be attentive to responses that may be perceived as dismissed and make efforts to be equitable in responses to questions or comments.

Microaggressions

Educators should have some beginning knowledge of the concept of microaggression. Microaggressions, defined by Sue et al. (2007) as "brief and commonplace verbal, behavioral, or environmental indignities, whether intentional or unintentional, that communicate hostile, derogatory, or negative racial slights or insults toward people of color" (p. 271), are reported to be common. In addition to race, they are reported to be perpetuated on the basis of gender, sexual orientation, and ability status. Refer to Table 17-3. The impact of continuing microaggressions on exclusion of the person of difference is real. Individuals experiencing these microaggressions have expressed feelings of lessened self-confidence and productivity (Mays, 2009). The implication is for educators to think about wording so as to eliminate statements that might be perceived as microaggressions. Educators must avail themselves of educational opportunities to attain the latest information and findings relating to inclusivity and equity in classrooms.

TABLE 17-3 Examples of Microaggressions

Culture and Learning	Statement or Behavior	Perceived Meaning of Statement
Ethnicity and Race	When I look at you, I don't see color.	Denial of individual's racial and ethnic experiences.
	There is only one race: the human race.	Denial of individual's ethnic and cultural being.
	Being ignored in the classroom.	Students from certain cultural groups are not valued.
Gender	Anyone can succeed, man or woman, if he or she works hard.	No acknowledgement of unfair benefits because of gender.
Ability	You are so articulate. You are a credit to your race and community.	People of color may perceive this statement as negative and demeaning rather than positive and uplifting.

Teaching International Students and English Language Learners

With an increase in admission of international students and others to nursing programs, the call is for faculty to be attentive to the behaviors and personal responses of these students (Xu & Davidhizar, 2005). There are reports of unconscious differential treatment in interactions with ELL students. Behaviors such as frowns, furrowed brows, and intense concentration have been reported. These may not be deliberate behaviors. Rather, their use may be related to reasons of trying to capture what is being voiced by the student. Nonetheless, these behaviors may have an impact on students' future participation in discussions and classroom interactions. They may refrain from participation or not respond to or ask questions because of the panicky feelings they may experience at having to speak in class.

Managing the Inclusive Classroom: Cultural Perspectives

The behaviors that are exhibited by students in the classroom may be related to culture. For example, there is a tendency for some students, because of their culture, to be passive (Morey & Kitano, 1997). Therefore these cultural perspectives must be considered by faculty. It is especially important for faculty to have an awareness of the adaptations that may be needed. Underrepresented students may feel isolated and uncomfortable in environments where they are among the minority. Faculty must be aware of the potential for these feelings and actions and strive to

enhance recognition of self-worth, as well as be sensitive to thoughts of isolation. In some cultures the teacher is viewed as holding a superior position in a hierarchy. This hierarchical perspective can affect the manner in which students respond to classroom activities. In Asian cultures the teacher is regarded as an authority who disseminates information. As a result, Asian students may passively listen and take for granted everything the teacher says without asking questions. In the United States students are expected to be active learners, to participate in group activities, to ask questions, and to openly express thoughts (Kataoka-Yahiro & Abriam-Yago, 1997). The responses of Asian students to classroom activities such as group exercises may not be highly regarded because the "authoritative figure" is not primary and center. Faculty can employ approaches to help these students understand cultural differences. One approach is to discuss the cultural differences in classroom dynamics in the United States in comparison with their own cultures.

Efforts can be made to address some of these differences by incorporating strategies to improve linguistic competence such as the use of assignments for reading with a study guide, for writing (including brief written assignments, accepting paper drafts, and ongoing writing), and for speaking and listening (Guttman, 2004). Faculty must also be knowledgeable about campus and community as referral resources that can be useful for assignments such as these.

Faculty can also devise strategies to facilitate active engagement in classrooms. For example, to enhance open communication in the classroom, start by using developmental approaches. Lou (1994) reports about the strategy of using structured group exercises and supporting small group involvement in developmental ways—for example, by permitting students to present written assignments verbally in small groups and progressing to the point at which the fear of participating in discussions is overcome. Games are another medium used to engage students and encourage participation.

The need to master the English language may also impede ELL students' participation in group and open discussion for fear of saying the wrong thing. Tucker-Allen (1989) contends that faculty must incorporate sensitive and innovative strategies into their teaching. Attention to techniques that are used for questioning may be useful—for example, asking "why" and "how" questions and encouraging and requesting students to "take risks" at no cost and to explore "possibilities." Questions framed in an open manner tend to be less intimidating than those that give the impression that only one answer is possible. Extending wait time for answers is also helpful; 10 to 12 seconds is acceptable. Especially for international students, this provides an opportunity for them to formulate and translate their thoughts from their native language to English. An additional way to engage students is to have an assignment that requires them to write a question related to the assignment each week and ask them to read the question in class. This activity has a high potential for opening dialogue, decreasing shyness, and enhancing community building with the class.

Faculty should also encourage ELL students to participate in student groups that reflect diversity (Doordan & Abriam-Yago, 1996). Peer support groups involving students of similar cultures help to eliminate feelings of isolation. Involvement of ELL students in group situations with diverse students can also be beneficial in that this facilitates development of communication and interpersonal skills (Kataoka-Yahiro & Abriam-Yago, 1997). Nonetheless, in planning group activities the teacher should sometimes intentionally divide students into groups and make selections of group members.

Furthermore, faculty must be willing to address students' affective issues that have an impact on their feelings about English. According to Halic, Greenburg, and Paulus (2009), graduate students from various countries outside the United States who participated in a phenomenological study about their language identity expressed major concerns about how faculty and peers perceived them as they developed a stronger grasp of the English language. Also, these students shared their own notions of English as a barrier and a "channel of access" given their interactions in classroom settings (Halic et al., 2009, p. 82).

Increasingly, support is being provided for the admission of students with disabilities to nursing programs. Special accommodations may be needed and faculty should be aware of available services, policies, and requirements for those accommodations.

Faculty (and students with disabilities) should be aware of available services. These services are varied and may range from special equipment to sign language interpreters, note takers, and audiotaped books (Maheady, 2003). Specific documentation from a health care professional is required and, according to the Americans with Disabilities Act (1990), such documentation mandates that all prescriptions are followed. Books focusing on success stories are available to enhance the understanding of nursing students with disabilities (Maheady, 2003; Serdans, 2002), and special equipment and technology are available for use by these students.

Environmental Support

The admission of diverse populations of students directly affects factors such as the learning environment of the educational unit (campus-wide and the school of nursing), the social environment, and recruitment (and retention). Therefore concerted efforts must be made to direct interventions that will have positive effects for all students. Refer to Table 17-4. Since it is not uncommon in informal settings for students to share personal feelings of exclusion or isolation, opportunities should provide for informal conversations outside of the classroom. The use of "gatherings" as a support strategy has been reported by ELL students, as well as other underrepresented students, to be beneficial (Stokes, 2003). This support initiative provides a forum for students to openly discuss issues and concerns in a supportive nonacademic environment. A resulting outcome can be increased confidence in abilities as well as facilitated and more frequent participation

TABLE 17-4 Environmental Support for Inclusion

Advertising Materials	Should be recruitment and diversity friendly; brochures, leaflets, pamphlets, bulletins, and websites should reflect diversity. Advertisement materials are frequently examined as students (family) and faculty are searching for a school or seeking employment.
Campus and Nursing Programs	Should promote services that are needed by diverse populations. Academic and student services should be welcoming and reflect the potential population for the campus or school.
	Variety of services including mentors and peer tutors. Writing centers, inviting study areas, libraries, equipment with representative population holdings.
	Gender-neutral and culturally appropriate language in policies.
	Recruitment and retention: faculty role models, diverse staff and student populations (including males). Academic services inclusive of mentors and peer tutors.
Classroom	Should be designed for multipurpose use and diverse ways of learning; movable tables, chairs, and desks are useful for peer-to-peer interaction and small group work.
Social Environment	Events planned to bring students of diverse populations together for socialization and learning. Bringing prominent and renowned speakers from a variety of ethnic groups and special program offerings.

in informal activities and in more formal classroom activities, including discussions.

Facilitating the Development of Cultural Competence in Students

The Sullivan Commission (2004) clearly points out the need for increasing diverse representation in the health care workforce. The increasing diversity of the American population provides a primary reason for students to understand their own culture and that of others. The American Nurses Association, National League for Nursing, and American Association of Colleges of Nursing continue to support the educational needs of faculty and students. Each has standards for increasing cultural competence of those who provide care. Preparing a culturally competent graduate is one goal of all nursing programs. To facilitate accomplishments of this goal, instruction and activities should be directed toward the meanings, development of cultural confidence, attributes, strategies, resources, and evaluation.

Definitions of Cultural Competence

Cultural competence has been discussed in the literature since the early 1980s. Over the past 2 decades, the concept has increasingly appeared in the literature from perspectives such as cultural awareness and cultural sensitivity. Continued work related to cultural competence reveals that *cultural awareness* and *cultural sensitivity* are distinct terms, and that they are indeed different than *cultural competence*. A review of the literature reveals multiple definitions of cultural competence. With these definitions, increasing attempts are being made to bring clarity to the concept (Burchum, 2002; Lister, 1999).

Among definitions of cultural competence are the skill of using multiple cultural lenses (Nunez, 2000) and the capacity to function effectively as an individual and an organization within the context of the cultural beliefs, behaviors, and needs presented by consumers in their communities. Purnell and Paulanka (2008) defined cultural competence as developing an awareness of one's own existence, thoughts, and environments without letting it influence others from different backgrounds; demonstrating awareness and understanding of the patient's cultural background; respecting and accepting cultural differences and similarities; and providing congruent care by adapting it to the patient's cultural health care beliefs, values, and norms. Campinha-Bacote, Yahie, and Langenkamp (1996) defined cultural competence as "a process, not an end point, in which the nurse continuously strives to achieve the ability to effectively work within the cultural context of an individual, family, or community from a diverse cultural and ethnic background" (pp. 1–2). In addition to these definitions, cultural competence has been described on a continuum (National

Alliance for Hispanic Health, 2001; Zimmerman, 2003). Each of these provides a beginning point for faculty as they direct efforts to facilitate cultural competence understanding among students.

These presentations of cultural competence not only define the concept, but also provide descriptions of actions, behaviors, and outcomes. These descriptions are powerful in facilitating clarity in relation to outcomes. For example, statements such as capacity to function effectively, awareness of one's existence (Purnell & Paulanka, 2008, 2009), and "*accepting* and *respecting* differences" (p. 2) and language provide clarity in terms of descriptions of cultural competence as well as expectations of a culturally competent person. Terms such as *demonstrate*, *develop*, and *provide* are distinct, crucial, and action-oriented. Terms such as *effective* (e.g., effective work within the context of the individual, family, and community), *respect*, and *appropriate* are outcomes that can be inferred from the context of behaviors.

While these definitions are presented in the context of health care (e.g., patient care provider), easy translation can be made to students and teachers. Teachers have a responsibility to facilitate the acquisition of knowledge and skills that reflect cultural competence. For example, for maximum outcome, teachers must be aware of the needs, learning styles, and culture of the students they teach. It is equally important for faculty to have an awareness and understanding of their personal beliefs and how these may affect teaching and learning.

An additional level of understanding that is needed relates to becoming a culturally competent person. Campinha-Bacote (1999) views cultural competence as a process rather than an end point. This implies that one continuously strives to achieve. Therefore it can be considered to be developmental as well as a journey. Faculty should have this understanding and convey to students that cultural competence is an outcome that will not develop overnight but over time.

A taxonomy of cultural competence has been identified by experts (Burchum, 2002; Lister, 1999). Work directed toward further defining cultural competence support process and development. Through a literature review, Burchum (2002) identified eight attributes of cultural competence: cultural awareness, cultural knowledge, cultural understanding, cultural sensitivity, cultural interaction, cultural skill, cultural competence, and cultural proficiency. Likewise, Lister (1999) identified seven terms that were classified as a taxonomy: cultural awareness, cultural knowledge, cultural understanding, cultural sensitivity, cultural interaction, cultural skill, and cultural competence. Wells (2000) proposed a model of cultural competence that incorporates two phases: cognitive and affective. The cognitive phase involves acquiring knowledge, whereas the affective phase relates to changes in attitudes and behaviors. Both of these are considered to be developmental. In viewing the concept on a continuum, there is progression from lack of or limited knowledge to cultural knowledge and then awareness. Characteristics of the affective phase are the development of cultural sensitivity, cultural competence, and cultural proficiency. The components of cultural competence are similar in each of these models.

Inherent in cultural competence is quality care for all human beings. One might propose that cultural competence is to quality care what multicultural education is to quality education. In working to facilitate learning for cultural competence, faculty can transform the curriculum to ensure that the concept is given in-depth attention. Using principles from Morey and Kitano (1997), such as opening the classroom to dialogue, providing opportunities for students to learn diverse perspectives (e.g., non-Western perspectives), and supplying opportunities for reflection, can greatly enhance students' learning, which can support the provision of quality care. To facilitate bringing students to this level, consideration must also be given to content, instructional strategies, assessment, and evaluation.

Criteria for Developing Cultural Competence

Three criteria are described to be essential to developing cultural competence: knowledge, skills, and attitudes (Kavanaugh & Kennedy, 1992). It is essential that these criteria be developed in a parallel fashion.

Knowledge is the attainment of information. The information may include cultural aspects of different ethnic groups and cultural differences (and similarities) between and among these groups. For example, the focus can be on health practices, beliefs, and traditions. There are numerous books, other printed material, and visual and auditory media devoted to providing information about ethnic cultural groups. Students should be directed to these as they are engaged in learning about cultural competence.

Skill relates to the ability to do something well. In the context of cultural competence, the skill may be the incorporation of health practices in plans of care or the effective communication with patients based on cultural norms. Acquisition of skills requires practice. Students must be provided with opportunities to engage in practice activities that will facilitate their acquisition of needed skills—for example, in interviewing, communicating, and interacting with patients or individuals from different cultural groups.

Attitudes are complex and are inferred from behavior. Attempts to assume attitudes may be hampered by factors such as a desire to please, political correctness, pressure from peers, ambivalence, and "just don't know." One difficulty with attitudes is that they are affective behaviors. One can choose an attitude (Langer, 1999). An attitude is personal. Covey (2004) asserts that all skills are important, but attitude is even more important. He further asserts that caring attitudes are essential for working effectively with people (Covey, 2004). It is important to remember that attitudes are conveyed in subtle ways, both verbally and nonverbally (e.g., body language, tone of voice, and choice of words). Therefore strict attention must be given to personal actions and reactions. It is important for teachers to be aware of how their attitudes affect teaching and learning. It is also essential to instruct students to examine their attitudes about their feelings and values and how these might affect others. For example, the display of a superior attitude can be easily conveyed in message deliveries and interpreted in ways that are not intended, are inappropriate, or are patronizing.

Knowing about diverse cultures without a change in attitude and behaviors by itself does not foster cultural competence. It is easy to provide avenues to enhance the knowledge base, but more challenging to change attitudes in regard to diverse patients (Todd, Lee, & Hoffman, 1994). Therefore it is essential to engage students in learning experiences that not only enhance knowledge and skills but also facilitate changing attitudes. Faculty must also model skills that are being taught so that students can learn them and realize the value of owning them.

Attributes of Cultural Competence Instructional Strategies, Resources, and Evaluation

In helping students understand cultural competence, faculty must ensure that students have in-depth knowledge of the dynamics of culture and the meaning of related terms and concepts such as *cultural group*, *ethnocentrism*, *ethnicity*, *ethnic group*, *ethnic culture*, *cultural care*, and *culturally competent*. When exploring students' understanding of these concepts, faculty should be alert to discussions that may indicate prejudice, stereotypes, and discrimination. At the outset, goals and specific objectives should be identified, assessment and instructional strategies should be established, and evaluation methods that will assist in making determinations of progression toward competence should be incorporated.

Teaching students about cultural competence should involve sharing information about the attributes of cultural competence. Several attributes have been identified: cultural awareness, cultural knowledge, cultural understanding, cultural sensitivity, cultural interaction, and cultural skills. A basic approach to understanding these concepts is facilitating students' understanding of the cultural self and the culture of others (Kai, Spencer, Wilkes, & Gill, 1999). This allows students an opportunity to learn that everyone belongs to a unique cultural group and with that come diverse perspectives in values, beliefs, lifestyles, and practices of individuals and family.

Cultural Awareness

Cultural awareness is the first step to cultural competence and the bridge to learning about other people. In planning activities for cultural awareness, a first step is for faculty to design assessment activities to facilitate students' awareness of self and others. Learning about oneself is important because it allows students an opportunity to learn that everyone belongs to a unique cultural group and with that come diverse perspectives in values, beliefs, lifestyles, and practices. Reflection is a key component of developing cultural awareness, and provides opportunities for students to examine personal biases, attitudes, and prejudices as well as communication patterns (verbal and nonverbal) and how they may be interpreted. A number of strategies and learning opportunities may be used—for example, having students write short papers describing themselves and then reflect on the descriptions. Encourage students to accept invitations to special events from individuals from a different ethnic or cultural group. These may include weddings, graduations, parties, rites of passage ceremonies, and visits to culturally diverse establishments such as ethnic restaurants and special museums. Students should take advantage of programs both on campus and in the community. When possible, faculty should accompany students to events and places so it is a shared, common experience and they can talk individually with students and explain what the student is seeing, learning, and experiencing. A list of cultural events and establishments can be identified and shared with students. Even better, the acquisition of this information can be an assignment for students.

Experiential learning projects are additional sources for gaining awareness (Dowling & Coppens, 1996; Lockhart & Resick, 1997). Examples of these are service-learning and immersion experiences. Encouragement to find resources on school and campus websites is another example. Faculty can alert students about upcoming cultural events occurring on the campus and in the community. In essence, these examples allow faculty and students to get to know others in order to learn about similarities and differences among ethnic and cultural groups.

An expected outcome for these kinds of activities should include students' ability to describe their own personal beliefs, values, attitudes, and prejudices and those of others. The use of reliable and valid instruments to measure cultural awareness has been researched. Rew, Becker, Cookston, Khosropour, and Martinez (2003) reported on a measure for cultural awareness that has an alpha coefficient of 0.91. In addition to the use of objective measures, qualitative information can be obtained by allowing students to reflect on specific instructional strategies and how they facilitated self-awareness and awareness of different cultural groups.

Cultural Knowledge

Cultural knowledge is the attainment of factual information about different cultural groups. Faculty can plan assignments for students to self-assess their knowledge base as well as facilitate them in finding answers to specific questions. Some questions could be related to (1) differences in health care practices, traditions, and health beliefs in different ethnic and cultural groups; (2) barriers to health care in specific populations; and (3) equity in treatment of nondominant groups in health care environments. Students' attendance at events that are universal to human experiences such as customs related to birth, developmental milestones, marriage, death, and special ceremonial occasions are useful for knowledge acquisition. Another approach is for faculty to identify conceptual models and frameworks to assist students in acquiring and processing information. For example, Giger and Davidhizar (2008) developed a transcultural assessment model that includes five components: communication, time, space, health beliefs and practices, and environment. Such a model can help students learn about themselves and other individuals by using these components as a framework for assessment, as well as for special assignments and points of reference in less formal conversations. Additional models designed for nursing are Leininger's (1993) Cultural Care Theory; Purnell and Paulanka's (2008) model for cultural competence; and Campinha-Bacote's (1999) model called The Process for Cultural Competence and Delivery of Healthcare Services, which incorporates cultural knowledge, awareness, skill, desire, and encounters. Spector (2009) has engaged in work that can be beneficial to faculty as they facilitate students' cultural competence journey. Readings from specific texts, articles, and popular books as well as the use of films can also be sources for acquiring information.

Both nonfiction and fiction books can be rich sources for information. Fiction sources can provide information about day-to-day lifestyles and events of people. In obtaining factual information from printed media, students should be encouraged to become critical readers. They must be encouraged to be alert to discrepancies, raise questions for clarification, and reflect on the content. Conversations with individuals from the specific ethnic groups can be arranged to discuss readings and find information about unanswered questions. The use of panel discussions with individuals from varied ethnic groups is an excellent way to facilitate knowledge acquisition. To facilitate the delivery of information desired by faculty and course objectives, an acceptable practice is to identify specific questions for panel members to use as a guide as the messages are delivered.

As information is shared and as students seek to learn new knowledge about specific cultural groups, faculty should make concerted efforts to ensure that students have knowledge of the concept of heterogeneity (e.g., variety, diversity, and differences in subgroups) as contrasted with the concept of homogeneity (sameness). While there is a tendency to classify individuals within an ethnic group as one group, the truth is that there are "multiple culturally similar" but not culturally homogeneous ethnic subgroups (Aponte, 2009, p. 3). In other words, there may be differences within groups because of the cultural heritage. Groups that are often used to illustrate this concept are Mexican Americans, Puerto Ricans, and Cuban Americans. These groups, according to Aponte (2009), come from three countries and have "developed a culture through interaction with Spain, but have developed one in part through its own unique ancestral heritage" (p. 3). The same is true for other groups such as African Americans and Asian Americans. An understanding of the differences must be manifested through the manner in which questions are phrased. The underlying point is to not make assumptions. In making cultural assessments, open-ended questions rather than direct questions should be phrased: "Tell me about your health practices . . . about food preferences" rather than "Do you believe in herb use? Do you eat beans?"

In addition to the examples of cultural information needed to enhance knowledge, there is related information that supports application. The support relates to the prevalence of multicultural and multilingual language within health care systems. One example is national standards, specifically the National Standards on Culturally and Linguistically Appropriate Services (CLAS) that were created by the Office of Minority Health (2001) to guide health care organizations and health care providers. These standards are organized around themes supportive of cultural competence. Faculty should apprise students of these standards, their mandates, and implications for their use within each component of the nursing process. Closely aligned to these is assuring students' knowledge of the use of interpreters and translators and their benefits to the care of patients with limited English proficiency, as well as options that are available to eliminate language barriers.

A knowledgeable student will show evidence of having learned information, as well as familiarity with the similarities and differences among ethnic and cultural groups. Students' cultural knowledge can be measured through the use of multiple-choice tests and essays, participation in case study discussions, the use and application of standards in patient care and virtual situations, responses to questions, observations of behaviors in role play (Shearer & Davidhizar, 2003), in clinical practice, and through the use of games and in virtual simulations. Faculty can be creative and self-design games for the purpose of knowledge assessment.

Cultural Understanding

Cultural understanding is the recognition that there are multiple perspectives, multiple truths, multiple solutions, and multiple ways of knowing. In other words, students develop insights and learn that "one culture does not fit all." To assess students' cultural understanding, faculty should plan activities that have the potential for students to demonstrate an understanding of different cultures. In addition to clinical practice, students can actively engage in discussion groups, for example, through case studies (Tomey, 2003), vignettes, role playing, essay writing, responses to questions, panel discussions, and game playing. A student who has an appropriate cultural understanding will recognize when values, beliefs, and practices of individuals are not compromised. As with other attributes of cultural competence, measurement for understanding can be sought through self-assessment, the use of multiple-choice tests, feedback from essays and other written assignments, role playing, and engagement in games.

Cultural Sensitivity, Cultural Interaction, and Cultural Skill

Cultural sensitivity develops as one comes to appreciate, respect, and value cultural differences. Clinical exchange experiences in a different part of the city or in different areas within the United States (e.g., reservations, U.S.–Mexican border, Appalachia) have been reported to facilitate the development of cultural sensitivity (Scholes & Moore, 2001). The extent of a students' sensitivity can be assessed through the use of role play, discussions and dialogue, evaluation of written assignments, and observations of behaviors. *Cultural interaction* relates to the personal contact, open discussion, and exchanges that occur between and among individuals of different cultures. A common contention is that one cannot develop cultural competence solely through reading or other intellectual exercises. Efforts should be made to actively engage with others and develop personal relationships with people who are from socioeconomic classes or cultural groups that are not the same as the students. In addition to encouraging interaction with others, faculty can provide leading questions or points that will help students feel comfortable engaging in conversations. Interaction and conversations can occur via e-mail (Kennell, Nyback, & Ingalsbe, 2005), in informal situations or during face-to-face informal chats (e.g., over lunch), or at special celebratory events and the like. Through continual cultural interaction, one can learn about customs and language (both verbal and nonverbal, such as body language, eye contact, touch, manners, and silence) and what each means. Cultural interactions can support the development of skills such as communication, cultural assessments, interviews, and interventions (AIDS Education & Training Centers, 2006). The interactions can occur in exchange and immersion experiences and in those described previously.

Cultural skill relates to effective performance, for example, in communicating with others. Skill development in the area of communication can be enhanced through the use of interviews (Morgan, 1996) and visual media, the latter of which can be shown in segments and as time permits for discussion and evaluation of the effectiveness and ineffectiveness of the communication or interview techniques. Faculty can provide feedback following role plays, small group exercises, discussions of case presentation, as well as permit students to self-assess. Evidence of skill development will be exhibited when beliefs, values, and practices are integrated into plans, when communication is effective, and when appropriate assessments and interventions are made.

Cultural competence is by nature a skill evidenced through skill sets. (Refer to page 202 for multiple definitions.) The process of becoming culturally competent involves the acquisition of specific knowledge, skills, and attitudes. Through the use of a variety of teaching–learning strategies, students can make significant strides on the journey. They must understand the need for continuing education through readings, workshops, seminars, conferences, and other educational engagements.

The expected outcomes should be clearly identified and should guide didactic content, student assignments, and testing. In this way, students' progress toward cultural competence can be monitored and assessed as students move through the curriculum. The curriculum provides a framework for mapping and a set of criteria for evaluation. The results of the evaluation should exemplify the attainment of specific knowledge, skills, and attitudes. Refer to Box 17-1 for specific questions that can be asked.

SUMMARY

The increasing enrollments of diverse student populations in nursing programs provide an avenue of opportunities for nurse educators to use current knowledge of multicultural education, equity pedagogy, and life experiences of diverse students to create a rich learning environment so that all students will have an equal chance to achieve academically. By directing attention to cultural factors—ethnicity, race, nationality (religion), language, socioeconomics, gender, age, sexual orientation, and life experiences—as well as factors relating to academics—needs and learning styles—positive learning outcomes can be facilitated and achieved. The use of teaching learning strategies that incorporate concepts of equity, inclusiveness, and active engagement can also affect positive learning. Cultural competence may be used as an exemplar for applying some of the principles of multicultural education while at the same time facilitating an understanding of its value in quality care. By exemplifying cultural competence as a process or a journey, both educators and students will realize that lifelong learning is inherent and a requirement for teaching, learning, and preparing graduates to work in a society that includes multiple diverse groups.

BOX 17-1 Assessing Personal Cultural Competence

Ask specific questions relating to each of the attributes.

Awareness	Am I aware of my personal biases, stereotypes, and prejudices toward cultures that are different than my own? To what extent am I aware?
Knowledge	Do I have factual information of the similarities and differences between and among varying cultural groups? Their health care practices, beliefs, and traditions?
Understanding	Do I understand that there are a variety of cultural factors that may contribute to why my patients may react the way they do? To what extent do I understand?
Sensitivity	Am I sensitive enough to convey to my patients that I appreciate, respect, and value their cultural differences? To what extent do I demonstrate sensitivity?
Cultural Interaction	Do I make deliberate efforts to make personal contact with individuals who are from a cultural group different than my own? Do I read books, articles, or watch movies, etc., and intellectually reflect on what I saw, read, or heard? To what extent?
	Do I take advantage of exchange programs in my school that would take me to environments of people within my community that have a culture different from my own? Study-abroad program? Mission trips? Do I frequent cultural establishments in my community?
Cultural Skill	Do I possess the skill sets to effectively communicate with my patients when I conduct a cultural assessment and a physical assessment that will provide evidence that I am appropriate, efficient, and safe? To what extent?
Cultural Competence	Do I demonstrate competence to the extent that I could (and my faculty would be able to) identify the following outcomes that provide evidence of:

- Facilitating or providing care that respects the values, beliefs, and health practices of the patient as well as being safe and satisfying care.
- Integrating cultural beliefs, values, languages, and health practices of others in assessment plans and actual care.
- Examining the impact of culturally tied beliefs and practices on individual health care needs.
- Meeting cultural needs of individuals and their families.
- Incorporating cultural aspects of health and illness during assessments and communication and in actual care.
- Applying national standards to facilitate the provision of appropriate care to individuals and families.

REFLECTING ON THE EVIDENCE

1. How can faculty assess their own readiness to develop and implement a multicultural and inclusive curriculum?

2. What is the state of the science for multicultural education in nursing?

3. Are instructional materials appropriate for a multicultural curriculum? To what extent do textbooks support inclusiveness? Are course materials reflective of diversity? Are tests free of gender, culture, religious, and ethnic bias? Can course policies be implemented fairly for all students?

4. To what extent are the instructional strategies evidence-based?

Personal Reflection

To what extent:
do textbooks, media, supplemental materials, and teaching–learning strategies support inclusive teaching (multicultural education)?
are materials (syllabi and other handouts) used in my class free of bias?
do I support diverse learning styles in my classroom?
do I seek to incorporate evidence-based teaching strategies?
do I encourage discussions from various perspectives?
do I embrace inclusivity in my pursuit of pedagogy?

REFERENCES

AIDS Education & Training Centers, National Resource Center. (2006). *Guiding principles for cultural competency.* Retrieved from http://aidsetc.org/

American Council on Education and American Association of University Professors. (2000). *Does diversity make a difference? Three research studies on diversity in college classrooms.* (Executive summary). Washington, DC: Author.

Americans with Disabilities Act. (1990). Public Law No. 101–136, 42 U.S.C. 1210.

Anderson, K. (2004). Teaching cultural competence using an exemplar from literary journalism. *Journal of Nursing Education, 43*(6), 253–259.

Aponte, J. (2009). Addressing cultural heterogeneity among Hispanic subgroups by using Campinha-Bacote's Model of Cultural Competency. *Holistic Nursing Practice, 23*(1), 3–12.

Bagnardi, M., Bryant, L., & Colin, J. (2009). Banks multicultural model: A framework for integrating multiculturalism into nursing curriculum. *Journal of Professional Nursing, 25*(4), 234–239.

Banks, J. (2007). *Educating citizens in a multicultural society* (2nd ed.). New York, NY: Teachers College.

Banks, J., & Banks, C. (1993). *Multicultural education: Issues and perspectives.* Boston, MA: Allyn & Bacon.

Banks, J. A. (2006). *Multicultural education: Goals and dimensions.* University of Washington, College of Education, Center for Multicultural Education. Retrieved from http://education.washington.edu/

Banks, J. A., & Banks, C. A. M. (2004). *Handbook of research on multicultural education.* San Francisco, CA: Jossey-Bass.

Billings, D. (2006). Journaling: A strategy for developing reflective practitioners. *Journal of Continuing Education in Nursing, 37*(3), 104–105.

Brennan, S., & Schulze, M. (2004). Cultural immersion through ethnography: The lived experience and group process. *Journal of Nursing Education, 43*(6), 285–288.

Burchum, R. (2002). Cultural competence: An evolutionary perspective. *Nursing Forum, 37*(2), 5–15.

Byrne, M. (2001). Understanding racial bias in nursing fundamentals textbook. *Nursing and Health Care Perspectives, 22,* 299–303.

Byrne, M., Weddle, C., Davis, E., & McGinnis, P. (2003). The Byrne guide for inclusionary cultural content. *Journal of Nursing Education, 42*(6), 277–281.

Caffrey, R., Neander, W., Markle, D., & Stewart, B. (2005). Improving the cultural competence of nursing students: Results of integrating cultural content in the curriculum and an international immersion experience. *Journal of Nursing Education, 44*(5), 234–240.

Campinha-Bacote, J. (1999). A model and instrument to address cultural competence in health care. *Journal of Nursing Education, 38*(5), 203–207.

Campinha-Bacote, J., Yahie, T., & Langenkamp, M. (1996). The challenge of cultural diversity for nurse educators. *Journal of Continuing Education in Nursing, 27*(2), 59–64.

Chang, M. J. (2002). The impact of an undergraduate diversity course requirement on students' racial views and attitudes. *Journal of General Education, 51*(1), 21–42.

Covey, S. R. (2004). *The 7 habits of highly effective people.* New York, NY: Free Press.

Craft, M. (2005). Reflective writing and nursing education. *Journal of Nursing Education, 44*(2), 52–53.

Doordan, A., & Abriam-Yago, K. (1996). Returning to school: LPN to BSN. *Minority Nurse,* 24–25.

Dowling, J., & Coppens, N. (1996). Understanding cultural and health practices through an experiential learning project. *Nurse Educator, 21*(6), 43–46.

Duarte, E. M., & Smith, S. (2000). *Foundational perspectives in multicultural education.* New York, NY: Longman.

Eliason, M., & Macy, N. (1992). A classroom activity to introduce cultural diversity. *Nurse Educator, 17*(3), 32–36.

Flowers, N. (2002). Inclusive teaching online. In D. Billings (Ed.), *Conversations in e-learning* (pp. 197–201). Boston, MA: Jones & Bartlett.

Giger, J., & Davidhizar, R. (2008). *Transcultural nursing: Assessment and intervention* (5th ed.). St. Louis, MO: Mosby.

Guttman, M. (2004). Increasing the linguistic competence of the nurse with limited English proficiency. *The Journal of Continuing Education in Nursing, 35*(6), 264–269.

Halic, O., Greenburg, K., & Paulus, T. (2009). Language and academic identity: A study of the experiences of non-native English speaking international students. *International Education, 38*(2), 73.

Helton, P. (2000). Diversifying the curriculum: A study of faculty involvement. *Diversity Digest,* Fall. Retrieved from http://www.diversityweb.org/

Hunt, R. (2007). Service-learning: An eye-opening experience that provokes emotion and challenges stereotypes. *Journal of Nursing Education, 46*(6), 277–281.

Kai, J., Spencer, J., Wilkes, M., & Gill, P. (1999). Learning to value ethnic diversity—What, why and how? *Medical Education, 33*(8), 616–623.

Kardong-Edgren, S., Bond, M. L., Schlosser, S., Cason, C., Jones, M. E., Warr, R., & Strunk, P. (2005). Cultural attitudes, knowledge, and skills of nursing faculty toward patients from four diverse cultures. *Journal of Professional Nursing, 21*(3), 174–182.

Kataoka-Yahiro, M., & Abriam-Yago, K. (1997). Culturally competent teaching strategies for Asian nursing students for whom English is a second language. *Journal of Cultural Diversity, 4*(3), 83–87.

Kavanaugh, K., & Kennedy, P. (1992). *Promoting cultural diversity: Strategies for health care professionals.* Newburg Park, CA: Sage.

Kennell, L., Nyback, M., & Ingalsbe, K. (2005). Increasing cultural competence through asynchronous web-based interactions between two nursing programs. *Journal of Nursing Education, 44*(5), 244.

Langer, N. (1999). Culturally competent professionals on therapeutic alliances enhances patient compliance. *Journal of Health Care for the Poor and Underserved, 10*(1), 19–26.

Leininger, M. (1993). Culture care theory: The relevant theory to guide nurses functioning in a multi-cultural world. In M. Parkes (Ed.), *Patterns of nursing theories in practice* (pp. 105–121). New York, NY: NLN Press.

Lister, P. (1999). A taxonomy for developing cultural competence. *Nurse Education Today, 19*(4), 313–318.

Lockhart, J., & Resick, L. (1997). Teaching cultural competence: The value of experiential learning and community resources. *Nurse Educator, 22*(3), 27–31.

Lou, R. (1994). Teaching all students equally. In H. Roberts, J. C. Gonzalez, O. Harris, D. Huff, A. M. Johns, R. Lou, & O. Scott (Eds.), *Teaching from a cultural perspective* (pp. 28–45). Thousand Oaks, CA: Sage.

Maheady, D. (2003). *Nursing students with disabilities: Change the course*. River Edge, NJ: Exceptional Parent Press.

Marchesani, L., & Adams, M. (1992). Dynamics of diversity in the teaching learning process: A faculty development model for analysis and action. In M. Adams (Ed.), *Promoting diversity in college classrooms: Innovative responses for the curriculum, faculty, and institutions* (pp. 9–20). San Francisco, CA: Jossey-Bass.

Marks, B. (2007). Cultural competence revisited: Nursing students with disabilities. *Journal of Nursing Education, 48*(2), 71–74.

Mays, R. (Presenter). (2009, December 4). *Multicultural education in nursing a* [Web seminar presented at the New Jersey Nursing Initiative, Faculty Preparation Program, Princeton, New Jersey: Robert Wood Johnson Foundation.] Merryfield, M. (2001). Moving the center of global education: From imperial world views that divide the world to double consciousness, contrapuntal pedagogy, hybridity, and cross-cultural competence. In W. B. Stanley (Ed.), *Critical issues in social studies research for the 21st century* (pp. 179–208). Charlotte, NC: Information Age Publishing.

Millon-Underwood, S. (1992). Educating for sensitivity to cultural diversity. *Nurse Educator, 17*(3), 7.

Morey, A. I., & Kitano, M. K. (1997). *Multicultural course transformation in higher education: A broader truth*. Boston, MA: Allyn & Bacon.

Morgan, C. (1996). The interview as a measure of cultural competence: A case study. *Language, Culture, and Curriculum, 9*(3), 225–243.

Morrison, J., Sullivan, F., Murray, E., & Jolly, B. (1999). Evidenced-based education: Development of an instrument to critically appraise reports of educational interventions. *Medical Education, 33*(12), 890–893.

National Alliance for Hispanic Health. (2001). *A primer for cultural proficiency: Towards quality health services for Hispanics*. Washington, DC: Estrella Press.

National League for Nursing. (2006). *Nursing data review academic year 2004–2005*. New York, NY: Author.

Nelson, C. (1996). Student diversity requires different approaches to college teaching, even in math and science. *American Behavioral Scientist, 40*(2), 165–175.

Nunez, A. (2000). Transforming cultural competence into cross-cultural efficacy in women's health education. *Academic Medicine, 75*(11), 1071–1075.

Office of Minority Health. (2001). *National standards on culturally and linguistically appropriate services*. Washington, DC: U.S. Department of Health and Human Services.

O'Grady, C. R. (2000). *Integrating service learning and multicultural education in colleges and universities*. Maluah, NJ: Lawrence Erlbaum.

Purnell, L., & Paulanka, B. (2008). *Transcultural health care: A culturally competent approach* (3rd ed.). Philadelphia, PA: FA Davis Company.

Purnell, L., & Paulanka, B. (2009). *Guide to culturally competent health care*. Philadelphia, PA: Davis.

Rew, L., Becker, H., Cookston, J., Khosropour, S., & Martinez, S. (2003). Measuring cultural awareness in nursing students. *Journal of Nursing Education, 12*(6), 249–257.

Sadker, M., & Sadker, D. (1994). *Failing at fairness: How America's schools cheat girls*. New York, NY: Macmillan.

Salter, D. (2004). *Gender bias in college classrooms: A study of the interactions between psychological and environmental types*. Available at http://www.ed.psu.edu/seta/NAWE.htm

Schoem, D., Frankel, L., Zuniga, X., & Lewis, E. (1995). *Multicultural teaching in the university*. Westport, CT: Praeger.

Scholes, J., & Moore, D. (2001). Clinical exchange: One model to achieve culturally sensitive care. *Nursing Inquiry, 7*(1), 61–71.

Serdans, B. (2002). *I'm moving on . . . Are u?* Philadelphia, PA: Xibris Corporation.

Shearer, R., & Davidhizar, R. (2003). Using role play to develop cultural competence. *Journal of Nursing Education, 42*(6), 273–275.

Smith, H., Parr, R., Woods, R., Bauer, B., & Abraham, T. (2010). Five years after graduation: Undergraduate cross-group friendships and multicultural curriculum predict current attitudes and activities. *Journal of College Student Development, 51*(4), 385–402.

Spector, R. E. (2009). *Cultural diversity in health & illness* (7th ed.). Upper Saddle River, NJ: Prentice Hall.

Stanley, C. A., Saunders, S., & Hart, J. M. (2005). Multicultural course transformation. In M. Ouellett (Ed.), *Teaching inclusively: Resources for course, department, institutional change in higher education* (pp. 566–585). Stillwater, OK: New Forums.

Stokes, L. (2003, July/August). Gatherings as a retention strategy. *Association of Black Nursing Faculty (ABNF) Journal, 14*(4), 80–82.

Stokes, L., Linde, B., & Zimmerman, M. (2005, 2008). *Instructional strategy for learning communities*. (Unpublished documentations).

Sue, D. W., Capodilupo, C. M., Torino, G. C., Bucceri, J. M., Holder, A. M. B., Nadal, K. L., & Esquilin, M. (2007). Racial microaggressions in everyday life. *American Psychologist, 62*(4), 271–284.

Sullivan Commission, The. (2004). *Missing persons: Minorities in the health profession* (Report of the Sullivan Commission on Diversity in the Healthcare Workforce). Washington, DC: Author.

Tate, D. (2003). Cultural awareness: Bridging the gap between caregivers and Hispanic patients. *The Journal of Continuing Education in Nursing, 34*(5), 213–217.

Todd, K. H., Lee, T., & Hoffman, J. R. (1994). The effect of ethnicity on physician estimates of pain severity in patients with isolated extremity trauma. *Journal of American Medical Association, 271*(12), 925–928.

Tomey, A. (2003). Learning with cases. *The Journal of Continuing Education in Nursing, 34*(1), 34–38.

Tucker-Allen, S. (1989). Losses incurred through minority student nurse attention. *Nursing and Health Care, 10*(7), 395–397.

Ukoha, R. (2004). Evidence-based multicultural teaching methods. *Nursing Educator, 29*(1), 10–12.

Underwood, S. M. (2006). Culture, diversity and health: Responding to the queries of inquisitive minds. *Journal of Nursing Education, 45*(7), 281–286.

U.S. Census Bureau. (2000). *The Hispanic population in the United States*. Washington, DC: Author.

Wells, M. (2000). Beyond cultural competence: A model for individual and institutional cultural development. *Journal of Community Health Nursing, 17*(4), 189–199.

Xu, Y., & Davidhizar, R. (2005). Intercultural communication in nursing education: When Asian students and American faculty converge. *Journal of Nursing Education, 44*(5), 209–215.

Zimmerman, M. (2003). *On the path to cultural competence*. (Unpublished manuscript).

Teaching in the Clinical Setting 18

Lillian Gatlin Stokes, PhD, RN, FAAN
Gail Carlson Kost, MSN, RN, CNE

The health care system is ever changing. Health care reform challenges faculty to prepare students for future roles and to practice in a health care system that is patient-centered, wellness-oriented, community- and population-based, and technologically advanced. Clinical settings within a variety of health care systems have also become highly complex. It is within these settings that students learn to use their acquired knowledge and skills as they think critically, make clinical decisions, and acquire professional values necessary to work in the practice environment. The purpose of this chapter is to describe the environments for clinical teaching and learning, how the curriculum relates to clinical teaching, roles and responsibilities of clinical teachers, and teaching methods and models that facilitate learning in clinical environments.

Practice Learning Environments

The environment for practicum experiences may be any place where students interact with patients and families for purposes such as acquiring needed cognitive skills that facilitate clinical decision making as well as psychomotor and affective skills. The practicum environment, referred to as the clinical learning environment (CLE), is an interactive network of forces within the clinical setting that influences students' clinical learning outcomes. The environment also provides opportunities for students to learn to apply theory to practice and to become socialized into the expectations of the practice environment, as well as the roles and responsibilities of health care professionals. To accomplish these outcomes, a variety of experiences are required in multiple settings. These settings may be special venues within schools of nursing or within acute care settings or communities. It is essential that practice environments be

supportive and conducive to learning so that students will develop the qualities and skill abilities needed to become competent professionals (Williams, 2001). The following section describes these settings. Included among these are practice learning centers such as learning labs, acute and transitional care, and community-based environments.

Practice Learning Centers

To foster a nonthreatening and safe learning environment, the practice learning center is used at several stages of students' learning. These centers encourage guided experiences that allow students to practice and perfect a variety of psychomotor, affective, and cognitive skills such as critical thinking and clinical reasoning before moving into complex patient environments. Simulation is one example of a teaching method used in the practice learning center. This method is increasingly used to evaluate knowledge acquisition as well as skill sets (Childs, 2002).

Simulation

According to Rush, Dyches, Waldrop, and Davis (2008), "Simulation is a strategy increasingly being used to promote critical thinking skills among baccalaureate nursing (BSN) students." Schiavenato (2009) also states, "The human patient simulator or high-fidelity mannequin has become synonymous with the word simulation in nursing education" (p. 388). Bremner, Aduddell, Bennett, and VanGeest (2006) believe that the incorporation of high-fidelity mannequin technology is one of the most important issues in nursing education today. Simulation may assist in supplementing didactic content in the classroom or it may be used to ensure that all students in a clinical course would experience a patient situation that may not be available during the regular clinical day. Schools across the country are increasingly using human patient simulators for teaching a part of a student's clinical nursing course. When evaluating the effectiveness of this teaching strategy, those involved need to determine what was learned and gained in the experience and what knowledge will be transferred to the real clinical setting, which will ultimately affect patient care. There are variations among Boards of Nursing as to the use of simulation in the curriculum. (See Chapter 20 for further discussion of simulations.)

Virtual Clinical Practica

Given the challenges of finding sufficient clinical experiences for students, faculty are exploring the use of virtual clinical experiences made possible by online technologies such as Second Life that can create virtual clinical environments (Schmidt & Stewart, 2009) and use existing technologies such as e-ICUs and telehealth capabilities to create opportunities for additional clinical experiences. According to Grady (2006), "Nursing education practices have changed little in response to massive and sweeping changes in the complex and dynamic health care environment" (p. 125). Research has been conducted to better define and "test leading-edge telehealth methods and technologies that can extend the reach of nursing in clinical areas as well as classroom settings" (p. 124). The Virtual Clinical Practicum (VCP) was designed to provide a live, clinical experience to nursing students from a distance. Students gain clinical experience and practice skills and clinical judgment using telehealth technologies in which students observe a nurse taking care of a patient in a clinical setting without going to the actual clinical site. The students can interact with the nurse and patient using telehealth technology. The VCP process was developed as a potential solution to expanding nursing school enrollment to accommodate the nursing shortage in the face of limited clinical practice sites as well as limited clinical experts, especially in rural areas. (See Chapter 21 for further discussion of virtual environments.)

Acute and Transitional Care Environments

Acute and transitional care environments provide clinical experiences for undergraduate and graduate students preparing for advanced practice roles. Experiences in these environments enable undergraduate students, in particular, to exemplify caring abilities and practice the use of cognitive, psychomotor, and communication skills as they interact with patients and their families. These environments have become increasingly more complex. The complexity relates to factors such as extensive use of technology (e.g., electronic record keeping), rapid patient and staff turnover, high patient acuity, and complex patient needs. Because of this complexity, there are increased safety risks for students, patients, faculty, and staff. Therefore safety must be enhanced through the use of creative teaching and learning strategies to ensure safe practice and the development of the student's ability to think critically while acquiring the competencies that facilitate attainment of curriculum outcomes. Examples of these strategies include assignment methodologies such as multiple assignments and teaching modalities (e.g., nursing grand rounds); simulated clinical scenarios; case studies; computer-assisted instruction; and the use of interactive CD-ROMs, shadow experiences, and virtual simulations (VCP, e-hospitals). Guided and focused small group sessions and selective capstone experiences also may facilitate students' acquisition of needed knowledge and skills.

The complexity of the environment also provides opportunities for faculty to become facilitators of learning, designers of clinical experiences, and developers of flexible skill sets that can be used across settings. Faculty must provide experiences to help students think, care, and act like nurses—and finally to be nurses (Tanner, 2002). For this to occur, the outcomes for specific learning experiences must be clearly identified and articulated.

Every health care environment and specific unit within these environments has a culture. The culture of the immediate environment affects teaching and learning. For example, the culture—or patterns of actions and behaviors—of the health care professionals can be observed in their attitudes, interactions, sense of support for each other, and commitment to quality patient care. These actions and behaviors can be influenced by staffing levels, acuity of patients, anxiety of staff, and workload. These aspects of the culture of the environment can in turn influence the time staff have to devote to students. The culture of the environment may also result in behaviors related to lateral violence. Lateral violence is often observed, witnessed, and verbalized by students. These verbalizations provide an opportunity for faculty to implement strategies and assist students with processing what they may be seeing, hearing, and feeling, and thus lessen the effects of these behaviors on students' learning. For example, faculty can hold debriefing sessions, listen to students' perceptions, and make concerted efforts to balance students' feelings and thoughts by using appropriate strategies to soften, yet not deny, the reality of the culture.

Community-Based Environments

The health care delivery system is continuing to shift from acute care hospital environments to the community. Several factors have facilitated this shift, including social, technological, and economic changes as well as the politics of health care. These changes have resulted in an increased use of community agencies such as ambulatory, long-term, home health, and nurse-managed clinics; homeless shelters; social agencies (e.g., homes for battered women); physicians' offices; health maintenance organizations; worksite venues (Schim & Scher, 2002), art galleries; day care centers; and schools (Buttriss, Kuiper, & Newbold, 1995; Chan, 2002; Faller, McDowell, & Jackson, 1995). Summer camps are also being used for special experiences (Totten & Fonnesbeck, 2002). Depending on the purpose of the camps, multiple objectives can be accomplished. For example, camps for children with health issues can be used for acquisition of targeted skills that could be obtained in acute care settings. Camps for healthy children could be used for acquisition of knowledge and skills relating to normal growth and development and communication.

The use of technology such as video conferencing, wireless remote communication, information systems, and online courses has made it possible for clinical experience to occur at a distance. The transition to community-based teaching requires faculty to adapt practicum skills to new technology, modify teaching methods, and adapt to methods of clinical supervision such as being accessible by pager or texting device.

Establishing appropriate and sufficient learning experiences in the community may be difficult and challenging. These challenges often relate to economic constraints and the nursing shortage, with a resultant lack of time for professionals to facilitate skill development and serve as role models. These challenges may require faculty to be creative in

their use and selection of resources within these environments and to consider establishing partnerships with the service agencies.

Selecting Health Care Environments

Regardless of the practice environment, faculty are responsible for selecting appropriate health care agencies and being aware of what particular systems are in place within the program to negotiate contracts that are congruent with the philosophies of the school of nursing and the agency, as well as those that specify the rights and responsibilities of both. Determinations must be made about accreditation status, adequacy of staff, the patient population for needed experiences, and expected course outcomes, whether or not the practice model is compatible for intended uses and curriculum needs. In addition, the adequacy and availability of physical resources (e.g., conference space) for students and faculty should be determined. Finding a practice environment that meets all specified needs is becoming a challenge due to factors associated with the delivery of health care. For example, rapid patient turnover often means faculty have to select available patients rather than those that best meet students' learning needs. This limitation in patient availability in turn creates opportunities for faculty to be creative in the manner in which learning experiences are selected and teaching strategies are used. Regardless of the limitation, the role of the faculty is to assist students in making learning connections.

Despite all efforts on the part of classroom and clinical faculty, there seem to be times of "great divide" between the two arenas. Benner, Sutphen, Leonard, and Day (2010) indicate that "even with faculty commitment to integration, all too often, nursing education is approached as if it has two discrete elements" (p. 159). Dual clinical and classroom assignments for faculty will assist in making those necessary connections between clinical and classroom. "The very strength of pedagogical approaches in the clinical setting is itself a persuasive argument for intentional integration of knowledge, clinical reasoning, and skilled know-how and ethical comportment across the nursing curriculum" (Benner et al., 2010, p. 159). Thus faculty have a significant role in helping students to make the necessary connections between clinical and classroom experiences.

Building Relationships with Personnel within Health Care Agency Environments

According to Piscopo (1994), "roles identify relationships and are interactional and reciprocal" (p. 113). The ability of the clinical faculty to facilitate students' learning can be enhanced when an effective working relationship is established within the clinical agency. Effective relationships begin with effective communication, which must be practiced in an ongoing manner to maintain relationships and facilitate learning (Lee, Krystyna, & Williams, 2002). This requires having an understanding of the environment and the roles of the individuals within the environment, and a realization that these do not exist in isolation but are patterned to dovetail with or complement other roles.

Information should be shared continually, clearly, and consistently about goals, competencies, and expected outcomes; the level of students; practice expectations; the clinical schedule; and related information. Such information enables the staff's ability to assist with identification of appropriate experiences for students.

Inasmuch as clinical faculty have the primary responsibility for teaching and guiding students in the clinical environment, others often assist in the process. Therefore the sharing of expectations with the staff is critical. Ensuring an orientation to the practicum environment and having students engage with staff early in the clinical experience promote positive student–staff interaction and provide opportunities for role clarification and the development of collegial relationships. A consistent demonstration of awareness of the mission and values of the agency through actions that are inherently respectful is crucial. Follow-up communication provides an avenue for those within the practice environment to keep abreast of changes.

Clinical Practicum Experiences across the Curriculum

Understanding the Curriculum

The curriculum, composed of a series of well-organized and logical entities, guides the selection of learning experiences and clinical assignments, organizes teaching–learning activities, and facilitates the measurement of student performance. The manner in which the curriculum is organized facilitates the planning of learning experiences in a logical, rational sequence. The curriculum is designed to build on prior knowledge and to reinforce learning. While this description of curriculum relates to process, this does not preclude faculty's use of creative and innovative methods in clinical environments. Creative methods have a high potential to motivate students and facilitate positive learning. As students progress and engage in varied practicum experiences, it is faculty's responsibility to interpret the curriculum and to describe the relationships between course competencies and practicum experiences.

Understanding the Student

Clinical experiences provide opportunities for students to practice the art and science of nursing, which enhances their ability to learn. To maximize these experiences, faculty must have full knowledge and understanding of each student (see also Chapter 2). The nursing student population is culturally diverse and includes members of varied age groups, many ethnic and racial groups, and an increasing number of males. This population is also likely to include persons with (or without) prior degrees from a variety of disciplines, as well as those who possess many different health care experiences and technological skill levels. In addition, students differ in their learning styles, levels of knowledge, and preferences for learning opportunities; therefore faculty must make concerted efforts to balance the students' learning needs, interests, and abilities when selecting clinical experiences without losing sight of the curriculum and expected competencies and outcomes. Such action can be facilitated by making an assessment of the knowledge, culture, and skills of the learner. Such an assessment helps the faculty determine whether students possess the cognitive, critical thinking, clinical reasoning, decision-making, psychomotor, and affective skills needed for the experiences.

Understanding the Clinical Environment

The clinical environment has been described as a place where students synthesize the knowledge gained in the classroom and make applications to practical situations. Chan (2002) describes the clinical learning environment as "the interaction network of forces within the clinical setting that influences student learning outcomes" (p. 70). A number of forces affect expected outcomes, including the increased complexity of care required by patients with higher acuity, the nursing shortage, the rapid pace, and multiple health care professionals and activities. These forces, coupled with the need to adjust to an environment that requires an integration of thinking skills and performance skills, often result in increased anxiety among students. Clinical strategies can be developed to reduce anxiety in clinical environments, especially where anxiety levels are high. Some strategies focus on the level of students. Two such strategies are (1) peer coaching, in which senior students coach beginning students (Broscious & Sanders, 2001), and (2) placement of students in long-term care settings.

Traditionally, clinical rotations have consisted of short blocks of time spent on a unit caring for a patient or two, mostly performing nursing skills with little or no time for integration of theory, application of critical thinking and clinical reasoning, or effective evaluation of the interventions performed. Faculty know that the clinical environment is not always conducive to student learning. Nursing staff are overworked, stretched thin due to consistently working in a short-staffed environment and caring for patients that are critically ill with multiple health care needs. Nurses intuitively want to be good role models and nurture students but often do not have the time to do so.

Regardless of location of the practice setting, faculty and staff should provide an environment in which caring relationships are evident. The clinical practice environment should be a place where students feel that they are accepted and that their contributions are appreciated by individuals with whom they interact (Chan, 2002). Attributes of staff such as warmth, support in obtaining access to learning experiences, and willingness to engage in a teaching relationship are considered helpful.

Faculty are responsible for accessing information systems such as websites, tutorials, structured meetings management, or orientation sessions within affiliating agencies and for shadowing staff in the immediate care area. The use of either of these techniques informs and facilitates decision making. Information should be reciprocal so that all parties (faculty, students, and staff) can learn.

Selecting Clinical Practicum Experiences

Practicum experiences refer to all activities in which students engage in the practice of nursing. Such experiences are essential for knowledge application, skill development, and professional socialization. Selection of practicum learning experiences requires all faculty to be knowledgeable about clinical education and have a sound understanding of the curriculum, the learners, and the learning environment.

Practicum experiences are selected and planned to provide students with opportunities to work across settings and manage care for varied populations with an emphasis on prevention and primary care. Through these experiences, nursing students can learn to work collaboratively with a variety of health disciplines. Therefore students should be provided with opportunities to work as members of interdisciplinary teams and in practice environments when interdisciplinary practice models are used for joint planning, implementation, and evaluation of outcomes of care. The goal of interdisciplinary education is to foster interprofessional relationships while enhancing contribution to each discipline.

Learning to collaborate with the many health care groups involved in patient care can be a daunting task. It is believed that the use of interdisciplinary simulations may assist students in health care disciplines such as nursing, medicine, pharmacy, and respiratory therapy to learn about the clinical management of a variety of patients. Rodehorst, Wilhelm, and Jensen (2005) indicated that the use of interdisciplinary learning helps to clarify the roles of each discipline and enhances learning from one another.

Nursing faculty are increasingly participating in teams and designing interdisciplinary clinical courses and learning experiences. Successful course development and implementation depend on faculty's commitment to the goal of interdisciplinary practice and a wide range of additional factors. For example, educators must demonstrate professional respect and role clarity. Educators must also have the ability to secure clinical facilities and develop schedules for clinical experiences that are compatible with the concurrent coursework and curriculum progression in each discipline. Other factors include identification of content and experiences with similarities, differences, and overlaps, as well as clarification of autonomy and role interdependency. Success depends on the ability to identify philosophical similarities and differences in clinical practice and to establish clear communication through avenues such as frequent interdisciplinary clinical conferences.

An expected outcome of interdisciplinary education is increased future collaboration among professionals. The assumption is that students who are taught together will learn to collaborate more effectively when they later assume professional roles in an integrated health care system. Rewards and benefits of interdisciplinary practice and education include clearer understanding of roles and better employment opportunities for graduates. The long-term outcome is improved access to care, quality care, and increased patient satisfaction and safety.

The practicum experiences should also help students prepare for outcomes in a progressive, developmental manner. Experiences with patients from diverse populations and with different levels of wellness should be provided. Faculty should take advantage of opportunities to use their creative talents, clinical skills, and expertise to ensure that all students have opportunities to interface virtually or directly with a variety of patient populations.

As faculty begin to plan the clinical experience, it is essential to determine the goal of the particular clinical experience for that day. For the beginning student, focused clinical experiences in which the student is to accomplish specific objectives and to achieve specific competencies and individual learning needs are appropriate (Gubrud-Howe & Schoessler, 2008). If that is the goal, faculty would plan for a *focused* clinical experience. Specifically, students may interview patients to work on communication skills, perform vital sign assessments to develop this particular skill set, observe in a specialty area, and give and receive reports. The focus of each experience is some needed skill set for students' or an individual's learning needs.

Other learning goals may emphasize facilitating students' ability to synthesize information, integrate didactic and clinical knowledge, develop clinical reasoning and judgment skills, and plan care for groups of patients (Benner et al., 2010; Tanner, 2010). Here, assignments that involve planning care for patients with complex needs and for multiple patients are appropriate. These *integrative* clinical experiences prepare students for transition to practice and typically occur toward the end of the program.

The selection of experiences should be consistent with the desired curriculum outcomes, which may be multiple and specific to the nursing program. For example, the expected outcomes for students in an undergraduate degree nursing program are different than those for students in a graduate degree program. Therefore the learning experiences that are selected and the practice opportunities that are provided for students should be congruent with the program outcomes.

Evaluating Experiences

Students are required to demonstrate multiple behaviors in cognitive, psychomotor, and affective domains. Consequently, clinical faculty must evaluate students in each of these areas. The evaluation must be both ongoing (formative evaluation), to assist students in learning, and terminal (summative evaluation), to determine learning outcomes. Constructive and timely feedback, which promotes achievement and growth, is an essential element of evaluation. For a discussion of clinical performance evaluation, refer to Chapter 27.

Scheduling Clinical Practicum Assignments

Although faculty schedule clinical practicum experiences to promote learning, there is ongoing dialogue about the best way to schedule experiences, with emphasis placed on the length of the experiences (hours per day, number of days per week, number of weeks per semester), the timing of the experiences in relation to didactic course assignments, and student needs. Porter and Feller (1979) examined the achievement of baccalaureate nursing students who either had clinical experience in two alternating clinical sites over a 16-week period or had experiences at one site for 8 weeks, followed by experiences at a second site for the last 8 weeks. No differences in scores on National League for Nursing Achievement Tests were found. Similarly, Dunn, Stockhausen, Thornton, and Barnard (1995) reported that no differences in clinical learning outcomes occurred when clinical assignments occurred either 1 or 2 days per week or in alternating 2-week blocks of time. Often students reported being frustrated by nonsequential clinical experiences because of the inability to form relationships with nursing staff and mentioned that they might provide an intervention in the morning but never are at clinical long enough to evaluate the effectiveness of that intervention. Schools are now rethinking the length of the clinical day and the need to experience a typical nurse's daily schedule.

When the learning goal is to integrate students into a clinical setting or when the students are working with a preceptor, students may work the same shift as the nurse with whom they are paired. Some acute care hospitals have a 12-hour shift option while others have only 12-hour shifts. Giving students the opportunity to work the 12-hour shift affords the full scope of practice in any given nurse's day. Students are able to quickly see and experience the role of the nurse. In one small study of senior nursing students in a second degree program working a 12-hour shift, Rossen and Fegan (2009) found that benefits included that students felt accepted by staff, had better socialization, and experienced a realistic work environment; disadvantages included decreased teaching time from the faculty.

While a shorter clinical day allows for skill acquisition, there is little time for the development of extensive critical thinking, clinical reasoning, and evaluation of care. According to Miller (2005), it is critical that students have adequate time on any given unit to progress beyond the minimum and to be exposed to the unit's structure, operations, and culture. Additionally, students described positive aspects of the clinical experience as having an experience at a particular organization, the clinical experiences, and the timing of assignments on work and family responsibilities (Dunn et al., 1995).

Although results of research about outcomes and student satisfaction with timing and scheduling of clinical experiences offer some guidance, faculty also must consider additional variables such as availability of patients, clinical facilities, course schedules, and student needs. Scheduling can also be influenced by the desire to have concurrent classroom and clinical experiences so that knowledge can be transferred and applied immediately. Clinical scheduling can be further complicated by the need to mesh schedules of students from more than one school of nursing. Thus ideal scheduling may not be a reality.

Effective Clinical Teaching

Clinical teaching involves the careful design of an environment in which students have opportunities to foster mutual respect and support for each other while they are achieving identified learning outcomes. Faculty who teach in practicum environments are the crucial links to successful experiences for students.

Research about clinical teaching over time consistently indicates that effective clinical teachers are clinically competent, know how to teach, have collegial relationships with students and agency staff, and are friendly, supportive, and patient (Hanson & Stenvig, 2008; Oermann, 1996; Sieh & Bell, 1994; Stuebbe, 1990). Morgan and Knox (1987) and Nehring (1990) found that the best clinical teachers exhibit expert clinical skills and judgment. Skills such as these have been described by students as being particularly important. Students tend to describe effective clinical teachers as those who demonstrate nursing competence in a real situation.

Being knowledgeable and being able to share knowledge with students in clinical settings are essential. Such knowledge includes an understanding of the theories and concepts related to the practice of nursing. Equally important is an ability to convey the knowledge in an understandable manner. Karuhije (1997) directs attention to three discrete teaching domains that will facilitate acquisition of the teaching skills needed to foster success in clinical settings: instructional, interpersonal, and evaluative. *Instructional* refers to approaches or strategies used to facilitate a transfer of knowledge from didactic to practicum. Strategies may include questioning and peer or patient teaching. Faculty should be cognizant that the type of questions can cover a range during exchanges with students. Faculty should also be mindful of the manner in which questions are constructed in order to facilitate positive effects on learning. Questions that ask students to analyze information result in more learning than simple recall. In clinical practice, factors such as the nature of the situation and available time are likely to influence the types of questions raised. Refer to Box 18-1 for examples.

Effective clinical teaching requires educators to facilitate students as they learn clinical reasoning skills. Clinical reasoning is a process that enables an individual to collect data, solve problems, and make decisions and judgments to provide quality nursing care in the workplace. Effective and efficient clinical reasoning requires knowledge, skills, and abilities grounded in reflection; is supported by an individual's capacity for self-regulation; and leads to the development of expertise (Kuiper, Pesut, & Kautz, 2009). Clinical reasoning occurs when an individual has the ability to reason

---

BOX 18-1 Guidelines for Questioning

Questions may fall in one of the listed categories. Their use should be guided by the need in a given situation. For example, if the need is for

1. Fact: Ask who, what, when, where, and how questions.
2. Interpretation: Ask questions that help students organize facts and ideas and discover relationships, such as compare and contrast.
3. Analysis: Ask questions that help students clarify reasoning. For example, what is your reason for thinking that? Share it with me.
4. Synthesis: Ask questions that help students come to a conclusion. For example, what decisions would you make? Tell me about the decision you would make.
5. Evaluation: Ask questions that help you make informed judgments based on a given standard. For example, what standards (criteria) would you (or did you) use to evaluate your action?
6. Application: Ask questions that help students use knowledge from one situation in another situation. For example, how would you apply this rule to situation A? Or, to your performance?

---

the details of a particular clinical situation. It is believed that students struggle with the ability to make sound judgments. The novice student does not have the ability to identify the subtle or relevant cues seen in a patient whose health condition is changing and for whom complications are beginning to occur. Faculty can assist students in identifying these subtle and relevant cues and start to collaborate with other health care professionals to provide the interventions needed to eliminate or treat these complications. See Box 18-2.

Interpersonal refers to relationships and interactions. *Evaluative* relates to making determinations about performance and achievement of goals. Feedback and debriefing are means for making these determinations.

Feedback, an essential element in teaching and learning, is described as information communicated to students as a result of an assessment of an action by students (Bonnel, 2008). Feedback, when properly delivered, has a high potential for learning and achievement. In clinical practice where assessments need to be made about the extent to which clinical competencies are met, clinical faculty have a variety of opportunities to offer feedback in response to performance behaviors relating to psychomotor as well as cognitive and affective actions. Regardless of the action, there are key considerations that should be practiced. These considerations are *specificity*, *timing*, *consistency*, *continuity*, and *approach*. Approach is important because of its capacity to alleviate anxiety and enhance engagement. Refer to Boxes 18-3, 18-4, 18-5, and 18-6 for information about the delivery of feedback.

Because of the variations in needs of students, each clinical experience provides opportunities for feedback. It is imperative that feedback not be given

---

BOX 18-2 Clinical Reasoning

Subtle Changes and Complications	Relevant "Cues"	Anticipated Collaborative Interventions	Anticipated Outcomes

Pulmonary edema	• Breath sounds (crackles, wheezing)
	• Coughing
	• BiOx % decreased
	• PaO_2 decreased
	• Shortness of breath
	• Cyanosis
	• Tachypnea
	• Orthopnea
	• Anxiety
	• Accessory muscle use
	• Blood-tinged sputum
	• Hypertension or hypotension
		• Semi- or high Fowler's position
		• Implement call orders related to low O_2
		• Using SBAR, contact physician to obtain orders
		• Anticipate the following:
		  • Diuretic: i.e., Lasix
		  • Chest X-ray
		  • Decrease IV fluids
		  • Give K+ if low
			• Decreased shortness of breath
			• Increase BiOx and PaO_2
			• Normotensive
			• Increased U/O
			• No accessory muscle use
			• Clear breath sounds
			• No arrhythmias associated with low K+

BOX 18-3 Descriptions of Domains of Teaching–Learning Actions and Components of Feedback

Domain	Description	Components across Domains
Cognitive	Actions indicative of critical thinking, reasoning, and judgment. Requires a knowledge base.	Specificity: Be clear and specific about the need for feedback with the realization that there may be a strong interrelation among the domains. Refer to student questions in teacher assessment. Research has demonstrated the value of specificity.
Psychomotor	Actions related to the performance of clinical procedures and tasks. Requires an integration of skill performance and effective communication and evidence of knowledge and thinking.	Time: Offer feedback as close to actions (or inactions) as possible. Timeliness has been documented to enhance learning effect. Delaying feedback—for example, by a week or until formal conference time (formative, summative)—will not have the same learning effect. Consistency: Offer feedback whenever a need is evident. Continuous: Offer feedback for exemplary as well as problem areas on an ongoing basis. Approach: The approach can be multiple depending on time constraints, nature of the situation, busyness, needs of other students, and available support. Always deliver the positive message first.
Affective	Actions related to feelings and attitudes. Requires application of principles of effective communication, caring, and concern.	Use approaches that can capture students' evidence of knowledge and critical reasoning. Use teacher behaviors that enhance learning and reduce anxiety—for example, caring, encouragement, and respect (for student and patient). Be engaging. Actively involve students. Provide opportunities for students to reflect and think as feedback is offered. For example, reflect on the situation and share what you think you did exceptionally well. Now, what are some areas for improvement? What was missing? Other considerations: Locale and environment for feedback. Offer feedback in an environment that exemplifies respect for both students and patients. Provide as much privacy as the environment will allow. The requirement is to move away from the patient's view and high-traffic areas.

BOX 18-4 Assessing Students

1. What did the student do or say, or not do or say?
2. How did the student perform?
3. Were application of principles of the specific task evident?
4. Was there evidence of critical thinking?
5. Was there congruency between verbal and nonverbal behaviors and communication?
6. What positives did I observe and hear?
7. Did the student verbalize learning?
8. Did the student indicate plans for preventing "a repeat"?

BOX 18-5 Teacher Assessment for Feedback

1. What did I observe and hear?
2. Was I specific and clear with the message?
3. When can I offer feedback?
4. What is the best time?
5. Where is the best place?
6. How should the feedback be framed?
7. Did I demonstrate each of the principles?
8. Did I offer the student a positive message first?
9. Did the manner of providing feedback exhibit caring, concern, and encouragement?
10. Was the message facilitating?

---

only at documented scheduled times for formative and summative evaluations. Faculty should be cognizant of those actions that require immediate interaction and those for which feedback can be delayed until a short time, but not too much, later. Methods must be identified to maintain data for timely sharing with students, for example, making brief written or electronic anecdotal or mental notes. The delivery of feedback can take multiple forms and will depend on the situation. Face-to-face, time-sensitive, brief conferences (e.g., a few minutes) or electronic conversations or dialogue are examples.

BOX 18-6 Application of Feedback Principles

Scenario: Student performs a simple or complex task without explaining it to or communicating with the patient.

"The procedure was performed perfectly. However, there was no communication with the patient during the procedure. Reflect on your performance and share with me what you could have communicated to the patient."

If the student is able to identify missing elements, respond positively and move forward.

Failure of the student to identify missing elements may require further questioning in a supportive way. It may be necessary to consider a different strategy, such as providing a brief written resource for the student to read or directing the student to an Internet resource. Continue the discussion after the reading is complete.

Engage in a conversation about goals for the future in relation to future performance.

Regardless of the method of delivery, guiding principles must be applied and the learning intent of feedback should be provided. Knowing how to give feedback regarding clinical performance and written clinical assignments is an important element of teaching. One method is to point out positive aspects of performance as well as areas that require improvement (see Chapter 27). Some situations may provide an opportune time to role-model. For example, if a student fails to integrate communication while performing a procedure, faculty can fill in the missing words. Such action may (or may not) alert the student to an "aha" learning moment: "I failed to communicate . . . " The faculty interjecting could have a lasting outcome.

Debriefing and guided reflections are forms of feedback often used immediately following a clinical experience, nursing rounds, or presentations to determine the extent to which expectations were met and any areas of concern (Overstreet, 2010). In the process of making determinations, the discussion often evolves into identifying areas needing improvement. While debriefing sessions generally take place in group settings (e.g., in clinical conferences), it is not uncommon for sessions to occur on a one-on-one basis. Faculty may take the lead by posing specific questions and listening to responses to guide further discussion. Students assume an active role in debriefing sessions and can take the lead in initiating the process.

Effective clinical teachers are expected to have expertise in the "art" of teaching. Equally important are teacher behaviors that facilitate learning and support students in their acquisition of nursing skills. There is empirical evidence that correlates specific teaching methods with enhanced student learning. Examples of such methods are use of objectives, effective questioning, and responses to questions. Krichbaum (1994) reported that student learning was significantly related to teacher behaviors, the use of objectives, and the provision of opportunities for practice. Facilitation of cooperative learning, active engagement, and the use of a variety of methods for learning has been reported to be highly effective (Wolf, Bender, Beitz, Wieland, & Vito, 2004). Common examples of cooperative strategies are peer teaching and pairing students for student-to-student instructions. Other effective behaviors include sharing anecdotal notes, being fair in evaluation, and communicating expectations clearly.

Massarweh (1999) contends that teachers can use motivational and critical thinking strategies in practicum settings to promote learning. Motivational strategies "foster increased productivity, vision, direction and excitement for the profession" (p. 45). Included among motivational strategies are discussing semester goals and relating them to the practicum arena, exhibiting enthusiasm about the profession, discerning student expectations, establishing reward systems, and trying new and different teaching strategies. Strategies that facilitate thinking modalities also include logic models (Ellermann, Kataoka-Yahiro, & Wong, 2006), case studies (Delpier, 2006), and concept mapping. A review of empirical studies of concept mapping indicates that this strategy improves students' critical thinking abilities and academic performance (Clayton, 2006). The above strategies can be used in the classroom as a way to prepare students for clinical practice and to bridge the gap between didactic courses and clinical learning experiences.

Teacher behaviors relating to interpersonal skills are reported to affect student outcomes. Behaviors such as showing respect for students and treating students with respect (Pardo, 1991), correcting mistakes without belittling (Sieh & Bell, 1994), and being supportive and understanding are reported to be effective. An additional point relates to teacher availability. In a study by Hanson and Smith (1996), students expressed the belief that teachers who were emotionally and physically available were able to facilitate students becoming an important part in the relationship.

Nursing students experience stress and anxiety in clinical learning situations (Elliott, 2002; Lo, 2002; Timmins & Kaliszer, 2002). Negative relationships with faculty can contribute to anxiety (Kleehammer, Hart, & Keck, 1990). The effective clinical teacher recognizes students' need for supportive and collegial relationships and develops an interpersonal style that promotes a collegial learning environment (Halstead, 1996). A safe learning environment has been created when students feel comfortable in speaking openly (Massarweh, 1999). Positive relationships are nurturing and can enhance learning. Caring behaviors and a caring environment are also essential.

The literature points to the importance of building relationships between students and teachers. It is believed that the quality of their interaction affects learning outcomes (Tanner, 2005). Concepts that facilitate the building of relationships may include the following: connections, caring, compassion, mutual knowing, trusting and respecting, availability, knowledge, confidence, and communicating (Gillespie, 2002). By knowing the students, faculty are prevented from making assumptions and eventually acting on them. Assumptions are perceived by students as being disrespectful. Making connections early in the relationship assists faculty in determining the elements needed to meet students' learning needs (Hanson & Smith, 1996).

Teacher confidence is another factor that enhances learning, and it is believed that teachers who lack confidence actually create distance between themselves and the students they teach (Crandall, 1993; Nehring, 1990). This hinders the sense of knowing and the possible connections that may have formed. A part of teacher confidence is foundation of knowledge. When clinical teachers use their expertise to support learning, the teacher–student relationship is strengthened.

Cook (2005) engaged in a study to explore perceptions of teacher behaviors that invite trust and student anxiety. The findings indicate that teachers need to be aware of how their behaviors can be negatively perceived by students, thus influencing the anxiety that occurs during the clinical experience and ultimately affecting learning. Senior clinical faculty should serve as role models and mentor junior clinical faculty to create a legacy of effective clinical teaching. Additional characteristics of effective teachers are listed in Box 18-7.

BOX 18-7 Characteristics of Effective Clinical Teachers

1. Create an environment that is conductive to learning that requires:
   - Knowledge of the practice area.
   - Clinical competence.
   - Knowledge of how to teach.
   - A desire to teach.
2. Be supportive of learners. Such support requires:
   - Knowledge of the learners.
   - Knowledge of the practice area.
   - Mutual respect.
3. Possess teaching skills that maximize student learning. This requires an ability to:
   - Diagnose student needs.
   - Learn about students as individuals, including their needs, personalities, and capabilities.
4. Foster independence and accountability so that students learn how to learn.
5. Encourage exploration and questions without penalty.
6. Accept differences among students.
7. Relate how clinical experiences facilitate the development of clinical competence.
8. Possess effective communication and question skills.
9. Serve as a role model.
10. Enjoy nursing and teaching.
11. Be friendly, approachable, understanding, enthusiastic about teaching, and confident with teaching.
12. Be knowledgeable about the subject matter and be able to convey that knowledge to students in their practice areas.
13. Exhibit fairness in evaluation.
14. Provide frequent feedback.

Preparing Faculty for Clinical Teaching

The preparation and development of faculty for clinical teaching are not as widely discussed and documented as the preparation of students for clinical learning. The need for such preparation and development is being voiced. Krautscheid, Kaakinen, and Warner (2008) indicate that the exposure of faculty to evidence-based teaching strategies and learning theory is minimal. As a result, these colleagues directed efforts to facilitate a reversal in this trend. A clinical faculty development program, developed to help faculty practice teaching by analogy and reflect on clinical teaching, was implemented. With this program, clinical teaching simulations were used to allow faculty to practice, teach, and receive immediate feedback. Scenarios were used to facilitate the process. Findings developed from participation in the scenarios were limited. However, significant outcomes from these engagements were faculty reports of being more reflective as teachers and practitioners and a realization of the value of simulation in facilitating learning in a safe practice environment, thus enhancing the ability of faculty to facilitate clinical learning in effective ways.

Expert clinicians often have a desire to teach in the practicum area. Some have been preceptors and believe that, to make the transition to a new role as clinical teachers, they need further instruction and guidance. Because clinical teaching is an acclaimed role, the desire can become a reality. Universities are challenged to meet the learning needs of new clinical faculty, especially those who maintain full-time clinical practices. These individuals should be encouraged and provided with information about where and how they can engage in activities that will facilitate their acquisition of the knowledge and skills required for the roles. Some schools have developed modules for that purpose.

One method for meeting the challenge of educating clinical teachers is to use an online course to orient clinicians who are making the transition from the role of expert clinician to that of clinical teacher (Vinten, Kost, & Chalko, 2003). Jarret, Horner, Center, and Kane (2008) developed a classroom curriculum to prepare staff nurses to serve as clinical faculty. The curriculum included topics such as teaching–learning theory, critical thinking, how to deal with challenging students, and making patient assignments. Because being an excellent clinical nurse does not mean that the nurse will be an excellent teacher, Cangelosi, Crocker, and Sorrell (2009) developed a Clinical Nurse Educator Academy to prepare clinicians for clinical teaching. After analyzing reflective papers at the end of the academy, the authors found that the nurses were enthusiastic about the educator role, but that the frustration from lack of mentoring indicates a need for ongoing development of the educator role.

In summary, effective clinical teachers are knowledgeable and know how to convey concepts to students in effective ways, are clinically competent, exhibit interpersonal skills that positively influence students' learning, and establish collegial relationships that often last well beyond a specific course or program. Clinical faculty also need to be oriented to and developed for the role. Research is likely to continue in this area.

Preparing Students for Patient Care

Teaching for patient care should involve orderly and logical actions taken to accomplish particular educational goals. The actual selection and use of a particular strategy should be based on expected outcomes, principles of learning, and learner needs. This section focuses on several strategies commonly used in clinical teaching: patient care assignments, clinical conferences, nursing rounds, and written assignments.

Students come to the health care environment not really understanding the culture of confidentiality. It is imperative that students know and understand the Health Insurance Portability and Accountability Act of 1996 (HIPAA) privacy and security regulations. It is the role of faculty to instruct students on the need to implement the HIPAA rules and regulations in all patient encounters. They are designed to protect the patient's right to privacy. Students should be informed of what they can and cannot do in relation to confidentiality, and these instructions must be enforced.

Patient Care Assignments

Patient care provides students with opportunities to integrate, synthesize, and use previously learned knowledge and skills. Some nursing courses require students to prepare in advance for their clinical experience. Advance preparation commences with making clinical assignments, which may be the responsibility of the clinical teacher, the teacher and student together (especially useful for beginning students), the student alone, the student with guidance from the teacher, or the nursing and health care staff or preceptors. When students are permitted some input into selecting clinical assignments, this encourages them to be self-directed as well as to choose experience on the basis of their personal learning needs. Refer to Box 18-8.

The selection of clinical assignments by students in collaboration with others has several benefits. It provides opportunities for students to select experiences that are based on personal learning needs, to experience a degree of control over their education,

BOX 18-8 Tips for Making Assignments

New faculty often are at a loss in knowing where to begin. The following tips should assist new faculty to enhance their comfort level in implementing this task.

- Come to the unit with knowledge of specific student needs.
- Have an assignment sheet with a list of the students for the given day.
- Get input from those in charge and from the staff nurses.
- Talk to the nurse in charge and ask for brief suggestions about the patients on the unit. This simple act of communication is one way to build a trusting, supportive relationship with the staff on the unit, as they can be very helpful in guiding what patients will make for a good assignment.
- Make rounds and talk to all of the patients and family you plan to care for on the following day. Just a few minutes chatting can assist you in deciding whether a patient will be appropriate for a student nurse.
- Obtain patient and family permission, as this may prevent early morning assignment changes because a patient refuses to have a student.
- Consider the specialty on your particular unit. Knowing the patient population will help determine when to make assignments. For example, if it is a surgical unit, you may want to make assignment later in the afternoon because patients may be admitted late to the unit following surgery. If you make an assignment too early, you may risk the problem of a patient being reassigned to a different unit or discharged.
- Be sure that students know who the charge nurse is in case the assignments need revision when faculty are not available. Establishing a protocol for this will lessen frustration among the staff.
- Always have a "backup plan." Add a couple of extra patients to the assignment sheet in case something changes when faculty are not available.

and to interact with practicing professionals during the process of selecting experiences. The extent to which students are permitted to self-select experiences depends on the goals or expected outcomes of the program, the philosophy of the specific clinical teacher, and the availability of resources in the clinical environment to assist students (i.e., to answer questions and provide guidance in patient selection).

Involvement of the clinical faculty is important when students select their experiences. For example,

faculty serve as resource advisers and sources of emotional support, communicate goals and intended outcomes, assist students in assessing the congruency between personal learning needs and course objectives, facilitate planning the experiences, collaborate with students as they strive to meet goals, and evaluate accomplishments. Making clinical assignments can be a challenge for clinical faculty. Novice faculty are often at a loss in terms of knowing where to begin. This is where the services of senior-level or expert faculty would be helpful.

Strategies for Implementing Clinical Assignments

Clinical assignments are an integral part of nursing practicum experiences. Several strategies for making clinical assignments have been adopted for clinical teaching. The strategy used in clinical instruction is often determined by factors such as the skill level of the student, the patient acuity level, the number of assigned students, and the availability of patients and resources, including the availability of technology. *Traditional* and *alternative strategies*, such as dual assignments, multiple assignments, and clinical conferencing, are discussed.

The *traditional strategy* is one in which nursing students are taught in a clinical setting with a varying faculty-to-student ratio. Ratios ranging from 1:8 to 1:10 are recommended (Schuster, Fitzgerald, McCarthy, & McDougal, 1997). The rationale for these ratios relates to the impact of increased numbers of students on patient safety (Becker & Neuwirth, 2002). From a student's perspective, this strategy involves the assignment of one student to one or two patients. The students assume responsibility for the nursing interventions needed in the care of the patient and may work alone in planning, implementing, and evaluating nursing activities.

There are two *alternatives* to the traditional method of clinical assignment: dual and multiple. The *dual assignment* strategy (Fugate & Rebeschi, 1991; Gotschall & Thompson, 1990) involves assigning two students to one patient. This alternative is useful when the level or complexity of care is beyond the capabilities of one student (deTornyay & Thompson, 1987). Because students must work closely to implement care, collaboration and communication between the students are requisites for effective use of this strategy. Refer to Box 18-9 for

---

> ### BOX 18-9 Benefits of Dual Assignments
>
> - An opportunity to further develop communication and time management skills
> - Opportunities to evaluate and improve skills in organization
> - Increased opportunities for faculty to assess the capabilities of each student and provide feedback
> - Opportunities for collaboration
> - Decreased number of patients for which the faculty member is responsible
> - Decreased level of anxiety among students

---

benefits that can be derived from the use of the dual assignment strategy (Meisenhelder, 1987).

When dual assignments are made, faculty have the responsibility of assuring that each student understands his or her specific responsibility. For 2-day clinical rotations, roles may be reversed on the second day of care (Gotschall & Thompson, 1990). Such reversal makes it possible for both students to direct care to the patient.

The strategy of *multiple assignments* is useful for beginning students and in situations where a limited number of patients are available. This strategy involves the assignment of three students per patient. Three roles are assumed: the doer, who provides the care; the information gatherer or researcher, who is responsible for obtaining information needed for the safe care of the patient; and the observer, who observes the student, the researcher, the student–patient interactions, the responses of the patient to his or her care, and the family members (VanDenBerg, 1976). The observer also makes suggestions for improving care. As with dual assignments, the roles for each student must be clearly defined. Adequate time must be made available for collaboration and discussion among students and faculty.

The multiple assignment approach must meet learning objectives. Glanville (1971) conducted a study to determine the effectiveness of this method as an approach to clinical teaching. Results revealed similarity in the extent to which objectives were met and in the levels of achievement for students assigned to the multiple assignment approach and those assigned to the traditional method. VanDenBerg (1976) randomly assigned 22 first-year associate degree students to two groups, traditional and multiple assignments.

Results showed that students assigned to the multiple assignment group demonstrated a significant increase in nursing knowledge compared to those assigned to the traditional group.

In light of the increasing complexity of learning environments and the instability of the patient census, consistent clinical assignments and multiple placement assignments were compared to determine learning outcomes (Adams, 2002). Here, *consistent* means that students were assigned to a unit for a specific time frame or used more than one unit during the period. Quantitative measures revealed no difference in the two methods of clinical rotation. However, the perceptions of the benefit of consistent clinical assignments were positive.

In summary, faculty, staff, and students play a significant role in determining assignments. Assignments are made according to a number of factors, including course objectives, learner needs, skill level, complexity of the clinical environment, and patients' acuity. The assignments may be implemented as solo or multistudent experiences. Each has been considered beneficial in enhancing learning.

Clinical Conferences

Clinical conferences are group learning experiences that are an integral part of the clinical experience. The use of clinical conferences in nursing is common. Conferences can provide meaningful learning experiences and excellent opportunities for students to bridge the gap between theory and practice. Through conferences students can develop critical thinking and clinical decision-making skills (Wink, 1995) and acquire confidence in their ability to express themselves with clarity and logic.

Successful clinical conferences are planned. Plans for conferences should take into consideration the curriculum and the learner. An identification of the purpose, topic, process, strategies, and methods of evaluation are essential if the teacher is to be instrumental in bridging the gap between theory and clinical practice.

Types of Conferences

The conferences can include traditional preclinical, midclinical, and postclinical conferencing. As a result of advancing technology, conferences may take place through electronic media. As such, the rules and regulations related to HIPAA and the Health Information Technology for Economic and Clinical Health (HITECH) Act apply to clinical groups that use clinical conferencing by electronic media. Student groups must be aware of maintaining patient confidentiality as the group presents patient data by electronic means. Using this form of conferencing is a means of using technology while supporting the needs of students. Some may be doing clinical assignments at different sites and electronic conferencing brings students together where debriefing can occur without having to travel to a central location.

Traditional Conferences

Preclinical, midclinical, and *postclinical conferences* by nature are small group discussion periods that immediately precede, occur during, or follow a clinical experience. Each provides opportunities for discussion. In preclinical conferences, students share information about upcoming experiences, ask questions, express concerns, and seek clarification about plans for care. Preclinical conferences also provide opportunities for faculty to correct student misconceptions, identify problem areas, assess student thinking, and identify student readiness to implement care.

Midclinical conferencing, in contrast to preclinical and postclinical conferencing, is another form of gathering students together to provide some form of midclinical debriefing. It has been found that, while doing a 12-hour clinical day, this gives students an opportunity to gather to share pertinent patient information and plan for further interventions, which may include patient teaching and discharge planning. This midclinical conference time also may help students collectively evaluate the efficacy of prior patient interventions. This exchange of data, in the form of a midconference, is a method of imparting knowledge and sharing common data with the intent of positively affecting patient care.

Postclinical conferences provide a forum in which students and faculty can discuss the clinical experiences, share information, analyze clinical situations, clarify relationships, identify problems, ventilate feelings, and develop support systems. In postclinical conferences there is interaction between the teacher and the students, which offers both a medium for learning and an exchange resulting in meaningful experiences.

Online Conferences

Online conferencing, occurring before or after clinical experiences, can assist students to come together in a virtual environment to exchange ideas, solve problems, discuss alternatives, and acquire information about issues of clinical care that occurred before or during the clinical experience (Vinten & Partridge, 2002). See Chapter 22 for further discussion of teaching in online learning communities.

Student and Faculty Roles during Conferences

Both students and faculty have specific roles in conferences. Student should be made aware of their role as active participants. As such, they should defend choices of care, clarify points of view, explore alternatives, and practice decision making. A student may also assume the role of group leader. Faculty serve as conference facilitators by facilitating behaviors identified in Box 18-10. As conferences are facilitated, efforts should be made to ask higher-level questions that assist students in applying knowledge to clinical situations (Wink, 1993). Conferences also provide opportunities for students to apply group processes and develop team-building skills.

Evaluating the Conferences

Conferences should be evaluated in light of their effectiveness and goal accomplishment. The teacher should obtain and provide feedback regarding the

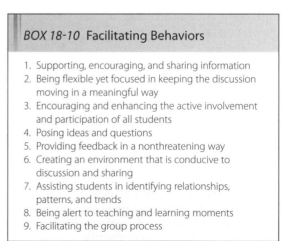

BOX 18-10 Facilitating Behaviors

1. Supporting, encouraging, and sharing information
2. Being flexible yet focused in keeping the discussion moving in a meaningful way
3. Encouraging and enhancing the active involvement and participation of all students
4. Posing ideas and questions
5. Providing feedback in a nonthreatening way
6. Creating an environment that is conducive to discussion and sharing
7. Assisting students in identifying relationships, patterns, and trends
8. Being alert to teaching and learning moments
9. Facilitating the group process

extent to which goals were accomplished, the effectiveness of the teaching methods or strategies, and the degree of learning achieved. The data from the evaluation can be used for planning future conferences.

In summary, traditional and electronic conferences play a significant role in facilitating students' learning. Conferences afford opportunities for enhancing critical thinking, clinical reasoning, and decision-making skills; for creating new meaning for care issues; and for enhancing group process and team-building skills. Successful conferences are planned. Inherent in planning are identifying the purpose, selecting topics, selecting teaching methods, and conducting and evaluating these methods.

Complementary Experiences

Nursing Grand Rounds

The practice of nursing grand rounds is a teaching strategy that uses the patients' bedside for direct, purposeful experiences. These experiences may involve demonstration, interview, or discussion of patient problems and nursing care. Rounds also afford an excellent opportunity for the exchange of ideas about patient care situations, which may involve clinical faculty, students, and staff.

The use of rounds as a teaching strategy requires planning. Planning includes obtaining permission from the patient and providing information about the nature of the rounds and the role the patient will play. After the session, patient participation should be acknowledged and some form of debriefing should occur, including planning for subsequent rounds.

Written Assignments

Written assignments generally complement clinical experiences and are considered to be useful in that they facilitate development of critical thinking and clinical reasoning and they promote an understanding of content. Such assignments may include short papers, clinical reasoning papers, nursing care plans, clinical logs, journals, and concept maps. Findings from research on the use of clinical logs indicate that their use provides opportunities for students to reflect on clinical experiences, communicate with the teacher, identify mistakes and

negative experiences, and learn from these experiences (Sedlak, 1992).

It is believed that faculty value assignments related to narrative writing that reflects on evaluating practice. According to Benner et al. (2010), narrative or first-person journaling is a means of chronicling clinical discoveries and areas of growth in the cognitive or psychomotor domains. Students articulate where learning has occurred or possibly where there are knowledge gaps. Some of the journaling questions may focus on those found in Box 18-11. These questions support a form of self-debriefing of the clinical day. Often journaling is not given an assigned grade but is assessed for completion. Faculty give students written feedback on the journaling, which allows for clarification and learning to occur.

Web-Based Technology

Electronic technology is increasingly being used to support clinical teaching. For example, online clinical courses have been designed to assist faculty with facilitating the development of clinical knowledge among students. Technology has been used to integrate content such as communication, collaboration, coaching, and cognitive strategies. Several advantages have been identified. Online discussions and live chat rooms promote peer support, idea sharing, and clarification of concepts. Students have opportunities to make inquiries about performance, thoughts, feelings, and experiences through the use of e-journals and e-boards, thus supporting reflection. Faculty can identify learning needs, misconceptions, and faulty patterns of critical thinking or clinical reasoning and judgment.

BOX 18-11 Sample of Journaling Questions

- What was the best part of your clinical day?
- If you could do your clinical day over, what would you do differently?
- What were you most concerned about as related to your patient's care?
- What goals do you have for your next clinical day?
- How did you feel about your clinical day?

Clinical Cases, Unfolding Case Studies, Scenarios, and Simulations

Simulated experiences that provide opportunities for students to integrate psychomotor, critical thinking, and clinical reasoning decision-making skills are equally valuable in assisting students to critically evaluate their own actions and reflect on skills. The use of the high-fidelity human patient simulator (HPS) is one example of using realistic scenarios to prepare students for clinical experiences, substitute for unavailable or unpredictable clinical experiences, or enhance clinical experiences in a safe environment. The use of HPS helps transition the student from the classroom to the practicum environment. Students' learning with the HPS method can be enhanced, patient care can be optimized, and patient safety can be improved. Additional benefits may include enhanced learning in a risk-free environment, promotion of interactive learning, repeated practice of skills, and immediate faculty or tutor feedback. (See Chapter 20 for additional discussion.) Cases, unfolding case studies, and scenarios are lower-fidelity strategies but equally helpful in preparing students for clinical experiences and bridging the gap between classroom and practice (Benner et al., 2010; Delpier, 2006).

Point-of-Care Technology

Nurses are increasingly using handheld devices, electronic health records, and other point-of-care technologies in the clinical setting, and faculty must provide opportunities for students to become familiar with their use. Simulated electronic health records can be embedded in clinical simulations as preparation for their use in the clinical agency or as a substitute for learning when agency policy precludes students' use of them in the agency. Personal digital assistants (PDAs) and smart phones equipped with reference software enable access to clinical information, care plans, and nursing, procedure, and evidence-based practice guidelines, and can provide access to skills videos and patient teaching materials (Zurmehly, 2010). In one study on the use of PDAs (Bauldoff, Kirkpatrick, Sheets, Mays, & Curran, 2008), faculty found that students who used PDAs were more confident in their knowledge and administered drugs more safely; they also appreciated not having to carry heavy textbooks. When using point-of-care technology in the clinical agency, faculty must assure compliance with HIPPA and other agency policies (White., 2005).

Models for Clinical Education

Several models for clinical education are used to educate nursing students. These models, alternatives to the traditional model, include preceptorship, associate model, paired model, academia–service partnerships, and adjunct faculty joint appointments. These models have evolved to increase capacity for clinical placements, manage faculty shortages, prepare graduates to be competent for practice, and foster closer ties with clinical agencies (Delunas & Rooda, 2009; Murray, Crain, Meyer, McDonough, & Schweiss, 2010; Neiderhauser, Macintyre, Garner, Teel, & Murray, 2010). Given the diversity of health care settings, faculty shortage, and the need for reduced faculty-to-student ratios, these models serve to enhance effective student learning, facilitate development of clinical skills, and promote role development.

Preceptorship

Preceptorship is a teaching model in which the student is assigned a nurse who serves as a preceptor. Preceptors are experienced nurses who facilitate and evaluate student learning in the clinical area over a specified time frame. Their role is intentionally implemented in conjunction with other responsibilities. The preceptor model is based on the assumption that a consistent one-on-one relationship provides opportunities for socialization into practice and bridges the gap between theory and practice. The preceptor model may be used at several levels. However, it is considered to be particularly useful for senior-level students and graduate students in advanced practice roles. Use at these levels provides opportunities for students to synthesize theoretical knowledge and apply information, including evidence-based research, in the practice environment. This method is also an excellent way for students to practice collaboration.

Theoretically, the preceptor provides one-on-one teaching, guidance, and support and serves as a role model. In one model (Billings, Jeffries, Rowles, Stone, & Urden, 2002) the preceptor, faculty, and student form a triad to facilitate the student's acquisition of clinical competencies. The preceptor may be assigned to a student on the basis of shared learning needs. The preceptor and student meet before the first clinical experience to discuss learning styles and goals for competency attainment and the desired outcome of the clinical experience. Although faculty have ultimate responsibility for the course and students' learning outcomes, the student and preceptor are empowered to conduct formative and summative evaluations of the student's clinical performance and learning outcomes. In the Integrative Clinical Preceptor Model (Mallette, Laury, Engelke & Andrews, 2005), the student assumes a proactive role, not only as a student, but also as a member of the health care team. In this model, the preceptor assumes responsibilities as a clinical teacher, mentor, and role model, while faculty serve as a role model and facilitator for the preceptor and the student as well as a consultant.

Preceptors are expected to be clinical experts, to be willing to teach, and to be able to teach effectively (Wright, 2002). Benefits that have been derived from preceptorships include enhanced ability to apply theory to practice, improvement in psychomotor skills, increased self-confidence (Letizia & Jennrich, 1998), and improved socialization (Collins, Hilde, & Shriver, 1993). Attributes of an effective preceptor are listed in Box 18-12.

In a preceptorship, the role of the nursing faculty is not lost. Preceptors and faculty work in a close relationship (Hsieh & Knowles, 1990). Faculty provide the link between practice and education. In providing this link, faculty monitor how well the students complete assignments and accomplish outcomes. Evaluation is a collaborative responsibility of faculty, students, and preceptors.

The use of preceptors requires that planning be done to ensure an understanding of their role. Ideally this is facilitated through strategically planned orientation and follow-up sessions; some schools of nursing offer workshops or courses to orient preceptors to their role (Smedley & Penney, 2009). These sessions provide a forum for sharing information related to the philosophical perspectives of preceptorship, expected outcomes, teaching strategies, and methods of evaluation.

Since roles change for faculty, students, and preceptors, all require orientation to new roles (Mallette et al., 2005; Trevitt, Graslish, & Reaby, 2001). One reported project included the use of two self-paced learning modules, one for students and one for preceptors, and a video. The reported outcome was that both students and preceptors felt more prepared for the experience.

The value of the preceptor model is generally related to providing a sense of independence for patient care and promotion of a sense of satisfaction. Satisfaction from the perspective of clinical faculty has been reported as positive (Zerbe & Lachat, 1991). Satisfaction is also reported as occurring on the part of the preceptor and the clinical agency that stands to benefit from hiring a well-prepared graduate (Happell, 2009). In one study (Wieland, Altmiller, Dorr, & Wolf, 2007), students, preceptors, and faculty reported that the students' knowledge and skills improved during the pregraduation practicum and that many of the students became integrated into the clinical agency's teams.

Clinical Teaching Associate

The clinical teaching associate (CTA) model involves a staff nurse who collaborates with a designated faculty member and instructs a specified number of students in the clinical area (Baird, Bopp, Schofer, Langenberg, & Matheis-Kraft, 1994; DeVoogd & Salbenblatt, 1989; Phillips & Kaempfer, 1987). Teaching responsibilities are assumed by the CTA, who also serves as a resource person and role model. A faculty member serves as lead teacher and is responsible for supervision and evaluation of clinical learning experiences, including assignment of grades and

---

BOX 18-12 Attributes of an Effective Preceptor

1. Knowledge of the patient care area
2. Effective communication skills (verbal and nonverbal)
3. Experience in a particular clinical area
4. Ability to relate to health care personnel and client
5. Honesty
6. Effective decision-making skills
7. Genuine caring behaviors
8. Leadership skills
9. Interest in professional development

Used with permission from Lewis, K. E. (1986). What it takes to be a preceptor. *The Canadian Nurse/L'infirmière Canadienne, 82*(11), 18–19.

collaboration with the CTA about assignments and experiences.

Results from a survey of nurse managers, CTAs, faculty, and students, conducted to determine the effectiveness of this model, were positive (Baird et al., 1994). Positive comments were presented in terms of student learning. Patient satisfaction with care was reported to be greater than with the traditional model. Nurses in the CTA role reported an increase in student confidence. Faculty reported that students were more relaxed and more self-confident. The effectiveness of the model was reported by students as allowing them to assume increased responsibility in comparison with the traditional model.

Paired Model

The paired model is designed to pair a student and a staff nurse for a practicum experience. It is an alternative to the one-patient, one-student model and is a variation of the preceptor model (Gross, Aysee, & Tracey, 1992). During the course, each student has a specified number of days in a paired relationship. The remaining time is spent acquiring experiences by using the traditional model. The staff nurse plans the learning experience; the faculty member oversees the experiences while creating a learning environment for students. However, most of the faculty member's time is spent in the traditional role with other students who have not been paired. To enhance the effectiveness of the paired model, it is essential that the staffing pattern be evaluated before making assignments.

The paired model has been viewed positively by students, faculty, and staff nurses in the service area. Earlier interaction, a sense of belonging in the practicum environment, feelings of being less anxious, and enhanced learning were reported by students as positive aspects of the model. The reasons for these positive outcomes were related to students being more comfortable in the practicum setting (Gross et al., 1992). Faculty were more effective as teachers. Staff nurses reported being challenged to think. Overall, the relationship between education and service was reported to be strengthened.

Academia–Service Partnerships

The clinical teaching partnership is a collaborative model shared by service and academia settings to enhance mutual goals of developing nurses competent for practice and creating safe practice environments. Partnerships are also formed to create new models of clinical instruction and increase student and faculty capacity in nursing programs (Delunas & Rooda, 2009). Although these partnerships take different forms, they are established collaboratively and result in redesigned clinical education experiences for students and faculty as well as for the nurses at the clinical agency.

In one early partnership model, the service institution shared the resources of nurses, a clinical nurse specialist (CNS), and an academic faculty member (Shah & Pennypacker, 1992). The CNS serves as an adjunct faculty member who provides patient assignments. The academic faculty member schedules the experiences. Jointly they collaborate in evaluating assignments and performance. Communication is reciprocal and essential to the success of this model. The faculty member shares information about problems that may influence students' performance. The CNS keeps the faculty member abreast of current student performance. Both schedule conferences to discuss anecdotal records of students.

Shah and Pennypacker (1992) have identified benefits of the model for the faculty and for the CNS. Benefits for the academic faculty member include increased time to pursue scholarly activities and a direct link with clinical staff for purposes of communication about policy and procedural changes and new equipment. Benefits for the CNS include joint involvement with academic and clinical settings, direct avenues for collaborative projects such as writing and publication, increased involvement in staff development, and satisfaction in observing student development.

Informal feedback from students about this model is positive. Reports indicate that students learned several roles assumed by nurses and different ways of performing clinical skills and that their ability to transfer theory learned in the classroom to clinical practice is enhanced.

Murray et al. (2010) report that students in their partnership model were better integrated into the clinical setting and increased levels of critical thinking and clinical decision making.

Adjunct Faculty

Adjunct faculty are health care professionals who are employed in the service setting and have a part-time academic appointment. Adjunct faculty may assume various roles, including those of preceptor, mentor, guest lecturer, and supervisor. These individuals may also collaborate on research projects. Faculty who are appointed in an adjunct capacity are registered professional nurses or professionals who are experts in areas such as clinical practice, research, leadership, management, legislation, and law.

Dedicated Education Units

Over the past decade, the Dedicated Education Unit (DEU) model has been implemented at various universities across the country (Edgecombe, Wotton, Gonda, & Mason, 1999). Moscato, Miller, Logsdon, Weinberg, and Chorpenning (2007) indicate that the "DEU offers a concrete strategy to more closely connect nursing units and education programs" (p. 32). DEUs involve new partnerships among nurse executives, staff nurses, and faculty for transforming patient care units into environments of support for students and staff nurses while continuing the critical work of providing quality care to acutely ill patients. Wotton and Gonda (2004) believe that the DEU model facilitates stronger relationship-building between nurses in academia and practice. Universities are implementing this strategy in a variety of ways. One Midwest university uses the term *Practice Education Partnership (PEP) units*. Extensive research is under way to measure the effectiveness of this PEP model as a strategy for teaching in the clinical area. The PEP unit is a hospital-based unit designed to provide the student with a strong partnership between the practice and education settings. The PEP model differs from the Australian DEU model in that it works to incorporate the culture of the unit and its clinical specialty into the availability of preceptors, level of patient acuity, and other influences on the education of the student. One of the unique aspects of the PEP model is that there is continuity and consistency among preceptors, faculty, and students as they partner to learn and grow together. Preceptors are coached on preceptor competencies by attending a full-day workshop. It is at this time that the partnership between the nurse and the faculty begins. This partnership is developed over time and ultimately the student learns the role of the nurse and together the student and preceptor provide exceptional patient care.

Residency Models

Recognizing that prelicensure programs may not be sufficient for preparing nurses for practice in complex health care settings, several studies and commissions (Benner et al., 2010; Institute of Medicine, 2010; Tanner, 2010) report on the need for postgraduate residencies and call for their increased use to improve transition to practice and development of leadership and population management skills. One 12-month program designed to develop a more competent nurse is being implemented and tested (American Association of Colleges of Nursing, 2010). Accreditation and regulatory standards have been developed for this approach to residency.

In another model, the residency is designed as a developmental model in which students, for three years, spend a significant portion of the educational experience in coursework, practice (e.g., lab and simulations), and field experiences. A work requirement is also an integral part of the model. In the final (senior) year, students engage in learning in the form of clinical immersions that are dedicated to performance and learning (Diefenbeck, Plowfield, & Herrman, 2006). Progressive in nature, students are admitted as freshmen in the nursing program whereby both nursing courses and science and liberal arts courses are taken. This pattern continues in the sophomore year with the addition of courses such as pathophysiology, research, pharmacology, clinical decision making, and others. Specialty courses are taught in the junior year. In the senior year, the clinical immersion experiences facilitate students' transition to professional practice. Students acquire experiences in specialty areas and are expected to function independently. The senior integration seminar, offered for the length of the final year, covers a wide range of topics, which allows students to have discussions in preparation for transitioning "to the world of work and/or graduate school" (Diefenbeck et al., 2006, p. 5). Field experiences are integral to the model, as is a work requirement. This model is being implemented and the expectation is that indicators will yield data that will provide evidence for its value (Diefenbeck et al., 2006).

Lee, Coakley, Dahlin, and Carleton (2009) have developed another form of residency program. It occurs after graduation and pairs a less experienced nurse with an experienced preceptor. The goal of this program is to enhance the effectiveness of care and improve outcomes for a specific population of patients.

In summary, several models for clinical education of student nurses exist. Alternative models, collaborative in nature, have evolved because of the increasing complexity of the health care environment. Among these models are preceptorships, the teaching associate model, the paired model, clinical teaching partnerships, and adjunct faculty. The nature of each model dictates the level of student that would benefit most. The paired and clinical associate models have been used for beginning students, whereas the preceptorship model is widely used for students in the upper level of their program and for graduate students. Empirical research on the effectiveness of these models has been sparse; there is a need for further evaluation of and research on these models in terms of their effectiveness on student learning and preparation for the workforce.

SUMMARY

Clinical teaching involves student–teacher interaction in experiential clinical situations that take place in diverse and often interdisciplinary practice environments. These environments may include laboratory, acute care, transitional, and community sites, including homeless shelters, clinics, schools, camps, and social service agencies. Faculty must have in-depth knowledge of behaviors that facilitate students' learning and development and have complete knowledge of the culture of the practice area as well as the health care provider. Effective clinical teachers are able to plan, facilitate, and evaluate experiences using instructive, interpersonal, and evaluative strategies. These strategies facilitate faculty's acquisition of the knowledge and skills required to become nurses.

A variety of teaching methods can be used to enable students to achieve desired outcomes. Patient assignments, clinical conferences, nursing grand rounds, and written assignments are among these. The skill level of students, patient's acuity level, number of students, and patient care resource availability will affect the method used. Among the models suggested for educating nursing students are the traditional one and alternatives to this model, including preceptorships, clinical teaching associates, teaching partnerships, and adjunct faculty. Information is also shared about a residency model planning, and ongoing contact with preceptors and agency personnel in the practicum setting is crucial to the success of any practicum experience. Practicum experiences prepare students for working in a health care system that is patient-centered. Teaching in the practicum setting blends faculty's clinical expertise with teaching skills to prepare nurses for current and future roles in an ever-changing health care system.

REFLECTING ON THE EVIDENCE

1. Choose a set of clinical teaching strategies for a group of students. What do you need to consider about the student, the setting, and the patients in order to make this decision? What evidence for practice will you draw on to make your decision?

2. What is the role of Internet-based teaching and learning in clinical teaching? Can clinical practice be learned in a fully online course?

3. What is the state of science about clinical teaching? What research questions are being asked? What methods are being used? What variables are included in the studies?

4. What are the best practices that are evidenced-based?

REFERENCES

Adams, V. (2002). Consistent clinical assignment for nursing students compared to multiple placements. *Journal of Nursing Education, 41*(2), 80–85.

American Association of Colleges of Nursing. (2010). UHC/AACN Nurse Residency Programs. Retrieved from http://www.aacn.nche.edu/education/nurseresidency.htm

Baird, S., Bopp, A., Schofer, K., Langenberg, A., & Matheis-Kraft, C. (1994). An innovative model for clinical teaching. *Nursing Educator, 19*(3), 23–25.

Bauldoff, G. S., Kirkpatrick, B., Sheets, D. J., Mays, B., & Curran, C. R. (2008). Implementation of handheld devices. *Nurse Educator, 33*(6), 244–248.

Becker, M., & Neuwirth, J. (2002). Teaching strategy to maximize the clinical experience with beginning nursing students. *Journal of Nursing Education, 41*(2), 89–91.

Benner, P., Sutphen, M., Leonard, V., & Day, L. (2010). *Educating nurses: A call for radical transformation.* San Francisco, CA: Jossey-Bass.

Billings, D. M., Jeffries, P., Rowles, C. J., Stone, C., & Urden, L. (2002). A partnership model of nursing education to prepare critical care nurses. *Excellence in Clinical Practice, 3*(4), 3.

Bonnel, W. J. (2008). Improving feedback to students in online courses. *Nursing Education Perspectives, 29*(5), 290–294.

White, A. Allen, P., Goodwin, L.,Breckinridge, D., Dowell, J., & Garvey, R. (2005). Infusing PDA technology into nursing education. *Nurse Educator, 30*(4) 150–154.

Bremner, M. N., Aduddell, K., Bennett, D. N., & VanGeest, J. B. (2006). The use of human patient simulators: Best practices with novice nursing students. *Nurse Educator, 31*(4), 170–174.

Broscious, S., & Sanders, H. (2001). Peer coaching. *Nurse Educator, 26*(5), 212–214.

Buttriss, C., Kuiper, R., & Newbold, B. (1995). The use of a homeless shelter as a clinical rotation for nursing students. *Journal of Nursing Education, 34*(8), 375–377.

Cangelosi, P. R., Crocker, S., & Sorrell, J. M. (2009). Expert to novice: Clinicians learning new roles as clinical nurse educators. *Nursing Education Perspectives, 30*(6), 367–371.

Chan, D. (2002). Development of the clinical learning environment inventory: Using theoretical framework of learning environment studies to access nursing students' perceptions for the hospital as a learning environment. *Journal of Nursing Education, 41*(2), 69–75.

Childs, J. C. (2002). Clinical resource centers in nursing programs. *Nurse Educator, 27*(5), 232–235.

Clayton, L. H. (2006). Concept mapping: An effective, active teaching–learning method. *Nursing Education Perspectives, 27*(4), 197–203.

Collins, P., Hilde, E., & Shriver, C. (1993). A five-year evaluation of BSN students in a nursing management preceptorship. *Journal of Nursing Education, 32*(7), 330–332.

Cook, L. (2005). Inviting teacher behaviors of clinical faculty and nursing students' anxiety. *Journal of Nursing Education, 44*(4), 156–161.

Crandall, S. (1993). How expert clinical educators teach what they know. *Journal of Continuing Education in the Health Professions, 13*(1), 85–98.

Delpier, T. (2006). Cases 101: Learning to teach with cases. *Nursing Education Perspectives, 27*(4), 204–209.

Delunas, L. R., & Rooda, L. (2009). A new model for the clinical instruction of undergraduate nursing students. *Nursing Education Perspectives, 30*(6), 377–380.

deTornyay, R., & Thompson, M. (1987). *Strategies for teaching nursing.* New York, NY: John Wiley.

DeVoogd, R., & Saldbenblatt, C. (1989). The clinical teaching associate model: Advantages and disadvantages in practice. *Journal of Nursing Education, 28*(6), 276–277.

Diefenbeck, C. A., Plowfield, L. A., & Herrman, J. W. (2006). Clinical immersion: A residency model for nursing education. *Nursing Education Perspectives, 27*(2), 72–79.

Dunn, S. V., Stockhausen, L., Thornton, R., & Barnard, A. (1995). The relationship between clinical education format and selected student learning outcomes. *Journal of Nursing Education, 34*(1), 16–24.

Edgecombe, K., Wotton, K., Gonda, J., & Mason, P. (1999). Dedicated education units: A new concept for clinical teaching and learning. *Contemporary Nurse, 8*(4), 166–171.

Ellerman, C. R., Kataoka-Yahiro, M. R., & Wong, L. C. (2006). Logic models used to enhance critical thinking. *Journal of Nursing Education, 45*(6), 220–227.

Elliott, M. (2002). The clinical environment: A source of stress for undergraduate nurses. *Australian Journal of Advanced Nursing, 20*(1), 34–38.

Faller, H. S., McDowell, M. A., & Jackson, M. A. (1995). Bridge to the future: Nontraditional settings and concepts. *Journal of Nursing Education, 34*(8), 344–349.

Fugate, T., & Rebeschi, L. (1991). Dual assignment: An alternative clinical teaching strategy. *Nurse Educator, 15*(6), 14–16.

Gillespie, M. (2002). Student–teacher connection in clinical nursing education. *Journal of Advanced Nursing, 37*(6), 566–576.

Glanville, C. (1971). Multiple student assignment as an approach to clinical teaching in pediatric nursing. *Nursing Research, 20*(3), 237–244.

Gotschall, L., & Thompson, C. (1990). Dual assignments: An effective clinical teaching strategy. *Nurse Educator, 15*(6), 6.

Grady, J. L. (2006). Faculty matters. *Nursing Education Perspectives, 27*(3), 124–125.

Gross, J., Aysee, P., & Tracey, P. (1992). A creative clinical education model. *Three Views, 41*(4), 156–159.

Gubrud-Howe, P., & Schoessler, M. (2008). From random access opportunity to a clinical education curriculum. *Journal of Nursing Education, 47*(1), 3–4.

Hanson, K. J., & Stenvig, T. E. (2008). The good clinical nursing educator and the baccalaureate nursing clinical experience: Attributes and praxis. *Journal of Nursing Education, 47*(1), 38–42.

Hanson, L., & Smith, M. J. (1996). Nursing students' perspectives: Experiences of caring and not-so-caring interactions with faculty. *Journal of Nursing Education, 35*(3), 105–112.

Happell, B. (2009). A model of preceptorship in nursing: Reflecting the complex functions of the role. *Nursing Education Perspectives, 30*(6), 372–375.

Hsieh, N., & Knowles, D. (1990). Instructor facilitation of the preceptorship relationship in nursing education. *Journal of Nursing Education, 29*(6), 262–268.

Institute of Medicine. (2010). *Future of nursing: Leading change, advancing health.* Retrieved from http://www.iom.edu/About-IOM.aspx

Jarrett, S., Horner, M., Center, D., & Kane, L. A. (2008). Curriculum for the development of staff nurses as clinical faculty and scholars. *Nurse Educator, 33*(6), 268–272.

Karuhije, H. F. (1997). Classroom and clinical teaching in nursing: Delineating differences. *Nursing Forum, 32*(2), 5–12.

Kleehammer, K., Hart, A. L., & Keck, J. F. (1990). Nursing students' perception of anxiety-producing situations in the clinical setting. *Journal of Nursing Education, 29*(4), 183–187.

Krautscheid, L., Kaakinen, J., & Warner, J. (2008). Clinical faculty development: Using simulation to demonstrate and practice clinical teaching. *Journal of Nursing Education, 47*(9), 431–434.

Krichbaum, K. (1994). Clinical teaching effectiveness described in relation to learning outcomes of baccalaureate nursing students. *Journal of Nursing Education, 33*(7), 306–315.

Kuiper, R., Pesut, D., & Kautz, D. (2009). Promoting the self-regulation of clinical reasoning skills in nursing students. *The Open Nursing Journal, 3,* 70–76.

Lee, S. M., Coakley, E. E., Dahlin, C., & Carleton, P. F. (2009). An evidence-based nurse residency program in geropalliative care. *The Journal of Continuing Education in Nursing, 40*(12), 536–542.

Lee, W. S., Krystyna, C., & Williams, A. (2002). Nursing students' and clinical educators' perception of characteristics of effective clinical education in an Australian university school of nursing. *Journal of Advanced Nursing, 39*(5), 412–420.

Letizia, M., & Jennrich, J. (1998). A review of preceptorship in undergraduate nursing education: Implication for staff development. *Journal of Continuing Education in Nursing, 29*(5), 211–216.

Lo, R. (2002). A longitudinal study of perceived level of stress, coping and self-esteem of undergraduate nursing students: An Australian case study. *Journal of Advanced Nursing, 39*(2), 119–126.

Mallette, S., Laury, S., Engleke, M. K., & Andrews, A. (2005). The integrative clinical preceptor model: A new method for teaching undergraduate community health nursing. *Nurse Educator, 30*(1), 21–26.

Massarweh, L. (1999). Promoting a positive clinical experience. *Nursing Educator, 24*(3), 44–47.

Meisenhelder, J. B. (1987). Anxiety: A block to clinical teaching. *Nurse Educator, 12*(6), 27–30.

Miller, T. W. (2005). The dedicated education unit: A practice and education partnership. *Nursing Leadership Forum, 9*(4), 169–173.

Morgan, J., & Knox, J. (1987). Characteristics of "best" and "worst" clinical teachers as perceived by university nursing faculty and students. *Journal of Advanced Nursing, 12*(3), 331–337.

Moscato, S. R., Miller, J., Logsdon, K., Weinberg, S., & Chorpenning, L. (2007). Dedicated education unit: An innovative clinical partner education model. *Nursing Outlook, 55*(1), 31–37.

Murray, T. A., Crain, C., Meyer, G. A., McDonough, M. E., & Schweiss, D. M. (2010). Building bridges: An innovative academic-service partnership. *Nursing Outlook, 58*(5), 252–260.

Neiderhauser, V., Macintyre, R. D., Garner, C., Teel, C., & Murray, T. (2010). Transformational partnerships in nursing education. *Nursing Education Perspectives, 31*(6), 353–355.

Oermann, M. H. (1996). Research on teaching in the clinical setting. In K. R. Stevens (Ed.), *Review of research in nursing education* (pp. 91–126). New York, NY: National League for Nursing.

Overstreet, M. (2010). E-chats: The seven components of nursing debriefing. *The Journal of Continuing Education in Nursing, 41*(12), 538–539.

Pardo, D. (1991). *The culture of clinical teaching.* (Doctoral dissertation). Available from UMI Dissertation Abstracts International (UMI No. AAT 9125. 50).

Phillips, S., & Kaempfer, S. (1987). Clinical teaching associate model: Implementation in a community hospital setting. *Journal of Professional Nursing, 3*(3), 165–175.

Piscopo, B. (1994). Organizational climate, communication, and role strain in clinical nursing faculty. *Journal of Professional Nursing, 10*(2), 113–119.

Porter, K., & Feller, C. (1979). The relationship between patterns of massed and distributed clinical practicum and student achievement. *Journal of Nursing Education, 18,* 27–34.

Rodehorst, T. K., Wilhelm, S. L., & Jensen, L. (2005). Use of interdisciplinary simulation to understand perceptions of team members' roles. *Journal of Professional Nursing, 21*(3), 159–166.

Rossen, B. E., & Fegan, M. A. (2009). Eight- or twelve-hour shifts: What nursing students prefer. *Nursing Education Perspectives, 30*(1), 40–43.

Rush, K. L., Dyches, C. E., Waldrop, S., & Davis, A. (2008). Critical thinking among RN-BSN distance students participating in human patient simulation. *Journal of Nursing Education, 47*(11), 501–507.

Schiavenato, M. (2009). Reevaluating simulation in nursing education: Beyond the human patient simulator. *Journal of Nursing Education, 48*(7), 388–393.

Schim, S., & Scher, K. (2002). Worksite "lunch and learn": A collaborative teaching project. *Journal of Nursing Education, 41*(12), 541–543.

Schmidt, B., & Stewart, S. (2009). Implementing the virtual reality environment. *Nurse Educator, 34*(4), 152–155.

Schuster, P., Fitzgerald, D. A., McCarthy, P., & McDougal, D. (1997). Work load issues in clinical nursing education. *Journal of Professional Nursing, 13*(3), 154–159.

Sedlak, C. (1992). Use of beginning logs by beginning students and faculty to identify student learning needs. *Journal of Nursing Education, 31*(1), 24–27.

Shah, H., & Pennypacker, D. (1992). The clinical teaching partnership. *Nurse Educator, 17*(2), 10–12.

Sieh, J., & Bell, S. (1994). Perceptions of effective clinical teachers in associate degree programs. *Journal of Nursing Education, 33*(9), 389–394.

Smedley, A., & Penney, D. (2009). A partnership approach to the preparation of preceptors. *Nursing Education Perspectives, 30*(1), 31–36.

Stuebbe, B. (1990). Student and faculty perspectives in the role of a nursing instructor. *Journal of Nursing Education, 19*(7), 4–9.

Tang, F. I., Chou, S. M., & Chiang, H. (2005). Students' perception of ineffective clinical instructors. *Journal of Nursing Education, 44*(4), 187–192.

Tanner, C. (2002). Clinical education, circa 2010. *Journal of Nursing Education, 41*(2), 51–52.

Tanner, C. (2005). The art and science of clinical teaching. *Journal of Nursing Education, 44*(4), 151–152.

Tanner, C. (2010). Transforming prelicensure nursing education. *Nursing Education Perspectives, 31*(6), 347–351.

Timmins, F., & Kaliszer, M. (2002). Aspects of education programmes that frequently cause stress to nursing students—Fact-finding sample survey. *Nursing Education Today, 22*(3), 203–211.

Totten, J. K., & Fonnesbeck, B. (2002). Camp communities: Valuable clinical options for BSN students. *Journal of Nursing Education, 41*(2), 83–85.

Trevitt, C., Graslish, L., & Reaby, L. (2001). Students in transit: Using a self-directed preceptorship pack to smooth the journey. *Journal of Nursing Education, 40*(5), 25–28.

VanDenBerg, E. (1976). The multiple assignment: An effective alternative for laboratory experiences. *Journal of Nursing Education, 15*(3), 3–12.

Vinten, S., Kost, G., & Chalko, B. (2003). *Orienting the clinical educator: Developing faculty competencies.* Paper presented at the Conference of the National League for Nursing, San Antonio, TX.

Vinten, S., & Partridge, R. (2002). E-learning and the clinical practicum. In D. Billings (Ed.), *Conversations in e-learning,* pp 187–196. Pensacola, FL: Pohl Publishing.

Wieland, D. M., Altmiller, G. M., Dorr, M. T., & Wolf, Z. R. (2007). Clinical transition of baccalaureate nursing students during preceptored, pregraduation practicums. *Nursing Education Perspectives, 28*(6), 315–321.

Williams, J. (2001). The clinical notebook: Using student portfolios to enhance clinical teaching learning. *Journal of Nursing Education, 40,* 135–137.

Wink, D. (1993). Using questioning as a teaching strategy. *Nurse Educator, 18*(5), 11–15.

Wink, D. (1995). The effective clinical conference. *Nursing Outlook, 43*(1), 29–32.

Wolf, Z., Bender, P., Beitz, J., Wieland, D., & Vito, K. (2004). Strength and weaknesses of faculty teaching performance reported by undergraduate and graduate nursing students: A descriptive study. *Journal of Professional Nursing, 20*(2), 118–128.

Wotton, K & Gonda J. (2004). Clinician and student evaluation of a collaborative clinical teaching model.*Nurse Educator Practice, 4*(2):120–7.

Wright, A. (2002). Preceptoring in 2002. *Journal of Continuing Education in Nursing, 33*(3), 138–141.

Zerbe, M., & Lachat, M. (1991). A three-tiered team model for undergraduate preceptor programs. *Nurse Educator, 16*(2), 18–21.

Zurmehly, J. (2010). Personal digital assistants (PDAs): Review and evaluation. *Nursing Education Perspectives, 31*(3), 179–182.

The Learning Resource Center

19

Kay E. Hodson Carlton, EdD, RN, ANEF, FAAN

The learning resource center (LRC) of today is a central hub of instructional activity for students, faculty, and professionals. Historically, the LRC was an area for psychomotor skills practice and performance. The contemporary LRC serves as a multifunctional teaching and learning center. The role of the LRC is becoming even more important with the increasing use of simulations, emerging media programs, and distance learning. This chapter describes the LRC's current and expanded functions and research on instructional issues, and introduces management and operational issues for the administration of an LRC.

The Learning Resource Center: Functions

Historically, the LRC evolved from psychomotor skills practice laboratories. The laboratories of the 1960s through the 1980s typically had a skills practice area with some inventory of task trainers and static manikins. Many of the practice laboratories were supported with a variety of audiovisual programs, such as slide-audiotape and filmstrip programs demonstrating nursing skills.

The LRC often served as a skills practice area for students in the introductory clinical nursing course at the undergraduate level. The evolution and expansion of LRCs began in the late 1980s with transformations in the methods of teaching and learning and the rapid changes in information and health care technologies. LRCs rapidly evolved from psychomotor skills practice laboratories to centers of learning that used the latest technologies

for learning. Learning also expanded from the psychomotor domain to the cognitive and affective domains.

Functions of the LRC, as well as its designation, still vary widely from institution to institution. *Learning resource center* or *learning resources center* is frequently used as the broad term for this teaching–learning support facility. Other examples of terms used to designate either the multifunctional facility or the associated clinical practice environment include *human patient simulation center, center for teaching and lifelong learning, information and learning technologies, educational resources, office of learning technologies, patient safety simulation laboratory, clinical learning resource center or lab, clinical simulation lab, nursing lab,* and *nursing skills laboratory* (Parr & Sweeney, 2006; Tarnow, 2005).

Regardless of the specific name of the instructional facility, a multitude of teaching and learning activities remain the primary goals of the LRC. The design and the role of the LRC should come from the curricular framework of the program(s). The facility and support services are a major indicator of institutional and program commitment, and resources and the LRC's quality and performance should be a component of annual program evaluation and curricular review.

The LRC facility is typically conceptualized as an emerging technologies environment where learners use visual, auditory, kinesthetic, and tactile abilities for the acquisition of cognitive, affective, and psychomotor skills for lifelong and interprofessional collaborative learning. The LRC can be a place for low-stress learning, role modeling, decision making and critical thinking, clinical judgment, independent and group study, and all levels of multimedia instruction and evaluation. Students

The author acknowledges the work of Pamela Carlisle-Worrell in the previous edition(s) of the chapter.

in fundamental clinical courses, as well as those preparing for advanced practice roles, are served by the LRC. In addition, enhanced functions of most LRCs around the country include all or some of the following:

- Operation of multimedia and computer laboratories and low- and high-fidelity simulation studios with a wide variety of task trainers and emerging technologies
- Technology and network services support for nursing and associated health care interprofessional users of the facility
- Multimedia and emerging technologies instructional design, development, and production
- Faculty development and consultation support for teaching and learning activities
- Coordination of distance learning for nursing and associated programs
- Nursing and associated health care disciplines clinical practice
- Consultation on research, evaluation, and administration of information and learning technologies
- Continuing and lifelong education
- Community and clinical agency resource facility

Teaching and Learning in the Learning Resource Center

Psychomotor Skill Instruction

It is not by chance that psychomotor nursing skill development and medication administration are essential teaching and learning foci of almost all LRC facilities. The Joint Commission (as cited in Koerner, 2003) claimed that inadequate training or orientation was the cause of threats to patient safety in 87% of cases. Medication administration and equipment use errors led the list of safety violations. Thousands of cases of injury or death were occurring annually, and one half of the errors were related to medication administration, with 62% of medication errors involving intravenous (IV) pumps. Subsequent developments have reinforced the critical role of nursing education in the preparation of competent caregivers who can provide safe and quality care.

The Institute of Medicine (IOM) report for nursing education proposed that newly registered nurses should be competent in five areas of professional nursing practice: patient-centered care, collaboration with interdisciplinary teams, awareness of quality standards, knowledge and use of evidence-based practice, and informatics and technology (Finkelman & Kenner, 2009). In addition, the Quality and Safety Education for Nurses (QSEN) (Cronenwett et al., 2007) project recommended that organizations ensure nurse competence based on standards of care and the use of evidence-based practice (Clark & Holmes, 2007; Finkelman & Kenner, 2009). The IOM has charged faculty in nursing programs with the preparation of competent practitioners in a broad range of skills. Therefore nurse educators have a responsibility to prepare students to function safely in practice.

Changes in the health care environment affect faculty capacity to prepare students adequately. First, as the severity of illness of hospitalized and home health care patients increases, students in clinical practice are confronted with providing more complex nursing care earlier in and throughout their undergraduate program experience. The traditional debate over whether it is ethical to teach students psychomotor skills in the practice setting or in the simulation laboratory is complicated by this increased severity of illness. Second, increased dependence on technology (e.g., medical equipment) requires that students and staff be trained to use a greater variety of equipment. Manufacturers' updates to equipment dictate the need for frequent retraining. Also, the increasing use of computerized systems for care and medication documentation adds to the complexity of clinical experiences. Third, turnover in staff, use of registry personnel, floating among assigned units, and a shortage of registered nurses (RNs) with extensive clinical experience can decrease the availability of competent preceptors for student nurses. The academic institution's role in teaching nursing skills has never been more salient than in today's dynamic health care milieu.

There is a continuing debate in nursing education over how to best teach psychomotor skills to undergraduates (Larew, Lessans, Spunt, Foster, & Covington, 2006; Lenchus, Kalidindi, Sanko, Everett-Thomas, & Birnvach, 2010). Implementation of the nursing process requires competency in a complex set of cognitive, social-emotional, and psychomotor skills. Psychomotor skill acquisition is now understood as a multidimensional learning event, yet evidence-based practice in this area, while increasing, is rudimentary.

The role of the LRC in nursing skill instruction has traditionally been to provide a setting in which students can observe and practice in a simulated environment. As others have indicated, the explosive continual expansion of simulation as an essential component of nursing education is broadening and transforming the traditional role of the LRC (Hyland & Hawkins, 2009; Kardong-Edgren & Oermann, 2009). The goals of instruction are to decrease anxiety and increase knowledge and skill through use of a simulated patient encounter before students have contact with patients in clinical practice. Teaching nursing skills in the transitioning LRC, with its focus on patient safety, interprofessional learning, and research outcomes, encompasses several evolving issues, which are summarized in Box 19-1.

Defining and Identifying Essential Nursing Skills

Defining psychomotor skills and identifying the essential skills to be taught in the undergraduate curriculum have been examined by several authors over the last two decades. In the 1990s, Oermann delineated three types of psychomotor skills: fine, manual, and gross. Fine motor skills were used for tasks that required precision. Manual skills were used in tasks requiring manipulation and possible repetition. Gross motor skills involved the large muscle groups and required more movement. Alavi, Loh, and Reilly (1991) categorized skills as fundamental, general therapeutic and diagnostic, and specialized therapeutic and diagnostic (Table 19-1).

BOX 19-1 Issues in Nursing Psychomotor Skill Instruction

- Defining and identifying essential nursing skills
- Implementing instructional strategies and evaluation
- Competency levels
- Integrating learning domains
- Simulations
- Traditional faculty role or self-directed, technology-enhanced model
- Student preferences and satisfaction
- Identifying conceptual and theoretical frameworks for instructional design
- Outcome measurement

Many psychomotor skills are involved in delivering nursing care (Boxer, Fallon, & Samuelson, 2001) and the identification of "essential" skills remains controversial. It is common to consult with staff in the practice setting to determine current skill sets in high demand, yet there is evidence that new graduate nurses are not adequately prepared to function independently without an extensive orientation period (Billings, 2008; Burns & Poster, 2008; Clark & Holmes, 2007; Hofler, 2008; Ironside, 2008; Ridley, 2008, Scott Tilley, 2008; Thomas, Ryan, & Hodson Carlton, 2011).

Implementing Instructional Strategies and Student Evaluation

Competency Levels

Another consideration in teaching psychomotor skills is competency level (Chase, 2005; Klein, 2006). Evaluation of competency skills can be particularly challenging due to the diversity of nursing education programs and practice standards in the United States (Allen et al., 2008). Educators are expected to prepare student nurses for transition to nursing practice and ensure competency (Billings, 2008; Cronenwett et al., 2007). Competency evaluation builds on a continuum of multifaceted dimensions: thinking in action, clinical decision making, and information retrieval for best practices. Competencies have been defined as the application of a range of skills that includes thinking in action and confidence and clarity in decision making. Some nurse leaders have recommended that a competency evaluation system be developed based on Benner's (1984) novice to expert model (Allen et al., 2008). Scott Tilley (2008) analyzed competency as a concept. In all domains of practice, competency was defined as the application of skills. Studies have identified competency skills for new graduates; however, further research needs to be conducted (Allen et al., 2008).

Nurse educators need guidance not only on content and skills that students are lacking, but also on methods for educators to adjust teaching strategies, especially in the areas of patient safety, evidence-based practice, self-confidence, and intradisciplinary communications (Tanner, 2006). Educators across the country are also reevaluating curricula and clinical education to increase the competency skills of students recommended by IOM and, more recently, by the report on QSEN

TABLE 19-1 Psychomotor Skill Categorization Scheme

Fundamental	General Therapeutic and Diagnostic	Specialized Therapeutic and Diagnostic
Mobilization	Inspection	Oxygen therapy
Range of motion	Auscultation of bowel, breath, and heart sounds	Oropharyngeal suction
Body mechanics	Palpation	Tracheostomy suction
Lifting		Stoma therapy
Showering	Percussion	Nasogastric tube
		Eye toilets
Bed-bathing	Ear, nose, and throat assessment	Eye irrigation and drops
Mouth care	Neurological assessment	
Hair care	Integrated physical assessment	Nose drops
Positioning	Specimen collection	Orthopedic applications
Pressure area care	Medication administration	Baby bath
Hand washing	Bandage application	Assessment of neonatal and child development
Bed making	Surgical asepsis	CVP measurement
Feeding	Wound drainage	Intercostal catheter care
Assisting with bedpan, urinal, or commode	Removal of sutures and staples	CPR
Assessment of TPR and BP	IV therapy	
Height and weight measurement	Isolation technique	
	Catheterization	
	Urinalysis	
	Cleansing enema	
	Suppositories	
	Hot and cold application	

Modified from Alavi, C., Loh, S. H., & Reily D. (1991). Reality basis for teaching psychomotor skills in a tertiary nursing curriculum. *Journal of Advanced Nursing,* 16(8), 957–965.

BP, Blood pressure; *CPR,* cardiopulmonary resuscitation; *CVP,* central venous pressure; *IV,* intravenous; *TPR,* temperature, pulse, and respiration.

(Cronenwett et al., 2007). Results from a regional study investigating nurse managers' perceptions of how well new graduate nurses met IOM competencies (Thomas, Ryan, & Hodson Carlton, 2011) supported findings from other studies that education and practice need a closer collaborative model (Allen et al., 2008).

In the LRC, a psychomotor skill performance guide has typically been used by the faculty and staff educator to evaluate competencies before the student performs the skill with a patient at a health care facility. Traditionally, skill performance guides have also been used to increase interrater reliability of evaluators and to communicate expectations to students.

The psychomotor skill performance guide items are generally derived from nursing textbooks, health care agency procedure manuals, and clinical practice guidelines. Methods for assessing continued competency of graduate nurses are varied, often incorporating simulation and virtual reality technology (Landry, Oberleitner, Landry, & Borazjani, 2006). When checklists are generated from various sources, the potential for discrepancy between service and educational settings is introduced. Variability in checklist design can compromise measurement of competency. In addition, the degree of detail of critical behaviors may vary from checklist to checklist. These discrepancies derive from a need to develop generic principle-based skills that students can take to any clinical setting. These skills should be based on evidence-based research.

Integrating Learning Domains

For the past few decades, many have advocated rethinking effective teaching strategies for psychomotor skills (Larew et al., 2006; Smith, 1992; Tanner, 2006). In the early 1990s, Oermann (1990) suggested that a psychomotor skill initially be broken down and the conceptual aspects be taught separately from the motor processes. However, psychomotor skills are not performed apart from the affective and cognitive components in patient care, and at some point students must have an integrated learning experience that simulates the clinical experience. For example, maintaining sterile technique while changing a dressing is a basic skill that requires demonstration of a minimal level of competence for the safety of the patient. However, the complexity of dressing varies. In addition, being able to communicate effectively to ease a patient's apprehension during a painful dressing change is an important skill. Changing dressings on a critically ill, ventilator-dependent patient with multiple trauma in an intensive care setting demands further competence. This more comprehensive approach to integration and evaluation of psychomotor, cognitive, and affective domains is attainable in a simulated environment.

Psychomotor skills need to be repeatedly practiced to maintain competence. For example, cardiopulmonary resuscitation (CPR) skills among nursing students were found to be maintained with as little as 6 minutes per month practice on a voice advisory manikin (Oermann & Kardong-Edgren, 2010). Lack of practice resulted in a significant loss of CPR skills in as little as 3 months. This research suggests that follow-up demonstration sessions of mandatory skills may benefit students.

Simulations

Simulations are a common and increasingly critical strategy used in the LRC to link multidimensional learning to practice and performance. Simulations can include the use of high- and low-fidelity simulators as well as a wide variety of task trainers for the practice of psychomotor skills, entire sequences of nursing clinical actions with computerized and virtual reality simulators, the use of emerging technologies, and human simulation with actors. Ziv, Small, and Wolpe's (2000) categories of simulation-based training provide a good basic framework for the discussion of integration of simulation in nursing skills. They are described here along with updates based on current and continued growth in emerging technologies. The categories include the following:

- Simple models or manikins
- Simulated or standardized patients
- Computer screen–based clinical case simulators
- Realistic high-tech procedural simulators or task trainers (RPSs)
- Realistic high-tech interactive patient simulators
- Virtual reality (VR)

Simple models or static manikins are relatively low-tech, low-cost simulators used to teach basic cognitive knowledge or hands-on psychomotor skills. Examples of these models, often referred to as task trainers, are the enema administration model, injection and IV arms, and abdominal suture models available from a variety of companies that produce medical and health care models used for educational purposes.

Simulated or standardized patients (SPs), individuals who are trained to play a scripted patient role, are now frequently used for undergraduate and graduate nursing student learning and assessment in history taking, physical examination, and communication skills, and to enhance manikin-based simulations. Anderson, Holmes, LeFlore, Nelson, and Jenkins (2010) describe one such successful use in nursing education. The use of SPs across levels of the curriculum in the undergraduate and graduate programs resulted in improved program quality and faculty and student satisfaction. The role of SPs has also been expanded to serve as family or caregivers with manikin-based simulations. Others have shared additional examples of successful experiences with the use of standardized patients as adjuncts for teaching pelvic examinations (Theroux & Pearce, 2006), for teaching and evaluating students on cultural competency (Rutledge, Garzon, Scott, & Karlowicz, 2004), for a simulated psychiatric clinical encounter (Robinson-Smith, Bradley, & Meakim, 2009), and for objective structured clinical examinations with advanced practice nursing students (Kurz, Mahoney, Martin-Plank, & Lidicker, 2009). Research results validate the teaching effectiveness of standardized patients (Becker, Rose, Berg, Park, & Shatzer, 2006).

The use of *computer screen–based clinical case simulators* proliferated in the 1980s with the emergence of the personal computer in nursing programs. Screen-based computer simulations continue to be available and are used for a wide variety of nursing clinical specialties. For example, DVDs, digitized video for mobile devices, interactive learning development, web conferencing, screen capture utilities, and other Internet tools are examples of computer screen–based simulators.

*Realistic high-tech procedural simulators (RPSs) or task trainer*s are described by Ziv et al. (2000) as instructional tools that enhance static models with audiovisual, touch–feel interactive cues, and sophisticated computerized software. Cardiology patient simulators, which present auscultatory and pulse findings of numerous cardiovascular conditions; an ultrasound system with a functional control panel, mock transducers, and a realistic patient-manikin; and laparoscopic high-tech surgery task trainers are examples of RPSs. Within the last decade, the explosive growth of technology has ushered in an era of high- and low-fidelity simulators. High- and low-fidelity simulation is discussed in further detail in Chapter 20.

Virtual reality (VR) is an evolving technology that is gaining dramatically in use in higher education (Ahern & Wink, 2010; Schmidt & Stewart, 2009). VR has become a "reality" in the practice setting and in nursing, allied health, and medical education (Simpson, 2003). VR is an emergent technology that holds significant potential for responding in areas where the nursing faculty shortage is critical and for training in underserved regions. Virtual reality is discussed in further detail in Chapter 21.

Another way to add realism to the simulated nursing care experience is to create a multibed simulated hospital unit within an LRC where a combination of simulated learning experiences are developed and implemented. For example, Bantz, Dancer, Hodson-Carlton, and Van Hove (2007) share experiences in the development, implementation, and evaluation of an eight-station clinical simulation day to help students transfer their classroom knowledge of labor and delivery, newborn infant care, and postpartum care into the clinical

setting. The initial focus of the simulation work was to develop a virtual clinical laboratory that prepared students to interpret normal findings in obstetrics and newborn care before they were posted to their different clinical placements; they were immersed in patient care scenarios depicting maternity labor and delivery, neonatal care, and infant care. Categories of simulation-based training included in the experience were the use of simple models and manikins, high-fidelity patient simulators, and computer screen–based clinical case simulation in addition to gaming and computerized clinical care documentation.

Advantages of using simulation strategies include the addition of realism and decision making to patient-like situations in the laboratory setting, teaching potential in cognitive and affective realms and psychomotor skill performance, the ability to control multiple extraneous variables present in the actual clinical environment, minimized ethical concerns, and evaluative possibilities. Positive outcomes for students when they use simulations include increased student organization and integration of separate skill modules, faculty identification of students' level of performance in clinical skills, increased student confidence, a ready vehicle to teach clinical judgment skills and clinical decision making, smoother transition from laboratory to health care setting, improved performance assessment, error management, improved safety culture, and new research possibilities (Arundell & Cioffi, 2005; Bearnson & Wiker, 2005; Bland & Sutton, 2006; Bremner, Aduddell, Bennett, & VanGeest, 2006; Cioffi, Purcal, & Arundell, 2005; Hyland & Hawkins, 2009; Johnsson, Kjellberg, & Lagerstrom, 2006; Long, 2005; Nehring, Lashley, & Ellis, 2002; Parr & Sweeney, 2006).

The most frequently cited disadvantage of simulations is the amount of time required for the design of the simulation. Other disadvantages include the time and staff needed to prepare, assemble, and maintain the supplies, space, and equipment required for the simulation; plans for and continual orientation of new and reassigned faculty to the simulations; and continual updating and revisions required for use of the simulation on a recurring basis. Nehring et al. (2002) point out the additional administrative consideration of maintenance expenses, including the purchase of equipment and compensation of faculty for training and practice. Addition of the role-playing element can also add managerial time, especially if nonstudent volunteers or individuals from outside the institution need to be scheduled and compensated for participation. Visible costs, especially with the more complex simulation tools, are relatively high, whereas cost benefits may be indirect, unsubstantiated, and long term (Seropian, Brown, Samuelson Gavilanes, & Driggers, 2004; Ziv et al., 2000).

Traditional Faculty Role or Self-Directed Technology-Enhanced Model

Two competing instructional strategies for teaching psychomotor skills have been the focus of most research on psychomotor skill instruction. One is the traditional faculty-mediated model of lecture and demonstration, followed by student practice and return demonstration to establish competence. The other model is student-directed learning that is enhanced through technology. Demonstrations and return demonstrations have been, and continue to be, a strategy commonly used in the LRC to develop and refine psychomotor skills and to develop decision-making skills related to psychomotor skill interventions, because of the ability to control the environment and simulate clinical practice. In an attempt to enhance learning and reduce student anxiety in traditional skill demonstration and return demonstration settings, instructors have explored alternative approaches to supplement some of the commonly used teaching strategies.

The alternative to the traditional faculty role is a self-directed approach, replacing the lecture and demonstration with technology and media. Instead of the traditional faculty role in lecture and demonstration, various forms of media—videotapes or DVDs, CD-ROM simulations, digitized video on mobile devices, Internet learning objects such as those found on MERLOT (www.merlot.org), and VR—are used, often in a modular format. Many institutions have designed and implemented modular learning approaches to the teaching and evaluation of nursing skills. In general, the "module" has a pretest and posttest (which may be computerized or offered on the Internet), specific objectives and outcomes, a listing of structured activities with designated resources, and a multimedia integration plan. Another variation of self-directed learning is the use of peers or videotape for obtaining feedback during practice and evaluation of psychomotor skills. The advantages of technology-mediated instruction include learners controlling the pace, consistent content, repetition as needed, multiple examples, and sensory input to meet the needs of different learning styles.

In research designed to compare traditional and technological approaches, three questions are typically included: (1) Are there differences in performance of the skill? (2) Are there differences in cognitive gains? (3) Are there differences in student satisfaction? Research findings reported in the literature have not indicated any consistent findings when comparing and contrasting the two approaches; this remains an area of nursing education that can benefit from further well-designed research.

Student Preferences and Satisfaction

Student responses to the incorporation of media and technology in the curriculum have been examined and found to be dependent on the questions being asked and when the data are collected. As with other aspects of nursing skills instruction, student preferences are complex and not clearly understood. Because students have a range of learning styles that include preferences for social interaction, responsiveness to criticism, and need for sensory input, the variability in student attitudes toward the type of instruction used and the degree of technology infusion should be anticipated. The addition of a measurement of learning style during comparison of instructional strategies would increase understanding of the variables influencing learner behavior and satisfaction.

Identifying Conceptual and Theoretical Frameworks for Instructional Design

Learning Theory

The foundation for nursing skill instruction can be grounded in social or observational learning theory (Bandura, 1986) and information processing theories of learning, regardless of the instructional design. There are four types of observational learning effects that can shape behavior. *Inhibition* occurs when a learner refrains from behaving in a particular way because he or she has observed the consequences that another experienced. *Disinhibition* occurs when a learner observes another behave in a socially unacceptable way and go unpunished. *Facilitation* is the result of seeing another who has behaved in a particular way being rewarded for that behavior in a manner that a learner values. Potential exists for facilitation, inhibition, and disinhibition when students observe peers in skill practice and return demonstration with faculty critique. The fourth type is *true observational learning* in which a behavior is learned by observation of a model and subsequent imitation. Although all four effects may occur when students learn nursing skills, true observational learning can form a foundation for instruction. According to Bandura (1986), attention, retention, production, and motivation are critical factors in observational learning. Information processing theories of learning use the computer analogy to explain learning (Snowman & Biehler, 2003). Analysis of instructional input can inform the selection of strategies for teaching nursing skills.

Attention to a model must occur for observational learning to take place. Research with social learning theory and information processing theory indicates that attention is more likely to occur when the following conditions are met:

- The model is perceived as competent.
- The model is respected.
- The consequences observed for executing the behavior are valued.
- The sensory register is not bombarded by unlimited input.
- Prior knowledge storage in long-term memory is adequate.
- Novelty exists.
- The teacher provides cues to important data.
- Accommodations for individual differences in learning style are made.

After observation, a behavior must be retained or remembered so that the student can imitate it. In addition to learning the process or steps involved in the behavior, a learner may have to remember other information, such as why or when the behavior is to be performed. For the information to be encoded in long-term memory and retrieved for later use, the learner must have opportunities to rehearse or actively think about it (Snowman & Biehler, 2003). Rehearsal encompasses not only repetition but also thinking about how new information is different from or similar to previous learning (Ausubel, Novak, & Hanesian, 1978). Retention is also enhanced when the information is organized in a meaningful way for the learner according to cognitive style. Cognitive style will influence retention and organization; some learners focus on the broad concepts and miss details while others miss the conceptual meaning and more easily learn the steps of a process. Factual information

such as the steps in a procedure, which have few meaningful links to prior knowledge, may be organized more efficiently by using memory strategies (mnemonics) such as rhymes, acrostics, acronyms, or loci methods (Snowman & Biehler, 2003). Retention can be facilitated by the following:

1. Actively rehearsing and organizing the information: note taking, summarizing, outlining, diagramming, telling, acting, teaching, performing, questioning, using mnemonic devices
2. Providing verbal, visual, and tactile or kinesthetic input and output
3. Offering rationales for why the behavior is important
4. Comparing and contrasting new information with previous learning

Production of a new behavior may be initially imitation; later, automatization or mastery occurs through practice with feedback on competence (Snowman & Biehler, 2003). Production is enhanced when there is limited time between observation and imitation. Learners are motivated to produce the behavior when they perceive the consequences to be rewarding. Feedback to reward accuracy or to correct errors is necessary and needs to be delivered within a limited amount of time after performance. The following are required to facilitate production of a new behavior:

1. Practice of skills
2. Immediate and accurate feedback
3. A valued consequence for completing the task

Bandura (1993) asserts that a learner's belief in his or her own ability to be successful, or self-efficacy, is an important motivational factor in observational learning. Self-efficacy is the result of previous learning attempts, persuasion by others that the learner is capable, emotional state, and seeing successful models whom the learner perceives as being like him or her. Learners with high self-efficacy have higher expectations of themselves, visualize themselves being successful, engage in more analytical and evaluative thought in problem solving, work longer at reaching their goals, and approach a new learning task with energy and curiosity. The implications for nursing psychomotor skill instruction include the following:

1. Stress and anxiety will affect performance.
2. Previous success and failure will affect feelings of confidence.
3. Students with a history of difficulty in developing psychomotor skills may need more encouragement, instruction, and positive feedback.

Faculty can design instruction with the use of these concepts to facilitate learning. These concepts would apply to both traditional faculty-directed instruction and media- or technology-mediated models and could be tested through research.

Expanded Functions of the Learning Resource Center

At many institutions the function of the LRC has expanded beyond the traditional focus on psychomotor nursing skills due to the rapid growth of technology in education. LRCs may now also incorporate technology support, development and production of technology, distance education, clinical practice, links to clinical practice, and lifelong learning.

Technology Support

As the use of technology in education and practice has evolved, so has the LRC as a place to support and develop the technology. Support for technology use in the nursing program can be a substantive responsibility of the LRC personnel. This often includes the provision of technical support for high- and low-fidelity simulation studios with the associated hardware and software; provision of academic software applications for electronic health records; operation and management of computer laboratories; support for wireless networks and mobile devices; and the design, development, and production of multimedia, web-based, and emerging technology products.

A common practice is the partnering of the nursing LRC with other technology services within or in partnership with the institution to provide this technology support or the development and production of multimedia emerging technology products. A case study example is the School of Nursing LRC at Ball State University (www.bsu.edu/nursing). Staffed with technology support personnel at the nursing academic unit level, the LRC is the initial point of technology service for students, faculty, and staff in the nursing program. However, a wide variety of institutional support services works in partnership with the school to offer more comprehensive services. These partnerships include personnel consultation, design, development and production staff, and financial support for the purchase of hardware and software at the unit level. In this case, institutional technology

support services partnering with the School of Nursing LRC include University Computing Services (www.bsu.edu/web/ucs), University Teleplex (www.bsu.edu/web/teleplex), University Libraries (www.bsu.edu/libraries), Innovation in Teaching, Assessment, and Scholarship (http://cms.bsu.edu/About/AdministrativeOffices/ITAS.aspx), Online and Distance Education (www.bsu.edu/distance), and Sponsored Programs Office (http://cms.bsu.edu/About/AdministrativeOffices/SPO.aspx). These partnerships often include external partners working with the nursing unit and the university. For example, mobilization of wireless mobile devices, such as handheld computers, or the development and implementation of emerging technologies, such as virtual reality, in the curriculum may necessitate academic unit and institutional partnerships with software and hardware vendors.

Distance Education

The coordination of distance education for the nursing program has been a natural evolution for some LRCs, especially those LRC units that have historically had technology support or the development and production of multimedia as one of their essential functions. Typically the nursing unit LRC partners with other institutional services in the support of distance education. The LRC director and staff are generally key support personnel for the development, implementation, and evaluation of the distance learning offerings, courses, and programs. In almost all cases, this function is done in close partnership with other institutional technology and teaching and support entities (e.g., library, extended or distance education, admissions, financial affairs, book services, telecommunications, computer services, and marketing). Resources that provide a comprehensive overview of the current status, strategies, support, and evaluation of distance education overall, and specifically in nursing education, are available (Bourbonnais, 2010; Johnson, 2008; Jones & Wolf, 2010; Weiner, 2008).

Clinical Practice and Electronic Documentation

The LRC is a vital link to the practice setting in various capacities. The LRC may serve as a center for clinical practice for faculty and students. For example, a physical assessment classroom or laboratory areas may be designed to serve as a clinic for providing health assessment services, or a simulated home health care room can serve as a place to teach families how to care for patients in the home. LRCs also can serve as resource centers for community groups (e.g., wellness programs or patient teaching) and clinical health care–related agencies and services. The LRC can therefore also offer an opportunity for providing services and teaching opportunities and generating income. The LRC may also be the point from which faculty and students provide health care services to patients at a distance. This may include telehealth applications, such as those described by Grady and Berkebile (2004) when faculty and students are linked from the LRC site to acute and home care agencies and patients.

Many LRCs are increasingly serving as a bridge, often virtual, to clinical practice. An example is the linkages some LRCs are implementing to teach electronic health record documentation. In the early 1990s Simpson (1990) first advised closing the rapidly expanding technological gap between the school and the automated environment of the health care workplace by integrating computer terminals at the bedside of each practice unit in the LRC and the functional networking of each of those terminals to a "real" hospital information system through a collaborative partnership with the vendor. The goal of this redesigned learning laboratory was to prepare the student to practice in the increasingly automated health care environment through use of and practice with the "real" automated tools of the health care workplace. This suggestion of the 1990s is now being implemented in many LRCs across the country, often with interprofessional partners and clinical agencies. The School of Nursing at Ball State University (www.bsu.edu/nursing) is one such case study example of a collaborative partnership among the university, a regional health care center, and a health care information system vendor to provide student orientation to computerized documentation in the LRC before practice at the health care agency (Melo & Hodson Carlton, 2008). A second similar practice–academic partnership example is that of the University of Saint Francis' link with Parkview Health System, an acute care facility, to integrate an electronic medical record system into the nursing curriculum (Lucas, 2010). It is expected that the need

for ongoing partnerships will become increasingly important as technology applications in acute care and home care clinical agencies continue to expand at a phenomenal rate.

Simulation centers of excellence have also been increasingly developed throughout the country. One such example is the Simulation Center at Fairbanks Hall in Indianapolis, Indiana, a facility jointly operated by Indiana University School of Medicine, Indiana University School of Nursing, and Indiana University Health (http://iuhealth.org/provider-portal/physician-education/simulation-center). The Smart Hospital at the University of Texas at Arlington School of Nursing is another such example (www.uta.edu/ra/real/editprofile.php?pid= 1307&onlyview=1). These facilities and others like them across the country have become LRCs dedicated to simulation-based education, training, and research. Such simulation centers, most frequently interprofessional in nature, typically have a variety of virtual clinical areas with an array of simulators and manikins, task trainers, medical and nursing equipment, and the associated multimedia and computer equipment, including electronic medical record and video recording systems to support student learning, faculty and health care–related staff development, product demonstrations, and new product beta site testing.

Lifelong Learning

Rapidly expanding electronic networks create the potential for the LRC to play a key role in the delivery of continuing education or lifelong learning. Health care and health care–related academic institutions and their health care organization partners now have World Wide Web and social media network home page sites, some with "virtual tour" and "virtual course" delivery, thus providing access to lifelong learning at the learner's time and place. Alumni and others may access continuing education programs and modules that provide just-in-time learning through the facilities of the LRC. With downsizing and outsourcing of education in health care facilities, the LRC may provide access to information and networking opportunities. Both computer technologies and interactive television may be used as delivery systems. There are also examples of partnerships with external organizations for the delivery of this continuing education. One example is the National League for Nursing's sponsorship of continuing education developed with various educational institutions (www.nln.org/facultydevelopment/index.htm).

Management and Operation of the Learning Resource Center

Physical Structure

The facility and physical layout of an LRC varies widely, depending on the scope of services and the particular institutional objectives for the unit. The central, organizational core of most LRCs is generally located within or near the nursing and health care programs. The physical dimensions of the LRC can vary dramatically. In 2002 Childs reported that 75% of 349 respondents from American Association of Colleges of Nursing schools indicated that the LRC facility was less than 4000 square feet, with the largest LRC size at that time reported as 15,000 square feet. However, today's LRC renovated with simulation studios, often in partnership with clinical agencies, may be significantly larger in physical space and virtual connections. Because of the continued phenomenal growth of the World Wide Web, the LRC also increasingly has a virtual space as well as a physical space dimension.

Considerations for physical space include use flexibility, conference room space, telecommunication infrastructure, storage and distribution space, current and future work space for staff and faculty, space for student and patient privacy, compliance with Occupational Safety and Health Administration (OSHA) and Americans with Disabilities Act (ADA) codes, custodial storage, space for a variety of changing work functions, viewing ability, maintenance and repair work space, and space for learning aids and display or bulletin boards. Additional checklist elements to add to this basic list are the hardware and software requirements for high-fidelity simulation studios including video conferencing and associated audiovisual and skill evaluation systems. Dimensions cited as important to include in considerations for virtual space remain computer-based technologies with Internet connections, access to patient database systems and institutional data sets, customer access from homes and work sites, access to a broadcast and receive site for technology-based conferences, capabilities for student–faculty contact from remote sites, connections to libraries

and electronic information distribution systems, and local and wide area networks.

There are contemporary examples of LRCs located in nursing programs across the country that illustrate the diversity in the physical design and size of today's resource centers. For example, the Clinical Simulation Lab at the University of Maryland is designed to replicate multiple clinical settings in one lab (i.e., a basic hospital unit and critical care, pediatric, maternity, and neonatal units). The facility maintains more than 25 clinical simulation labs, including remote sites, and operates a clinical education and evaluation laboratory, a joint venture of the University of Maryland's School of Nursing and School of Medicine. Other examples are located at the University of Texas at Arlington, the Temple College Health Sciences Center, and the Indiana University School of Nursing's Resource Center for Innovation in Clinical Nursing Education.

Learning Resource Center Administration and Personnel

There is wide diversity in the administrative position titles and organizational structure, academic qualifications, and salaries of LRC directors from institution to institution. These differences are often related to the mission of the institution and the role the LRC plays in meeting the institution's mission. Some LRC administrators may be full time and tenured with full academic rank and governance and curriculum roles. Others may be part time with other teaching and administrative roles. Increasingly, this position is considered to be a key administrative position within the institution, and individuals who provide leadership in LRCs are expected to be skilled in the use of technology and engaged in the scholarship of teaching.

Responsibilities of the LRC administrator role vary widely depending on institutional goals and support. Support for teaching and learning activities has traditionally been the predominant role of the LRC administrator. This role generally includes assisting faculty and students with curriculum development and implementation and integration of technology; coordination of unit activity with other institutional and extra-agency technology support areas; and fiscal, personnel, hardware, and software management, including grant writing and teaching functions. Other responsibilities can include participating in or leading committees, conducting remedial programs for students, consulting with faculty or other departments, evaluating student performance, managing classroom media services, coordinating technology resources in the school or program, managing distance learning support services, acting as a resource for the community and alumni, and producing multimedia.

In recent years, dimensions of the role and responsibilities of the LRC administrator have exploded as the functions of the LRC have expanded and diversified. As Kardong-Edgren and Oermann (2009) have pointed out, the addition of a high level of simulation and technology complexity calls for additional skills. These skills can include technology expertise, grant writing, research, and evaluation. Hyland and Hawkins (2009) have also emphasized the transformation (i.e., role of educators, teaching strategy innovations, and workload and budget reconfigurations) that is occurring in nursing LRCs based on the expansion of the use of high-fidelity human simulators.

Student staffing is also a critical personnel component of many LRC units. Students can perform a wide range of work responsibilities, including serving as core staff during evening and weekend hours, setting up supplies and equipment for teaching and learning activities, cleaning equipment and the practice and evaluation area, teaching skills, serving as student mentors, and assisting other LRC staff members in the operation and maintenance of the facility.

Professional staff positions may also be allocated as LRC support for technical, computer networking, secretarial, and psychomotor skill and simulation supervision and scenario development. Some institutions have successfully employed faculty or RN staff as preceptors in the LRC to provide assistance and feedback to students who are practicing skills. Often these individuals will also evaluate the students' performance of psychomotor skills before performing the skill in the health care setting.

There can be frequent turnover in LRC personnel because of the lack of standardization of LRC administrative responsibilities, qualifications, and benefits from institution to institution; wide variations in LRC unit staff composition; and the heavy dependence of the position's stability on the administrative prerogative of the chief executive officer of the institution. However, stability and the presence of high-quality personnel in this position are increasingly important as the pervasiveness of technology in the profession continues. The effective use of this position and the LRC staff composition can have far-reaching benefits for the institution in terms of effective and efficient technology integration and use at the unit level and successful internal and external resource collaborative efforts.

Fiscal Management: Budget and Operating Costs

Significant variations exist in budgetary allocations and the fiscal management policies of LRCs. Budgets for the LRC may range from very limited available funds for the nursing unit LRC, managed by the administrative officer of the entire unit, to budgets in excess of $1 million, managed by the LRC director. The primary source for funding of the majority of LRCs across the country remains the supporting institution, often augmented by student clinical or technology fees. On the other hand, there is the emergence of multiphase and multidisciplinary simulation centers, such as the LRC at University of Texas at Arlington's School of Nursing or the Simulation Center at Fairbanks Hall in Indianapolis, Indiana, both of which have required a large initial and continuing financial investment in the development of significant state-of-the-art simulation centers.

Regardless of the individual variations, a key trend is the movement toward internal and external collaboration and partnerships for the most effective use of resources and, in some cases, revenue generation. Nassif, Herrington, Delaney, Carr, and Deshotels (2003) described such experiences in sharing laboratory space between nursing and pharmacy technician students. Burgess (2007) described the development of a collaborative regional laboratory with pooled resources from the rural area. Another example is the nursing unit that uses an institutional computer laboratory rather than obtaining support for the personnel, equipment, and supply expenditure for this laboratory from the unit budget. Revenue for the nursing unit LRC may also be generated by costing out services and equipment to other units through the collaborative sharing of skill practice laboratory or computer laboratory space and resources. Several models of fee for services have now been developed across the country, as the evolving state-of-the-art learning resource and simulation centers have a fee schedule for outside users of the facilities, equipment, and services. As technology continues to evolve at a rapid rate, it is a continuing challenge to keep the LRC current so that students perceive their learning experience as "real world."

Additional Learning Resource Center Operational Issues: Safety, Evaluation, and Networking

Additional LRC issues are important to consider in the operation of the facility. The following discussion focuses on three dimensions: safety, evaluation, and professional networking opportunities.

The operation of a nursing psychomotor skills practice area, typically the most common function of the majority of LRCs in the United States, must include consideration of safety issues typical of clinical experiences in health care institutions and community health experiences. In their discussion of ways in which educators can reduce the risk of injury to students and potential litigation charging educational negligence, Goudreau and Chasens (2002) and Redford and Klein (2003) provided dimensions that may be used to develop a proactive

plan to ensure student safety in the skills laboratory. Some of the dimensions of such a proactive plan with suggestions to promote laboratory safety are summarized in Table 19-2.

Although evaluation is increasingly a critical component of success and continuing functionality of any entity, there are no specific standards for the evaluation of LRCs. Guides and recommendations related to evaluation of the nursing LRC from a cost-benefit analysis or program–instructional service perspective have also been scarce in the literature. Available reports usually focus on one aspect of LRC operation, such as budgetary analysis, rather than providing a comprehensive evaluation of the entire LRC operation (i.e., curriculum, faculty and student support, and fiscal accountability). Areas deemed critical for inclusion in an evaluation plan are learning outcomes, benefits to students, adequacy of resources, and value for money.

In summary, it appears that the area of LRC evaluation needs more attention, especially in an era of soaring costs, budget reductions, and demand for measurable outcomes. Until LRC comprehensive performance and outcome standards are established, it is recommended that, at a minimum, existing units

---

TABLE 19-2 Proactive Plan: Promoting Safety in Skills Laboratories

Potential Risks	Suggestions to Reduce Injury Risk
Use of dangerous materials and equipment such as needles, sharp instruments, biohazards, electrical equipment, and crutches outside of faculty-supervised times	Student instruction on safe operation of equipment is part of new student orientation.
	Lock areas where needles are stored.
	Require students' yearly attendance at OSHA in-service.
	Develop guidelines for using needles, syringes, and sharp instruments that students must sign.
	Partner with institution's environment specialist for compliance with use and maintenance of biohazardous materials, electrical equipment, and supplies.
Malfunctioning equipment such as electric beds, wheelchairs, and other electronic equipment	Contractual agreement with associated clinical facility or commercial vendor for annual maintenance checks and repairs as needed.
Latex allergy	Partner with institution's Office of Disabled Student Development.
	Obtain medical verification of physical impairment.
	Provide accommodation compliance with ADA and the Rehabilitation Act of 1973.
Back injuries	Provide supervised practice in transferring patients, emphasizing both student and patient safety.
Bloodborne pathogens	Use same protective measures in skills laboratory as would be used in clinical setting (e.g., use of gloves).
	School maintains documentation of student training in standard precautions.
Student live participation in procedures versus simulation	Student who volunteers to undergo or perform procedure is asked to sign consent and release from liability form that discloses risks and hazards.

use evaluation questionnaires or surveys for their diverse on-site and virtual customers.

As diverse as LRCs are across the country, there have been increasing efforts toward developing professional networking among LRC directors during the last four decades. In the early 1980s a few LRC directors identified the need for a periodic LRC national conference at which LRC directors from across the country could collaboratively explore the issues of teaching and learning in LRCs and network with each other about operational issues of the unit. In 1996 this national conference was broadened to include an international perspective and it has become a biennial event held in different regions of the country. Although a planning committee of LRC directors from across the country originally developed the programs for these conferences, a merger of this interest group with the International Association for Clinical Nursing Simulation and Learning (INACSL), established in 2002, enables the combination of LRC and simulation interests. The mission of INACSL is to promote and provide the development and advancement of clinical simulation and LRCs, and INACSL is committed to and supports collaboration, application of resource management concepts and integration of teaching strategies, research, and scholarship and information dissemination. In 2011 INACSL renewed its affiliation agreement with the Society for Simulation in Healthcare (SSH). Joint membership expands an individual's ability to network and provides access to the SSH journal as well as to INACSL's journal, *Clinical Simulation in Nursing*. The International Nursing Simulation/Learning Resource Centers Conference is an important biennial meeting for LRC directors and faculty interested in the development and operation of LRCs.

Membership in INACSL also provides access to an electronic discussion list communication. A great deal of information is exchanged in the electronic discussion communication, including tips on the use of simulations, comparative equipment pricing and recommendations, and ideas for teaching and learning in the skills laboratory. In summary, the management and operational issues for the administration of an LRC are complex and often vary widely depending on institutional goals and budget allocation for the facility. Dimensions of managing the LRC can vary widely and include physical and virtual space, personnel composition, qualifications, responsibilities, and funding allocations. One of the

areas of management that requires further exploration is the development and implementation of comprehensive evaluation. Positive trends during the last 4 decades have been increased professional networking among LRC administrators, the development of collaborative service–academia partnerships, and the continued evolution and integration of technology nursing and health care–related education.

SUMMARY

The LRC remains an integral part of nursing education programs for the purpose of nursing skills instruction and holds the potential for enhanced functions with the integration of technological supports and bridges to clinical practice and collaborative partnerships. The range of uses for LRCs across nursing programs is due to variability in operational budgets and institutional and unit goals. Budget constraints affect media and technology infusion, faculty involvement and responsibilities, administration and staffing, and the design of the physical space and virtual presence. Budget allocations often reflect the institution's philosophy and goals regarding the importance of teaching psychomotor skills within the curriculum or the willingness to assume responsibility for technology management.

Agreement on essential clinical nursing skills and minimal levels of behavioral competencies has yet to be achieved in nursing. The intellectual skills and motor processes that allow a student to think critically about the how, why, and what while actually performing continue to be underestimated in both research and instructional design. A lack of national standardization in identifying and measuring essential nursing skill competencies has the potential effect of minimizing the importance of dedicating resources to an LRC. For example, if accrediting agencies were to stipulate nursing skill competencies or proficiencies for best practice, the instructional methods and evaluation practices would need to be organized and standardized under the management of an academic unit such as an LRC. Laboratory practice, the use of media and technology, psychomotor skill demonstrations and return demonstrations, and simulations are common elements in nursing skill instruction. Infusion of technology into instruction adds another dimension for study. Initial research indicates that faculty-mediated instruction and media and technology instruction produce similar skill performance and that self-directed, media and technology forms of instruction can yield higher cognitive gains. In the future, using conceptual frameworks from observational learning theory and information processing can enhance the design and evaluation of instructional strategies for teaching nursing skills. The functions of the LRC offer many opportunities for the scholarship of teaching, and this is an increasingly important area of nursing education in which to focus research and evaluation efforts.

REFLECTING ON THE EVIDENCE

1. Think about the operation of the learning resource center (LRC) at your nursing program. How do the operation and functions of the LRC support student learning and faculty development? Identify some internal and external partnerships that might enhance the services and facilitate the resources of the LRC.

2. Identify some of the "essential" psychomotor skills for the nursing clinical course you are teaching. Develop a plan for how you can partner with the LRC personnel to facilitate students' performance of these skills in the simulation laboratory before the clinical laboratory. How will you incorporate a teaching–learning framework and an evaluation plan?

3. Identify three research questions that should be asked related to the design and evaluation of instructional strategies for teaching nursing skills in the next 2 years. How do your research questions relate to improving the clinical judgment and clinical decision making of the nursing student?

REFERENCES

Ahern, N., & Wink, D. (2010). Virtual learning environments: Second life. *Nurse Educator, 35*(6), 225–227.

Alavi, C., Loh, S. H., & Reilly, D. (1991). Reality basis for teaching psychomotor skills in a tertiary nursing curriculum. *Journal of Advanced Nursing,16* (8), 957–965.

Allen, P., Lauchner, K., Bridges, R. A. , Francis-Johnson, P., McBride, S.G., & Olivarex, A. (2008). Evaluating continuing competency: A challenge for nursing. *Journal of Continuing Education in Nursing 39* (2), 51–52.

Anderson, M., Holmes, T. L., LeFlore, J. L., Nelson, K. A., & Jenkins, T. (2010). Standardized patients in educating student nurses: One school's experience. *Clinical Simulations in Nursing, 6*(2), e61–e66.

Arundell, F., & Cioffi, J. (2005). Using a simulation strategy: An educator's experience. *Nurse Education in Practice, 5*(5), 296–301.

Ausubel, D. P., Novak, J. D., & Hanesian, H. (1978). *Educational psychology: A cognitive view* (2nd ed.). New York, NY: Holt, Rinehart, & Winston.

Bandura, A. (1986). *Social foundations of thought and action: A social cognitive theory.* Englewood Cliffs, NJ: Prentice-Hall.

Bandura, A. (1993). Perceived self-efficacy in cognitive development and functioning. *Educational Psychologist, 28*(2), 117–148.

Bantz, D., Dancer, M., Hodson-Carlton, K., & Van Hove, S. (2007). A daylong clinical laboratory: From gaming to high-fidelity simulators. *Nurse Educator, 32*(6), 274–277.

Bearnson, C. S., & Wiker, K. M. (2005). Human patient simulator: A new face in baccalaureate nursing education at Brigham Young University. *Journal of Nursing Education, 44*(9), 421–425.

Becker, K. L., Rose, L. E., Berg, J. B., Park, H., & Shatzer, J. H. (2006). The teaching effectiveness of standardized patients. *Journal of Nursing Education, 45*(4), 103–111.

Benner, P. (1984). *From novice to expert: Excellence and power in clinical nursing practice.* Menlo Park, CA: Addison-Wesley.

Billings, D. (2008). Quality care, patient safety, and the focus on technology. *Journal of Nursing Education, 47*(2), 51–52.

Bland, A., & Sutton, A. (2006). Using simulation to prepare students for their qualified role. *Nursing Times, 102*(22), 30–32.

Bourbonnais, F. F. (2010). Transitioning a master's of nursing course from campus to on-line delivery: Lessons learned. *Nurse Education in Practice, 10*(4), 201–204.

Boxer, E., Fallon, A., & Samuelson, A. (2001). Critical skills for new graduate nurses. *Nursing Monograph, 17–23.*

Bremner, M. N., Aduddell, K., Bennett, D. N., & VanGeest, J. B. (2006). The use of human patient simulators: Best practices with novice nursing students. *Nurse Educator, 31*(4), 170–174.

Burgess, C. (2007). Developing a collaborative regional nursing simulation hospital. *Teaching and Learning in Nursing, 2*(2), 53–57.

Burns, P., & Poster, E. C. (2008). Competency development in new registered nurse graduates: Closing the gap between education and practice. *Journal of Continuing Education in Nursing, 39*(2), 67–73.

Chase, T. (2005). Get in the game! Essential skills for SCI patient education. *SCI Nursing, 22*(3), 146–149.

Childs, J. C. (2002). Clinical resource centers in nursing programs. *Nurse Educator, 27*(5), 232–235.

Cioffi, J., Purcal, N., & Arundell, F. (2005). A pilot study to investigate the effect of a simulation strategy on the clinical decision making of midwifery student. *Journal of Nursing Education, 44*(3), 131–134.

Clark, T., & Holmes, S. (2007). Fit for practice? An exploration of the development of newly qualified nurses using focus groups. *International Journal of Nursing Studies, 44*(7), 1210–1229.

Cronenwett, L., Sherwood, G., Barnsteiner, J., Disch, J., Johnson, J., Mitchell, P., & Warren, J. (2007). Quality and safety education for nurses. *Nursing Outlook, 55*(3), 122–131.

Finkelman, A., & Kenner, C. (2009). *Teaching IOM: Implications of the Institute of Medicine reports for nursing education.* Silversprings, MD: Nursesbooks.org, American Nurses Association.

Goudreau, K. A., & Chasens, E. R. (2002). Negligence in nursing education. *Nurse Educator, 27*(10), 42–46.

Grady, J. L., & Berkebile, C. (2004). Nursing telehealth applications initiative: A research project for nursing education and practice. *Home Health Care Technology Report, 1*(6), 81, 86, 96.

Hofler, L. D. (2008). Nursing education and transition to the work environment: A synthesis of national reports. *Journal of Nursing Education, 47*(1), 5–13.

Hyland, J. R., & Hawkins, M. C. (2009). High-fidelity human simulation in nursing education: A review of literature and guide for implementation. *Teaching and Learning in Nursing, 4*(1), 14–21.

Ironside, P. (2008). Safeguarding patients through continuing competency. *Journal of Continuing Education in Nursing, 39*(2), 92–94.

Johnson, A. E. (2008). A nursing faculty's transition to teaching online. *Nursing Education Perspectives, 29*(1), 17–23.

Johnsson, A. C. E., Kjellberg, A., & Lagerstrom, M. I. (2006). Evaluation of nursing students' work techniques after proficiency training in patient transfer methods during undergraduate education. *Nurse Education Today, 26*(4), 322–331.

Jones, D. P., & Wolf, D. M. (2010, Spring). Shaping the future of nursing education today using distant education and technology. *The ABNF Journal, 21*(2), 44–47.

Kardong-Edgren, S., & Oermann, M. H. (2009). A letter to nursing program administrators about simulation. *Clinical Simulation in Nursing, 5*(5), e161–e162.

Klein, C. J. (2006). Linking competency-based assessment to successful clinical practice. *Journal of Nursing Education, 45*(9), 379–383.

Koerner, J. (2003). The virtues of the virtual world: Enhancing the technology/knowledge professional interface for life-long learning. *Nursing Administration Quarterly, 27*(1), 9–17.

Kurz, J., Mahoney, M. K., Martin-Plank, L., & Lidicker, J. (2009). Objective structured clinical examination and advanced practice nursing student. *Journal of Professional Nursing, 25*(3), 186–191.

Landry, M., Oberleitner, M. G., Landry, H., & Borazjani, J. G. (2006). Education and practice collaboration: Using simulation and virtual reality technology to assess continuing nurse competency in the long-term acute care setting. *Journal for Nurses in Staff Development, 22*(4), 163–171.

Larew, C., Lessans, S., Spunt, D., Foster, D., & Covington, B. G. (2006). Innovations in clinical simulation: Application of Benner's theory in an interactive patient care simulation. *Nursing Education Perspectives, 27*(1), 16–21.

Lenchus, J. D., Kalidindi, V., Sanko, J. S., Everett-Thomas, R., & Birnvach, D. J. (2010). Critical elements to advance procedural instruction: Knowledge, attitudes, and skills. *Academic Internal Medicine Insight, 8*(1), 14–15, 18.

Long, R. E. (2005). Using simulation to teach resuscitation: An important patient safety tool. *Critical Care Nursing Clinics of North America, 17*(1), 1–8.

Lucas, L. (2010). Partnering to enhance the nursing curriculum: Electronic medical record accessibility. *Clinical Simulation in Nursing, 6*(3), e97–e102.

Melo, D., & Hodson Carlton, K. (2008). A collaborative model to ensure graduating nurses are ready to use electronic health records. *CIN: Computers, Informatics, Nursing, 26*(1), 8–12.

Nassif, D., Herrington, K., Delaney, M., Carr, C., & Deshotels, D. (2003). Introducing interdisciplinary collaboration to nursing and pharmacy technician students. *American Journal of Health-System Pharmacy, 60*(9), 951.

Nehring, W. M., Lashley, F., & Ellis, W. E. (2002). Critical incident nursing management using human patient simulators. *Nursing Education Perspectives, 23*(3), 128–132.

Oermann, M. H. (1990). Psychomotor still development. *Journal of Continuing Education in Nursing, 21*(5), 202–204.

Oermann, M. H., & Kardong-Edgren, S. (2010). HeartCodeTM BLS with voice assisted manikin for teaching nursing students: Preliminary results. *Nursing Education Perspectives, 31*(5), 303–308.

Parr, M. B., & Sweeney, N. M. (2006). Use of human patient simulation in an undergraduate critical care course. *Critical Care Nursing Quarterly, 29*(3), 188–198.

Redford, D.S.& Klein, T. (2003). Informed consent in the nursing skills laboratory: An exploratory study. *Journal of Nursing Education 42* (3), 131–133.

Ridley, R. T. (2008). The relationship between nurse education level and patient safety: An integrative review. *Journal of Nursing Education, 47*(4), 149–156.

Robinson-Smith, G., Bradley, P. K., & Meakim, C. (2009). Evaluating the use of standardized patients in undergraduate psychiatric nursing experiences. *Clinical Simulation in Nursing, 5*(6), e203–e211.

Rutledge, C. M., Garzon, L., Scott, M., & Karlowicz, K. (2004). Using standardized patients to teach and evaluate nurse practitioner students on cultural competency. *International Journal of Nursing Education Scholarship,1* (1), 18–26.

Schmidt, B., & Stewart, S. (2009). Implementing the virtual reality learning environment: Second life. *Nurse Educator, 34*(4), 152–155.

Scott Tilley, D. D. (2008). Competency in nursing: A concept analysis. *Journal of Continuing Education in Nursing, 39*(2), 58–64, 65–66, 94.

Seropian, M. A., Brown, K., Samuelson Gavilanes, J., & Driggers, B. (2004). Simulation: Not just a manikin. *Journal of Nursing Education, 43*(4), 164–169.

Simpson, R. L. (1990). Technology: Nursing the system: Closing the gap between school and service. *Nursing Management, 21*(11), 16–17.

Simpson, R. L. (2003). Welcome to the virtual classroom: How technology is transforming nursing education in the 21st century. *Nursing Administration Quarterly, 27*(1), 83–86.

Smith, B. E. (1992). Linking theory and practice in teaching basic nursing skills. *Journal of Nursing Education, 31*(1), 16–23.

Snowman, J., & Biehler, R. (2003). *Psychology applied to teaching* (10th ed.). Boston, MA: Houghton Mifflin.

Tanner, C. A. (2006). Thinking like a nurse: A research-based model of clinical judgment in nursing. *Journal of Nursing Education,45* (6), 204–211.

Tarnow, K. G. (2005). Humanizing the learning laboratory. *Journal of Nursing Education, 44*(1), 43–45.

Theroux, R., & Pearce, C. (2006). Graduate students' experiences with standardized patients as adjuncts for teaching pelvic examinations. *Journal of the American Academy of Nurse Practitioners, 18*(9), 429–435.

Thomas, C., Ryan, M., & Hodson Carlton, K. (2011). Competency skills of new graduate nurses: Perceptions of nurse managers. *Nursing Management* (in press).

Weiner, E. E. (2008). Supporting the integration of technology into contemporary nursing education. *Nursing Clinics of North America, 43*(4), 497–506.

Ziv, A., Small, S. D., & Wolpe, P. R. (2000). Patient safety and simulation-based medical education. *Medical Teacher, 22*(5), 489–496.

20 Clinical Simulations: An Experiential, Student-Centered Pedagogical Approach

Pamela R. Jeffries, PhD, RN, FAAN, ANEF

John M. Clochesy, PhD, RN , FAAN, FCCM

Clinical simulation offers nurses, students, and health professionals the opportunity to learn in varied situations that are comparable to actual patient encounters while maintaining a safe learning environment for students (Dobbs, Sweitzer, & Jeffries, 2006; Katz, Peifer, & Armstrong, 2010). Simulation technology provides a risk-free, controlled learning setting that supports the learners' transfer of classroom and skills laboratory knowledge to realistic patient interactions (Halstead, 2006; Medley & Horne, 2005). In many areas, nurse educators have been challenged to find appropriate clinical sites and clinical experiences for nursing students to meet curricula competencies, and thus nurse educators are exploring alternative strategies for clinical preparation for nursing students. Clinical simulation technology is rapidly expanding and nursing programs are making large investments in equipment and learning space. As simulations and related teaching and learning strategies move into nursing programs, the nurse educator must be prepared to teach using this methodology. This chapter discusses clinical simulations as an experiential, student-centered pedagogical approach. The chapter begins with an overview of types of simulation—the purposes, challenges, and benefits of clinical simulations—and concludes with information about planning, implementing, and evaluating simulations as they are integrated into courses and curricula. Emphasized are (1) the types of clinical simulations being developed and implemented in nursing programs; (2) challenges and benefits to student learning, thinking, and practice; (3) a framework and steps to consider when developing and using clinical simulations; and (4) the evaluation component to consider when implementing simulations in the teaching–learning environment.

Simulations

Simulations are activities or events that mimic real-world practice (Seropian, 2003). Simulations are used when real-world training is too expensive, occurs rarely, or puts participants (or patients) at unnecessary risk. Simulations provide the opportunity for students to think critically, problem-solve, use clinical reasoning, and care for diverse patients in a non-threatening, safe environment. Today's learners must be prepared for the complexity and fast pace of the care environment, able to solve problems quickly by making appropriate assessments and decisions and to intervene to achieve desired outcomes. Incorporating simulations into a nursing curriculum as a teaching and learning strategy offers nurse educators the opportunity to support learners' educational needs by providing them with an interactive, practice-based instructional strategy.

Simulation Nomenclature

There are various types of simulations. The terms used to describe various aspects of the simulation experience are described here. The simulation nomenclature matrix includes learning domains and tool and environmental realism. Tool and environmental realism can be categorized into types of fidelity—low, medium, and high—and the context of the fidelity as partial or full.

The authors acknowledge the work of Marcella Hovancsek, MSN, RN, in the previous edition of the chapter.

Fidelity

Fidelity, or the realism of simulations, is described along a continuum—from low fidelity to high fidelity—relative to the degree to which they approach reality.

- *Low fidelity.* This type of simulation experience includes written case studies to educate students about patient situations or the use of a partial task trainer (e.g., plastic model arm to learn how to perform a venipuncture) to allow students to perform a task or skill. Some realism, but at a low level, is present; however, principles and concepts can still be learned using this type of simulation.
- *Medium fidelity.* This type of simulation is technologically sophisticated in that the participants can rely on a two-dimensional, focused experience to solve problems, perform skills, and make decisions during the clinical scenario. Examples include VitalSim Anne® and VitalSim Kelly®. These are manikins with less sophistication than the high-fidelity patient simulators.
- *High fidelity.* This type of simulation involves full-scale, high-fidelity human patient simulators that are extremely realistic and provide a high level of interactivity and realism for the learner. Examples include SimMan® 3G, iStan, and METI HPS®, all of which permit the student to listen to various body sounds and can be programmed to talk and to respond to interventions performed by the students.

Partial or Full-Context Simulations

The context of simulations can be partial or full.

- *Partial task trainers.* Partial task trainers are those simulations in which a body part, plastic model, or partial manikin is used to depict a certain function and on which a student can practice a particular psychomotor skill. Examples of partial task trainers include intravenous (IV) cannulation arms and low-technology manikins that are used to help students practice specific psychomotor skills integral to patient care such as inserting urinary catheters or nasogastric tubes.
- *Full-context simulations.* These simulations include the full context of a scenario, an event, or an activity that replicates reality. For example, a static manikin with limited functions such as VitalSim Kelly® is full context but medium fidelity. The full context of an event can be represented using this type of simulation in a low-fidelity manner. High fidelity, full context would be a simulated learning experience using a high-fidelity simulator and immersing the participants in a realistic mock code situation.

Full-scale patient simulations using sophisticated, high-fidelity patient simulators provide a high level of interactivity and realism for the learner. Less sophisticated, but still educationally useful, are computer-based simulations in which the participant relies on a two-dimensional, focused experience to solve problems, perform skills, and make decisions during the clinical scenario. Studies have shown that the two-dimensional experience has merit in terms of positive learning outcomes and skill acquisition (Jeffries, Woolf, & Linde, 2003). Partial task training devices such as IV arms and haptic (force feedback) IV trainers are used in simulations for psychomotor skills. The learner is able to practice a skill repeatedly before performing it on a real patient. The partial task trainers typically ensure a satisfactory rate of achievement of objectives and benefit to the participant. Studies have shown that after having used these task trainers, participants demonstrate a psychomotor skill and use that skill set in the real patient environment (Engum & Jeffries, 2003). Programs or courses in which the task trainers are used include clinical laboratory courses and modules during which specific skill sets and goals need to be obtained. Another approach to learning is the use of two-dimensional CD-ROMs to provide interactive practice with skills.

Types of Simulation Technologies

Simulations variously involve role playing, standardized patients (actors), interactive videos built on gaming platforms, and manikins to teach procedures, decision making, and critical thinking in realistic environments (Ryan et al., 2010). There are a variety of technology-based simulations to support student and novice nurses. They include computer-based interactive simulations, haptic partial task trainers, and digitally enhanced manikins. Haptic trainers use force feedback to provide opportunities to develop psychomotor skills. In addition to types of simulations categorized by the equipment or manikin used, there are simulations categorized by the type of pedagogy used when implementing the simulations. These types of simulations are described below.

Hybrid Simulations

A hybrid simulation is the combination of a standardized patient and the use of a patient simulator in one scenario to depict a clinical event for the learner. For example, the simulation scenario may begin with the student performing a health history on a standardized patient who has just arrived in the emergency department after having been involved in a motor vehicle accident. As the case evolves, the activity shifts to a patient simulator because of the clinical symptoms that need to be demonstrated by the manikin to reflect reality. This is a hybrid simulation because the history is being performed on a standardized patient and then the scenario shifts to a patient simulator, where the patient is now experiencing "hypovolemic shock" that is being reflected in the vital signs and other clinical findings of the manikin.

Unfolding Case Simulations

Another type of simulation is the unfolding case. Unfolding cases evolve over time in an unpredictable manner. An unfolding case may include three to four events that build on each other, providing students with a view across a clinical event, a hospitalization, or a view across the life span (Page, Kowlowitz & Alden, 2010). Purposes of unfolding cases vary, but a few include:

1. To demonstrate hierarchal order so the learner can view the health disruption progression and symptom management. For example, the first scenario demonstrates the patient being admitted with a head injury due to a fall; focused neurological assessment is needed. The unfolding case leads to a second scenario, in which the patient experiences specific neurological signs (e.g., severe headache, widening pulse pressure). The third case occurs postcraniotomy and involves care of the patient after the subdural hematoma was removed.
2. To visualize and prioritize hospital trajectory and care of a patient that progresses. For example, the patient is admitted through the emergency department, with the learner performing an assessment. The second scenario depicts the patient being admitted to the progressive care unit and the third scenario is designed for the learner to prepare the patient with discharge instructions.
3. To provide the learner with a view across the life span, showing the impact of the health disruption or disease process and nursing interventions required for a particular patient. For example, the first scenario depicts a patient newly diagnosed with chronic obstructive pulmonary disease (COPD). The second scenario progresses to the patient having compromised gas exchange related to COPD, and then the third scenario depicts end-stage disease with a focus on end-of-life care.
4. To serve as a mechanism to include a variety of important assessments and findings where one event leads to another. For example, the first scenario focuses on hypotension and subtle findings of sepsis and the second scenario centers on the critically ill patient with sepsis and hypotension.

Several organizations have developed unfolding case studies related to particular topics that are available at no cost to faculty. Four unfolding cases that focus on older adults and address the complexity of decision making about their care can be found at http://www.nln.org/facultydevelopment/facultyresources/ACES/index.htm; unfolding cases related to patient safety can be found at the Quality and Safety Education for Nurses site at http://www.qsen.org.

Standardized Patients

Standardized patients are live actors trained to portray the role of a patient according to a script or to clinical scenarios written by the faculty. The actors become the patients, demonstrating clinical symptoms and responses of real patients. A variation of the standardized patients instructional strategy is the use of these types of simulations to evaluate physical assessment skills, history taking, communication techniques, patient teaching, and types of psychomotor skills or objective structured clinical examination (OSCE).

In Situ Simulations

In situ simulation is a type of simulation that involves training performed in a real-life setting where patient care is commonly provided (Dismukes, Gaba, & Howard, 2006). The aim of this type of simulation is to achieve high fidelity (realism) by performing the simulations in actual clinical settings. Typically, the simulation-based experiential learning focuses on interdisciplinary professional teams. Practicing professionals are well versed in their particular field, possess a fair amount of experience, and prefer their learning to be problem-centered and meaningful to their professional lives. Adults learn best when they can immediately apply what they have learned. Traditional teaching methods (e.g., a teacher imparts facts to the student in a unidirectional model) are not particularly effective in adult learning because it is important for adults to make sense of what they experience or observe.

Virtual Simulations

Simulations can also take place in virtual environments. One commonly used environment is Second Life, a virtual world accessible by the Internet that enables its users, called residents, to interact with each other through avatars. In this simulated world, residents can explore, meet other residents, socialize, participate in individual or group activities, and create services for one another or travel throughout the world. The software is a three-dimensional modeling tool that attempts to depict reality for the users. Second Life is used as a platform for education by many institutions, such as colleges, universities, libraries, and government entities. For the top 10 health care–related virtual reality applications, go to http://scienceroll.com/2007/06/17/top-10-virtual-medical-sites-in-second-life/.

Purpose of Simulations

Clinical simulations in nursing education can be used for many purposes, for example, as a teaching strategy or for assessment and evaluation. However, one of the most important reasons that educators use simulations is to provide experiential learning for the student. Students can be immersed in a simulation, where they can actually portray the primary nurse, a newly employed nurse in orientation, or whatever role within the scope of practice of nursing the learner is assigned.

Experiential Learning

The use of simulation corresponds with a shift from an emphasis on teaching to an emphasis on learning (Dunn, 2004; Jeffries, 2005) in which the faculty facilitate learning by encouraging students to discover, or construct, knowledge and meaning. David Kolb (1984) and others (Sewchuck, 2005; Svinicki & Dixon, 1987) suggest that the experiential learning cycle is a continuous process in which knowledge is created by transforming experience. Individuals have a concrete experience, they reflect on that experience (reflective observation), they derive meaning (abstract conceptualization) from the experience, and they try out or apply (active experimentation) the meaning they've created, thus continuing the cycle with another concrete experience.

When making a shift in approach from a focus on teaching to a focus on learning, goals of the educational program serve as the framework for the development of specific learning activities. For example, both nursing students and nurses entering professional practice find it difficult to transfer learning into clinical practice. The use of simulation allows students to experience the application of theory in a safe environment where mistakes can be made without risk to patients.

The use of highly realistic and complex simulation is not always an appropriate educational approach. The literature suggests the use of low-fidelity and noncomplex simulated experiences with beginning students (Janes & Cooper, 1996; Schumacher, 2004). In simulation centers, beginning students can use low-fidelity simulation to work on attainment of foundational skills, including effective communication with patients, psychomotor skill performance, and basic assessment techniques. With task trainers or standard manikins, students can practice procedural skills and caregiving in a safe environment that allows them to make mistakes, learn from those mistakes, and develop confidence in their ability to approach and communicate with patients in the clinical setting. In addition, students benefit from the opportunity to work with technologically sophisticated equipment such as clinical information systems and hemodynamic monitoring systems in the educational setting before encountering such equipment in the clinical setting.

Advanced nursing students benefit from high-fidelity simulations that are complex, realistic, and interactively challenging experiences that support them in developing and practicing teamwork and decision-making skills. With patient simulators, for example, students can practice complex assessment skills involving a wide range of complex cardiac rhythms, variations in QRS morphology, changes in blood pressure, normal and abnormal breath sounds and patterns, heart sounds, pulses, bowel sounds, and computer-generated sound and vocalizations that provide *subjective* information. Faculty can create scenarios and program equipment to simulate serious clinical situations such as respiratory arrest or aberrant cardiac rhythm that may require an emergent response. More recently, the use of simulation in mental health situations has increased (Brown, 2008; Kameg, Howard, Clochesy, Mitchell, & Suresky, 2010; Kameg, Mitchell, Clochesy, Howard, & Suresky, 2009). As students respond to these situations, they demonstrate their abilities to establish priorities, make decisions, take appropriate action, and work successfully as part of a team (Reese, Jeffries, & Engum, 2010). Within the simulated environment, advanced students can demonstrate application of learning because they are no longer merely acquiring knowledge and skills. Students learn from the simulated practice without the need for faculty stepping in to correct and control the situation. High-fidelity simulation allows all students the opportunity to experience a baseline set of clinical scenarios, including those that are uncommon or rare. Students can practice a scenario repeatedly and use simulations for remediation, which enhances their preparation for clinical practice.

Clinical Simulations as a Teaching–Learning Strategy

With the advent of technologically advanced approaches, learning resource centers and clinical simulation centers have been developed to better prepare students for and maximize their learning experiences with patients in the clinical setting (Bearnson, 2005). Experiential learning through simulation affects patient care, health, and safety. Interactive experiences through the use of clinical simulations engage students through participation, observation, and debriefing (Rothgeb, 2008).

Forces Influencing Emergence of Simulation in Nursing Education

Nurse educators have used low-fidelity simulation such as manikins, role play, and case studies for decades. The introduction of high-fidelity simulation (in the form of affordable, portable, and versatile human patient simulators) in the late 1990s transformed health care education and appears to be one of the technologies of the future. Using simulation in nursing education as an instructional strategy is supported not only by a constructivist approach to education but also by lessons learned from those preparing pilots, military special forces teams, and students preparing for administering anesthesia or performing surgery. Across disciplines, unpredictable situations cause critical thinking challenges, including making the right assessment, taking timely action, and performing competently (Macedonia, Gherman, & Satin, 2003). Simulation has the advantages of posing no safety risks to patients and not provoking ethical dilemmas because it provides a wide range of experiences.

The dynamics of the hospital environment make it a less than ideal educational setting. Increased severity of illness of patients, decreased length of stay, heightened technology, patient safety initiatives, and workforce shortages all decrease the ability of staff nurses, even if expert, to mentor students. With increased enrollment in schools of nursing, nurse administrators are unable to accommodate all requests for student placements. To identify and resolve threats to patient safety, simulation has been used to identify latent threats to patient safety and to test potential resolutions (Hamman et al., 2010; Henneman et al., 2010). In a recent study, it was discovered that nursing students relied heavily on automated devices to obtain vital signs (Shepherd, McCunnis, Brown, & Hair, 2010). The use of simulation allows for a reliable way to assess students' skill at obtaining vital signs over a wide range of values. Clinical learning using simulation has emerged because of all of these forces.

Simulations Used for Assessment and Evaluation

With the rapid advancement of simulation technologies, the potential of using simulations for assessment and evaluation has expanded greatly. While more traditional forms of assessment continue to be employed—for example, pretesting and posttesting using multiple-choice tests—simulation-based assessments have gradually worked their way into the evaluation process, both in a formative manner, as part of an educational activity or training, or in a summative manner, as part of a certification process or licensure obtainment (Boulet, 2008; Boulet et al., 2003).

When simulations are being used for assessment or evaluation, the activities fall into two broad categories—"low-stakes" and "high-stakes" situations—depending on the significance of the evaluation (Boulet & Swanson, 2004). Low-stakes assessments are situations in which the simulation is used by the learner and faculty to mark progress toward personal, course, or program learning goals. High-stakes assessments include licensing and certification examinations, credentialing processes, and employment decisions (Jeffries, Hovancsek, & Clochesy, 2005). Simulation technologies used for assessment range from case studies and standardized patients (e.g., OSCEs) to haptic task trainers and high-fidelity human simulators.

As with any type of assessment, faculty must consider the issues of validity and reliability (Boulet et al., 2003; Clauser, Kane, & Swanson, 2002). For assessments in low-stakes or learning situations, construct and concurrent validity should be addressed. Construct validity is the degree to which an assessment instrument measures the dimensions of knowledge or skill development intended. Concurrent validity is determined by evaluating the relationship between how individuals perform on the new assessment (in this case a simulation) and the traditional (standard) assessment instrument (Pugh & Youngblood, 2003). An assessment with high concurrent validity, for example, is one in which the learner's simulator assessment score is comparable to his or her score when performing the same examination on a standardized patient scored by using a checklist.

Predictive validity is required for simulations used in assessments in which licensure, certification, or employment are at stake. Determining predictive validity in high-stakes assessment is a complex process. Predictive validity is the extent to which performance on a particular simulation predicts future performance, such as clinical decision making or psychomotor skills. Evaluating predictive validity requires that, in addition to current performance, the clinical skill or decision making of specific individuals be tracked over time. There has been little research and evidence-based information specifically focused on quantifying the impact of simulation-based assessment activities on student or practitioner learning.

Simulations also are being used to assess and evaluate students' clinical skill competencies and clinical decision-making capabilities. Using standardized patients to assess the clinical skills of medical students and residents has become widespread (Chambers, Boulet, & Gary, 2000). OSCEs are clinical examinations that vary in format but mostly include a set period of time for the student to assess and interact with a standardized patient, an actor or actress hired to portray a certain type of patient with a specific diagnosis and clinical symptoms. Wilson, Shepherd, and Pitzner (2005) used the low-fidelity human patient simulator to acquire and then assess nurses' health assessment knowledge and skills. The use of the low-fidelity manikins proved to be an effective tool to assess for health assessment skills. Miller, Leadingham, and Vance (2010) used the human patient simulator to meet learning objectives across core nursing courses.

When using simulations as an assessment mechanism, the nurse educator should also consider the improvement in the use of standardized patients, the sophistication of computer-based evaluation techniques, the use of newer physiological electromechanical manikins, and the fidelity of immersive haptic devices. Because of these advances, nurse educators are now better able to assess learning, promote a better educational effort, improve academic courses and programs, and ultimately prepare students to give quality and safe patient care.

Challenges and Benefits of Using Clinical Simulations

Simulations can offer nurse educators and health care providers a significant educational method that meets the needs of today's learners by providing them with interactive, practice-based instructional strategies. Implementing and testing the use of simulations in educational practice has both challenges and benefits.

Most of the challenges of using clinical simulations center on educators' preparation for using simulation. Before using simulations as a learning strategy, the faculty must have:

1. A firm foundation in experiential learning
2. Clear learning objectives for the simulation experience
3. A detailed design taking into account that an educator facilitates learning (versus tells the learner)
4. Sufficient time for learners to experience the simulation, to reflect on the experience, and to make meaning of the experience

5. Faculty development in the area of simulation pedagogy; the teaching strategy is student-centered, which for many is a paradigm shift in teaching

The benefits of using clinical simulations include:

1. *Active involvement of students in their learning process.* By interacting with the simulation, examples, and exercises, the learner is required to use a higher order of learning rather than simply mimicking the teacher role model. Decision-making and critical thinking skills are reinforced through this teaching modality.

2. *More effective use of faculty in the teaching of clinical skills and interventions.* In a simulated experience, faculty members have an opportunity to observe students more closely and to allow students to demonstrate their potential more fully. The feedback or debriefing by faculty is a powerful learning tool.

3. *Increased student flexibility to practice based on their schedules.* The learner can access the simulation at his or her convenience and would not be required to practice the skills in front of an instructor, although that option would remain available for those who need extra instruction or reinforcement. The learner can revisit a skill several times in an environment that is safe, nonthreatening, and conducive to learning.

4. *Improved student instruction.* Student instruction is improved through better consistency of teaching; increased learner satisfaction in both the classroom and the clinical setting; the opportunity for safer, nonthreatening practice of skills and decision making; and a state-of-the-art learning environment.

5. *Effective competency check for undergraduates, new graduates, or new nurses going through orientation.* The simulation experience would provide a competency check of the participants' knowledge, skills, and problem-solving abilities in a nonthreatening, safe environment.

6. *Correction of errors discussed immediately (Medley & Horne, 2005).* Students can learn by being immersed in their learning experience and then being debriefed after the encounter on what was right and what needed to be done differently.

7. *Standardized, consistent, and comparable experiences for all students.* Educators can create consistent, standardized teaching activities so that all students in a clinical course can experience an important clinical event, assessment activity, or other essential clinical learning encounter.

As educators are incorporating simulations into their courses and into the nursing curriculum, major challenges and benefits have been noted. Faculty must consider both challenges and benefits as the simulation pedagogy is adopted into courses and the nursing curriculum.

Planning to Use Clinical Simulations

Using simulations in classroom or clinical teaching requires advance planning. Planning should consider the need for resources and the needs of the student, faculty, and curriculum.

Resources

A staff dedicated to simulation is essential for its successful integration into nursing curricula. Kyle (2004) offers the simile that dedicated staff (or simulation professionals) are like the chef, manager, and staff of a restaurant who conceive and organize a meal. Teachers are essential to the success of using alternative learning experiences such as simulation activities. However, unlike in the traditional classroom setting, instruction when using simulations is no longer teacher-centered, but rather is student-centered, with the teacher playing the role of a facilitator in the student's learning process. The educator's role during the simulation process will vary, depending on whether the simulation is being conducted for learning or evaluation purposes. In the teaching or facilitating context, teachers must provide learner support as needed throughout the simulation and debriefing at the conclusion of the experience. If the simulation is being conducted for evaluation purposes, the teacher's role is that of an observer.

When using simulations for the first time, faculty must feel comfortable with the simulations they are using. Faculty may require assistance with simulation design, use of the technology, and setting up equipment for the activity. Whei Ming and Juestel (2010) found that novice faculty members needed assistance to operationalize the critical thinking learning objectives in a clinical simulation. To assist faculty, the educators developed a series of questions that provide direction about the specific thought processes involved in the application of the nursing process through the use of clinical simulations (Table 20-1).

The use of simulations in a nursing curriculum has the potential to assist students, faculty, and the overall nursing program. The following describes the needs that can be met when using simulations in the teaching–learning environment.

Student Educational Needs

The integration and use of simulations in nursing programs can assist with various students' learning needs. For example, simulations may offer a flexible, accessible opportunity to practice skills and interventions when student schedules permit. The learner can access the simulation at his or her convenience and not be required to practice the skills in front of an instructor, although that option can remain available for those who need extra instruction or reinforcement. Simulations also offer an opportunity to practice a selected skill set a number of times in an environment that is safe, nonthreatening, and conducive to learning. According to Brannan, White, and Bezanson (2008), the human patient simulator can be used as a tool for experiential learning, providing a mechanism by which students can participate in clinical decision making, practice skills, and observe outcomes of clinical decisions made. Most importantly, simulations can provide exposure to real-life clinical experiences for students before caring for a specific type of patient in a specific type of clinical setting.

Faculty Educational Needs

Using simulations in a nursing course can assist faculty to use more effective methods to facilitate the learning of clinical skills and to measure skill competency or problem-solving abilities before taking students to a clinical unit. Simulations can provide an innovative, experiential approach to teaching that actively involves students in their learning process. By interacting with simulations, the learner is required to use a higher order of learning than simply mimicking the teacher role

---

TABLE 20-1 Critical Thinking Learning Objectives and Core Questions to Ask in Clinical Simulations

Critical Thinking Learning Objectives	Core Questions
Assess client to collect relevant data. • Identify cues and make inferences. • Validate data.	• What are the possible problems in this situation that need to be solved? On what evidence have you based your inferences? • Is your evidence valid? What factors may alter the accuracy of the data? How would you validate each item of evidence? • Why are these items relevant? How are they related?
Diagnose actual and potential client health needs. • Cluster data. • Draw diagnostic conclusions.	• Are the clustered data sufficient to support each diagnosis? What additional data do you need? • Are there different possibilities for clustering these data? Are there other alternative diagnoses that may fit different ways of clustering? • What other data are needed to rule in/out these possibilities?
Plan care based on identified client health needs. • Set priorities. • Predict outcome criteria. • Generate solutions (interventions).	• What are the most important problems that need solved? On what criteria did you base your decision? • What are the expected outcomes of the problem? • What are the possible interventions for the problem described? • What are the possible risks/benefits involved in each intervention?
Implement plan of care. • Test solutions.	• When do you assess the client's response to each intervention? What are the desired responses to the intervention?
Evaluate progress toward attainment of outcomes. • Perform a criterion-based evaluation.	• If an adverse reaction happened, what would you do next? Why?
Self-critique thinking strategies used to reach decisions. • Self-regulate thinking.	• What were the factors influencing your thinking? • What would you do differently in a different situation?

From Whei Ming, S., & Juestel, M. (2010). Direct teaching of thinking skills using clinical simulation. *Nurse Educator, 35*(5), 197–204.

model. Decision-making and critical thinking skills are required and implemented by the student when using this teaching modality. The use of simulations in the instructional process can improve student learning outcomes and allow for more consistency in clinical and didactic instruction, more learner satisfaction in the classroom and clinical setting, and learning in a safe, nonthreatening environment.

Curricular Needs

A competency-based curriculum may require accurate documentation of critical behaviors and selected skill sets. Simulations can serve as a vehicle to validate skill competency for undergraduates, new graduates, or individuals going through orientation; the simulation experience could serve as a mechanism to measure students' knowledge, skills, and problem-solving abilities in a nonthreatening, safe environment. The use of simulations can serve as an educational model for clinical education that is interactive and promotes a higher order of thinking and decision making. The incorporation of simulations into the nursing curricula can serve as a new experiential model for these expectations.

Designing Clinical Simulations

Simulations should be carefully planned. The process of designing, implementing, and evaluating a simulation to support learning in nursing education is best done using a systematic, organized approach. To help nursing educators and researchers in this developmental process, a simulation framework (Jeffries, 2005) has been developed to identify the components of the process and their relationship to guide the design, implementation, and evaluation of these activities.

The Simulation Model

A framework (Fig. 20-1) has been designed by a national group organized by the National League for Nursing to assist educators in outlining the first steps of simulation development, to provide a consistent and empirically supported model to guide the design and implementation of simulations as well as the assessment of learning outcomes when using simulations (Jeffries, 2005). Within the framework, five design features for developing a clinical simulation scenario are described. A simulation template used as a guide to develop the

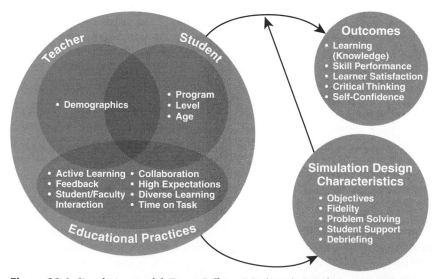

Figure 20-1 Simulation model. From: Jeffries, P.R. (2007). *Simulations in nursing education: From conceptualization to evaluation.* New York: National League for Nursing. (Included with permission.)

clinical simulations can be found at the Simulation Innovative Resource Center (SIRC) website at http://sirc.nln.org/. When developing the scenario, the design features are considered within the development process. For example, problem-solving components are considered in the scenario progression writing. Faculty can consider one or two problem-solving components designed in the scenario to be implemented by the novice students and three or four decision-making components for the more senior advanced student, perhaps to facilitate and emphasize prioritization at this level. After the simulation template is completed, it is advised that the scenarios be peer reviewed by content experts to ensure that evidence-based practices are being incorporated into the scenario and to confirm accuracy and that the content is up to date for today's health care world. Finally, the scenario must be pilot-tested with targeted end users so that educators can be assured that the scenario is at the correct level for the learner and can review the scenario for sufficient decision-making points and cues to engage the students in the simulation. A variety of resources exist to provide educators with knowledge and skills on developing simulation scenarios, including regional and national workshops, conferences, instructor courses, and several publications (Campbell & Daley, 2008; Guhde, 2011; http://sirc.nln.org; Jeffries, 2007).

Debriefing and Reflection

Debriefing is one of the key design features when developing a simulation (Fig. 20-1). Debriefing is a process by which educators facilitate learners' reflection or reexamination of clinical encounters (Dreifuerst, 2009). Debriefing, in the context of simulation, usually involves reflective observation and abstract conceptualization. Reflective observation has its roots in Gestalt psychology and in the works of Kurt Lewin (1951), Donald Schön (1987), Diefenbeck, Plowfield, and Herrman (2006), and David Kolb (1984). Kolb (1984) and others (Sewchuck, 2005; Svinicki & Dixon, 1987) suggest that the experiential learning cycle is a continuous process in which knowledge is created by transforming experience. Individuals have a concrete experience, they reflect on that experience (reflective observation), they derive meaning (abstract conceptualization) from the experience, and they try out or apply (active experimentation) the meaning they have created, thus continuing the cycle with another concrete experience.

The role of faculty in facilitating simulation exercises is to support participants in the reflection and debriefing process. Table 20-2 describes one approach using different components of debriefing (Overstreet, 2010). Faculty members coach students to reflect on what they saw, heard, smelled,

---

TABLE 20-2 Components for Debriefing Nursing Students Using the Ee-Chats

Debriefing Component	Educator Action/Activity/Strategy
E – Emotion	Faculty need to address learners' emotions that have been stimulated during the simulation encounter; encourage the students to translate emotions into words.
e – Experience	Faculty can briefly share their experiences or stories; inform the students how the expert would have handled the situation—but be brief, this is only one small part of debriefing.
C – Communication	Educators should talk less and students more; students also can observe your verbal and nonverbal messages; the debriefing should be a positive experience.
H – Higher Order of Thinking	Students should be encouraged to reflect in, on, and beyond the simulation encounter they have experienced; how will this experience translate into the clinical one?
A – Accentuate the Positive	Educators need to be positive when conducting a debriefing—reframe and rephrase your questions into inquiry-time ones, not blaming. Focus on behaviors that are professional and essential.
T – Time	Allow students time to formulate their responses and reflections. Embrace silence.
S – Structure	Debriefing time should focus on the encounter, the events, actions, and behaviors demonstrated in the simulation.

From Overstreet, M. (2010). Ee-chats: The seven components of nursing debriefing. *The Journal of Continuing Education in Nursing, 41*(12), 538–539.

and touched. Faculty also encourage students to reflect on internal sensations "in their hearts and in their guts." Advances in neuroscience show increased recall of conceptualizations that are tied to visceral sensations or experiences (Bransford, Brown, & Cocking, 2000). The key for faculty during this phase is not to provide more information or to lecture on the "correct" way or answer but to guide students along the path of reflection.

Faculty members using this approach often find it useful to have another faculty member shadow them to provide feedback regarding their coaching of the learners. Many find the S-E-I-A (or statement, evidence, impact, action/plan) approach to providing feedback useful in this setting.

Implementing Clinical Simulations

Once the simulation is designed, faculty members are ready to implement it into the nursing course. The following guidelines may be useful to educators implementing simulations into their nursing courses:

1. Make sure specific objectives match the implementation phase of the simulation. When faculty design a simulation, the objectives and nature of the simulation should be clearly defined for the students. Furthermore, if the simulation is designed, for example, around the care of an insulin-dependent patient, then the scenario should be created using problems typically encountered and the problem-solving skills needed for that patient's care. The simulation should focus on the objectives and not on potential co-morbidities or extraneous issues.

2. Set a time limit for the simulation and the debriefing encounter and then adhere to it. Too often instructors observe that in simulations students are immersed for a specific time limit but are not able to accomplish all of the assessments and interventions the instructor had desired. At times instructors may let the scenario proceed beyond the specific time frame; however, if the simulation is scheduled for 20 minutes, the encounter needs to be 20 minutes. If students do not achieve the objectives desired, the reflective observation time can be spent on their experiences and the meaning they make of them.

3. Make assignments so students know their specific roles during the simulation. Unless developing or testing team leadership skills, students need roles (e.g., nurse, observer, family member) assigned before encountering the simulation in order to bring organization to the experience. If roles are not assigned, students waste time trying to decide what role to play.

4. Avoid interrupting the simulated encounter when students are trying to problem-solve on their own. Ideally, faculty would observe a simulation remotely, either behind a one-way mirror or via closed-circuit television, so students cannot see facial expressions, hear comments, or see other nonverbal gestures. It is best for faculty to discuss the points of concern, prioritization, and problem-solving issues during the debriefing that typically follows immediately after the simulation event.

5. Involve a limited number of learners in the simulation experience in addition to one or two observers or recorders of the encounter. Typically, two to six students are each assigned a role in the simulation experience. The roles within the simulation need to be identified before and recognized during the simulation. For example, students can wear name tags or labels and appropriate clothing for particular roles or have certain props available to help delineate the roles. When an educator has more students than are needed to participate in the simulation, these students can be assigned an observer role.

6. Ensure that the simulation is appropriate for the learners' skill levels and cognitive ability. Although a prominent design feature when developing simulations is fidelity, simulations need to be realistic to the degree that matches the learning level of the student group. Beginning students benefit from the low fidelity offered by practice with standard manikins, equipment, and task trainers as they focus on skill and knowledge acquisition. More advanced learners benefit from a higher level of fidelity, including challenges found in a complex environment such as simulated emergent events that require them to cooperate and collaborate with the health care team to achieve a common goal. Simulations assist students at the application level of learning to practice their decision-making, problem-solving, and team member skills in a nonthreatening environment. The environment needs to be sufficiently realistic to

allow for suspension of disbelief, so that the transition of knowledge from theory to practice can be stimulated.

7. When planning to incorporate simulations into the course or curriculum, ensure that faculty development is included in the planning. Faculty need to know how to conduct a simulation and achieve the desired outcomes with the teaching–learning strategy. Faculty need to be prepared to design and conduct simulations in the educational setting before they are actually placed in the learning laboratory or clinical practicum with students in a simulation situation. All faculty members using this type of strategy in their classroom or clinical instruction need to be aware of and clear about the purpose of the simulation activity. At the end of the simulation, a clear summary and highlights need to be included by all instructors, particularly if there are several educators using the same simulation in a course. Discussion about simulations and how to implement them and clarity on learning outcomes for the simulation are needed and must be agreed upon by faculty before implementation of the simulation.

Integrating Simulations into Courses and Curricula

Simulations can be integrated into nursing courses, laboratory experiences, and clinical courses to promote more active and experiential learning at most schools of nursing (Katz, Peifer, & Armstrong, 2010). As more schools adopt clinical simulations in their courses and curricula and as actual clinical experiences are becoming more difficult to obtain, some faculty and their state boards of nursing are supplementing or substituting clinical time with simulations. Studies are being conducted on the use and amount of simulations being substituted for clinical time, with a landmark study being conducted by the National Council of State Boards of Nursing (NCSBN) in the fall of 2011 (www.ncsbn.org).

Faculty have integrated simulations in a variety of courses. Thomas, Hodson-Carlton, and Ryan (2010) used clinical simulations in a senior leadership course to better prepare and facilitate new graduates to clinical practice. Clinical scenarios were developed that incorporated students, faculty, staff, and community volunteers who role-played situations that students may encounter upon graduation. Some of the issues embedded in the scenarios include staffing problems, physician interactions, patient and family communications, and crisis interventions.

Hamilton (2010) used clinical simulations during academic and clinical experiences to equip students with the skills necessary to productively cope with the stressors faced in difficult end-of-life situations. Using the End-of-Life Nursing Education Consortium (ELNEC) materials, the educator found simulations to be an effective teaching strategy to identify anxiety levels prior to clinical experience and as a venue for exploring learning and coping styles.

Maternity simulators have been used to teach students about maternal and child health. Undergraduate faculty from a large Midwest nursing program implemented a 6-hour laboratory and virtual clinical experience for students in the maternal–newborn health rotation that incorporated various simulations (Bantz, Dancer, Hodson-Carlton, & Van Hove, 2007). This experience consisted of eight stations, including assessment of the postpartum fundus, newborn assessment and care (with SIM baby), newborn nutrition, labor and birth (with the Noelle birthing simulation manikin), fetal heart rate assessment and interpretation, Leopold's maneuvers, and computerized charting. According to Bantz et al. (2007), the majority of students who participated in this clinical laboratory experience indicated that they felt better prepared to provide nursing care to newborns and their mothers in the clinical site.

DeBourgh and Prion (2010) used a quasi-experimental, pretest and posttest study of 285 prelicensure students to teach students fall prevention and patient safety using clinical simulations with standardized patients. The results of the teaching and research conducted concluded that the simulation learning experience provided students with knowledge and skill gains they could apply to clinical practice.

Thompson and Bonnel (2008) integrated the use of high-fidelity simulation in an undergraduate pharmacology course to provide an applied learning experience where students could make connections between learned content and clinical application. An experience of safe medication administration has been added to both pharmacology course simulations and any simulation in which the "patient" is to receive medications.

As distance education course formats proliferate in nursing curricula, simulation has been recognized as a potentially rich learning strategy. Nelson and Blenkin (2007) used online role-play simulation to provide students with the opportunity to learn professional and personal relationships in an online environment. The online learning platform provided students with a learning opportunity to deal with difficult behavior and to manage violence, abuse, and patients with dementia. To initiate the learning activity, the authors built what was called a "kickstart" episode, in which students would have to react to a significant event, for example, a patient dying. Participating students logged in and played their assigned roles, which ranged from long-term care residents to facility staff members. During the computer-based event, students role-playing as health care professionals could enter into an "interaction space (ispace)" where a threaded discussion could occur about the patient's problem. Several resources were available to students within the online simulation environment, including instruction sheets and video clips to assist the students with the care of these selected patients. Students immersed themselves in the online simulations and believed that the level of realism paralleled clinical nursing practice and offered a relevant student learning experience.

Unfolding case simulations are gaining more attention in nursing programs. Durham and Sherwood (2008) used unfolding simulated cases to teach quality and safety concepts and how these concepts are integrated into nursing practice. In addition, Batscha and Moloney (2005) used online unfolding case studies to facilitate nursing students to analyze, organize, and prioritize in novel situations. Finally, Azzarello and Wood (2006) suggest that unfolding cases can be used to evaluate students' changing mental models since they offer a practical strategy for revealing flaws in students' problem solving that would otherwise not be obvious.

Evaluation Considerations when Using Clinical Simulations

Evaluation of the Design and Development Phase of Simulation

To evaluate the design and development of simulations created by nurse educators, Jeffries (2005) developed the Simulation Design Scale (SDS). The purpose of this tool is to provide the educator with information and feedback that can be used to improve the simulation design and implementation.

The SDS is a 20-item tool that the learner completes after participating in a simulation to provide feedback on whether the intended simulation design features were present. These features include the objectives and information, support, problem solving, feedback and debriefing, and fidelity. These are referred to as *simulation design features* because they define what a quality simulation requires if it will have a positive impact on learning outcomes. Content validity of this instrument was determined by a panel of nine nurse experts. Cronbach's alpha was computed to assess internal consistency reliability for each scale. The coefficient alpha for the overall scale was 0.94. Table 20-3 briefly describes the SDS's five components.

Evaluation of the Implementation Phase

When simulations are implemented, particular components need to be included to ensure good learning experience, student satisfaction, and good learner performance. According to Chickering and Gamson (1987, 1991), incorporating the Principles of Best Practice in Education assists educators to implement quality teaching activities and improve student learning. As a component of the simulation model (Jeffries, 2005), those educational practices are considered very important in the implementation of simulations in the students' learning environment. To measure this component, the Educational Practices in Simulation Scale (EPSS) was developed. The EPSS is a 16-item tool that the learner completes after a simulation. This tool measures whether the best practices in education, according to Chickering and Gamson (1987), are being used in the simulation. All seven educational practices in simulation are being evaluated; however, after conducting a factor analysis on the scale, four factors were identified and several of the factors were collapsed into these four components of the scale. Therefore the elements being evaluated in the EPSS are active learning, diverse ways of learning, high expectations, and collaboration, as shown in Table 20-4. The questionnaire was tested for validity and reliability. Content validity was established through a review by nine nursing experts. The coefficient alpha was 0.92.

TABLE 20-3 Simulation Design Scale Components

Concept/Design Features	Description of Concept
Information/objectives	Clear objectives and timeframe for the simulation is information needed by the student before the simulation begins.
Problem solving/complexity	The simulation needs to be designed with problem-solving components embedded in the written scenario or case. The level of problem solving needs to be considered, for example, simple tasks and decisions if students are in a fundamentals course versus more complex tasks if students are in an upper-level course and are 6 months away from graduating.
Student support/cues	Student support in a simulation is offered before, during, and after. Support includes providing information and direction to the student before the simulation.
Fidelity	A simulation should be as close an approximation as possible to the real event or activity that is being modeled to promote better learning outcomes.
Guided reflection/debriefing	Guided reflection reinforces the positive aspects of the experience and encourages reflective learning, which allows the participant to link theory to practice and research, think critically, and discuss how to intervene professionally in very complex situations.

From Jeffries, P. R. (2007). *Simulations in nursing education: From conceptualization to evaluation.* New York: NY: The National League for Nursing. (Included with permission.)

TABLE 20-4 Educational Practices in Simulation Scale (EPSS)

Components of the EPSS	Description of Components within the Scale	Examples
Active learning	Through simulation, learners are directly engaged in the activity and obtain immediate feedback and reinforcement of learning. Learning activities can range from simple to complex.	A case scenario in which an intubated patient is restless, agitated, and coughing, affecting his oxygenation status. Students can be asked to select the most appropriate intervention and describe the rationale for the intervention.
Diverse styles of learning	Simulations should be designed to accommodate diverse learning styles and teaching methods and allow students and groups with varying cultural backgrounds to benefit from the experience.	Design a scenario that has visual, auditory, and kinesthetic components.
High expectations	High teacher expectations are important for the student during a learning experience because expecting the student to do well becomes a self-fulfilling prophecy.	Set up a scenario with multiple patient problems to challenge the learner and to advance learning and skill application to the next level.
Collaboration	Collaboration is pairing students in a simulation to work together. Roles are assigned so that students jointly work on the problem-solving and decision-making skills within the simulation together.	Assign a student the role of a primary nurse and a third-year medical student the role of a physician. Place the two students in a setting where they will be confronted with a patient having post-operative complications that requires quick assessments and efficient decision-making skills to intervene appropriately with the patient.

From Jeffries, P. R. (2007). *Simulations in nursing education: From conceptualization to evaluation.* New York: NY: The National League for Nursing. (Included with permission.)

Evaluation of Learning Outcomes

As discussed previously, learning outcomes can be measured through low-stakes and high-stakes simulations. Outcomes are defined for the learning activity and can be measured by a well-designed clinical simulation. Research in this area is growing as educators measure the outcomes of the simulation activity desiring to close the knowledge and skills gap within academe and practice.

SUMMARY

Educators use simulations to enhance learning outcomes and promote safe patient care environments. Nursing organizations, commissions of higher education, accrediting bodies, academic institutions, and schools of nursing are seeking answers to questions about simulation design and development, teaching and learning practices, implementation processes, and associated learning outcomes. Educators and researchers must join forces to develop more rigorous research studies testing simulation outcomes. National, multisite simulation studies by nurse educators are currently being conducted to enhance understanding of the educational usefulness of nursing simulations. For example, when simulations are used as a teaching–learning intervention, are learning outcomes improved? When developing a simulation, what are the important design features of a well-executed simulation in nursing education? How can simulations be used to prepare for or replace clinical experience? How does the use of simulations contribute to advancing nursing into the next generation? Educators need to make certain they are informed about the possibilities of simulations, their usefulness in enhancing student education, and the progress of educational research efforts conducted to develop and test new models of using simulation in nursing education.

REFLECTING ON THE EVIDENCE

1. What evidence is available on the effectiveness of using simulation in support of learning?

2. When using a simulation framework, how would you construct a research project to test the framework?

3. Identify three research questions that might be addressed when studying reflective observation.

4. What is the optimal balance of simulated versus actual clinical practice in nursing education?

REFERENCES

Azzarello, J., & Wood, D. E. (2006). Assessing dynamic mental models: Unfolding case studies. *Nurse Educator, 31*(1), 10–14.

Bantz, D., Dancer, M., Hodson-Carlton, K., & Van Hove, S. (2007). A daylong clinical laboratories: From gaming to high fidelity. *Nurse Educator, 32*(6), 274–277.

Batscha, C., & Moloney, B. (2005). Using Powerpoint to enhance unfolding case studies. *Journal of Nursing Education, 44*(8), 387.

Bearnson, C. S. (2005). Human patient simulators: A new face in baccalaureate nursing education at Brigham Young University. *Journal of Nursing Education, 44*(9), 421–425.

Boulet, J. (2008). Summative assessment in medicine: The promise of simulation for high-stakes evaluation. *Society for Academic Emergency Medicine, 15*(11), 1017–1024.

Boulet, J., Murray, D., Kras, J., Woodhouse, J., McAllister, J., & Ziv, A. (2003). Reliability and validity of a simulation-based acute care skills assessment for medical students and residents. *Anesthesiology, 99*(6), 1270–1280.

Boulet, J. R., & Swanson, D. B. (2004). Psychometric challenges of using simulations in high-stakes assessment. In W. F. Dunn (Ed.), *Simulation in critical care and beyond* (pp. 119–130). Des Plains, IL: Society of Critical Care Medicine.

Brannan, J. D., White, A., & Bezanson, J. (2008). Simulator effects on cognitive skills and confidence levels. *Journal of Nursing Education, 47*(11), 495–500.

Bransford, J. D., Brown, A. L., & Cocking, R. R. (Eds.). (2000). *How people learn: Brain, mind, experience, and school.* Washington, DC: National Academies Press.

Brown, J. F. (2008). Applications of simulation technology in psychiatric mental health nursing education. *Journal of Psychiatric and Mental Health Nursing, 15*(8), 638–644.

Campbell, S., & Daley, K. (2008). *Simulation scenarios for nursing educators: Making it real.* New York, NY: Springer Publishing.

Chambers, K., Boulet, J., & Gary, N. (2000). The management of patient encounter time in a high-stakes assessment using standardized patients. *Medical Education, 34*, 813–817.

Chickering, A. W., & Gamson, Z. F. (1987). Seven principles for good practice in undergraduate education. *AAHE Bulletin, 39*(7), 3–7.

Chickering, A. W., & Gamson, Z. F. (1991). Applying the seven principles for good practice in undergraduate education. *New Directions for Teaching and Learning, 47.* San Francisco, CA: Jossey-Bass.

Clauser, B., Kane, M., & Swanson, D. (2002). Validity issues for performance-based tests scored with computer-automated scoring systems. *Applied Measurement in Education, 15*(4), 413–432.

DeBourgh, G. A., & Prion, S. (2010). Using simulation to teach prelicensure nursing students to minimize patient risk and harm. *Clinical Simulation in Nursing, 6*(1), e1–e210.

Diefenbeck, C. A., Plowfield, L. A., & Herrman, J. W. (2006). Clinical immersion: A residency model for nursing education. *Nursing Education Perspectives, 27*(2), 72–79.

Dismukes, R. K., Gaba, D. M., & Howard, S. K. (2006). So many roads: Facilitated debriefing in healthcare. *Simulation in Healthcare, 1*(1), 23–25.

Dobbs, C., Sweitzer, V., & Jeffries, P. (2006). Testing simulation design features using an insulin management simulation in nursing education. *Journal of International Nursing Association Clinical Simulation, 2*(1), 1–9.

Dreifuerst, K. (2009). The essential of debriefing in simulation learning: A concept analysis. *Nursing Education Perspectives, 30*(2), 109–114.

Dunn, W. F. (2004). *Simulators in critical care and beyond.* Des Plaines, IL: Society of Critical Care Medicine.

Durham, C., & Sherwood, G. (2008). Education to bridge the quality gap: A case study approach. *Urological Nursing, 28*(6), 431–438.

Engum, S., & Jeffries, P. R. (2003). Intravenous catheter training system: Computer-based education versus traditional learning methods. *The American Journal of Surgery, 186*(1), 67–74.

Guhde, J. (2011). Nursing students' perceptions of the effect on critical thinking, assessment, and learner satisfaction in simple versus complex high-fidelity simulation scenarios. *Journal of Nursing Education, 50*(2), 73–78.

Halstead, J. (2006). Evidence-based teaching and clinical simulation. *Journal of International Nursing Association of Clinical Simulation, 2*(1), 1–6.

Hamilton, C. A. (2010). The simulation imperative of end-of-life education. *Clinical Simulation in Nursing, 6*(4), e131–e138.

Hamman, W. R., Beaudin-Seiler, B. M., Beaubien, J. M., Gullickson, A. M., Orizondo-Korotko, K., Gross, A. C., . . . Lammers, R. L. (2010). Using simulation to identify and resolve threats to patient safety. *American Journal of Managed Care, 16*(6), e145–e150.

Henneman, E. A., Roche, J. P., Fisher, D. L., Cunningham, H., Reilly, C. A., Nathanson, B. H., & Henneman, P. L. (2010). Error identification and recovery by student nurses using human patient simulation: Opportunity to improve patient safety. *Applied Nursing Research, 23*(1), 11–21.

Janes, B., & Cooper, J. (1996). Simulations in nursing education. *Australian Journal of Advanced Nursing, 13*(4), 35–39.

Jeffries, P. R. (2005). A framework for designing, implementing, and evaluating simulations used as teaching strategies in nursing. *Nursing Education Perspectives, 26*(2), 96–103.

Jeffries, P. R. (2007). *Simulations in nursing education: From conceptualization to evaluation.* New York: NY: The National League for Nursing.

Jeffries, P. R., Woolf, S., & Linde, B. (2003). Technology-based vs. traditional: A comparison of two instructional methods to teach the skill of performing a 12-lead ECG. *Nursing Education Perspectives, 24*(2), 70–74.

Jeffries, P.R., Hovancsek, M. T. & Clochesy, J. M. (2005). Using clinical simulations in distance education. In J. M. Novotny &R/J/ Davis (Eds_. Distance education in nursing (2nd ed) (pp 83-99). New York: Springer Publishing.

Kameg, K., Howard, V. M., Clochesy, J., Mitchell, A. M., & Suresky, J. M. (2010). The impact of high fidelity human simulation on self-efficacy of communication skills. *Issues in Mental Health Nursing, 31*(5), 315–323.

Kameg, K., Mitchell, A. M., Clochesy, J., Howard, V. M., & Suresky, J. (2009). Communication and human patient simulation in psychiatric nursing. *Issues in Mental Health Nursing, 30*(8), 503–508.

Katz, G. B., Peifer, K. L., & Armstrong, G. (2010). Assessment of patient simulation use in selected baccalaureate nursing programs in the United States. *Simulation in Healthcare, 5*(1), 46–51.

Kolb, D. A. (1984). *Experiential learning.* Upper Saddle River, NJ: Prentice-Hall.

Kyle, R. R. (2004). Technological resources for clinical simulation. In W. F. Dunn (Ed.), *Simulators in critical care and beyond* (pp. 95–113). Des Plaines, IL: Society of Critical Care Medicine.

Lewin, K. (1951). *Field theory in social science.* New York, NY: Harper & Row.

Macedonia, C. R., Gherman, R. B., & Satin, A. J. (2003). Simulation laboratories for training in obstetrics and gynecology. *Obstetrics & Gynecology, 102*(2), 388–392.

Medley, C., & Horne, C. (2005). Using simulation technology for undergraduate nursing education. *Journal of Nursing Education, 44*(1), 31–34.

Miller, C. L., Leadingham, C., & Vance, R. (2010). Utilizing human patient simulators (HPS) to meet learning objectives across concurrent core nursing courses: A pilot study. *Journal of College Teaching & Learning, 7*(1), 37–43.

Nelson, D. L., & Blenkin, C. (2007). The power of online role-play simulations: Technology in nursing education. *International Journal of Nursing Education Scholarship, 4*(1), 1–12.

Overstreet, M. (2010). Ee-chats: The seven components of nursing debriefing. *The Journal of Continuing Education in Nursing, 41*(12), 538–539.

Page, J. B., Kowlowitz, V., & Alden, K. R. (2010). Development of a scripted unfolding case study focusing on delirium in older adults. *Journal of Continuing Education in Nursing, 41*(5), 225–230.

Pugh, C. M., & Youngblood, P. (2003). Development and validation of assessment measures for a newly developed physical examination simulator. *Journal of the American Informatics Association, 9*(5), 448–460.

Reese, C., Jeffries, P. R., & Engum, S. (2010). Learning together: Using simulations to develop nursing and medical student collaboration. *Nursing Education Perspectives, 31*(1), 33–37.

Rothgeb, M. K. (2008). Creating a nursing simulation laboratory: A literature review. *Journal of Nursing Education, 47*(11), 489–494.

Ryan, C. A., Walshe, N., Gaffney, R., Shanks, A., Burgoyne, L., & Wiskin, C. M. (2010). Using standardized patients to assess communication skills in medical and nursing students. *BMC Medical Education, 10*(24), 1–8.

Schön, D. A. (1987). *Educating the reflective practitioner.* San Francisco, CA: Jossey-Bass.

Schumacher, L. (2004). Simulation in nursing education. In G. E. Loyd, C. L. Lake, & R. B. Greenberg (Eds.), *Practical health care simulations* (pp. 169–203). Philadelphia, PA: Elsevier.

Seropian, M. (2003). General concepts in full scale simulation: Getting started. *Anesthesiology and Analgesia, 97*(6), 1695–1705.

Sewchuck, D. H. (2005). Experiential learning—A theoretical framework for perioperative education. *AORN Journal, 81*(6), 1311–1318.

Shepherd, C. K., McCunnis, M., Brown, L., & Hair, M. (2010). Investigating the use of simulation as a teaching strategy. *Nursing Standard, 24*(35), 42–48.

Svinicki, M. D., & Dixon, N. M. (1987). The Kolb model modified for classroom activities. *College Teaching, 35*(4), 141–146.

Thomas, C., Hodson-Carlton, K., & Ryan, M. (2010). Preparing nursing students in a leadership/management course for the workplace through simulations. *Clinical Simulation in Nursing, 6*(1), e1–e6.

Thompson, T. L., & Bonnel, W. (2008). Integration of high-fidelity simulation in an undergraduate pharmacology course. *Journal of Nursing Education, 47*(11), 518–521.

Whei Ming, S., & Juestel, M. (2010). Direct teaching of thinking skills using clinical simulation. *Nurse Educator, 35*(5), 197–204.

Wilson, M., Shepherd, C., & Pitzner, K. J. (2004). Assessment of a low-fidelity human patient simulator for the acquisition of nursing skills. *Nurse Education Today, 25*(1), 56–67.

Creating Interactive Learning Environments Using Media and Digital Media

Enid Errante Zwirn, PhD, MPH, RN

Alexander Muehlenkord, MBA

The current generation of students—those who are the "millennials," the Net Generation, and mobile learners—learns in digital environments and has a high degree of digital literacy. Media and electronically mediated (digital) technologies are increasingly used to support and enhance the teaching and learning that occur in institutions of higher education and their schools of nursing. These media create learning communities that are convenient, accessible, and student focused. The purposes of this chapter are to define and provide an overview of the various types of media, to present a systematic course of action to guide the selection and use of media and the environments in which they are used, and to describe how the roles of faculty and students change when they use media or multimedia and adopt technology-rich learning environments.

Media, Digital Media, and Multimedia

The term *media* refers to the models, images, and audio or video aids used to convey messages; *digital media* refers to media that use digital codes and are deployed through electronic formats for use on computers, netbooks, and handheld web-accessible devices and thereby extend the classroom to the learning resource center, clinical agency, home, and wherever the student chooses to interact with learning materials. *Multimedia* refers to any combination of video, audio, text, and graphics. The strengths of several media can be combined to appeal to a variety of learning styles and to facilitate learning. The benefits of using multimedia include reduction in the cost of teaching and learning, and improved learning effectiveness as a result of increased learner motivation, improved retention of learning, interactivity, satisfaction, and opportunities

for peer and faculty collaboration (Gleydura, Michelman, & Wilson, 1995). Each type of media accomplishes specific purposes and has advantages and disadvantages (Table 21-1).

Instructional media are typically categorized as follows: (1) realia and models, providing visual, tactile, auditory, kinesthetic, and sometimes olfactory channels for learning; (2) still visuals (nonprojected and projected), providing information to be carried visually to a more concrete level than the level of verbal symbols alone; (3) moving visuals, providing for motion and the manipulation of temporal and spatial perspectives for learning; and (4) audio media, providing for the recording and transmission of information that can be accessed aurally. Each of these categories of instructional media is discussed with consideration for use.

Realia and Models

Realia are actual objects such as medical equipment that provide the learner with the most concrete learning experiences, whereas models "are three-dimensional representations of real objects . . . [that] may be larger, smaller, or the same size as the object it represents" (Smaldino, Russel, Heinich, & Molenda, 2005, p. 215). Models have some advantages over realia in that they can be modified to accentuate certain details or disassembled to provide interior views. Realia and models are used in classroom demonstrations or in learning resource centers to provide students with an opportunity to practice nursing skills and simulate patient care. Models can also be displayed in digital formats and manipulated in virtual reality environments.

Whether they are using realia or models, students should be encouraged to handle and manipulate

TABLE 21-1 Advantages and Disadvantages of Various Types of Media and Multimedia

Category	Advantages	Disadvantages
Realia and models (manikins, models, medical equipment, patients)	• Represent reality • Can be manipulated • Facilitate simulating psychomotor skills • Models decrease risk to patients	• Expensive • Difficult to use with a large audience
Nonprojected still visuals (photographs, diagrams, graphics, posters, cartoons, handouts)	• Inexpensive to produce • Can be developed by students • Easy to transport or distribute	• Difficult to display to a large group • Graphic materials have high cultural specificity
Projected still visuals (diagraphs, charts, anatomic images)	• Easy to produce with presentation software • Quick way to project enlarged materials	• Requires use of projector and screen display • Room must be darkened
Moving visuals (Internet video, digital videodiscs)	• Effective way to show motion and sound • Can be used independently by students	• Requires projection equipment and/or computer
Audio (CDs, VoiceThread, digital audio)	• Inexpensive • Easy to use and store • Facilitates self-paced and independent study • Portable	• Requires equipment (compact disc player, MP3 player) • May be erased accidentally
Multimedia (Internet, World Wide Web, computer-assisted instruction, CD-ROM, podcasts, interactive videodiscs, virtual reality)	• Engages all senses • Facilitates interactive, collaborative, and independent learning • Cost-effective when used with large numbers of students	• Expensive to produce and purchase • Requires specific hardware to use

each object. To facilitate easy student access, the instructor may need to provide more than one of the same item to a group of students. Another suggestion is for the instructor to place a series of different objects, with their supportive texts and instructions, around the classroom and have learners visit each station in turn. Learning resource centers that house realia and models provide students with opportunities for individual or group learning during scheduled class periods or at other times convenient for the students (for additional discussion, see Chapter 19).

Still Visuals

Nonprojected Still Visuals

Nonprojected visuals do not require projection onto a screen for viewing. These graphic materials include still pictures, drawings, charts, graphs, posters, and cartoons designed specifically to communicate a message to the viewer. Some of these materials may be posted or distributed during class meetings; others may appear in prepared course handouts or viewed as PowerPoint handouts or links to images at a particular website. Nonprojected still visuals offer

high resolution at low cost. However, the cost of reproduction must be considered as well as a limited viewing audience.

Graphic materials often include verbal and symbolic visual cues and, as forms of communication, are becoming more important within a global society in helping to overcome language and other barriers to communication. Faculty should be aware that visual symbols can mean different things to students from different cultural groups, and sometimes students misinterpret the intended meaning (Fleming & Levie, 1978; Heinich, Molenda, Russell, & Smaldino, 1996; Teague, Rogers, & Tipling, 1994).

Still pictures are "photographic (or photograph-like) representations of people, places and things" (Smaldino et al., 2005, p. 241). Still pictures are readily available, often in digital formats, easy to use, and relatively inexpensive; however, the size of a still picture may limit its use with a group unless multiple copies of the same picture are obtained or the picture is enlarged or posted to a website. Still pictures also provide only a two-dimensional representation; pictures of the same objects, taken from different angles, offset this problem.

Drawings, sketches, and diagrams "employ the graphic arrangement of lines to represent persons, places, things, and concepts. Drawings are, in general, more finished and representational than sketches, which are likely to lack detail" (Smaldino et al., 2005, p. 241). Additionally, drawings are more likely than photographs to be correctly interpreted, because drawings are less detailed and their pertinent attributes can be more easily seen. During presentations, faculty and students can use drawings, sketches, and diagrams to enhance specific instructional content.

Graphs improve the ability to communicate numerical information efficiently and effectively. Graphs can also show "relationships between units of the data and trends in the data" (Smaldino et al., 2005, p. 242). Types of graphs include circle graphs, which show percentages or portions of a whole; bar graphs, which show relative performance of one or more items against one or more factors; line graphs, which provide for an overview of continual trends; and picture graphs, which are variations of bar graphs in which symbols depicting the items represented in the data are used. Graphs can be made easily by faculty and students using presentation software.

Posters "incorporate visual combinations of images, lines, colors, and words. They are intended to catch and hold the viewer's attention at least long enough to communicate a brief message, usually a persuasive one" (Smaldino et al., 2005, p. 242). Posters should communicate a single idea "and when kept on display, are a continuing reminder of information being used" within an instructional setting (Teague et al., 1994, p. 8). The most effective posters convey a single, simple message. Posters can be designed by nursing students or faculty to stimulate interest in new topics, to increase motivation, to promote safety, and to promote good health practices. By designing their own posters, students can be encouraged to select and present key concepts (Moneyham, Ura, Ellwood, & Bruno, 1996; Sorenson & Boland, 1991). Posters that depict successful community partnerships or clinical research efforts are often designed for and displayed at nursing conferences. Faculty and students can easily construct posters by employing electronic templates and digital poster construction services to develop sophisticated visuals.

Cartoons are simple line drawings. These rough caricatures of real or imagined persons or sentient animals are among the most widely available of the visual formats. Cartoons, through their wit and wisdom, appeal to all age groups. However, cartoons that fall outside the intellectual and experiential range of students or patients may not be understood or appreciated.

When editorial cartoons are used, it is important to remember that people tend to project their own feelings and prejudices onto cartoons. Thus cartoons that are easily interpreted and well received by one group of learners may not be meaningful, or might even be offensive, to another group. Students can be encouraged to draw their own cartoons relating to a wide variety of subjects—including student life, community health issues, and health promotion—to reinforce instruction.

Projected Still Visuals

Projected visuals are . . . media formats in which still images are enlarged and displayed on a screen. Such projection is usually achieved by passing a strong light through transparent film (as in overhead transparencies), magnifying the image through a series of lenses, and casting this image onto a reflective surface. (Smaldino et al., 2005, p. 246)

Not only are new developments in the projection of computer-generated visuals onto a reflective surface becoming more common in nursing education, but the projection equipment itself is also becoming smaller and even portable. ELMOs (electricity light machine organizations) attach to a laptop computer and allow faculty and students to "present images of virtually anything, to anyone, anywhere, at any time" (ELMO, 2010). As nurse educators develop greater expertise with integration of desktop video, documents, and digital cameras, as well as whiteboards, these technologies will join the ranks of overhead and slide projectors in ease of use.

Moving Visuals, Video, and Animation

Moving visuals add motion to the projected visual image and present a process more effectively than do other media. Moving visuals permit safe observation of phenomena that might be hazardous to view directly. Faculty can also use moving visuals to dramatize events and situations, explore personal and social attitudes, enhance problem-solving instructional situations, and teach the subtleties of unfamiliar cultures. Finally, moving visuals serve as a method of gaining student attention to the topic and cue the learner to the most relevant components of instruction. Moving visuals are commonly stored and made available through technologies such as the World Wide Web, compact discs (CDs), USB flash drives, digital versatile disks (DVDs), and Blu-ray discs.

It was the medium of film that was first to contribute the attributes of changing space and time. Spatial perspectives could be modified by "zooming in" or "zooming out." Time compression or expansion could be realized though time-lapse photography or filming in slow motion.

The limitations of film (size, weight, expense, and technical complexities) have been overcome by the adoption of newer video-related technologies, but its positive attributes continue to provide unique features for teaching.

- *DVD technology:* This technology can be categorized as either still or moving visual media. DVD technology offers the capacity to provide motion video, a combination of motion and still video, or still video alone. DVD is a "high density mass storage medium . . . capable of storing large amounts of information due to improvements in recording density and use of multiple layers per side" (Mehlinger & Powers, 2002, p. 311). DVD technology is now coupled with computer-managed instruction, providing the learner with ready access to textual, numerical, and graphic instructional material. The advantage of the DVD over the CD is the capability to store more data (4.7 gigabytes [GB] compared with 700 megabytes [MB]). The next evolutionary step in high-density mass storage media is the movement from DVDs to Blu-ray discs. For example, Blu-ray drives are rapidly replacing CD-ROM and DVD drives as standard hardware in many new personal computers, providing faculty with a fivefold increase in data storage and resulting in much higher resolution of instructional videos depicting patient procedures.
- *Mass storage devices:* The emergence of additional portable mass storage media contributes to the increased possibilities of using stored large data files such as video and audio. USB flash drives, also called "thumb drives," are typically small and lightweight, easily removable devices using the USB mass storage standard. By means of flash drives, users are able to easily carry storage media ranging from 8 MB to several GB (up to 256 GB in 2010) on their key chains (Microsoft Corporation, n.d.).

The advantages of the flash drive compared to CDs, DVDs, and Blu-ray discs are easy handling, plug-and-play functionality, and the option to rewrite the drive over and over again.

- *Handheld video camcorders:* Handheld video cameras found on most smart phones have the capability of files being directly uploaded and shared using a USB port. The video files can be attached to an e-mail or posted to a website, learning management system, or video-sharing site ("7 Things . . . flip camcorders," 2008). These small cameras can be used by students and educators to videotape skills performance, role play, and presentations.
- *Videocapture:* The action on a computer screen itself can be recorded, even without a camera. There are different tools for capturing, recording, and replaying full-screen demonstrations of computer applications (e.g., spreadsheet, PowerPoint, or whiteboard content) for educational purposes on the market. Camtasia, ECHO360, ScreenR.com, and Adobe Captivate are among the options of choice. Adobe Captivate (first created by RoboDemo, then Macromedia) automatically records all on-screen actions and instantly creates what is known as an interactive flash simulation. To do this, the faculty member can add text or narration at any point in the recording (Adobe Systems, Inc., 2010). ScreenR is an online application that allows faculty to designate a portion of the screen to be recorded and narrated. The content then can be shared immediately on YouTube or can be downloaded to the personal computer for further editing or other use. For example, a video can be integrated as a movie file into a PowerPoint presentation for students.
- *Video sharing:* With the advent of video-sharing websites such as YouTube, the ability to access and use video has increased exponentially along with videos particularly applicable to nursing, which can be located using the search engine on the website (Agazio & Buckley, 2009). The videos can be used in the classroom, viewed on web-accessible handheld devices for just-in-time learning, or assigned for use by students at their convenience. Students and faculty can also generate their own videos for sharing. As with using any video, videos from video-sharing websites can be used to provide content, stimulate discussion, create community, and offer opportunities for reflective learning.

Audio Media

Audio media include the use of sound for instructional purposes. Audio media tend to be inexpensive, simple to use, easily adapted, and portable. Audio media can be used in nursing education for self-paced instruction, mastery learning, drill and practice, interview skills, or performance evaluation.

- *Audio recordings*: Digital audio (a method of encoding analog audio signal into digital bits of information) can be easily produced and used by students to tape lectures in the classroom for repeated listening and study. Audio recordings have also been used to tape dialogue with clients and used for reflection, feedback, and evaluation (Sorenson & Dieter, 2009). Learners wishing to revisit a recorded lecture can listen to the digital audio recordings at their own pace, either faster or slower than the rate at which it was recorded, without altering either the pitch or the intelligibility of the original. Digital media players, such as the stand-alone MP3 player (iPod), or computer software applications, such as Windows Media Player, offer several settings to variably increase the speed of the playback of the recording. Among the many audio file formats available, the audio compressing format MP3 has become the standard for delivering audio files via downloads using the World Wide Web, digital storage media, or streaming audio.
- *Podcasts:* These are "feeds" that contain digital audio and/or video files. This new instructional medium builds on the popularity of the increased use of distributing CD-quality audio over the Internet to devices such as Apple's iPod. Users subscribe to feeds (a difference between podcasting and real-time streaming or simple downloads) and instructors apply software that periodically assesses and provides new content automatically (Skiba, 2006a). The necessary tools are available online for free (Podcasts from PBS, n.d.). Universities publicize podcasts on their websites and faculty at numerous schools of nursing include podcasts in their classes as an additional learning opportunity. (See Chapter 22 for additional information.)
- *Voice threads*: VoiceThread is a software application that enables audio recordings to accompany visual media ("7 Things . . . VoiceThread," 2009). For example, nursing faculty and students can add a voice thread to a visual image of a particular piece of equipment, which they describe or critique, and upload it to the web for sharing. VoiceThread software can also be used in online courses to accompany a photo of each student who is introducing himself or herself or as a way of making a short presentation using audio and visual media.

Electronically Mediated Learning

Computer-Based Instruction

Computer-based instruction, computer-assisted instruction, computer-assisted learning, and *computer-based training* refer to the use of the computer to guide learning and create learning communities. The computer programs (software) can be used as tutorials, simulations, and tests or to enrich or remediate learning. In a computing environment in which students work on a network that provides access to software, files, and electronic mail, computer-mediated learning promotes dialogue, inquiry, collaboration, and shared interactive learning experiences. These networks create virtual classrooms and knowledge communities that can be accessed at any time and any place.

Tutorials teach new concepts to students. A tutorial program assumes that the student has little or no prior knowledge of the particular subject matter. Generally, tutorials present facts and principles; ask the student to interact with the content by answering questions; and then, on the basis of the student's response, provide feedback and move on to the next component of the lesson.

Testing by computers gives the faculty member the opportunity to develop, administer, grade, and perform statistical measurements of an examination (item analysis, standard deviation, mean, median, and mode) with ease. A wide variety of computerized test development software programs is available to facilitate the development and administration of tests and is included in most learning management systems (see Chapter 22). Computer-based testing can also be used to assess learning needs and learning styles, administer pretests and posttests to determine mastery, or simply to provide the student with an opportunity to practice taking tests related to specific content areas for self-evaluation of learning. A variety of commercial computer-based testing services are available for use by nursing programs to assess nursing program applicants or current students for such characteristics as learning readiness, critical thinking abilities, and learning styles. Computer-based testing services are also used throughout the curriculum to assess student's mastery of course concepts and readiness for taking the licensing exam and for predicting student success.

A combination of previously mentioned methods can come together in a "learning management system," or LMS. The University of New Orleans online glossary for distance education defines an LMS as

> Software that tracks student progress in a course and indicates completions. At the least, learning management systems track individual student progress, record scores of quizzes and tests within an online learning program, and track course completions. At the most, learning management systems transfer this information to other record management software, such as PeopleSoft, so permanent educational records reflect progress in online learning. (Glossary, n.d.)

Most LMS solutions support the standard SCORM for their stored learning content, materials that would be made available to learners in online courses. SCORM (sharable content object reference model) is a collection of specifications that enables interoperability, accessibility, and reusability of web-based learning content (Advanced Distributed Learning, n.d.). In short, SCORM-compliant courses can be accessed and shared by different LMSs without need for modification. Through the use of SCORM-compliant courses, faculty across different schools of nursing can collaborate and share in course development and distribution, though the costs per student remains prohibitive for many institutions.

Virtual Reality and Virtual Worlds

In virtual reality, learners immerse themselves in multimedia, computer-based, three-dimensional simulated environments in which they can interact, demonstrate professional behaviors, practice skills, manipulate equipment, and learn teamwork and collaboration. Virtual worlds in nursing and health care (Second Life is one common virtual reality space) are simulated health care environments such as a clinical agency (Skiba, 2009), an operating room, or a community (Curran, Elfrink, & Mays, 2009; Giddens, Shuster, & Roehrig, 2010) that also include the patients, families, groups, and health care team who are members of the virtual world being portrayed. The student, using an avatar that can be either created by the student or precreated by the developer of the virtual world, enters the three-dimensional environment, assumes the role of the nurse, and participates in solving clinical problems.

Virtual worlds can also be designed as classrooms and meeting spaces for students and faculty (Schmidt & Stewart, 2009). Here, students and faculty conduct discussions, ask and answer questions, show media, and share or develop documents such as creating a database or executing statistical analyses. Experiences in virtual worlds can be used as adjuncts to online courses, experiences with high-fidelity manikins, or actual clinical experience (Schmidt & Stewart, 2009).

Participation in the virtual worlds can occur individually or in groups during a synchronous role play. The faculty can assume roles of facilitator, instructor, and coach or take part in the role play as a patient or health team member.

The advantages of using virtual reality include providing a replicable learning experience for each student, creating the opportunity to manipulate equipment and perform procedures in a safe environment, and simulating a clinical experience when it is difficult or not possible for a student to have that experience. Net Generation students find learning in a virtual reality environment appealing due to their experience with online games that use a similar approach (Skiba, 2009).

There are also disadvantages to using virtual reality, the most significant one being expense. The cost of purchasing or creating the virtual world can be prohibitive; other costs include development time and orientation for students and faculty to learn to work within the environment (Schmidt & Stewart, 2009). Using virtual reality also requires the use of a computer offering graphic processing capability not available on entry-level computers affordable to some students. Faculty have a choice to develop or employ existing case studies and scenarios for the student to use and plan the debriefing and evaluation that follows participation in the virtual world. For some users there is a sense of discomfort and invasion of privacy while in the virtual world (Skiba, 2009).

Selecting Media

Regardless of type and attributes, media should be selected to facilitate teaching and learning in a given learning environment. Several principles can be used to guide selection.

Media should be selected for the learner's level of readiness. As instructional technologies become more complex, students must be oriented to their appropriate use. Faculty should build orientation sessions into each course that is using complex digital media or have available support staff who can assist students on demand.

Media should be selected for use in an environment that is conducive to learning. The environment for learning should be accessible, physically comfortable, and emotionally supportive and should encourage students to be active participants.

Media should contain information relevant to the learner's interest and use. Relevance and motivation are closely linked.

Media should be appropriate for the audience. It is known that more effective communication occurs when the source and the receiver are similar. To enhance communication, faculty might choose pictorial examples that reflect the composition of the intended audience (Fleming & Levie, 1978). Males and females, young and older adults, persons of many ethnic backgrounds, and persons wearing or not wearing identifiable uniforms may all be depicted as nursing students. A visual with outdated styles of uniforms or equipment will quickly cause students to question the competence of the content being presented.

Media should provide learners with opportunities to apply knowledge. Media should never stand alone. Application—whether by answering questions, manipulating models, or identifying application in patient care—helps students integrate the content presented.

Media should be selected to support the learning experience. Edgar Dale (1969) has arranged various teaching methods into a hierarchy of lesser to greater abstraction—from the most concrete experiences to the most abstract experiences—in the form of a cone (Fig. 21-1). As the teaching methods move away from the cone's base, they become more and more abstract. According to Dale (1969), the learner is able to more profitably apply the more abstract instructional content only after having experienced that content on a more concrete level that would give meaning to the abstract representation of reality. Faculty, cognizant that instructional media provide different degrees of abstraction, can choose media that match the level of experiential concreteness desired within a teaching–learning experience. For example, learning in a real situation may include direct experiences in clinical agencies. Learning through interpretation of a real situation may include demonstrations, simulations, role playing, or dramatizations held after an incident has taken place. Learning through vicarious representations of the real situation may include listening to audio recordings, interacting with computer programs, or watching videos. Learning through verbal descriptions of the real recorded situation may occur through listening to live lectures, participating in discussion sessions, or reading about the situation.

Media carry messages from the sender or transmitter (a human being or an inanimate object) to the receiver. Faculty should first identify the content of the lesson and the information the learner should receive, and only then match media choice to the particular lesson content or the objectives of the lesson. Several media alternatives for presenting the instruction, providing for practice, or evaluating student performance could be made available.

If the messages are to be informational only (the receiver of the information is not held responsible for measurable, specific actions or performance), *a medium providing one-way or unidirectional communication is sufficient.* These applications may be viewed primarily as presentation media and technology, and lend themselves well to formal presentations. Examples of one-way communication media include printed handouts, traditional textbooks, audiotapes or videotapes, materials available in reference centers, and dial-access retrieval systems.

If the messages are to be instructional (the receiver of the instruction is to give demonstrable proof that he or she has learned), *two-way communication is required between the source and the receiver.* These applications can include interactive media and technology that are designed for individual use but may be used in group learning settings as well. Examples of two-way communication include a lecture followed by exercises, computer-mediated instruction, programmed texts, and tests (Teague et al., 1994).

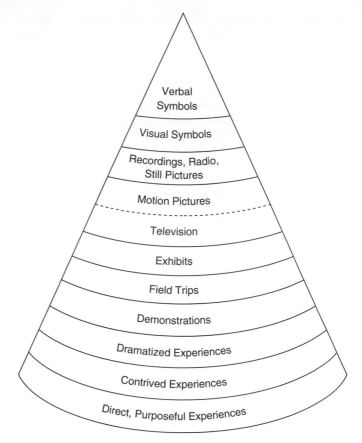

Figure 21-1 Dale's cone of experience. From *Audio-Visual Methods in Teaching*, Third Edition, by Edgar Dale, Copyright 1969 by Holt, Rinehart and Winston, Inc., reprinted by permission of the publisher.

Verbal
Symbols

Visual Symbols

Recordings, Radio,
Still Pictures

Motion Pictures

Television

Exhibits

Field Trips

Demonstrations

Dramatized Experiences

Contrived Experiences

Direct, Purposeful Experiences

Learners become accustomed to receiving messages from the types of media to which they are frequently exposed. By looking at the typical forms of instruction used at institutions of higher learning, faculty can rapidly determine those media traditionally used. Such observation should not deter the nurse educator from trying something new, because the novelty of a different instructional medium often receives increased learner attention.

Cost, preferred learning styles, and preferred teaching styles play important roles in media selection. Media must be eliminated from consideration if their costs cannot be justified. Cost-effective media achieve objectives at lower cost when capital and running costs (costs incurred during use) between alternative media are compared. Fortunately, even with all the considerations noted previously, nurse faculty members have many media choices that can be used to satisfy the demands of the messages that need to be transmitted.

Romiszowski (1981) suggests that faculty follow two rules when attempting to match media with the level of specificity required by the established behavioral objectives. The first rule states: "if you expect a certain behavior from the learner after instruction, you should give him opportunities to practice that behavior during instruction" (p. 348). Instructional media should be provided to the learner in locations where practice of the behavior is possible. Although auditory or visual instruction may initially help guide the learner, materials to which the learner can apply the new learning directly must be made available. Learning laboratories in which learners can first watch instructional videos, then go to the materials or simulations where the skills can be practiced, follow this rule.

Romiszowski's second rule states that faculty should "use the most appropriate sensory channels for communicating the information to be learned"

(1981, p. 349). Sensory channels include vision, sound, touch, smell, taste, and kinesthetics. If the objectives include psychomotor behaviors, instructional media that provide learning in that sensory channel (i.e., realia, models, or simulations) are most desirable. If the objectives include only recognition of sounds, a medium providing sound transmission only, such as an MP3 player, should suffice.

In summary, media selection is based on three important considerations: What are the learning objectives? What are the learner's special needs? What are the instructional strategies selected by the faculty? The selection of appropriate media may be initially challenging and time consuming. However, learner acceptance, dependence, and expectation for technological applications used in their learning environments change over time and are increasing. Nursing faculty who familiarize themselves with and select (often with student input) appropriate media will find that presentation of information, provision for student practice, and evaluation of student performance are not only facilitated but also enriched.

Using Media

Once faculty and students have selected appropriate media, they are ready to integrate media into the course or assignments. Using media involves planning, requires preparation, and demands that the faculty member develop skills of showmanship.

Planning for Using Media

A procedural model should be followed when systematically planning for learning experiences using media. The acronym ASSURE can help faculty plan learning experiences by following these six steps (Smaldino, 2010):

1. Analyze learners for general characteristics, specific entry competencies (knowledge, skills, and attitudes about the topic), and learning styles.
2. State objectives or learning outcomes as specifically as possible. Objectives should be stated behaviorally (what the student will be able to do, the conditions under which the student's performance is to take place, and the criteria established for success).
3. Select, modify, or design instructional materials.

4. Use those materials and follow them up with class discussion, small group activities, or individual projects and reports.
5. Require learner response to help process the knowledge or skills and obtain feedback before formal assessment takes place.
6. Evaluate the media used for their impact and effectiveness.

Nurse educators will find it especially useful to attend to those three areas of media application most often overlooked: the initial analysis of learner characteristics, the reinforcement of correct learning by requiring learner response before formal assessment, and the final evaluation of chosen media in aiding the learner's attainment of stated objectives.

Preparing and Using Media

Using media requires careful preparation. Teague et al. (1994) suggest the following five-step procedure for faculty and students when they are preparing to use instructional media:

1. *Preparing yourself:* Carefully review the instructional materials to be used for content appropriate to the established objectives. If a study guide is provided with the medium, the instructor should identify which related audience preparation or suggested follow-up activities might be explored. Sometimes only a portion of the instructional materials should be used, and that portion should be identified.
2. *Preparing the environment:* The environment must often be adjusted for use of the media. Tasks may include rearrangement of seating for optimum viewing, hearing, and accommodation of individuals with mobility challenges; setting up and testing the necessary equipment; and controlling ventilation and available room light.
3. *Preparing the audience:* Preparing the audience for instruction is the most crucial step in the entire process of using media. Bring the audience to the point at which they are ready to learn. This may be accomplished by presenting a broad overview of the content of the presentation, by pointing out specific content to which the learner is to pay special attention, or by defining unfamiliar vocabulary or visual cues. Learners can also be provided with a guide or set of questions to be answered during

or after use of the materials. When learners are well prepared, they are more likely to be active participants and see relevance of the media to the topic being presented.

4. *Using the media:* Faculty and students who have prepared themselves well are confident that their learners will experience the planned outcomes when the media are used. They will demonstrate technical ease with the equipment and be able to "troubleshoot" common technical breakdowns. Last, they understand that they, too, "are an instructional medium" and apply effective media use practices.

5. *Combining the media with other learning:* Instructional media are components of planned sequences of learning activities and must be integrated with the entire instructional design process to be maximally effective. Since media should never stand alone, it is important that content presented within instructional media be connected to content provided by other sources, such as reading materials, other students, and faculty.

Presentation Skills

Media are often a component of courses and presentations; thus faculty should consider presentation factors that must be performed effectively if a presentation is to be successful. Faculty behaviors, such as body position and movement, should be considered, as well as media projection principles.

Body Position and Movement

If the front of the classroom is thought of as a stage, the position directly centered and closest to the audience is the most dominant, grabbing the attention of the audience. Thus if the audience is to focus on a model or screen, the model or screen should be placed "front and center," with the presenter standing off to the right side of the stage, in a less dominant position. Many speakers, for emphasis or to signal the beginning of a new topic, successfully use movement. If the presenter moves from a less dominant to a more dominant position in front of the learners, the point being made at that time is likely to be underscored. Movement toward a centered visual (e.g., the screen) adds dramatic emphasis to that visual and increases learner interest. Movement may be excessive, however, if it distracts the learner from the points

being made. The presenter should also avoid distracting physical or verbal mannerisms. Such mannerisms may remain unknown to the presenter unless he or she has had an opportunity to be videotaped during a presentation. Videotaping and other similar forms of feedback allow the presenter to become aware of nervous movements, such as throat clearing, or oft-repeated and unnecessary phrases, such as "you know" or "um."

Body positions assumed by the presenter have been rated for strength. The full-front body position is the strongest. The three-quarter full-front position is the second strongest. The one-quarter view, with the back nearly turned toward the audience, is the weakest position. Thus for the strongest presentation, when pointing to an aspect of a projected image, a faculty member should point with the arm closest to the screen, while facing front, rather than make a one-quarter turn away from the learners.

Speaker Amplification

Literature shows that using audio amplification, even in smaller classrooms, enhances learning. People in the back of the room feel closer to the speaker, students are less distracted by their peers, and the speaker can speak in more natural tones.

Projecting Media

Projection principles are applied to a wide variety of projected media to increase legibility and visibility. The "two and six rule" suggests that the closest a viewer should be placed to a projected image is two times the width of the screen. Conversely, the farthest a viewer should be placed from a projected image is a distance no greater than six times the width of the viewing screen (Motion-picture technology, 2010). The projected image should fill the screen, and the bottom of the projected image should be at the viewer's eye level. The projection equipment or the presenter should not block the view of learners, if possible.

The projection equipment should be placed parallel to the screen to prevent "keystoning" (a projected image that is trapezoidal rather than rectangular). Correction of keystoning, to maintain a parallel relationship between the projection equipment and the screen, may require moving the projection equipment or moving or tying back the bottom of the screen. New models of projection equipment also offer a software-driven option to manage a keystone effect by manipulating the setup using the available menu functions of the projection apparatus.

One last consideration for projected images is the placement of the screen. A screen placed in the corner of a classroom allows for simultaneous use of a projected image and the dry erase board. To lessen the amount of ambient light that reaches the screen and reduces image brightness, the presenter should place the screen in front of the windows that have the greatest light leakage.

An effective presenter engages the audience by being natural and enthusiastic. A relaxed environment with wise use of humor and unexpected conclusions keeps the energy level high. The light source should be moved from the projected visuals to the presenter when the visuals are no longer the focus. Presentation skills are not difficult to learn and the faculty member or student who follows effective presentation guidelines provides for a more enjoyable, smoother, and stronger learning experience.

Designing Media

With the advent of low-cost, easy-to-use computer presentation systems, flip camcorders, desktop publishing, and authoring software, as well as technical and design support from instructional media and learning resource centers on many campuses, more instructional material and courses are being developed by nursing faculty for their own and their colleagues' use.

Designing DVDs and Video Clips

Because of the availability and ease of use of video cameras, students and faculty are increasingly developing their own digital videos. For example, faculty make short videos as an introduction to their web course, post video clips to video-sharing websites such as YouTube, and develop DVDs (Fleming, Reynolds, & Wallace, 2009) or vodcasts (see Chapter 22) of skills demonstrations that students can access on a web-accessible handheld device as needed.

Nursing students can also develop and use instructional materials for patient instruction or class presentations or to make short videos of skills proficiency for self and faculty feedback and to insert into electronic portfolios of competency attainment.

Sorenson and Dieter (2005) tested the feasibility of using student- and faculty-generated videos for use in an online physical assessment course. Students produced videos of themselves conducting a physical assessment as a prerequisite for entry into the course, while faculty developed video vignettes to simulate concepts of family dynamics in the course. Faculty found that using the videos was helpful in identifying students who required remediation with skills and that students scored higher on exams. Green and Hope (2010) had students in small groups make patient education videos to post in a private class site on YouTube as a way to synthesize course materials while creating a usable patient education product. Faculty must solve issues of privacy of students and patients as well as use of copyrighted material when making assignments of videos that will be publicly displayed.

Designing Graphic Materials

Graphic materials, whether generated by faculty or students, are becoming both more visually sophisticated and ubiquitous in learning environments. As presentation design software, such as PowerPoint, allows for more powerful manipulation of graphic materials, it remains important to attend to the basic design principles of balance, emphasis, simplicity, and unity.

- *Balance*, a form of equilibrium, provides a sense of coherence. To reduce a ragged text line, left-justify bullet points. To provide for uninterrupted text space, do not center graphics; instead place the graphic on the left side of the slide to lead the viewer's eye to the text.
- *Emphasis* helps the student identify the main theme. Increasing the font size or bolding certain words helps those words to stand out.
- *Simplicity* makes it easier for students to identify key elements. Avoid text overload by limiting text to six words per line and six lines per page. Each screen should contain only a small amount of information, allowing the presenter to provide elaboration. Faculty should also use restraint with fonts, choosing only a few that are familiar. Within the same presentation, all slides should retain the same background.
- *Unity* provides for continuity of thoughts and ideas. Items supporting the same theme can be grouped, shown within a border, and even color-coded.

Other considerations for development of graphic materials include the visual elements of space, size, lines, shapes, color, contrast, and texture.

- *Space* without any text or graphics on a slide is referred to as "negative" or "white" space. An uncomplicated slide with abundant negative space can help to visually focus the student's attention to the "positive" space filled with text or images.
- *Size* attracts attention to certain elements of a visual. Larger size usually gains greater attention. The text of slide headers should be larger than the text on the rest of the slide; conversely, images or text containing equal value should be of equal size.
- *Lines* direct the student to a specific area or object. In a still projected visual, lines can also depict movement, calmness, and even radiating heat or light.
- *Shapes* may be geometric, symbolic, or abstract representations of familiar objects. The same geometric shapes can be used as borders to enhance unity. Shapes can also be used across cultures to provide clearer visual communication, but must be tested for meaning before implementation.
- *Color and contrast*, if harmonious, unify a design and enhance visual attractiveness. Strong and contrasting colors produce emphasis. On the one hand, when producing materials in hard copy, dark text should be printed on a light background. On the other hand, projected text should be light in color on a semi-dark background. Critical contrasts should not use the colors of red and green to accommodate those viewers who are red-green color-blind. Always check the color on the projection equipment to be used, as what looks good on a computer screen may project as unreadable in the classroom.
- *Texture*, the variations of lines and dots producing a pattern, may take on a characteristic of cloth or other material forms and can provide emphasis to certain parts of a visual. A textured background should not be used under text or graphic visuals, as legibility is lessened.

In addition to making decisions about the design of projected materials, slides, or visuals to be used alone or with other media, the *effectiveness* of the visuals must always be considered. "The effectiveness of visuals is measured by the degree of learner recall of its content" (Teague et al., 1994, p. 257); thus whatever visuals are used should attract attention and hold the interest of the student, but not be so excessive that the key points to be shared are overwhelmed by the visual and aural capabilities of the software program. Even attractive presentations may fail their intended purpose. It is not the medium that is the message, it's the information contained within the medium. Remember, "Just because you can, doesn't mean you should."

Current Shifts in the Teaching–Learning Environment

As early as 1991 Collins proposed that integration of digital media into courses would lead to eight major shifts in teaching and learning. Many of these proposed shifts have been implemented to varying degrees in nursing education.

1. The shift *from lecture and recitation to coaching.* If the direction for the content is provided by means of interactive technologies, faculty will be able to spend more of their time facilitating student learning.
2. The shift *from whole-class instruction to small-group instruction.* Students need no longer move in lockstep through material. Faculty, interacting more with individual students and small groups of students, can address student misunderstandings and assess learning.
3. The shift *from working with better students to working with weaker students.* The faculty member is freed to identify and target student populations at risk and devote more time to those students who need more help.
4. The shift from every student learning the same thing to *different students* being recognized, and perhaps being rewarded for *learning different things.*
5. The shift toward *more engaged students.* With interactive technology, attention is ensured because instruction comes to a halt when there are no responses from learners.
6. The shift toward *assessment on the basis of products and progress* rather than test performance. Nursing students are assessed on projects that include realistic tasks that incorporate what is being learned and show how these concepts and principles are applied to new areas.
7. The shift *from a competitive to a cooperative goal structure.* Students will share their own

work, developed from extensive databases, through networked communication systems. Faculty will generate new methods of assessment according to the collaborative nature of student products.

8. The shift *from the primacy of verbal thinking to the integration of visual and verbal thinking.* Multimedia has the capacity to engage a variety of senses. The visual support for learning will supplement the auditory (listening) mode, and learners will integrate and use both channels.

High-Tech Classrooms

If located on campus, the shifts that Collins (1991) mentions often occur within spaces variously referred to as *high-tech*, *mediated*, *technology-rich*, *"smart,"* or *technology-enabled* classrooms. A convergence of technologies has produced teaching–learning environments in which actively engaged students, using high-tech communications equipment, can participate in desktop experiments, collaborative learning activities, and student–faculty dialogue.

Technologies may differ in classrooms considered "high-tech." The usual technologies that might be found in high-tech classrooms include ceiling-mounted video projectors, an instructor workstation with video conferencing and World Wide Web interactivity, multiple interactive student workstations, multiple student microphones, a document camera, an electronic whiteboard, and networked printers.

Use of Audience Response Systems

Another example for the use of technology in the classroom is the integration of an audience response system (ARS), also called classroom participation systems and "clickers." Faculty members are able to poll the students in attendance and get immediate feedback. The responses are transmitted as students use remote controls and are instantly tabulated and shown to the audience as an automatically generated PowerPoint slide. ARS allows the faculty to keep students engaged and involved in the classroom, to receive feedback, and to check whether students understand the material. ARS also allows students to work actively in small groups and provides students opportunities to practice test taking skills (Moredich & Moore, 2007; Skiba, 2006b) and

take quizzes. In a small study of the effect of ARS on students' perception of learning, Porter and Tousman (2010) report that students were positive about the use of ARS and believed that the system helped them better understand course concepts due to the discussion that followed the posting of the questions and responses. Smith and Rosenkoetter (2009) surveyed students in an undergraduate ethics course and found that 95% of students supported the use of ARS and that younger and female students preferred its use more than older and male students. When ARS was used for quizzes, 95% of students also agreed that having a hard copy of the quiz submitted was important.

Some universities have equipped the majority of their classrooms with ARS technology (Wong, 2005); others require students to purchase their own systems and then track students' participation in an electronic gradebook. ARS technology itself is not new, but its added wireless capabilities are a recent development.

Another recent development in the ARS field is the integration of additional channels to collect audience responses. Online participants can submit their responses via web forms hosted on Internet sites or via smart phones (cell phones) by texting their responses to a online service provider that is accumulating the feedback and presenting it in real time to all participants. Polling questions embedded in video conferencing programs are yet another way to use ARS concepts. Response devices can also be used in courses offered at a distance (Berry, 2009). Berry found that when students in her course used audience response devices, students were more actively engaged and final course grades were higher for the class that used the devices when compared to the class in the previous semester that did not.

Back-Channel Communications

In addition to ARS, other technologies such as e-mail, text messaging, and Twitter can be used within or outside the classroom to engage students. Back-channel communication ("7 Things . . . backchannel communication," 2010), the communication that supports constant communication links between learners and faculty, can occur within (via an Internet relay chat channel specifically set up to talk about what is happening in the presentation) or outside the course structure to support communities of practice.

Back-channel communication can be useful for clarifying and collaborating on assignments, seeking or providing help with technology tools, and developing social bonds. Back-channel communication technologies range from talking on landline phones to collaborative editing (e.g., Google Docs) to video sharing (e.g., YouTube). See Chapters 22 and 23 for additional information.

Wireless Access and Use of Computers, E-readers, and Handheld Devices

Going "wireless" is a main trend changing the way users can access the World Wide Web or other networks. A wireless network is often called a *hotspot* or a *Wi-Fi area.* Microsoft ("7 Tips . . . wireless hotspots," n.d.) describes a "hotspot" as "a wireless local area network (LAN) that provides high-speed Internet and virtual private network (VPN) access in public locations, such as coffee shops, libraries, hotels, and even some airports." Mobile devices may also use the cellular data network to access the Internet. These devices include laptop computers; Apple iOS devices of the iPhone, iPad, and iPod Touch; as well as many other smart phones using the Android and Windows Phone operating systems. At many universities, faculty and students can access the network from anywhere on campus, accessing campus information, offering and taking interdisciplinary and nursing courses, and grading and working on course assignments. These mobile devices make learning content accessible almost anywhere and at any time. One example would be the access to a recorded or live streaming class or lecture via a student's iPhone. The student can switch, for example, between the display of the PowerPoint slides, the "talking head" of the lecturer, and the chat window to exchange information with other students or the teaching assistant.

The use of computers and handheld devices in the classroom is increasingly common and also controversial. While using computers and handheld devices can help students learn how to access and critique information, take notes, and participate in collaborative learning teams, purchase and technical support are expensive when required and can be a distraction when students use the devices for nonclass-related purposes (Mennenga & Hendricks, 2008). Establishing norms about use and including them in the syllabus is one way to minimize the negative aspects of using wireless devices in the classroom (see Chapter 10).

Students may also bring their textbooks to the classroom in an electronic format. Most textbooks and resource books such as drug guides and laboratory test manuals are available in electronic formats that can be downloaded to a personal digital assistant (PDA), computer, or e-reader ("7 Things . . . e-readers," 2010; Williams & Dittmer, 2009). Students can use these resources to look up information for just-in-time learning, to participate in team and group work in the classroom, and to make annotations during the class.

Designing and Using Classrooms to Facilitate Interactive Learning

With easy access to media and digital media and the pervasive presence of computers and web-accessible handheld devices, faculty have the opportunity to engage students in lively and interactive learning. To take advantage of the ability to use the media, the classroom should have innovative seating arrangements to encourage students to take more active and collaborative roles in the learning process (Graetz & Goliber, 2002; Skill & Young, 2002). For example, the Massachusetts Institute of Technology (Brehm, 2001) has transformed some traditional classrooms with chairs on one level into amphitheater-style rooms with fixed tables and loose chairs to encourage group work. Arizona State University has some classrooms with team-based seating where the instructor has the ability to project student work onto main screens. The Rose-Hulman Institute of Technology, with its completely networked campus environment, requires that every student purchase a specified laptop computer at the time of enrollment. Also at Rose-Hulman, many classrooms are equipped with network and power connections with which students can access software and applications for individual or group work. At Texas A&M University, in large classes of approximately 100 students, one computer is provided for every two students. Students at Texas A&M sit in teams (for collaborative work), at rectangular tables that are *perpendicular* to the placement of the faculty workstation (for ease of faculty observation), and may observe projected materials on screens on both sides of the classroom (so students do not have to turn from side to side) (Cordes & Froyd, 2002).

Furniture should "facilitate learning, not just be a place to sit" (Cornell, 2002, p. 37). In high-tech classrooms, one no longer sees rows of single chairs with armrests. Furniture is selected that "[helps] the instructor and student achieve their goals using the methods and tools of their choice" (Cornell, 2002, p. 37). Cornell, in the chapter titled "The Impact of Changes in Teaching and Learning on Furniture and the Learning Environment," speaks to five aspects of furniture functionality that support the emerging paradigm of teaching and learning. Rooms must be able to be *readily reconfigured* from lecture to small group setups and unused equipment must be able to be easily stored ("fold-n-go"). Ubiquitous *access to technology* should be available to students and faculty ("plug-n-play"). *Presentation, modification, recording, and retrieval of information* for both faculty and students must be supported ("say-n-see"). The environment must *provide for both individual student concentration and student collaboration* ("relate-n-reflect"). Last, Cornell emphasizes that the teaching–learning environment should be *"fun, energetic, and enjoyable"* ("inspire-n-invite").

Chism and Bickford (2002) contrast new assumptions about learning space design with the old assumptions and share implications for current educational design practices. These implications include designs that (1) consider the whole campus as a potential learning space, (2) facilitate social interaction, (3) expand per-student space allocation, (4) amplify both faculty and student input, and (5) foster broad participation and collaboration among "multiple actors" in the design process. For example, at the University of Pittsburgh stakeholders (faculty and learners) were part of the planning process in the design of a learning space, a classroom when completed, that increased user engagement (Britnell, Andriati, & Wilson, 2009).

Social Media and New Roles for Faculty and Students

Goldberg (1999), in *Overcoming High-Tech Anxiety*, states: "historically people have always flourished when offered the opportunity for exploration and settlement of new frontiers. The electronic frontier offers such a world of opportunities and possibilities" (p. xv). Higher education is experiencing a paradigm shift from teaching to learning; the previous paradigm is no longer seen as having the "capacity to solve problems and generate a positive vision of the future" (Barr & Tagg, 1995). Media have the potential to support and enhance learning experiences, and the use of media by both nursing faculty and students will help them find ways to build knowledge and to communicate that information.

One example is the increasing use of social media. Social media networks have been created for the purpose of distributing and sharing user-generated content. A study published by Pearson (Sociable professors..., 2010) found more than 30% of faculty communicate with students using social networks such as Facebook. For further discussion of social media, see Chapter 23.

The shift from content-centered presentations to shared quests between students and faculty to use existing information to answer questions and solve problems will facilitate modeling, foster creativity, and enhance active and collaborative learning. Recognition of, and respect for, individual competencies, needs, and interests will make it possible for each student to travel a unique route to successful education in nursing. Faculty who remain open to change and become familiar with tools that foster student engagement and participation (supported by administrators who anticipate and support whatever forms education might take in an age rich in instructional media) will find themselves sometimes anxious, many times challenged, but always growing.

SUMMARY

This chapter explored the use of media, multimedia, and technology-rich, interactive learning environments in educational settings for nurses. By gaining an understanding of the basic precepts of designing and using digital media that support a student-centered learning paradigm, learning experiences for nursing students and faculty will become more fruitful, effective, and fulfilling as students gain the art, science, and spirit of nursing.

REFLECTING ON THE EVIDENCE

1. Think about your presentation style. In what ways do you already engage learners? How and where do you see yourself trying new approaches? How will you evaluate the success of these new strategies?

2. Identify all of the interrelated components of media and multimedia integration during the teaching–learning experience. Place these components in order of consideration and identify those areas to which you will pay particular attention. Why have you chosen those areas?

3. You have chosen to develop projected still visuals for class presentation. What popular software package are you likely to employ? Identify and describe five visual attributes that serve as design guidelines.

4. As uses of multimedia technologies increase in nursing education, there are likely to be intended and unintended consequences. Describe and discuss three research questions that you would like to see answered regarding multimedia applications in the next 5 years.

REFERENCES

Adobe Systems, Inc. (2010). *Adobe Captivate 5*. Retrieved from http://www.adobe.com/

Advanced Distributed Learning. (n.d.). *SCORM*. Retrieved from http://www.adlnet.gov

Agazio, J., & Buckley, K. M. (2009). An untapped resource: Using YouTube in nursing education. *Nurse Educator, 34*(1), 23–28.

Barr, R., & Tagg, J. (1995). From teaching to learning—A new paradigm for undergraduate education. *Change, 26*(6), 13–25.

Berry, J. (2009). Technology support in nursing education: Clickers in the classroom. *Nursing Education Perspectives, 30*(5), 295–298.

Brehm, D. (2001). New classrooms offer high-tech education in physics, mechanical engineering. *MIT TechTalk*. Retrieved from http://web.mit.edu/newsoffice/

Britnell, J., Andriati, A., & Wilson, L. (2009). Learning space design with an inclusive planning process promotes user engagement. *Educause Quarterly, 32*(4). Retrieved from http://www.educause.edu

Chism, N. V. N., & Bickford, D. J. (2002). Improving the environment for learning: An expanded agenda. In N. V. N. Chism & D. J. Bickford (Eds.), *The importance of physical space in creating supportive learning environments: New directions for teaching and learning* (pp. 91–97). San Francisco, CA: Jossey-Bass.

Collins, A. (1991). The role of computer technology in restructuring schools. *Phi Delta Kappan, 73*(1), 28–36.

Cordes, D., & Froyd, J. (2002). *Engineering classrooms before and after innovation*. Paper presented at Pedagogical Network for Engineering Education, Copenhagen, Denmark. Retrieved from http://www.foundationcoalition.org

Cornell, P. (2002). The impact of changes in teaching and learning on furniture and the learning environment. In N. V. N. Chism & D. J. Bickford (Eds.), *The importance of physical space in creating supportive learning environments: New directions for teaching and learning* (pp. 33–42). San Francisco, CA: Jossey-Bass.

Curran, C. R., Elfrink, V., & Mays, B. (2009). Building a virtual community for nursing education: The town of Mirror Lake. *Journal of Nursing Education, 48*(1), 30–35.

Dale, E. (1969). *Audio-visual methods in teaching* (3rd ed.). Austin, TX: Holt, Rinehart, & Winston.

ELMO. (2010). Retrieved from http://www.elmousa.com/

Fleming, M., & Levie, W. H. (1978). *Instructional message design: Principles from the behavioral sciences*. Englewood Cliffs, NJ: Educational Technology.

Fleming, S., Reynolds, J., & Wallace, B. (2009). Lights . . . camera . . . action! A guide for creating a DVD/video. *Nurse Educator, 34*(3), 118–121.

Giddens, J. F., Shuster, G., & Roehrig, N. (2010). Early student outcomes associated with a virtual community for learning. *Journal of Nursing Education, 49*(6), 355–358.

Gleydura, A. J., Michelman, J. E., & Wilson, C. N. (1995). Multimedia training in nursing education. *Computers in Nursing, 13*(4), 169–175.

Glossary. (n.d.). The University of New Orleans, Office of Registrar. Retrieved from http://registrar.uno.edu

Goldberg, B. (1999). *Overcoming high-tech anxiety*. San Francisco, CA: Jossey-Bass.

Graetz, K. A., & Goliber, M. J. (2002). Designing collaborative learning spaces: Psychological foundations and new frontiers. In N. V. N. Chism & D. J. Bickford (Eds.), *The importance of physical space in creating supportive learning environments: New directions for teaching and learning* (pp. 13–22). San Francisco, CA: Jossey-Bass.

Green, B., & Hope, A. (2010). Promoting clinical competence using social media. *Nurse Educator, 35*(3), 127–129.

Heinich, R., Molenda, M., Russell, J. D., & Smaldino, S. E. (1996). *Instructional media and technologies for learning* (5th ed.). Englewood Cliffs, NJ: Merrill.

Mehlinger, H. D., & Powers, S. M. (2002). *Technology and teacher education: A guide for educators and policymakers*. Boston, MA: Houghton-Mifflin.

Mennenga, H. A., & Hendricks, L. (2008). Faculty concerns about requiring laptops in the classroom. *Nurse Educator, 33*(4), 151–154.

Microsoft Corporation. (n.d.). *Microsoft USB flash drive manager (standard)*. Retrieved from http://www.microsoft.com

Moneyham, L., Ura, D., Ellwood, S., & Bruno, B. (1996). The poster presentation as an educational tool. *Nurse Educator, 21*(4), 45–47.

Moredich, C., & Moore, E. (2007). Engaging students through the use of classroom response systems. *Nurse Educator, 32*(3), 113–121.

Motion-picture technology. (2010). In Encyclopædia Britannica Online. Retrieved from http://www.britannica.com/

Podcasts from PBS. (n.d.). Public Broadcasting Service (PBS). Retrieved from http://www.pbs.org/

Porter, A. G., & Tousman, S. (2010). Evaluating the effect of interactive audience response systems on the perceived learning experience of nursing students. *Journal of Nursing Education, 49*(9), 523–527.

Romiszowski, A. J. (1981). Media selection. In A. J. Romiszowski (Ed.), *Designing instructional systems* (pp. 339–359). New York, NY: Nichols.

Schmidt, B., & Stewart, S. (2009). Implementing the virtual reality environment. *Nurse Educator, 34*(4), 152–155.

7 Things you should know about backchannel communication. (2010, February). Educause Retrieved from http://www.educause.edu/

7 Things you should know about e-readers. (2010, March). Educause. Retrieved from http://www.educause.edu/

7 Things you should know about flip camcorders. (2008, November). Educause Learning Initiative. Retrieved from http://www.educause.edu/

7 Things you should know about VoiceThread. (2009, June). Educause Learning Initiative. Retrieved from http://www.educause.edu/

7 Tips for working securely from wireless hotspots. (n.d.). Microsoft at work: Working remotely. Retrieved from http://www.microsoft.com/

Skiba, D. J. (2006a). The 2005 word of the year: Podcast. (Article excerpt). *Goliath Business Knowledge on Demand.* Retrieved from http://goliath.ecnext.com/

Skiba, D. J. (2006b). Got large lecture hall classes? Use clickers. *Nursing Education Perspectives, 27*(5), 278–279.

Skiba, D. J. (2009). Nursing education 2.0: A second look at Second Life. *Nursing Education Perspectives, 30*(2), 129–131.

Skill, T. D., & Young, B. A. (2002). Embracing the hybrid model: Working at the intersections of virtual and physical learning spaces. In N. V. N. Chism & D. J. Bickford (Eds.), *The importance of physical space in creating supportive learning environments: New directions for teaching and learning* (pp. 23–32). San Francisco, CA: Jossey-Bass.

Smaldino, S. E. (2010). *The ASSURE model: Creating the learning experience.* Retrieved from http://wps.prenhall.com/chet/_smaldino_instruct_8/223/6319/1617894.cw/navbar/index.html

Smaldino, S. E., Russel, J. D., Heinich, R., & Molenda, M. (2005). *Instructional technology and media for learning* (8th ed.). Upper Saddle River, NJ: Pearson Merrill.

Smith, D. A., & Rosenkoetter, M. M. (2009). Effectiveness, challenges, and perceptions of classroom participation systems. *Nurse Educator, 34*(4), 156–161.

Sociable professors: First-of-its-kind survey finds college faculty increasingly using social media. (2010, May 4). *Pearson: Press releases.* Retrieved from http://www.pearsoned.com

Sorenson, D. S., & Dieter, C. (2005). From beginning to end, video-based introductory, instructional, and evaluation applications. *Nurse Educator, 30*(1), 40–43.

Sorenson, E. S., & Boland, D. (1991). Use of the poster session in teaching research critique to undergraduate nursing students. *Journal of Nursing Education, 30*, 334–340.

Teague, F. A., Rogers, D. W., & Tipling, R. N. (1994). *Technology and media.* Dubuque, IA: Kendall/Hunt.

Williams, M. G., & Dittmer, A. (2009). Textbooks on tap: Using electronic books housed in handheld devices in nursing clinical courses. *Nursing Education Perspectives, 30*(4), 220–225.

Wong, W. (2005). Students and professors click with technology. *EdTech: Focus on Higher Education*, Winter. Retrieved from http://www.edtechmag.com/

22 Teaching and Learning at a Distance

Barbara M. Friesth, PhD, RN

Technological advances in computers and broadband connectivity have opened up new ways for nursing faculty to connect with their students and deliver media-rich content at a distance. Increasingly, students want to learn in more flexible programs that maximize their time and other life commitments (Connors, 2008; Maring, Costello, & Plack, 2008). At the same time, higher education programs are recognizing the need to increase student access to distance-accessible programs (Allen & Seaman, 2007). Distance education offers the ability to bring practitioners to rural and underserved areas (Effken & Abbott, 2009). By educating those who already live in rural areas, there may be a greater likelihood that they will remain and practice in their home towns upon completion of their studies (Effken & Abbot, 2009).

There is a current faculty shortage in nursing schools, and this trend is expected to worsen in the coming years with advancing faculty age and looming retirements (American Association of Colleges of Nursing, 2010). Distance education programs offer a means to reduce the faculty shortage and connect specific student learning interests with faculty expertise, despite the distance between the two (Billings, 2010; Mancuso-Murphy, 2007). Distance education delivery systems that encourage innovation and flexibility have the potential for maximizing use of institutional infrastructure, improving access to credit courses, and providing consistency for learning at multiple locations.

Distance education is broadly defined as students receiving instruction in a location other than that of the faculty. This separation of teacher and student could be as close as within the same community or campus or as far away as across states or continents. The options of available delivery systems to implement distant academic courses or continuing education opportunities have become increasingly competitive and are frequently defined by cost, administrator, and faculty knowledge, acceptance, and readiness. Additionally, computers and computer-based communication systems continue to have a positive and dramatic effect on teaching and learning, thus becoming invaluable tools for distance instruction. Because many different instructional delivery systems are available, faculty should find the specific material presented in this chapter useful.

Distance education delivery systems are undergoing rapid change. In most cases, technologies have merged with others to form a blend of delivery or are being replaced by new and innovative delivery options. Obsolescence of existing media within the next 5 to 10 years will be commonplace, as the changes in technology continue at a very rapid pace. However, the concepts related to leading, planning, using, supporting, administering, and evaluating student learning remain applicable. The virtual classroom, defined for this purpose as the learning environment occurring wherever the student can access information, has become more common as colleges and universities endeavor to offer efficient and effective higher education opportunities to students anyplace and at any time.

Online education is continuing to grow at a rate that is faster than the overall higher education market in general (Allen & Seaman, 2007). Numerous studies in distance education continue to support that learning at a distance is at the very least equivalent to traditional face-to-face courses, and in fact there are data to suggest that blended methods may produce the best outcomes overall (U.S. Department of Education, 2009; Zhao, Lei, Lai, & Tan, 2005). Blended, or hybrid, approaches use a combination of online and face-to-face formats. Synchronous video technologies offer a way to deliver blended courses to students at a distance, without requiring the time and expense associated with travel to the host site. The use of blended approaches in higher education is expected to increase in the coming years (Kim & Bonk, 2006). The technologies available today offer a wide variety in strategies for delivering blended approaches at a distance.

Distance learning tends to capitalize on a constructivist, or problem solving, approach to learning. This approach is in direct contrast to Gagné and Briggs's (1979) distinct learning groups, which are based on a hierarchy of complexity and the need for mentoring and role modeling. However, distance learning seems to support Piaget's (2001) position that learning is not just inherent or just experiential in nature, but a combination of both. Driscoll (2004) identifies constructivism as becoming more popular with the increased interest in computers as an educational tool. Although other instructional media are not excluded from this consideration, computers and networked learning have had a huge impact on the learner's ability to construct and manage his or her own learning environment. Distance learning and computer-based instruction have created a newfound independence.

The variety of options available to support distance instruction continues to increase as technologies improve and the transformation from a teacher-centered focus to a learner-centered focus becomes more prominent (Billings, 2007; Connors, 2008). Use of distance learning technologies requires planning and development of materials long before the course begins (Connors, 2008). State-of-the-art resources for faculty development of instructional materials must be available. Training and support for faculty to develop and use the new technology must be present. In addition, support for students must be provided in the use of the technology. With proper resources for development and support, faculty can deliver distance-accessible programs that meet the educational needs of students enrolled in online courses.

Online course management software, commonly called a *learning management system* (LMS), has had an impact on distance learning. Learning management systems provide an instructional environment that incorporates a support system for course management. This includes course information, announcements, communication for synchronous and asynchronous collaboration, and assessment. The LMS used in conjunction with synchronous and asynchronous strategies opens up the realm of possibilities for connecting with students and providing media-rich content.

With the shift toward computer-based instruction, the number of courses offered exclusively in the form of face-to-face instruction is decreasing substantially. However, many courses offer a blended, or hybrid, approach with other technologies such as video conferencing, audio conferencing, video streaming, podcasting, and other specialized web-based computer applications. Some technologies use *synchronous* technologies, or technologies that connect people simultaneously, or at the same time. Other technologies use *asynchronous* approaches, allowing learners to access materials without the constraints of a specific time or place. This chapter covers selected strategies used in educating students who are geographically dispersed and separated from the main campus of instruction, and both synchronous and asynchronous approaches. An overview of delivery systems, their advantages and disadvantages, and other pertinent information specific to each medium are also presented in Table 22-1.

Synchronous Technologies

With expected continued growth in the blended format of higher education programs, there is a growing need to use technology to provide face-to-face interactions for students at a distance. Synchronous technologies offer a way to deliver blended courses to students at a distance, without requiring travel to the host site. Synchronous video technologies discussed in this chapter include institutionally based video conferencing systems, institutionally focused web conferencing solutions, and one-on-one or small group web conferencing programs. Synchronous audio-only technologies include audio conferencing, over either existing telephone lines or Voice over Internet Protocol (VOIP) systems.

Audio Conferencing

Instruction transmitted over telephone lines is a delivery strategy commonly referred to as *audio conferencing*. A teacher located at the origin site, not necessarily a classroom, interacts with students in one or more receiving sites. Some distance teaching

TABLE 22-1 Instructional Delivery Systems

Type	Advantages	Major Disadvantages	Costs Related to Technology
Institutionally based video conferencing systems	• Highest quality audio and video • Easy to use • Multiple sites possible • Students attend classes in groups at their respective sites • Remote sites must have high-speed Internet access but students do not need it in their homes	• Requires hardware at all remote sites • Requires technical support at all remote sites • No ability to provide spontaneous breakout sessions for small group work • Students required to attend at a video conference site and are not able to participate from home	• Very expensive with need for centralized bridge access at the institution level • Hardware units required at host and all remote locations • Support staff at host and remote locations
Institutionally focused web conferencing software (two-way)	• Interactive video from multiple participants • Desktop and document sharing with polling capabilities • Ability to have multiple spontaneous breakout groups concurrently for group projects	• Finite limit to number of participants • Video quality decreases with increased number of participants • High-speed Internet required for all participants	• Institutionally purchased software • Cost of computer, web camera, headset with mic, and access to high-speed Internet for both host and recipients • Support for audio and video difficulties
Webinar	• Real-time video over Internet to personal computers • Screen-sharing capabilities • Requires minimum technical assistance for recipients • Numerous participants possible	• One-way video • Response back may be audio or instant message • High-speed Internet required for all participants	• Institutionally purchased software • Cost of computer, web camera, headset with mic, and access to high-speed Internet for host • Recipients require computer and high-speed Internet • Support for audio and video difficulties
Individual or small group web conferencing	• Very low cost or free software • Easy to install and use	• Limited to one on one or to very small number of interactive video participants	• Proprietary networks require line fees • High demand on network bandwidth • Salaries to provide scheduling and technical support
Audio conferencing	• Learner centered • Low cost • Can be taught from or received at any location that has telephone or high-speed Internet access	• Calls may be joined from remote classrooms or homes • Styles of class presentation may need to be altered • Visual learners and students with hearing limitations may be at a disadvantage	• Long-distance telephone toll charges • Audio conferencing equipment at receive sites, if more than one student is enrolled • Service provider fees • Salaries for site coordinators
Podcast, enhanced podcast, vodcast	• Learner centered • Access anywhere • Real-time and anytime delivery • Engaging across learning styles • Portable • Inexpensive • Fun	• Requires iPod or other mobile device to use in mobile format • Need for faculty to learn new technology • Potential compatibility issues across platforms	• High-speed Internet access • Personal player or computer required • Production staff salaries • Support staff salaries

universities and colleges incorporate audio conferencing in a blended manner with other technologies, such as webinars. Existing phone conferencing services may be used for the audio conferences; however, increasingly, VOIP software is used to connect the audio of numerous participants. VOIP software allows one to make phone calls, or conference calls, using software and high-speed Internet, thus eliminating teleconferencing or long-distance charges. Some learning management systems have VOIP audio conferencing capabilities built into their software, but freely available software such as Skype and Google Voice Chat can be used as well.

If the blend of instruction does not include a visual component, photographs or video of the instructor and students may be shared by electronic or other means at the beginning of the course. In addition, students should be encouraged to identify themselves and their location when they speak during the audio class sessions to facilitate a feeling of classroom community. For the best audio experience, students should be instructed to use a headset with a built-in microphone. Participants not currently speaking should be encouraged to "mute" their lines to eliminate distractions and extraneous noises during the conference call. Activities that provide opportunity for some student socialization should also be incorporated into early class sessions at the same time that students are provided orientation to use of the technology. Because the teacher is unable to identify nonverbal cues, teaching strategies should include more questioning to determine class understanding of content being addressed. Methods of drawing students into discussion should be planned and appropriately incorporated into classes throughout the course. One common strategy to engage students at remote sites is to call on students on a rotational basis.

Institutionally Based Dedicated Video Conferencing Systems

Many educational institutions, businesses, and health care systems are using dedicated Internet Protocol (IP) video conferencing systems (such as Polycom or Tandberg) to connect with one or multiple sites. Simultaneous video conferencing of three or more systems, also known as multipoint video conferencing, is conducted via use of multipoint control units. These multipoint control units, or bridges, allow video connections from multiple sources and control the throughput of the audio and video to each site. A dedicated video conferencing unit is required at any site wishing to participate in the video conference. One or many participants may be present at any given site. Current state-of-the-art systems are employing the use of high-definition cameras, resulting in very high-quality video. This high-quality video enables the participants to experience and see details of facial expressions and body language. The cameras can be controlled remotely to zoom in or out and to focus on one or many participants.

Video output from the conference is typically displayed using flat-panel high-definition televisions (HDTVs) in the case of very small classrooms or high-definition video projectors in larger classrooms. An important feature of these dedicated video conferencing systems is sophisticated audio handling. The dedicated units use echo cancellation technology, which eliminates problems where the remote parties may hear their own voices speaking back to them over the system (echo) and reverberation or audio feedback. The video output from the conference can be customized to display one or multiple parties on the screen. When using a single-view option of remote sites, the bridge will automatically switch video signals to display the site that is currently speaking. These institutionally based units have the highest quality audio and video available on the market today and are typically very easy to use.

A very high-fidelity version of institutionally based video conferencing is "telepresence." Telepresence video conferencing uses a combination of life-size, high-definition video technology and special acoustic mics, speakers, and soundproofing to deliver an experience of near lifelike quality (Educause, 2009). Special attention is given to placement of embedded cameras at eye level, to give the illusion of being able to look the remote participants in the eye. Furniture is configured to match at each location, and the participant visually perceives the remote site as if they were looking across the table at a person in the same room. Currently, telepresence technologies are very expensive to install; however, as technology costs decrease over time, this type of technology may become a more viable and affordable option for more sites.

Institutionally Focused Web Conferencing Solutions

For institutions that are unable to leverage regional and institutionally based video conferencing units where the target students are located, webcasting or web conferencing offers an alternative for distance students. Institutionally focused web conferencing software allows connection of two or more individuals simultaneously. Examples of such software include Adobe Connect Professional, Elluminate Live, Wimba Live Classroom, and Saba Centra. Some web conferencing software requires installation of software on each participant's part, while others are strictly web-based applications and require no installation to join. Some of the software solutions are built directly into institutionally deployed LMSs. Each individual who is connecting to the web conference does so via a computer connected to high-speed Internet. Participants may receive audio and video from others, but in order to share their own video, they must also have a web camera. Web cameras have become standard equipment on newer laptops and many newer computers. To avoid audio feedback problems, all participants should have headphones with a built-in microphone.

While it is possible to see all participants who have web cameras, the actual size and quality of the video may vary greatly based on the number of participants and the quality of the bandwidth. With the addition of each participant, the size of each displayed video stream will be reduced. With as few as 10 students in a class, the scaled size of the images may not give sufficient detail to view facial expressions.

Most web conferencing software has the ability to share desktops, thus sharing presentations or papers from either the host or participant computers. Many also have polling software and instant messaging available. Web conferences can be recorded and made available for students to view later or for students who miss a particular class session to review at a later date. Some of the systems allow students or faculty to create breakout group areas, allowing for small group collaboration among participants working on group projects. In addition to using the web conferencing for face-to-face class sessions, office hours may be scheduled using the software, thus enabling a face-to-face interaction for students desiring to take advantage of such support.

Another version of web conferencing is "webinars," which are typically one-way broadcasting of actual video. The actual software used to deliver webinars is the same as that used for web conferencing, and the capabilities of displaying slides and desktop applications are similar. There are several advantages of webinars over interactive two-way video conferences. One advantage is the possible number of participants. Since video is broadcast in only one direction, broadband limitations are generally not affected by multiple participants, and it is possible to have more than 100 participants in any given webinar. Participants may still engage during live sessions, but will do so via polling mechanisms, chat, and audio only. Webinars still require high-speed Internet access, though a web camera is not necessary for participation at remote locations. The obvious disadvantage to webinars is the loss of the face-to-face interaction with the remote sites.

Individual or Small Group Web Conferencing

While many institutions may subscribe to professional-level web conferencing software solutions, software also exists for connecting one-on-one or in small groups for no, or very little, charge. Examples of this software include Skype, Microsoft Office Communicator, iChat, and Google Video Chat. Most of these web conferencing solutions are offered as a free download with the creation of an account for their service. The software is very easy to use and requires a computer with web camera, headphones with microphone, and high-speed Internet access.

Most of these types of software also allow for instant messaging and a "status indicator" to let people know if you are available for web conferencing or messaging. While not designed to allow multiple video connections at one time, such software is a cost-effective way to enable one-on-one, face-to-face interactions between faculty and students or between small student groups. Such software may be used to facilitate face-to-face tutoring sessions or to bring groups together for project work across geographic locations. Instructors can also use the software to host office hours with students, by posting their availability to students and being available at specified times each week. This software may also be used to bring a guest content expert to your classroom virtually, without the expense and time involved with actual travel. Some of the software allows for desktop sharing but overall the robustness of sharing features is limited compared to institutionally focused web conferencing solutions. Nonetheless, given the inexpensive cost to use these products, these tools offer a valuable way to connect with students.

Support and Strategies for Synchronous Connections

Each medium has identifiable differences specific to the technology but the similarities of required support, planning, and implementing use of technology in the classroom and online represent the major focus. Virtual classroom teaching requires faculty to carefully plan the best strategies for learning over a distance. Within this overall process, students must be oriented to the technology and clear expectations must be communicated to the learners. Student outcomes can be influenced by both process and content of learning. Clear and concise orientation is an important step toward improved academic self-concept. Strategies that have been developed in the past for adapting teaching strategies for television delivery are still applicable today in the video conferencing arena. A summary of adapting strategies specifically for teaching via interactive video is given in Table 22-2.

As with other instructional delivery strategies, it is imperative that marketing, site selection, effective communication, and ongoing course coordination be managed efficiently. The teacher and administrators must work together closely to ensure that these components of the total educational plan are in place.

TABLE 22-2 Teaching with Television, Interactive Video Conference, and Video Stream: Adapting Teaching Strategies

Strategy or Use in TV Courses	Teaching Strategies
	LECTURE
Provides an efficient method of presenting much factual information in a short period	• Lectures "come alive" through presentation of bits or chunks of material (10- to 15-minute segments) interspersed with some type of feedback, such as live or web-based question-and-answer forum.
	• Provide a variety of material by using interactive communication with other strategies.
	• Strive to get audience to interact mentally with the material being presented; give them pretests to motivate; use organizers to focus on central ideas.
	• Enhance lecture with web- and computer-based materials, graphs, charts, and other media such as slides, video, and computer graphics.
	• Be certain guest speakers are aware that this is an interactive video class. Instruct them to adapt their presentation for this medium of instruction.
	DISCUSSION
Generates feeling that all learners are important	• Bring in multiple points of view and experiences; students enjoy the variety of perspectives of others.
Facilitates collaborative process	• Preassign individuals to give specific reports that enhance discussion.
Provides a change of pace and a chance for all to participate	• Call on students frequently; establish a dialogue between reception sites.
Includes stimulating questions and develops critical thinking skills	• Allow sufficient time for students at all sites to respond to questions and enter the discussion.
	• Ask open-ended questions.
	• Repeat and rephrase question while waiting for students to prepare a response.
	• Encourage all reception sites to participate.
	• Encourage participation from reception sites by looking into the camera or focusing camera with a close-up on the site (two-way video).
	INTERVIEW
Experts or clients bring additional information or viewpoints to the class in an interview format	• Segments can be prerecorded with guest "live" for questions or available by telephone.
	• Moderator should make frequent summaries and clarifications and keep interview moving and to the point.

Continued

TABLE 22-2 Teaching with Television, Interactive Video Conference, and Video Stream: Adapting Teaching Strategies—cont'd

Strategy or Use in TV Courses	Teaching Strategies
	PANEL DISCUSSION
Helps bring in a wide range of informed opinions	• Students should be prepared by previous assigned reading. • Four panel members is optimum. Be sure that wide-angle camera can show the entire panel. • Panel members can be at different locations—live and online—but be sure to guide discussion to all panel members. • Moderator's summaries are crucial to bring out important points, because presentation is not as orderly and systematic as it is in the on-campus classroom. • Encourage panel to develop visual aids.
	ROLE PLAYING
Adds variety to teaching strategies Encourages collaboration and student involvement	• Role playing can be recorded ahead and shown during class. • Prepare learners ahead of time, because there is less spontaneous activity than in a classroom. • Encourage response from students at all reception sites. • Use role playing in groups at local sites or as a prerecorded "vignette." • Keep role-playing segments short so that other students can react. • Follow up role playing with discussion to bring out important learning, feelings, and so on. • Role playing can be used to follow up a previous assignment such as "What would you do in this situation?"
	REACTOR PANEL
Stimulates audience participation by "getting the ball rolling" through the use of an audience reaction team, made up of a few members of a large audience who act as representatives of the group to react to a speaker	• Preassign a number of individuals to fill this role; they can be at the same or different locations. • Encourage others at reception sites to participate. • Use with large groups when network time will not allow much participation by students to allow "audience interaction" with the speaker.
	BUZZ GROUPS
When group is too large at an individual site for discussion or when topic to be discussed is facilitated by off-the-air discussion groups	• Sites with large enrollment should divide into groups of 5 to 10 for discussion purposes. • Give buzz groups explicit instructions as to the task to be accomplished, such as "develop one question" or "agree on one disadvantage"; keep instructions clear and simple. • Have groups report back on the air.
	QUESTION AND ANSWER
Question-and-answer periods can be built into classes to provide feedback to both speaker and participant Stimulates discussion Keeps student attention	• Participants should be encouraged to make note of questions or comments as the program goes along so they are ready to respond. • Respect for individuals' questions is necessary; provide opportunity through computer, live stream, or 800 number to answer questions from individuals who did not have a chance to participate during the class session.
	CASE STUDY SIMULATION
Helps individuals to weigh and test values, separate fact from opinion, and develop critical thinking skills	• Case studies should be sent as part of advance materials so the learners can identify the facts and issues and prepare responses. • If oral case studies are presented, they can add a change of pace; keep these short (5 to 10 minutes) so that others in the group can assimilate the details. • Use slides, video, or computer-assisted instruction to enhance the case study.
	GROUP WORK SESSIONS
Provides opportunity for practical work sessions in a collegial and collaborative environment Encourages participation and builds group rapport at local sites	• Give clear directions for group work activities; teach and develop collaborative learning skills before use with activity; monitor effectiveness of work groups at all sites. • Use team-building skills to develop collaborative learning. • Activities can be organized or guided by local group leaders or site coordinators. • Variety increases interactivity and critical thinking.

TABLE 22-2 Teaching with Television, Interactive Video Conference, and Video Stream: Adapting Teaching Strategies—cont'd

Strategy or Use in TV Courses	Teaching Strategies
	DEMONSTRATION
Shows steps of procedure efficiently, in shorter time, with visual reinforcement	• Plan ahead so camera positions are appropriate. • Use text to highlight or focus attention on key points. • Speak and demonstrate slowly and repeat as needed.
	DEBATE
Clarify points and positions	• Plan ahead and give clear directions.
Helpful for values clarification and developing critical thinking and communication skills	• Have groups develop criteria for judging. • Be sure students at all sites can hear points; repeat as needed.
Supports learning in the affective domain	• Can preassign positions to be debated to specific groups.
	MULTIMEDIA, GRAPHICS, SLIDES
Provides visual clarity and close-up view of selected material	• Keep graphics simple. • Use "horizontal" or "landscape" aspect. • Use large letters. • Use contrasting background and foreground (blue, gray, and pastel are best as background colors).

Adapted with permission from Billings, D. (1995). *Guide to teaching on television.* (Unpublished manuscript). Indiana University School of Nursing, Indianapolis, IN.

Selection of a Synchronous System

The selection of any video conferencing solution for a given institution will vary based on existing resources and the student population. Whether there are existing regionally based video conferencing units in the locations desired will certainly factor into the decision. Collaborative relationships or rental of remote equipment is also possible in some cases. The regional video conferencing model gives remote students a chance to get to know others geographically close to them, since they come together in remote classrooms. In rural areas or areas with poor broadband access, video conferencing units located at regional hospitals or small town libraries may be one way to accommodate access to the virtual classroom, particularly when students do not have access to broadband in their homes.

In areas where students do have access to high-speed Internet, use of a web conferencing solution offers great flexibility for access to the virtual classroom. Many institutions subscribe to a particular product, and use of the institutionally available product will be most cost effective. It is important to note that the quality of the video may not result in the ability to see facial expressions and detail; however, you will have some of the benefits of a face-to-face interaction. When considering web conferencing, one must also consider the potential number of students expected at remote sites. With large numbers of participants, switching to a webinar format may be preferred, though this option must be weighed against the loss of two-way interactive video. One area expected to grow significantly in the near future is the ability to connect handheld mobile devices such as smart phones and other small form factor computer devices to web conferences (Educause Evolving Technologies Committee, Bentley, & Collins, 2007). Currently some systems are capable of reception, but as cameras are added to the mobile devices the possibility to share mobile video will be present as well.

Asynchronous Technologies

Podcasts

A popular tool for receiving streaming media over the Internet is a podcast. *Podcast* was a term originally derived from Apple's portable music player, the iPod (Podcast, n.d.) and involves the broadcast of audio using a Really Simple Syndication (RSS) format of the Extensible Markup Language

(XML) for distribution of content on the World Wide Web. The most common file type for distribution of audio-only podcasts is MP3 files. Typically, a series of audio files will be updated and distributed periodically via the RSS feed. Students will "catch" the feed with an RSS aggregator, or podcatcher, designed to automatically retrieve new media files. One of the best known podcatcher software is iTunes, which integrates seamlessly with iPod devices. In addition, many learning management systems have podcasting capabilities built into their system, allowing faculty to send out feeds and students to catch them directly into their online class site.

One popular form of podcasting is to capture live, face-to-face lectures. An easy way for faculty to capture lectures for podcasting is with portable flash-memory audio recorders that record directly in the MP3 format. Use a lapel microphone for higher audio quality. The recording can be made at a low bit-per-second rate (32 kbps is recommended) that reduces file size without much compromise in audio quality. Be sure to state the name and date of the class at the beginning to help students know the topic of the audio file. These files require no post-class processing except for changing the name. Files can be uploaded to a course management system such as Blackboard or Desire 2 Learn or even can be e-mailed directly to students.

Advantages of this style of podcasting include making content available for additional student review to increase the understanding of difficult concepts and allowing additional note-taking time for items missed during class. An archive of lectures can be created and used for inclement weather dates or in case of faculty illness for future classes. The major disadvantage of this form of podcasting is that some students may perceive an opportunity to miss class periods. Strategies such as using interactive class elements or in-class quizzes can help discourage this behavior. Another disadvantage of this form of podcasting is that it does not add any additional information to the class.

Another form of podcasting involves replacing lecture time with prerecorded podcasts. A study comparing performance on exams after podcasted lectures and face-to-face lectures found no significant differences in the two formats (Vogt, Schaffner, Ribar, & Chavez, 2010). While overall satisfaction with the podcast format was good, the majority of students did not prefer podcasts to live lectures.

Podcasting supplementary materials to students is another strategy in the use of podcasting. Podcasting supplementary materials allows students to explore topics in greater depth and extend their learning beyond what was received in the classroom. Ideas for podcasting include addressing most common questions from the week, bringing guest lecturers to students, weekly review of top topics, or creating a "precast" of materials prior to class to allow better preparation for in-class periods (Indiana University, n.d.). A precast of materials can also allow faculty to deliver lecture content via the podcast and then use face-to-face class time for application and active learning activities.

Enhanced Podcasts

Enhanced podcasts are audio podcasts that include still images that are synced with the audio narration. One common format of an enhanced podcast in education is PowerPoint-style slides with voice-over narration. The slides and audio are synced together, delivered via the RSS stream, and made playable on computers and some mobile devices. The most common file format for enhanced podcasts is the Advanced Audio Coding–encoded audio file. Another popular format is Adobe Presenter, which results in a pdf or Flash-based output file. It is important to note that not all mobile players can play every format of file and the capabilities of mobile devices change rapidly. If your institution has a handheld or mobile device requirement, targeting file formats that are most compatible with those mobile devices is important. Computers and laptops are capable of playing any of the file types.

In a study using enhanced podcasts to deliver general surgery content to medical students, the authors reported that students who had prior experience with audio-only podcasts preferred the enhanced podcasts (Shantikumar, 2009). Interestingly, nearly half of the students in the study watched the enhanced podcasts on their computers rather than on a mobile device. The statistic of roughly half of individuals choosing to view the podcast at a computer instead of via a mobile device is consistent with Forbes and Hickey's (2008) findings. A contributing factor to this finding may be that compatibility across mobile devices is less ubiquitous when using files other than audio-only formats (MP3).

Vodcasts

A video podcast, or *vodcast*, is a podcast that includes video. This video may include enhanced material, such as slides with synced narration, but typically it includes live action film of the speaker or speakers. Similar to podcasts and enhanced podcasts, vodcasts are distributed and made available for streaming or download on a routine basis by subscription (Brittain, Glowacki, Ittersum, & Johnson, 2006). One cautionary note on video formats, similar to enhanced podcasts, is that there is less compatibility across devices. For example, Adobe Flash, one of the Internet format standards for *streaming* video, is not playable on the most popular mobile devices, such as the iPod. The more common format for iPod devices is MPEG4 video, or specifically H.264 codec, used for video compression. HTML5 is another emerging video format that is touted to use less power on mobile devices and result in smaller file sizes. All vodcast files tend to be relatively large and therefore careful attention should be given to whether video is a necessary component to the delivery of the material. If video is essential, using shorter clips (less than 5 or 10 minutes) is desired to limit the size of the file download. The size of the playback window can also be reduced to make smaller file sizes for distribution.

Podcast and Vodcast Creation Tools

Simple audio-only files are easy to capture and may be created with a variety of portable recorders. For the most professional results, the use of a sound-proof booth and special microphone will result in the best quality of sound (Stoten, 2007). Editing of audio files can be done with software such as GarageBand (Mac platform) or Audacity (Mac or PC) that is available for free via the Internet. In addition, some universities are making automated podcast systems available in special classrooms to capture live lectures (Educause Evolving Technologies Committee et al., 2007). This takes the time needed for recording and posting the files out of the individual faculty member's responsibilities and automates the process with technical setup and support ahead of time.

Creation tools for enhanced podcasts include the iLife suite of applications, such as GarageBand, Keynote, and iMovie, on the Mac platform. In addition, a very popular and easy to use tool for creation of enhanced podcasts is PowerPoint and Adobe Presenter. Using the Adobe Presenter plug-in within PowerPoint, faculty can create voice-over narrations of their slides and can output the file as streaming video (Flash), a self-contained pdf file, or a movie file. As noted earlier, not all file types are compatible with mobile players, so it is important to target formats that fit the student profile in your institution.

Creation of vodcasts involves cameras to capture the live video, and postproduction software to edit the video. Video may be captured simply by using a basic handheld video camera (such as a Flip camera) or built-in web cameras, or may be more professionally done with professional video cameras and microphones. Use of professional equipment will result in higher-quality audio and video in the final product. Software needed to edit and process such files includes Adobe Premiere, Adobe Presenter, and iMovie. If extensive editing of video files is required, it is recommended to have support staff skilled in the use of such software provide assistance in this area, as learning to use video-editing software with proficiency can be time consuming. Similar to enhanced podcasts, it is important to understand your user group when making vodcasts available and either to provide multiple file formats or to target those most used by your student group.

Emerging Technologies for Distance Education Clinical and Telehealth

Along with the advances and changes in technology that have enabled students to attend courses from a distance, similar technology has allowed for nursing care at a distance (Grady & Schlachta-Fairchild, 2007). *Telehealth* involves the use of electronic communication equipment to share clinical and health-related information (American Telemedicine Association, 2008). *Telenursing* is the use of these electronic communication devices and equipment to deliver, manage, and coordinate care from a distance. Many nursing faculty have little knowledge of telehealth (Gallagher-Lepak, Scheibel, & Gibson, 2009), yet a recent study of nurses working in telehealth supported that telehealth technologies should be included in undergraduate curriculums (Grady & Schlachta-Fairchild, 2007). The same technologies that are used to provide care and monitoring to remote locations might also be used in monitoring students at remote sites. Such technologies include video and audio conferencing, computers, and specialized remote monitoring equipment. One strategy is to have students serve as patients and care providers in role-playing activities, using telehealth technologies. Winters and Winters (2007) used a similar format with undergraduate nursing students assigned to complete a neurological exam and teaching. Students were able to perform the assessments and teaching activities at a distance using two different formats for connecting (high versus low bandwidth). Overall student satisfaction with the experience was positive. As the need for health care in the home increases, the need for students educated in the use of telehealth technologies will also increase.

Adapting Teaching for Distance Education

Although there are differences in the technology and intricacies of various distance education delivery systems, there are commonalities that should be considered regardless of the medium to be used. Primary to teaching through a distance delivery system is the understanding that there must be modifications to the style of teaching and to the materials used (Connors, 2008; Jones & Wolf, 2010). Planning as a team rather than individually, emphasizing content rather than process, and using a syllabus to cohesively link content are important elements of the distance education planning process. Faculty will take on the role of a facilitator or a guide in distance education (Lewis & Price, 2007). While extensive supports are needed to help faculty in the use of technology, faculty must still possess a baseline in technological capabilities (Connors, 2008) as well as organizational planning (Jones & Wolf, 2010).

Needs Assessment

Before a distance education program is initiated, the need for its introduction into the proposed geographic area should be determined to ensure adequate student participation. Nursing education administrators have embraced distance learning because there is perceived need and demand for it. A move forward with the curriculum implies a commitment from the university that students will

be able to complete a significant portion, if not all, of the academic or continuing education program through distance instruction. In addition, the target audience needs to be considered in regards to the availability of technology and access to high-speed Internet. Since so many of the current distance technologies rely on high-speed Internet, knowing where your potential users have broadband access will dictate to a certain extent the strategies that will be selected. Requiring students to have a minimum level of high-speed Internet connection is one way to ensure that students will be able to use the latest technologies deployed. Marketing a course or program in a new geographic area is usually effective for ensuring adequate registration. Once the program has been initiated, student satisfaction serves as the best method of promoting the program.

Electronic Classroom: The Teacher's View

The classroom remains an essential component of distance education delivery. However, the increasing number of web-based courses and online supplements is changing how the classroom is used for distance instruction. When electronic classrooms are needed to support all or portions of a course, the commitment to technology and the site must be considered as a long-term investment because the cost of equipping the facility will be substantial. A newly designed classroom may comprise complete multimedia systems including computerized presentation systems and wired and wireless high-speed data networks. Visual presentation can be at the touch of a button from a single touch-panel control module. Camera control, digital video recorder (DVR), DVD, Blu-ray DVD, CD, electronic whiteboard, and other computer-based presentation devices are typically integrated into the classroom design for quick and easy access (Suvajian, 2003). In addition, portable video conferencing and audiovisual equipment that can be moved to different locations gives flexibility for use in a wide variety of instructional spaces, while still using state-of-the-art technologies.

While the need for advanced classroom technology is still present, particularly with programs that blend on-site delivery with remote delivery or use of institutionally based video conferencing, increasingly faculty can teach many portions of their content from their offices or even from home. To teach from alternate locations requires that the faculty member still have access to state-of-the-art computers with audio and video capabilities, high-speed Internet access, and technical support. With such supports in place, the faculty member may choose to teach from literally anywhere.

When the opportunity to select a totally new site within a geographic area exists, its location should be considered with respect to its centrality to population, access to public transportation, and relationship to library and computing resources. However, universities generally opt to have the origin site located on an existing campus, although the selection of the building in which a traditional classroom will be converted to an "electronic origination classroom" can become a political quagmire within the institution.

When there is a commitment to online delivery, there must also be a financial commitment to infrastructure, including data networks and computing resources for hardware, software, and instructional media. Personnel for technical support must also be included in this plan.

Electronic Classroom: The Student's View

When distance education technologies that include off-site learning facilities are used, a site coordinator, carefully selected to provide support to faculty and students, is essential to having the program run smoothly. Moore (1995, pp. 1–5) suggests the following "five Cs" of this resource person's role:
1. A willingness and ability to *communicate* effectively
2. *Competence* in handling technical needs and serving as an instructional assistant
3. *Control* of events that helps instill student confidence in the system
4. *Caring* demonstrated for student achievement and success
5. *Continuity* of role from one semester to the next

It is apparent, from the multiple tasks that must be accomplished at each distant site to ensure a smoothly delivered program, that a site coordinator, not necessarily a nurse, is an invaluable resource who serves as the extended arm of the teacher (Moore, 1995).

For programs where students attend virtual classrooms from their homes, centralized support systems must be in place to troubleshoot technology at a distance. Students using web conferencing

equipment in their homes need to test and practice using such technology prior to the start of the program. Ongoing support during all class sessions is also necessary, to ensure that faculty can concentrate on instruction while support personnel assist remote learners with technical problems. Support personnel and time availability can be given to students along with options for contacting them for help via telephone, live chat, or e-mail.

Logistics of ensuring availability of library, computer, and audiovisual resources must be handled by administrative and support staff. Such resources are essential to successful course delivery; however, teaching faculty should not be expected to coordinate the plethora of other relevant activities. Support efforts to ensure efficient registration; advising; locating physical resources; hiring of technicians, site coordinators, or proctors; handling of syllabi and other course materials; obtaining copyright permissions; arranging travel (if a part of the instruction design); and providing other similar services are essential to the success of any distance education delivery program. Support needs will vary depending on the medium being used.

Clinical Site Development

Creating collateral clinical experience for distance learners can be a challenge for health care educators. It may be necessary to replicate all aspects of clinical practice to meet curriculum mandates for successful skill development and competence. This requires coordination with health care agencies for creation of consistent, high-quality clinical experiences. Site visits may be required to ensure accuracy and calibration with instruction at the main campus. Preceptors and clinical coordinators may need to be hired to act as mentors to distant students, to ensure adequate skill development, and to support the alliance between programs and agencies.

Distance video conferencing technologies can also be implemented to provide for interactive consultation. These technologies, along with other telecommunication systems, make it possible for faculty to work with students remotely, when it has been traditionally done in person. Electronic document transfer, online evaluation instruments, and collaboration over interactive networks have made it feasible to assess student performance at a distance and to guide the student's clinical experience.

Preparing Faculty

Orientation to technology and ongoing development are needed for faculty teaching distance education courses. This is a way to create new understanding and to advance existing expertise to new levels of pedagogical effectiveness. Faculty must intricately understand the delivery mechanism to give full attention to the learners instead of the technology. Formative development is a desired approach because it improves specific instructional strategies and ensures strong learning focus.

If they are given an orientation early in their commitment to teaching the course, faculty will have time and opportunity to incorporate innovative tactics into their design and presentation style and to modify teaching materials appropriate to the technology. For example, presentation software, images, and printed copy used for television delivery should be altered for better accommodation to a video screen format. Likewise, graphics, interactive activities, and multimedia need to be carefully developed and evaluated for web-based courses.

Continuous and formative updates during the course of instruction ensure that strategies are being implemented appropriately and that learning focus is maintained. The formative nature of these updates allows for adjustments and modifications to both teaching and learning so faculty and students can maintain good social presence in the learning environment for the duration of the course.

Course Enhancements and Resources

Three factors have been identified as having positive outcomes for distance education courses: "instructor involvement, media involvement, and types of interactions" (Zhao et al., 2005, p. 1861). Blended models that have incorporated a mix of synchronous and asynchronous technologies have been associated with the best student outcomes (U.S. Department of Education, 2009). In addition, conditions in which learners spend more time on task are also associated with more positive learning outcomes (U.S. Department of Education, 2009).

In a blended approach to distance education, the learning value of the course is increased through supplemental media and several adjunct resources

that support instructional delivery. Electronic document exchanges, e-mail, instant messaging, and audio and video interactions are necessary enhancements. Through use of these tools, faculty and students have increased opportunities for communication throughout the term of instruction. Some universities have made available toll-free telephone numbers for enrolled students' use to facilitate their communication with faculty, registrar, financial aid advisers, and other home campus support services. Additionally, many universities are moving forward with a "portal" that will provide a personalized online interface to all university and educational activities.

Evaluation

Ongoing evaluation of student learning will provide the best measure of learning success and will provide faculty with information to improve teaching strategies and the use of technology for distance learning. Evaluation of distance education delivery systems should also occur both formatively and summatively. Formative evaluations are extremely important for the success of the online instructor as well as the online student. These evaluations can be used to determine the student's understanding of the content as well as the instructor's effectiveness. Simply asking the student, "What have you liked the most so far in this online class?" or "What have you liked the least so far in this online class?", is an effective way to obtain valuable feedback. Summative evaluations can also be done at the end of the course using a variety of survey technologies or sites such as surveymonkey.com. More in-depth information related to formative and summative evaluation can be found in Chapter 23.

Peer evaluation of the course by other educators familiar with technology and blended learning environments is important. Peer evaluation may occur at the local level by individuals from the school or institution, or nationally through a program such as Quality Matters. Quality Matters is a national organization that conducts peer reviews of both online and blended courses, using a team of faculty reviewers and an evidence-based rubric (Quality Matters, n.d.).

Student and faculty perceptions of the technology and delivery efficacy should be explored, as well as the rate of student success within the course. Reasons for student attrition should be researched and constructs should be designed to reverse negative trends.

Evaluation data should also include the cost of the course to the university. Factors considered will include salaries or wages for faculty, technicians, site coordinators, and other support staff; equipment; potential lease fees for facilities and communication systems; travel costs for faculty; mailing or courier charges; and other resources needed for course implementation. All expenditures must be evaluated against the income generated through tuition and provided by other financial support sources.

SUMMARY

Increased opportunities for access to higher education are becoming more readily available for students who live and work in areas remote from a central campus, as well as within a wired or wireless central community. Informational and educational technologies are regularly used to reach undergraduate and graduate nursing students, as well as registered nurses seeking nonacademic continuing education. As technology improves and increased research provides greater direction for use of selected paradigms, nursing faculty will find additional challenges to propel curricula and curricular applications far into the future.

Leaders must carefully assess data collected about distance education to set new parameters for future learning. For nursing education, it will be necessary to determine the extent to which distance delivery will be a part of the educational process. Will it become the single most important process? Will it be used to support other more traditional processes? Will it provide additional opportunities to extend learning in a more collaborative way with other organizations and institutions of higher education? Without a doubt, the advancement of computer-based data networks, innovative design of instruction, and creative leadership will provide a solid platform for distance learning environments in the future.

REFLECTING ON THE EVIDENCE

1. Identify issues of concern that could prohibit or significantly delay implementation of one or more instructional delivery systems in your institution.

2. How do information and distance technologies allow for innovative and extended experiences for faculty teaching to a group of geographically disperse students?

3. Which methods of distance education delivery systems are available for your use? How might you adapt your course to be taught through that medium?

4. Reflect on the cost factor for various approaches to teaching via technology. Consider both the origin and the receive sites. How might costs be minimized yet not impede effectiveness of the course delivery?

5. Design a research study that would evaluate effectiveness of a selected distance education course.

REFERENCES

Allen, I. E. & Seaman, J. (2007). *Online nation: Five years of growth in online learning.* Retrieved from http://sloanconsortium.org/publications/survey/pdf/online_nation.pdf

American Association of Colleges of Nursing. (2010, September 20). *Nursing faculty shortage.* (Fact sheet). Retrieved from http://www.aacn.nche.edu/

American Telemedicine Association. (2008). *Telehealth nursing: A white paper developed and accepted by the Telehealth Nursing Special Interest Group.* Retrieved from http://www.americantelemed.org/

Billings, D. (2010). Distance education in nursing: 25 years and going strong. *CIN: Computers, Informatics, Nursing, 25*(3), 121–123.

Brittain, S., Glowacki, P., Ittersum, J., & Johnson, L. (2006). Podcasting lectures. *Educause Quarterly, 29*(3). Retrieved from http://www.educause.edu/

Connors, H. (2008). Beyond the classroom: Considering distance education approaches. In B. Penn (Ed.), *Mastering the teaching role: A guide for nurse educators* (pp. 163–175). Philadelphia, PA: F. A. Davis.

Driscoll, M. (2004). *Psychology of learning for instruction* (3rd ed.). Needham Heights, MA: Allyn & Bacon.

Educause. (2009, September). *7 Things you should know about telepresence.* Retrieved from http://net.educause.edu/

Educause Evolving Technologies Committee, Bentley, K., & Collins, S. (2007, October 11). The evolution of web conferencing. Retrieved from http://net.educause.edu/

Effken, J., & Abbott, P. (2009). Health IT-enabled care for underserved rural populations: The role of nursing. *Journal of the American Medical Informatics Association, 16*(4), 439–445.

Forbes, M., & Hickey, M. (2008). Podcasting: Implementation and evaluation in an undergraduate nursing program. *Nurse Educator, 33*(5), 224–227.

Gagné, R., & Briggs, L. (1979). *Principles of instructional design* (2nd ed.). New York, NY: Holt, Rinehart & Winston.

Gallagher-Lepak, S., Scheibel, P., & Gibson, C. (2009). Integrating telehealth in nursing curricula: Can you hear me now? *Online Journal of Nursing Informatics, 13*(2), 1–16.

Grady, J., & Schlachta-Fairchild, L. (2007). Report of the 2004–2005 international telenursing survey. *CIN: Computers, Informatics, Nursing, 25*(5), 266–272.

Indiana University, Center for Teaching and Learning. (n.d.). *Tips for academic podcasting.* Retrieved from http://ctl.iupui.edu/common/uploads/library/CTL/CTL34951.pdf

Jones, D., & Wolf, D. (2010). Shaping the future of nursing education today using distant education and technology. *The ABNF Journal, 21*(2), 44–47.

Kim, K. & Bonk, C. (2006). The future of online teaching and learning in higher education: The survey says. *Educause Quarterly, 4*, 22–30.

Lewis, P., & Price, S. (2007). Distance education and the integration of e-learning in a graduate program. *The Journal of Continuing Education in Nursing, 38*(3), 139–143.

Mancuso-Murphy, J. (2007). Distance education in nursing: An integrated review of online nursing students' experiences with technology-delivered instruction. *Journal of Nursing Education, 46*(6), 252–260.

Maring, J., Costello, E., & Plack, M. (2008). Student outcomes in a pathophysiology course based on mode of delivery: Distance versus traditional classroom learning. *Journal of Physical Therapy Education, 22*(1), 24–32.

Moore, M. G. (1995). The five C's of the local coordinator (Editorial). *The American Journal of Distance Education, 9*(1), 1–5.

Piaget, J. (2001). *The psychology of intelligence* (2nd ed.). (M. Piercy & D. E. Berlyne, Trans.). New York, NY: Routledge.

Podcast. (2010, October 8). Retrieved from http://en.wikipedia.org/

Quality Matters. (n.d.). Retrieved from http://www.qmprogram.org/

Shantikumar, S. (2009). From lecture theatre to portable media: Students' perceptions of an enhanced podcast for revision. *Medical Teacher: An International Journal of Education in the Health Sciences, 31*(6), 535–538.

Stoten, S. (2007). Using podcasts for nursing education. *The Journal of Continuing Education in Nursing, 38*(2), 56–57.

Suvajian, J. (2003). It's all in the presentation at URI. *Syllabus, 16*(11)), 33–34.

United States Department of Education. (2009). *Evaluation of evidence-based practices in online learning: A meta-analysis and review of online learning studies.* Washington, DC: U.S. Department of Education, Office of Planning, Evaluation and Policy Development, Policy and Program Studies Service. Retrieved from http://www2.ed.gov

Vogt, M., Schaffner, B., Ribar, A., & Chavez, R. (2010). The impact of podcasting on the learning and satisfaction of undergraduate nursing students. *Nursing Education in Practice, 10*, 38–42.

Winters, J., & Winters, J. (2007). Videoconferencing and telehealth technologies can provide a reliable approach to remote assessment and teaching without compromising quality. *Journal of Cardiovascular Nursing, 22*(1), 51–57.

Zhao, Y., Lei, J., Lai, B., & Tan, H. (2005). What makes the difference? A practical analysis of research on the effectiveness of distance education. *Teachers College Record, 107*(8), 1836–1884.

Teaching and Learning in Online Learning Communities

23

Judith A. Halstead, PhD, RN, ANEF, FAAN

Diane M. Billings, EdD, RN, FAAN

Online education is assuming an increasingly prominent role in higher education within the United States. Allen and Seaman (2010), in the 2009 Sloan Consortium online education survey, reported that in fall of 2008 more than 4.6 million college students were enrolled in at least one course where 80% or more of the content was delivered online. This represents an increase of 17% from the previous year's survey. More than one in four college students report taking at least one online course during their time in higher education (Allen & Seaman, 2010). The growing influence of online learning has global significance as well, creating interconnected learning communities that span the world. Bonk (2010) references the "Web of Learning," in which the use of web technology is enhancing how people learn worldwide and empowering them to take advantage of learning opportunities that previously did not exist for them.

The online courses and programs offered on today's college campuses are just as likely to attract students who are living on campus as those who live at a distance. This increased use of online learning in higher education has occurred for a number of reasons. The learners of today expect ready access to course offerings and flexibility in scheduling to meet their educational needs (Parker & Howland, 2006). The current generation of college students, many of whom have been raised in the digital age (Lahaie, 2007a) and have already grown accustomed to learning in ways that are supported by technology, is seldom intimidated by the computer and fully expects faculty to incorporate technology into their classroom learning activities. The nursing shortage, the improving quality of available technology, and existing evidence that learning outcomes from in-class courses and online courses are similar are other factors that have contributed

to the proliferation of online learning (Baldwin & Burns, 2004).

Online learning has a significant presence in nursing education with an ever-expanding number of programs being offered online, especially for those students who are seeking BSN completion degrees and graduate degrees. Providers of continuing education programs are also using online technology to reach larger audiences of health care professionals who appreciate the flexibility and convenience of having their educational needs met in their own homes. Many nursing faculty are integrating aspects of online learning into courses that are primarily taught in the classroom in "real time," thus creating blended or hybrid courses that maximize the use of web-based learning resources. Online learning has revolutionized higher education and continuing education, erasing place and time boundaries for institutions, students, and faculty. As such, online learning is emerging as one strategy that can be used to effectively facilitate interprofessional education in the health professions (Luke et al., 2009). Online learning is also facilitating the development of an international learning community within the nursing profession, as nurses from around the world can access educational offerings to meet their learning needs.

Even with the increasing presence of technology and online education in higher education, teaching in online learning communities (OLCs) remains a new experience for many nurse educators. Engaging successfully in online learning requires faculty and students to reconceptualize their roles as teachers and learners in the teaching–learning process. In addition, multiple institutional issues must be considered when the decision is made to implement online education. This chapter defines online learning; identifies factors that must be considered in the planning, implementation, and evaluation of online learning; and describes online course design issues. In addition, this chapter discusses the implications of online learning for the teaching–learning process, as well as the development needs for faculty and students. The chapter concludes with evidence of the effectiveness of online teaching and learning.

Online Learning Communities

Online learning uses the Internet paired with the capabilities of learning management system (LMS) software to create a learning environment in which a community of learners and educators, as well as other content experts such as clinicians and patients, gather for the purposes of teaching and learning (Babenko-Mould, Andrusyszyn, & Goldenberg, 2004; Jafari, McGee, & Carmean, 2006). Online learning takes place in a virtual learning environment that is created by learning management systems (e.g., WebCT, Blackboard eCollege, Desire2Learn, Moodle). These learning management systems use software to manage teacher–student interactions through the use of such integrated features as discussion forums, chat rooms, audio and video streaming capabilities, e-mails, announcement pages, posting of course documents (e.g., syllabi, assignments), and shared workspaces. E-learning environments have capabilities to integrate podcasts and vodcasts, multimedia, wikis, web logs (blogs), voice threads, and Short Message Service (SMS) tools (instant messaging) (Dell, 2002; Jafari et al., 2006) (see Chapters 21 and 22 for further discussion of these online tools and products). These virtual learning environments are designed to enhance collaboration and interaction through use of shared workspaces and mobile wireless devices and to provide a full complement of learner support through access to academic advisers, mentors, preceptors, and librarians. The learning management systems also typically include assessment and evaluation software such as test generation and administration software, plagiarism detection software, portfolio management software, and online grade books with grade calculation. Additionally, the online learning environment is becoming more integrated with campus services such as the bursar and registrar, thus enabling students to register for courses and receive grades and transcripts (Nelson et al., 2006).

In nursing education, online learning is frequently used to offer individual courses and complete degree programs for academic credit. In clinical settings, online learning may be used to facilitate orientation to clinical practice, meet requirements for mandatory continuing education, and create learning communities to support career development, mentoring, and coaching programs for nurses (Billings et al., 2006; Pullen, 2006). Online learning is a popular means by which nurses participate in lifelong learning and obtain continuing education contact hours.

Educators and learners use the capabilities of online learning in various ways. For example, content may be developed in self-contained *learning modules*, or tutorials. Online learning modules typically contain objectives, learning outcomes, learning activities, and an evaluation component. Because of their self-contained nature, learning modules are flexible and lend themselves to multiple uses. For example, learning modules are useful for providing access to information that can be learned without interaction with faculty or classmates and colleagues. Learning modules can also be used to provide clinical updates, "mandatory" education required in clinical agencies, or background material in preparation for higher-order application in a classroom or clinical setting. Modules are often integrated into classroom or online courses as *reusable learning objects (RLOs)*, predeveloped content with objectives, content, and evaluation that can be used in courses as required or optional learning activities. It is increasingly common for RLOs to accompany textbooks as ancillary teaching materials; they are also available from web-based learning resource repositories such as MERLOT (http://merlot.org).

Online learning can occur in a variety of configurations to support learning in a course. The courses may be designed to be offered fully online, as *full-web courses*, in which faculty and students do not meet in person. Typically these are courses that include primarily didactic content, but increasingly clinical courses with a preceptor are offered fully online. The preceptor is usually a qualified clinician in the student's geographic region who facilitates application of the course concepts in a clinical setting.

Online courses can also be developed to integrate with face-to-face meetings in classrooms or clinical practice. These *blended* courses, also referred to as *web-enhanced*, *web-supported*, or *hybrid courses*, combine the benefits of face-to-face, classroom, or clinical experiences with the online learning community (Bonk & Graham, 2005). Here, the educator uses online assignments such as pretests or case studies to assess student knowledge and facilitate learning course concepts before students participate in face-to-face classroom activities. The educator may even decide to deliver a short online video or audio stream on selected course concepts prior to class. Students can receive feedback about their learning before they come to the classroom, and thus faculty and students are better prepared to use classroom time to clarify misunderstood concepts or focus on more complex problems such as those related to developing clinical decision-making skills. Blended courses can use a combination of technologies to meet the needs of students. For example, for those students who are enrolled in the course but live far away from the campus, one-way or two-way web-based video conferencing may be used to "connect"

students to the class during the times of on-campus class meetings. The goal of blended learning is to take advantage of faculty expertise, the learning management toolkit, and just-in-time learning to provide learners with opportunities to learn and apply content, practice and receive feedback, think critically, and assume the role of the nurse across all domains of learning. The educator must make well-thought-out decisions as to which experiences should be held in the classroom and which should be held in the OLC. Table 23-1 offers suggestions for blending learning in classroom, clinical, and laboratory settings with an online learning environment.

Interactions in online learning may occur asynchronously or synchronously, depending on the desired nature of the interaction. *Asynchronous* interactions are those that are not dependent on time and place. E-mail, threaded discussions in discussion forums, podcasts, and archived video and audio streams are examples of interactions that

---

TABLE 23-1 Blending Online Teaching with Various Learning Environments

Classroom, Clinical, or Laboratory Learning Environments	Online Learning Environment
Demonstration of psychomotor skills and clinical decision-making skills with simulated or standardized patient scenarios	Assessment and evaluation of student learning through self-testing, practice testing, administration of summative tests Use of simulated and virtual case studies; problem-based learning scenarios Video streams of clinical skills, including students' own return demonstration
Discussion of difficult-to-learn content; clarification of assignments	Discussion forums in which students can lead or manage the application of content without direct guidance from the faculty Peer review of work, where students provide feedback to each other Study guides
Clinical practice (with or without preceptor or faculty)	Reflective learning assignments, such as journaling or follow-up debriefing after simulated or actual clinical experiences Written care plans, concept maps Written assignments requiring synthesis of clinical concepts and experiences
Demonstration of verbal and nonverbal communication skills requiring interpretation and feedback; modeling of professional values and behaviors; evaluation of student presentation style and abilities	Preparation for class by completing mastery test or worksheet Reaction and reflection papers following classroom discussion or laboratory demonstration Personal application of course concepts in response to a focused question Follow-up to in-class assignments
Panel discussions with guest speakers when online presentations are not feasible	Preparation for panel discussion through reading assignments, study guides Reflection on classroom discussion and application of content to own nursing practice Online debates on topic
Clinical practice situations requiring feedback to prevent or reverse an error	Active learning strategies designed to focus on fostering culture of safety and prevention of errors such as root cause analysis, case studies, debate, one-minute papers, and self-paced learning modules
Administration of high-stakes examinations and psychomotor skills competency validation	Self-evaluation activities; optional learning activities for testing or enhancing learning; remediation learning options

are asynchronous. Participants involved in an asynchronous interaction can choose to access or respond to the communication at a time that is convenient for them. *Synchronous* interactions are those that occur in "real time" and require participants to be available at a specific time to participate in the discussions. Class meetings using live video conferencing, chat rooms, or webcasts (use of Internet to share information on a desktop through the use of web-based conferencing software) are examples of synchronous interactions. It is also possible to use e-mail or instant messaging in a synchronous fashion, if those involved in the e-mail messaging prearrange the time for sending and responding to the messages. Electronic "office hours" during which the faculty member is available to promptly answer any student e-mails sent during that period is an example of using e-mail in a synchronous fashion.

Regardless of the type of online course the faculty member is teaching, it is important to remember that it is the use of educational practices such as interaction between students and faculty, interaction among classmates, opportunity to receive feedback while learning, and respect for diverse ways of learning that will promote interaction, prevent isolation, and ultimately determine students' satisfaction with the learning experience and the attainment of intended outcomes. The remainder of this chapter provides information that will help faculty to successfully plan, implement, and evaluate learning experiences that will promote the development of online learning communities.

Institutional Planning for Online Learning

Many institution and program issues must be considered when the decision is made to engage in online education. To successfully plan, implement, and evaluate online education, institutions and individual programs must identify how the needed infrastructure for online education will be sustained and how faculty and student development and support needs will be met. It is common for planning committees consisting of administrators, technology staff, student support personnel, and faculty to be charged with addressing and monitoring these issues. The various perspectives of each of these individuals are important when designing a model for online education that can be sustained

within the institution. Policies and procedures specific to online education may need to be developed within the institution.

Before implementing online education, the institution and program needs to give some consideration to how offering online courses or programs fits with the mission of the institution. Administrators and faculty need to be clear about the forces that are driving the desire to offer online education. Is the institution or nursing program interested in offering online education primarily to serve and retain the current student population or to extend course or program offerings to a wider target audience, maybe even serving a global market? An understanding of the reasons for engaging in online education will help guide marketing decisions. Before an online course or program is developed, it can be helpful to conduct an environmental scan to gauge the market and identify which other universities are offering online education and the nature of the courses offered online. What niche does the proposed course or program fill that is not being met by another institution? A needs assessment can also be conducted among prospective students to identify the level of interest in enrollment in an online course or program and the reasons for their interest in online education, as well as the level of computer skills and availability of Internet access present within the targeted population. Having this information before an online offering is planned can help ensure that the learners' educational needs will be met.

It is also important to acknowledge that some of the most strategic marketing of online education may need to occur "internally" within the institution (Billings, 2002). Online education is still new to many faculty, students, and administrators. Faculty who are "early adopters" of technology and online education will need to communicate the potential advantages of online learning to faculty who are more skeptical.

Institutions have reported that using benchmark standards helps ensure quality in online courses (Leners, Wilson, & Stizman, 2007; Little, 2009). To promote the development of quality online education courses and programs, quality indicators and benchmarks have been established by professional organizations and accrediting bodies for institutions to use when planning online programs and courses. Most states have established guidelines for the delivery of distance education through the government bodies that regulate higher education. Examples of frequently referenced quality indicators include those established by the Sloan Consortium (Moore, 2005) and the Institute for Higher Education Policy (2000). The quality indicators and benchmarks espoused by these two organizations are similar in nature in that they identify essential elements that must be addressed to ensure quality in online education: institutional support and commitment; effective course design and teaching–learning principles, faculty development, support, and satisfaction; student support and satisfaction; and outcome evaluation related to learning effectiveness. How each institution decides to address these elements will vary depending on the resources available to the institution and the specific needs of educators and learners.

Accrediting agencies expect that online courses and programs will provide learners with access to learning experiences that achieve the same learning outcomes of traditional "in-class" courses and programs. The two professional nursing accrediting bodies, the Commission on Collegiate Nursing Education (CCNE) and the National League for Nursing Accrediting Commission (NLNAC), have also established standards for distance education programs that state the expectation that learner outcomes will be evaluated using appropriate methodology and with the same rigor associated with traditional face-to-face courses. In addition, many institutions have internal approval processes that must be followed to approve a course or program for online delivery before it can be offered to students. Faculty should familiarize themselves with the guidelines that apply to their particular state, institution, and program as they undertake the planning of online learning programs.

Institutional Planning and Commitment

At the institutional level, decisions must be made about the institution's commitment to online education in terms of human, fiscal, and physical resources. Organizational and administrative infrastructure, funding sources, technology support services, and student support services are areas that will need to be addressed. For example, who within the institution's organizational structure will provide administrative oversight for the development, implementation, and evaluation of online education? Does the institution already employ the technical and instructional design personnel needed to provide course design and delivery support or will additional positions need to be created and funded? A decision will also need to be made as to which of these services will be centralized within the institution or decentralized to the respective academic units.

How the development, implementation, and evaluation of online courses and programs will be funded is another crucial area in which decisions will need to be made. While many online nursing programs are initially developed with the use of grant funds, it is important that sustainability of grant-funded initiatives be addressed. It is likely that student technology fees or distance education fees will need to be assessed in addition to tuition fees to sustain online education within the institution. If such technology or distance education fees are collected by the institution, further decisions will need to be made about how the funds will be dispersed across the academic and service units within the institution.

Reliable and effective technology support for faculty and students is essential for delivering quality online education. As mentioned previously, a decision will need to be made about which technology support services will be centralized within the institutional structure and which will be decentralized in the individual schools and programs. A combination of centralized and decentralized support may be a more effective support model. Outsourcing support services is another option to be considered, and may be more economically feasible depending on the extent of technology expertise that already exists within the institution. The level and extent of technology support that the institution will provide to faculty and students will also need to be determined (Halstead & Coudret, 2000). Many institutions have found it necessary to provide around-the-clock support services to faculty and students to limit undue frustration and "down time" related to technology issues. Faculty and student satisfaction with online learning is frequently related to their satisfaction with technology support services.

The acquisition and maintenance of the hardware and software necessary to support online education and facilitate access is another area that must receive serious institutional attention. Is the institution's current computer network system and bandwidth capable of providing online access to large numbers of simultaneous users with speed and reliability, or are upgrades required? Do faculty have convenient access to the hardware and software needed to support teaching online? Is there a plan to replace computer hardware and software on a regular schedule in faculty offices and student computer clusters to maintain access to adequate technology resources? Do students have access to broadband Internet services in their geographic region? If not, online courses will have to be developed with these bandwidth constraints in mind and content delivery options that require large amounts of bandwidth, such as video streaming, will need to be minimized or avoided (Richard, Mercer, & Bray, 2005).

It is also important for the institution to make a decision about which LMS software will be used to support the delivery and management of online courses. There are a variety of commercial vendors and learning management systems from which to choose. Some of the larger university systems have chosen to design and support their own course management systems. Using an LMS to deliver online courses provides faculty with a relatively easy-to-use, consistent template on which to build their courses. It also provides students with a consistent learning environment with which they can become familiar, transferring this knowledge from course to course. There are advantages and disadvantages associated with each of the various commercial programs available; each institution needs to evaluate the programs to determine which will best meet the needs of the university's faculty and students.

The institution will also need to consider the means by which ongoing faculty and student development for teaching and learning with technology will be provided. Faculty development issues that will need to be addressed include intellectual property policies and ownership of any developed online courses; policies related to providing additional compensation and release time, if any, for faculty who design and teach online courses; and the amount and type of resources that will be provided to help facilitate faculty designing online courses and transitioning to online teaching. The institution or program may also wish to consider questions about what the average student enrollment numbers should be in online courses. Student development issues are primarily related to ensuring that students have the technology access and skills needed to participate in online

learning and facilitating student transition to online learning.

Adequate institutional planning to address questions similar to those raised in the preceding paragraphs is essential to ensuring the success of any online education efforts. It is also important that an institutional infrastructure be established that allows for such planning efforts to be ongoing and include input from all stakeholders, as constant advancements in educational technology will need to be monitored for the institution to stay current and informed about developing trends in online education.

Faculty Development and Support

When implementation of online learning is initiated, faculty development needs will likely be focused on the following areas: instructional design and course development, technology management, workload and time management, role reconceptualization, student–faculty interactions, and assessment and evaluation of learner outcomes (Halstead & Coudret, 2000; Lahaie, 2007b). Before faculty begin any online course development, it is important to assess their knowledge and comfort level regarding conversion of traditional classroom courses into online courses and identify what level of instructional design support will be needed. Developing expertise in online teaching is usually a gradual learning process for faculty and initially may be intimidating even for experienced faculty (Zsohar & Smith, 2008). Faculty who are expert teachers in the classroom suddenly find themselves in the role of a novice when it comes to teaching online (Ryan, Hodson-Carlton, & Ali, 2004). Faculty will need to reconsider their role in the learning process and redesign their pedagogical strategies to facilitate student learning (Ali et al., 2005; Richard et al., 2005; Ryan, Hodson-Carlton, & Ali, 2005; Zsohar & Smith, 2008) and will benefit from mentoring during this adjustment. Scheduling an ongoing series of educational sessions focused on such topics as technology and time management, developing online courses that promote active learning and foster student–faculty interactions, and evaluating learner outcomes throughout the academic year can help faculty acquire the knowledge and skills necessary to successfully design and teach online courses. These topics are covered in more depth later in this chapter.

Learner Development and Support

Introducing online education into a program will have a major impact on the delivery of learner support services, especially if the introduction of online education affects more than just a few individual courses. All aspects of the institution's student support services will ultimately be affected and need to be reconsidered to best serve the needs of students who are geographically distant from the campus, as well as those who are on campus (Mills, Fisher, & Stair, 2001; Nelson, 2007). It is a requirement of national higher education accrediting bodies, as well as nursing accrediting bodies, that the academic support services for online students be similar to those available for on-campus students (Baldwin & Burns, 2004). Student support that will need to be reconsidered and redesigned for students who enroll in online programs include academic advising, tutoring, financial aid, library, and bookstore services. Ensuring that all online experiences are accessible to students with disabilities is another important institutional consideration (Nelson, 2007). The admission and registration processes may also need to be restructured so that students who live at a distance will be able to accomplish these tasks without being physically present on campus.

The decision to deliver online education will also result in the need for the institution to make financial decisions regarding tuition costs and any additional student technology or distance education fees. Many universities or colleges automatically charge students on-campus usage fees, such as activity fees and parking fees. Will these fees be waived for students who never come to campus? These decisions and others related to the delivery of student support services will require the consideration and collaboration of numerous departments in the institution so that students will have a quality learning experience.

Faculty should proactively address the development needs of students engaging in online learning. Learners who are new to online learning frequently need some initial guidance in how to manage their time when they are taking online courses. The relatively independent nature of online education requires students to understand that they are assuming responsibility for their own learning to an extent with which they may be unaccustomed (Johnston, 2008). They are moving from the structure of the traditional classroom to a more unstructured learning environment that does not necessarily include the physical, face-to-face presence of faculty and peers and the weekly time commitment to attend class. Some students may assume that an online course will be "easier" than a traditional course, a notion that is usually quickly dismissed after the course begins and they become overwhelmed with the independence that an online course allows them in managing their own time to meet their learning needs. It is easy for students to underestimate the amount of self-direction and self-pacing that is needed to be successful in online learning.

Faculty can help students by clearly identifying expectations for participation and due dates for assignments (Beitz & Snarponis, 2006; Zsohar & Smith, 2008). If weekly online discussion is expected, this should be stated in the course syllabus. During the first 2 to 3 weeks of the course, those students who are not participating in the course should be actively sought out. The lack of participation is likely due to technology issues or the inability to be self-directive in learning (Halstead & Coudret, 2000). Reaching out to the student at this critical point in the course may make a difference in whether the student will be successful in completing the course.

Students will also require an orientation to the course management system and any other technology that they may be required to use in their coursework. Although orientation to technology can occur face to face or using printed materials, Carruth, Broussard, Waldemeirer, Gauthier, and Mixon (2010) developed a 5-day online orientation course for graduate students who lacked sufficient technological skills to be effective learners in their online course. Evaluations indicated that the students had improved technology proficiency and, because attrition for students who did not have the necessary technology skills was reduced, the course is now required. The institution needs to consider how it can provide orientation to technology for distant learners, as well as technology support when students encounter problems.

In addition to an orientation to support services, students who enroll in online programs also need an orientation to the institution, school, and program. The institution needs to consider how best to establish relationships and "create a sense of presence" (Nelson, 2007, p. 188) with students who may attend the institution only from a distance yet will obtain a degree and become alumni. Effective use of websites, social networking, and virtual tours of the campus can help form connections that will lead to satisfactory student–institution relationships.

Assessment and Evaluation of Online Learning

Faculty and administrators also need to give consideration to how online courses and programs will be assessed and evaluated to determine whether curriculum and program outcomes are being met, as well as for the purpose of continuous quality improvement (Billings, 2000). Effectiveness of online courses and programs can be measured using a variety of methods. As mentioned previously, quality indicators and benchmarks, as well as accreditation standards, provide guidelines for measuring program quality. A systematic evaluation plan can be established that will foster continuous, ongoing quality improvement efforts in all aspects of program delivery: institutional support, faculty satisfaction, student satisfaction, adequacy of technology and student–faculty support services, and effectiveness in meeting expected learner outcomes, including a comparison to traditional course offerings. Data regarding student enrollment numbers, academic progression, and graduation can be compiled to address retention concerns. Data related to established program outcomes can be collected to demonstrate effectiveness of selected pedagogical strategies (Broome, Halstead, Pesut, Rawl, & Boland, 2011; Hunter & Krantz, 2010). Rubrics can also be established to assist faculty with their own and peer review of their online courses (Blood-Siegfried et al., 2008).

Faculty Role in Online Learning

The faculty member's role as an educator undergoes a change when he or she is teaching online courses (Halstead, 2002). First of all, real-time, face-to-face interaction with students becomes more limited, with many interactions occurring asynchronously. Most important, in online courses the educator is less likely to be the primary source of information for students. Instead, the educator's role becomes one of facilitating students' learning experiences. Students assume more responsibility for identifying

their own learning needs and being self-directed in how they choose to meet identified learning outcomes. For some faculty who are new to online teaching, this results in feeling a loss of control over the learning process. Teaching online may require faculty to rethink long-held beliefs about the role of the educator in the teaching–learning process and explore new paradigms of teaching (Shovein, Huston, Fox, & Damazo, 2005).

Becoming a "facilitator" of learning, however, does not lessen the need for the educator or the importance of the educator's role in the learning process. The educator retains responsibility for identifying the expected outcomes of the course, designing learning activities that will promote active student involvement in the learning process and higher-order thinking, and evaluating student performance. Facilitating online discussion is another important role for faculty who are teaching online, as is providing timely feedback to students, so that students will know whether they are achieving the desired learning outcomes.

Two common concerns of faculty who are engaged in online teaching for the first time are related to how to facilitate and manage asynchronous online discussion and how to manage time most effectively. Faculty have indicated that their workload increases when they engage in online teaching (Ryan et al., 2005). In their comparison of faculty workload in web-based and face-to-face graduate nursing courses, Anderson and Avery (2008) found that while the amount of faculty teaching time did not increase in a statistically significant manner in online courses, there were differences in the amount of time spent in course preparation and student contact time, with those faculty teaching online courses reporting more time devoted to each of these activities. More research is needed to more fully understand the demands on faculty workload created by online teaching.

Managing Online Discussion

Time management frequently becomes an issue for faculty teaching online courses because of the amount of student communication generated within the course. The communication generated by students in online courses can be overwhelming if the educator has not given some prior thought to how to manage it. Successful management of asynchronous discussion requires the educator to initially identify the purpose of the discussion and to be sure that all students are contributing to the discussion (Halstead, 2002). As the online discussion unfolds, the educator may find it necessary at times to change the direction of the discussion or to correct any factual errors students may have made in their postings. However, faculty usually serve as discussion facilitators (Zsohar & Smith, 2008). It is not desirable to respond to every comment made by students in online discussion; faculty should strive to avoid dominating the conversation, reserving their comments to emphasize or summarize key concepts, praise students and provide feedback as appropriate, and make other similar contributions.

Because online courses promote student flexibility and convenience in learning, students tend to access the course, post comments, and send e-mails to faculty at all hours of the day, 7 days a week. That is why it is essential to implement time management strategies before the course begins. By having a plan in place, faculty can respond to student comments in a timely manner while still retaining a sense of control.

Some strategies for managing online communication that have proven helpful include (1) deciding how quickly to respond to student inquiries (e.g., within 48 hours) and informing students of this time frame so that they will know when to anticipate an answer; (2) establishing individual student electronic file folders in which to retain a record of course communication; (3) using a separate e-mail account or the learning or course management system e-mail option for student communications, so that student e-mail is automatically separated from other professional or personal correspondence; (4) establishing "electronic" office hours to interact with students; and (5) creating and saving standardized responses to the most commonly asked questions that can be quickly accessed and individualized for students. Faculty may also find it helpful to "block out" scheduled amounts of time each week to devote to the online course.

Another means of managing online communication is to have students provide peer feedback to postings in the discussion forums. Students can critique posted assignments, lead and summarize group discussions, and participate in collaborative group learning activities. Students can be responsible for synthesizing and analyzing the responses in the forum, thus providing faculty

and classmates from other groups an opportunity to respond to summarized work. Faculty can appoint and rotate student discussion leaders to provide opportunities for all students to experience a leadership role. Not only do these techniques foster timely feedback and reduce sole reliance on the faculty for feedback, but they also promote active learning (Phillips, 2005). These strategies also work to effectively manage discussion in classes that have larger enrollments.

Managing Large Enrollments in Online Courses

Because of educator shortages, increased student enrollment, and pressures to admit additional students to nursing programs, faculty are teaching classes with larger enrollments, including online courses. Although there is no evidence to indicate that the quality of teaching and learning is less in larger classes such that students are dissatisfied, faculty are responsible for assuring quality learning experiences in their courses and need to consider strategies for facilitating learning when course enrollment increases.

What is a large class? The answer to this question depends on the nature of the student (beginner or advanced, graduate or undergraduate); the type of content (simple or complex, easy to learn or difficult to learn, applied in similar or novel circumstances); the experience of the faculty (novice or expert); and the design of the course (first time, in draft form and well designed, tested and revised). Current evidence indicates that, in general, an online class size of 20 can be taught by one faculty member (Colwell & Jenks, 2006). Some authors have indicated 25 students to be an appropriate enrollment for an online course (Lahaie, 2007b). Some institutions have established a maximum enrollment for online courses because of the increased time commitment for the faculty. Policies regarding class size vary among institutions.

When teaching an online course with large enrollments, faculty must ensure that the course is designed for maximum learning, educational practices are designed to promote learning, and discussion forums are managed to foster higher-order learning. For courses in which enrollment surpasses 15 or so students, it may be more effective to divide the students into smaller discussion groups. These smaller groups encourage interactions among students while allowing faculty to focus on the outcomes of individual and group work.

The amount of time spent providing feedback to and grading students' work increases as class size increases. Faculty can choose teaching and evaluation strategies that promote learning while limiting the faculty time required to respond to nonsignificant issues. Fewer carefully designed assignments that prompt practice and feedback and foster higher-order learning are preferable to more assignments that require the faculty or students to process information in lower levels of the cognitive or affective domains. As described earlier, faculty can also create opportunities for feedback that students themselves and their classmates are capable of providing. Faculty can also use "sampling" strategies for grading, whereby faculty read only selected portions of student writing during formative development of written work or read only selected (but varied) portions of care plans, reflection papers, journals, and other written work that is in formative development. Finally, the use of grading rubrics makes expectations clear to students, maximizes the likelihood of success on the assignment, and simplifies the grading process for faculty.

Teaching assistants may be used to help manage the communication generated by larger classes (Parker & Howland, 2006). Depending on the knowledge and preparation of the teaching assistant, teaching assistants can grade papers, facilitate discussion, provide feedback to drafts, answer questions, and assist students with technology problems. Teaching in an online course as a teaching assistant or teaching practicum is one way to prepare nurses and students for future roles as educators.

Despite the potential increase in time demands for faculty who teach online, faculty do experience the same convenience and flexibility in teaching online courses as students enrolled in online courses do. With careful planning, faculty can incorporate their responsibilities for online teaching into their schedules at a time that is most convenient for them. Faculty can remain in contact with their students even when they are traveling and attending professional conferences. Online teaching helps to promote maximum flexibility in balancing the demands of the various aspects of the faculty role: teaching, scholarship, and service.

Designing Courses and Learning Activities

Offering a module, course, or academic program fully or partially online provides faculty an opportunity to reconceptualize the way the course or program is designed and sequenced. Evidence for best practices indicates that course design influences how students learn and how well the course influences time on task and productive use of students' learning time (Palloff & Pratt, 2003). Ideally, faculty have access to course design specialists such as instructional designers, graphic artists, and web technicians. Ultimately, however, faculty are responsible for the design and integrity of courses that are moved to the OLC and must be aware of course design basics.

Nurse educators should develop their online courses according to theories of teaching and learning and instructional design (Bolan, 2003; Hollingsworth, 2002a; O'Neil, Fisher, & Newbold, 2004; Sternberger, 2002). These theories suggest that students learn when actively engaged, interact in a social and applied context, and reflect on their practice. See Chapters 10, 11, and 12 for foundational information about theories of teaching and learning, developing courses, and selecting learning experiences.

When developing online courses, faculty first will need to consider whether the course, the course content, and the needs of the students can be best met in a fully online course; in synchronous or asynchronous modes; or with a mix of online activities, on-campus meetings in a classroom or laboratory, or clinical practica. At this time, faculty also need to consider what learning or course management tools and online resources are available or need to be acquired to support the pedagogical goals.

Course development should also be guided by frameworks and models that assure attention to all steps of the teaching–learning process (Sternberger, 2002; Zsohar & Smith, 2008). Course development should also be guided by the use of good practices in education (Chickering & Gamson, 1987), as well as by evidence of best practices (Billings, Skiba, & Connors, 2005; Suen, 2005). These practices include high expectations, active learning, feedback, interaction with faculty, interaction with classmates, time on task, and respect for diverse ways of learning (Table 23-2).

TABLE 23-2 Educational Practices in Online Courses

Educational Practice	Examples in Online Courses
High expectations	Communicate learning outcomes and expectations in several places in the course; expect success; online learning is not easier than or less than classroom expectations
Active learning	Use case studies; problem-based learning; discussion; round robin; critical thinking vignettes
Rich, prompt feedback	Create self-graded activities; structure learning activities that require students to produce work for review by self, students, and faculty
Interaction with faculty	Use online office hours; use course e-mail for individual communications; be available to answer noncourse-related questions; share examples of faculty work; participate in socialization activities
Interaction with classmates	Use group projects to promote collaborative work; structure communication tools for small group work, learning circles, chats; create opportunities for students to share reflections and experiences; ensure places for public and private communication for class members
Time on task	Time spent on learning activities should be reasonable; allow sufficient time between assignments; structure online classroom so students are not reading voluminous and nonessential postings and online time is productive and related to course outcomes; create separate "social spaces" as options for participation
Respect for diverse ways of learning	Create options for learning and evaluation; present choices for content and learning activities; encourage diverse opinions while creating norms of respect; use reflective journals to assist students to assess their own needs, styles, and values

Basic principles of course design are discussed below. However, we suggest that faculty work with an instructional design team when developing courses for the first time.

1. *Start with the learner.* The student is the focal point for designing online courses. Educators must assess student learning styles, learning needs, current knowledge, motivation, and adaptive needs (see Chapter 2). While not all students prefer learning online or have well-developed self-directed learning skills that are essential to success in an online learning community, most students can adapt and draw on strengths and resources that facilitate their learning when online coursework is required. Educators must also understand the current generation of "m-learners," those students who use mobile, wireless devices and who are accustomed to multitasking and acquiring and processing information just as they need it and in a context that meets their needs (Alexander, 2004). Faculty should also understand the learner's technology skills and provide learner support and adequate resources, particularly when online courses are offered for the first time.
2. *Define learning outcomes, objectives, and competencies.* Specifying learning outcomes is a curricular process and should be completed within the context of course and curriculum development (see Chapters 9 and 10). Outcomes in all domains of learning can be facilitated within online courses, and the course design can accommodate a variety of learning domains and levels within the domains.
3. *Organize content into short, logical units such as lessons or modules.* Courses designed for the classroom are typically planned for the semester and class hour schedule of the institution. With web-based courses, however, there is more flexibility in scheduling, and thus the content can be organized with additional attention to pedagogical principles. Storyboards and course plans facilitate the organization of modules and courses (Hollingsworth, 2002a). Each unit should include an overview, outcomes and objectives, learning activities, readings and assignments, and evaluation (Zsohar & Smith, 2008).
4. *Integrate educational practices.* Educational practices such as those listed in Table 23-2 provide a foundation for developing the course and related learning activities. Mounting evidence indicates that the use of these educational practices enhances outcomes such as learning, socialization, student satisfaction, and transition to practice, as well as a sense of caring and social presence in the course

(Billings et al., 2006; Brownrigg, 2005; Burruss, Billings, Brownrigg, Skiba, & Connors, 2009; Diekelmann & Mendias, 2005; Pullen, 2006; Sitzman & Leners, 2006).

5. *Provide students with opportunities to practice and apply course principles in context.* Additionally, learning activities should be designed for the higher levels of the cognitive domain to assist the students in moving from comprehension to synthesis and evaluation and to connect the learning to clinical practice (Benner, Sutphen, Leonard, & Day, 2010).

The course should begin by establishing clear and *high expectations.* These are communicated in the full syllabus (see Chapter 10).

Learning activities should require *active learning and participation*—interaction with the content, course, classmates, and the teacher. In repeated studies of teaching in courses conducted fully or partially online, findings demonstrate the importance of selecting effective teaching strategies and well-designed learning experiences (Billings, Connors, & Skiba, 2001) to foster active student learning. In general, teaching practices used in the classroom are also effective for promoting discussion and active learning in the online environment. These educational practices (see Table 23-2) have been derived from work by Chickering and Gamson (1987) and adapted for use in the online classroom (Beitz & Snarponis, 2006; Chickering & Ehrmann, 1996; Daroszewski, Kinser, & Lloyd, 2004a; Edwards, Hugo, Cragg, & Peterson, 1999; Kirkpatrick, 2002; Phillips, 2005).

A variety of learning activities such as debates, games, concept maps, WebQuests, case studies, questions, treasure hunts, or written work such as papers and reflective journaling and projects engage the student in active learning. Most nursing textbook publishers have created virtual environments and interactive learning activities that accompany the textbook; faculty can integrate these rich resources into the course design to provide students opportunities for active and self-directed learning. Other sources for learning activities include reusable learning objects that are self-contained modules with learning outcomes, learning activities and an assessment component, websites that have developed no-cost learning activities for specific content such as quality and safety (http://www.qsen.org), and consortia that have developed low-cost modules on a variety of topics (Wink, 2009).

Assignments that foster active learning at higher levels are those that promote analysis or critique of a concept. These include concept clarification, case studies, and debates. Identifying a challenging clinical problem or ethical health care issue and having students brainstorm solutions or debate the pros and cons of a given solution to the problem are other examples of higher-level discussion techniques that promote discussion and interaction. It is relatively easy for students to identify real-life issues in nursing practice that can be used to generate online discussion. See Box 23-1 for an example of a discussion forum showing the use of a variety of teaching–learning strategies used to promote active learning.

Students must receive *feedback* while they are learning. Feedback in online courses can include acknowledgement, for example, by recognizing that students have submitted work; information, by giving information or direction; and evaluation such as making judgments about students' work and offering information for improvement (Bonnel, 2008). Feedback can come from students themselves, classmates, and the faculty. Bonnel (2008) recommends creating a multitude of opportunities for feedback during the course design stage. These can include use of automated responses and computer-graded practice tests. Self-graded case studies are simple ways for students to check their own progress. Peer review on written work or small study and discussion groups provides students an opportunity to learn from each other. Faculty must provide feedback at every step of the learning process by monitoring student work, correcting errors, and providing examples of expected outcomes. The faculty role also includes developing the students' own capabilities for self-reflection.

Interaction is essential in online learning. Students must have opportunities to work with each other, share ideas, collaborate, and work in groups. When students work together there is a sense of social presence and being connected to the course (Brownrigg, 2005). The isolation often attributed to online courses can be overcome by course design that encourages interaction. As noted earlier, faculty, too, must be actively engaged and "present" in the course by responding to students' questions, providing feedback, and establishing a collegial learning environment (Diekelmann & Mendias, 2005). Faculty can demonstrate caring by providing feedback, responding to students in a timely

BOX 23-1 Discussion Forums

INTRODUCTIONS

Introduce yourself: Tell us where you work, why you are taking this course, and anything else you want us to know about you!

MODULE 1: FOCUS ON THE LEARNER

Post a description of your learners, how you will assess their needs, and what support they need in your web course.

MODULE 2: DEBATE

Question: Should *all* nursing courses be designed to be offered only on the Internet? Participants with last names A–M will argue the affirmative; participants with last names N–Z will argue the negative. Participant with first last name starting with the letter A, summarize the affirmative; person with first last name starting with the letter Z (or last of alphabet) summarize the negative.

MODULE 3: TREASURE HUNT

In this course, find the various strategies used to inform learners about the course expectations and learning outcomes to be attained. Post your findings and comment on the value of each strategy.

MODULE 4: ROUND ROBIN

Post a response to the question "How can we assist learners in web courses to obtain feedback?"

MODULE 5: CHAT SUMMARY

Summarize the work of your chat room discussion.

MODULE 6: ONE-MINUTE PAPER "ONLINE LEARNING COMMUNITIES"

Write a "one-minute paper" describing what helped you become a member of the online learning community in this course.

MODULE 7: MUDDIEST POINT

What is still not clear to you at this point in the course? Post your questions and all (faculty and participants) will try to clear up your muddiness.

STUDENT LOUNGE

This is the place to kick back and relax.

QUESTION OFFICE

Post your questions about the course content, process, or technical aspects here. Answers will be provided within 24 hours.

fashion, demonstrating support for the student in the interaction, and conveying a sense of empathy (Sitzman & Leners, 2006). The use of social networking software, web conferencing, and other Web 2.0 tools can be used to facilitate interaction and collaboration.

Online courses must also be designed to *respect the diversity* of ways that students learn and the diversity of the learners themselves. This occurs by providing options for participating in the course, for ways of learning course material, and for assessing and evaluating learning outcomes. Because of the increasing racial, ethnic, generational, and language diversity of students in nursing schools, faculty must also design courses and communicate expectations for respecting differences of opinion and ways of learning.

1. *Create assessment, evaluation, and grading plans.* The evaluation and grading criteria should be clearly stated. A variety of strategies for evaluation can be adapted for use in online learning environments (see Chapter 25). These include tests, case studies, simulations, journals, debates, discussion, and portfolios. Many classroom assessment techniques (CATs) have been modified as "e-CATs" and are effective for both students and faculty to assess learning (see Chapter 16). Evaluation strategies should be selected to provide formative feedback to students while they are learning and also to evaluate learning outcomes at the end of the module, lesson, or course. The faculty must indicate the grading plans and guidelines to the student at the outset of the course.

2. *Use graphic design principles.* Course design is improved by the use of colors, fonts, and visual images (Hollingsworth, 2002b). The use of colors and fonts must meet design standards and the use of images must not infringe on copyright; faculty are well served by working with design experts. The course designer should integrate media such as videos, audio, and visuals thoughtfully (see Chapter 21).

3. *Respect copyright laws.* Because of the easy availability of graphics, text, and video media, it is tempting to include many of these resources in online courses. Faculty and instructional designers, however, must work within the guidelines of the U.S. Copyright Act and the Technology, Education and Copyright Harmonization Act (TEACH Act). Rhoads and

White (2008) advise faculty to be familiar with these laws and consider that copyright works can be used only for educational purposes, for "fair use," and with permission of the copyright holder.

Creating Community

Because of the absence of face-to-face communication in the online community, faculty must use specific strategies to overcome the sense of distance and create a learning environment in which students feel connected and have a sense of the presence of each member.

At the beginning of each course, the educator can establish a learning community through activities that promote personal student interaction and allow the class to get acquainted with each other as individuals. Sharing pictures, using "icebreaker" activities, and posting brief introductory messages during the first week of the course are just a few examples of some activities that can promote interaction among the students before discussion of course content begins. It is equally important for faculty members to share information about themselves; faculty can use a photograph or a short video introduction to help students learn more about the faculty. Establishing a discussion forum that can be used by students to ask course questions and promote student dialogue without faculty presence can also be helpful in promoting a learning community. Some faculty elect to schedule periodic face-to-face interactions to promote a sense of community, but this is not always possible or even necessary. A learning community can be successfully built online without the participants ever meeting each other.

Caring and Social Presence

Palloff and Pratt (1999) identify six elements that are essential to building communities and promoting interaction: honesty, responsiveness, relevance, respect, openness, and empowerment. For meaningful participation to occur, students must be able to expect that they will receive honest, respectful, constructive feedback and prompt responses from faculty and students. The subject matter and discussion need to be relevant to real life. Respecting students as equal participants in the learning process and empowering them to be self-directed,

responsible learners are also important. Finally, students need to feel free to share their thoughts and feelings without fear of retribution in the form of lower grades.

It is also important for faculty to create a sense of caring in the course. In the on-campus classroom, caring is facilitated by expressing concern, being genuine, and the use of facial expressions and body language; different strategies are needed when the classroom is online. Sitzman and Leners (2006), in a small study of students in an online course, asked students to identify the factors that created a caring learning environment. These researchers found that caring occurred when there was frequent feedback, when there was participation and response to postings, and when the faculty member conveyed concern or empathy by asking about the students' welfare. In a subsequent study with a larger sample, Sitzman (2010) further clarified student-preferred caring behaviors and noted that students appreciated clarity in expectations and directions, timeliness in response to postings and e-mails, having faculty who were an empathetic presence, and being fully engaged and available to students. In a replication of the study with graduate students, Leners and Sitzman (2006) found that along with knowing the faculty on a personal level, students also wanted affirmation and encouragement from both classmates and the faculty.

Other researchers refer to the need to create a sense of social presence, an awareness of other persons in the class (Brownrigg, 2005), and to reduce transactional distance, the space of potential misunderstandings between the student and faculty (Patillo, 2007). When students do not feel connected to the members of the class, motivation and engagement decrease (Lahaie, 2007a). Strategies to overcome these barriers include increasing the amount of dialogue, interaction, and collaboration in an online course and establishing small discussion groups. Other strategies are to use web conferencing software (webinars) to facilitate synchronous class meetings; assigning projects that require collaboration and interaction among students; using polling features of the course management system; and increasing the amount of contact students have with faculty through e-mail, communication technologies such as Skype, and, as needed, face-to-face meetings. Emoticons can also be used to convey an affective dimension to the dialogue, although they should be used with caution as they are open to varied interpretation (Lahaie, 2007a).

Social Networking

Another strategy for promoting community in online courses is to use social networking, the use of Web 2.0 tools such as Facebook, YouTube (see Chapter 21), Twitter, wikis, and blogs to facilitate information and media sharing, collaborative work, and professional development. These tools, most of them already a part of students' daily lives, also can be used in the on-campus or online classroom to promote interaction among faculty and students. Suggestions for using these tools for instructional purposes are provided below with the caveat that when used in courses there must be clearly defined instructional purposes and measurable outcomes; communication in the community must be restricted to the members of the online community with safeguards such as passwords; communication must not violate school or university policies or legislation that prohibits public sharing of private information; and there must be an agreement that all members will respect diversity of the opinions shared within the community and observe course norms for appropriate professional behavior.

Social networking sites (for example, Facebook and Twitter) are websites in which members create a profile and add "friends" with whom they wish to share information. Facebook can be used in courses by having students create a Facebook page to introduce themselves to each other, share class notes, and work on class projects; some faculty create a Facebook page for a manikin in the learning resource center and then class announcements and assignments come from the manikin's "Facebook page" (Skiba, 2010). One of the advantages of using Facebook is that many students already have accounts and are accustomed to sharing information in this format. Twitter allows users to send short (140-character) messages ("tweets") to an individual or a group in the social network (Bristol, 2010; Skiba, 2008). The messages are retrieved from an Internet website. Faculty and students can use Twitter to post challenge questions to students, to update assignments, or to share information from a conference. Faculty also use Twitter during a class session to receive responses to questions posed in class.

Social writing tools (for example, wikis and blogs) promote collaboration and can be used to develop thinking and writing skills (Billings, 2009). A wiki is a single document developed by a group; the software facilitates adding, deleting, and editing members' contributions as well as attaching photographs, video, and audio clips. Wikis can be used for writing group reports or papers, posting the summary of a community assessment, hosting a journal club, or holding "grand rounds" in which each student presents his or her patient and others contribute to the care plan. A blog (web log) is a document composed of sequential postings by members of the learning community. Blogs can be used as reflective journals, with each student posting individual reflections throughout the course. Blogs are also an easy way to illicit comments about a controversial topic, to conduct focus groups, and to share examples of a particular concept.

Professional networking sites (for example, Ning and LinkedIn) establish interest-focused communities, typically for the purpose of establishing and expanding a list of professional contacts and networking for seeking employment and professional development. Students can use these sites to market themselves and explore employment opportunities.

Clinical Teaching

Although the clinical practice experiences with clients required in nursing cannot be provided online, the tools and strategies that are the strengths of the OLC can be used to support clinical experiences for students and nurses (Babenko-Mould et al., 2004; Billings et al., 2005; DeBourgh, 2001; Lashley, 2005; Vinten & Partridge, 2002). Several types of clinically focused courses lend themselves to being offered in an online environment. For example, Lashley (2005) found that in a physical assessment course students could learn the clinical skills and clinical decision making that were the outcomes for the course. Faculty can use e-mail and chat as well as discussion forums to link students to their instructors, classmates, preceptors, expert nurses, health care professionals, and clients in the broader community of professional practice.

In the clinical teaching environment, the knowledge learned in the didactic course is applied. Here apprenticeship strategies, use of preceptors, and interaction with colleagues facilitate knowledge transfer. For example, Nesler, Hanner, Melburg, and McGowan (2001) found that precepted clinical experiences for students in online courses were important components for professional role socialization, and Billings et al. (2001) found that use of good education practices within the online course correlated highly with socialization and preparation for real-world work. Stewart, Pope, and Hansen (2010) used clinical preceptors in an online program for students seeking an accelerated BSN degree; students who worked with clinical preceptors during five courses reported being well prepared for the real world of nursing practice.

When the clinical courses use preceptors, orientation of the preceptor is imperative and should include information about teaching and evaluating, as well as information about the course and course procedures (Billings et al., 2006; Stewart et al., 2010). In the triad model in which the student, preceptor, and faculty collaborate to promote student learning, the preceptor may be invited to participate in the online course and thus share clinical insights and connect clinical practice to concepts being taught in the online classroom.

The online learning environment has also been used for preconference and postconference discussions associated with a particular clinical experience (Babenko-Mould et al., 2004; Daroszewski, Kinser, & Lloyd, 2004b). For courses in which students are dispersed throughout a range of clinical experiences, the online environment provides an ideal setting for bringing students together to share experiences and apply content to demonstrate attainment of clinical learning outcomes. For example, when directed journaling and reflection were used following a clinical experience in an advanced practice community health course, Daroszewski et al. (2004b) found that students used critical thinking, demonstrated socialization, and had increased understanding of course content. Babenko-Mould et al. (2004) found that students' self-efficacy for nursing competencies improved when they participated in an online computer conference associated with a clinical practicum.

Increasingly, the online learning environment has become a resource environment for students and practicing nurses. Here, links to research findings, evidence for practice, and access to information about drugs and therapeutic interventions provide the basis for informed practice. As students acquire the skills, knowledge, and values of the profession rather than memorize facts, online resources and their access to them by way of mobile devices will become increasingly important.

Evaluating and Grading Learning Outcomes

Evaluation is as important in online courses as it is in the classroom or clinical practice environment. Best practices indicate that evaluation begins with clearly stated and communicated learning outcomes or competencies; provides students with an opportunity to learn and practice the expected behaviors and receive feedback during the learning process; and concludes with judgment or "grading," indicating the degree to which learning has occurred. Special considerations for these evaluation practices as they pertain to the online environment are discussed here.

Timing of Evaluation

Evaluation in online courses, particularly those courses that are fully online, assumes greater significance because of the asynchronous nature of the course and the potential lack of face-to-face communication. Faculty must therefore be deliberate about the timing of the evaluation and thoughtful in choosing evaluation strategies and providing feedback throughout the course.

Formative evaluation occurs during the course and is essential to learning in online courses. Case studies, critical thinking vignettes, and self-tests provide students with opportunities to practice and receive formative evaluation when teaching feedback is included in the test or scenarios. Adapting CATs (see Chapter 15) to the online learning environment is another way to help both students and faculty gauge students' understanding of course concepts. For example, a CAT such as an online "muddiest point" or electronic survey early in the course can help faculty to modify the course or teaching strategies as the course progresses. Taking advantage of the features of an online gradebook will help students keep track of their own progress.

Summative evaluation occurs after students have had the opportunity to learn and apply course content. Evaluation strategies that work well in the classroom usually work well in online courses (see Chapter 24). Strategies that are particularly effective include written work, games, debates, discussion, portfolios, electronic poster presentations, and tests (Bloom & Trice, 1997; Reising, 2002; Rossignol & Scollin, 2001).

Evaluation in online courses should take advantage of the course management tools such as discussion forum, e-mail, testing, and portfolio management. Online gradebooks assist students in tracking their own progress and, to the extent possible, in determining when they are ready for summative or final evaluation such as taking a final examination.

Academic Integrity in Online Courses

Academic integrity must be observed and protected in the online community, as well as in the classroom. Policies may need to be written to include online courses or may need to be adapted to be more inclusive of or specific to the online course. In addition, norms of respect for individuals and their ideas must be observed. All expectations must be communicated to the student in the syllabus (see Chapter 10).

Recent concern about the reported lapses in academic integrity in higher education has prompted faculty to reconsider how to manage plagiarism and cheating on tests in their on-campus and online classrooms. Plagiarism involves using the work of another without attributing credit to the original author. The electronic environment provides students with easy access to papers and projects from students throughout the world, as well as from students in similar or previous courses within the same school. Faculty have a responsibility to assist students in learning the conventions of citing published work and to be proactive in offsetting the potential for plagiarism. Simple measures include developing an honor code statement, requiring students to submit copies of all cited references, selectively altering assignments each semester, and choosing assignments that can be completed only by using original work such as a care plan for a specific patient. More complicated and expensive measures include purchasing plagiarism detection software that faculty can use to check students' written work for similarities to other student papers or published works.

Cheating on tests offered in the online environment can occur because students may be able to print tests and share them, use textbooks or Internet sites to answer questions, sit together in a computer cluster and assist each other in answering test questions, or have someone else take the test for them (Hart & Morgan, 2009). However, as Hart and Morgan (2010) also point out, in one small study of students in an RN to BSN program, cheating was more prevalent in the on-campus classroom and occurred more frequently among younger students in the traditional classroom. Nonetheless, faculty have responsibility for creating a culture of academic integrity and test security. As in the classroom, methods for ensuring test security can be simple and low cost or they may be complicated and involve additional human and fiscal resources (Reising, 2002). Easy-to-manage security in online tests includes having students log in with a user name and password, using timed tests, adding new questions to each test, giving "open book" tests, and using test software features to scramble test answers or generate alternative versions of examinations. Faculty can also design evaluation and grading plans that use a variety of evaluation methods that are not solely dependent on testing. Most faculty ask students to sign academic honesty pledges, and Hart and Morgan (2009) recommend making consequences clear; others find that indicating to the student that it is easy for faculty to track and compare student responses on online examinations is a sufficient deterrent.

More complex measures to prevent or track cheating include tracking Internet Protocol (IP) addresses for the computers on which students are taking a test, hiring proctors to observe students while taking the test, and purchasing browser security products (Hart & Morgan, 2009). Some faculty have used video cameras to monitor students while they are taking an online test. Students use small cameras on their computers that are monitored by faculty or a proctor. In one study (Mizra & Staples, 2010) researchers found that the experience of being observed on the camera was uncomfortable for the students, and that the students themselves believed it would be easy to cheat because the camera did not view the entire testing area. New advances in proctoring technology use analysis of keystroke rhythms along with web cameras.

Finally, faculty can require students to take the test or skills check-off in a proctored classroom on campus or in the clinical agency. Ultimately, and particularly for high-stakes examinations, faculty are responsible for providing examination security and must take reasonable means to create a secure environment for all students.

Effectiveness and Continuous Quality Improvement

The use of online learning in nursing education continues to increase, particularly as doctorate in nursing practice (DNP) and PhD programs seek to make their programs distance accessible. There is a growing body of evidence about the effectiveness of online courses and programs and various pedagogical approaches to designing courses and teaching then online. These findings can be used to guide current practice and improve existing courses.

Effectiveness of Online Courses and Programs

Studies of the effectiveness of online courses reveal that *student achievement* is similar in online courses and in the classroom (Bata-Jones & Avery, 2004; Coose, 2010; Leasure, Davis, & Thievon, 2000; Leners, Wilson, & Sitzman, 2007; Little, 2009; Mancuso-Murphy, 2007; Mills, 2007). In different studies, Coose (2010) and Mills (2007) compared achievement of course goals and found student grades to be comparable in online and on-campus courses. Buckley (2003) reported that there were no differences in learning outcomes between a classroom, a web-enhanced, and a web-based nutrition course for undergraduate nursing students. Pullen (2006) found that online learning, when used for continuing professional development, increased learning and knowledge outcomes and that participants also reported improvement in clinical practice.

In other studies, students report *satisfaction* with online learning (Billings et al., 2001) and favor the online format (Wills & Stommel, 2002). DeBourgh (2003) found that student satisfaction with computer-mediated distance education is most associated with the perceived quality of the instruction and the effectiveness of the instructor. Ali, Hodson-Carlton, and Ryan (2004) found that graduate nursing students were satisfied with the flexibility and convenience of online learning and that timely feedback from faculty was a very important indicator of student satisfaction. Doctoral students in a study conducted by Leners, Wilson, and Sitzman (2007) reported satisfaction with the access to the doctoral program and the ability to enroll in a doctoral program while continuing their employment.

Other researchers examined the *effectiveness of the educational practices* within web courses. For example, Billings et al. (2001) found that the use of active learning strategies and ample opportunity for interaction within the course were correlated with outcomes such as student satisfaction, socialization, and preparation for real-world work. Leners, Wilson, and Sitzman (2007) also found that students believed they were being prepared for professional practice and, because of mentoring in the online course, were becoming socialized. VandeVusee and Hanson (2000) found that faculty could facilitate active learning by carefully structuring the discussion forums that were used to promote outcomes of critical thinking. Billings et al. (2005) found that the educational practices in online courses influenced outcomes, but there were differences between undergraduate and graduate students' perceptions of the educational practices within the course.

Continuous Quality Improvement

As with all course development and teaching, faculty must obtain feedback from students and colleagues about their work and use it to continuously improve course quality (Chao, Saj, & Tessier, 2006). Obtaining course evaluations from students is one important way to determine how the course is working for them and to obtain suggestions for improvement (see Chapter 27 for information about course evaluation).

Peer review of web courses is another way to receive feedback about the course design and the impact on student learning (Cobb, Billings, Mays, & Canty-Mitchell, 2001). Peer review may include informal review of the course and teaching by colleagues and integrating suggestions for improvement. Zsohar and Smith (2008) suggest that peer reviewers have experience and expertise teaching online as well as the necessary content expertise and use preestablished criteria for evaluating the course and instruction. Another review method is to invite colleagues outside nursing but with online teaching experience to review the course. More formal review occurs when peers review courses for promotion, tenure, or teaching awards.

Nurse educators should continue to monitor the effectiveness of the use of technology, the educational practices within the OLC, and the outcomes of the courses and educational programs in which online teaching and learning occur. Using the opportunities of new learning environments will continue to challenge assumptions about teaching and learning and in the long run will result in improvement of pedagogical practices.

SUMMARY

Online learning and the use of online courses has become an accepted educational practice in nursing education. While evidence continues to indicate that online courses are as effective as on-campus courses, the focus of inquiry has shifted to gathering evidence for the best practices for designing full web and blended courses, for using the appropriate mix of classroom and online learning experiences, for using the emerging technologies for maximum effectiveness, and for promoting learning for the students who are enrolled in these courses. Nurse educators are leaders on university and college campuses in implementing online education and will continue to be in the forefront of identifying the best practices for designing, implementing, and evaluating online courses and programs.

REFLECTING ON THE EVIDENCE

1. What is the state of the science about teaching and learning in online learning communities?

2. What are strategies to promote social presence and caring in online courses?

3. What learning activities can be used in an online course to facilitate socialization to the profession, ethical comportment, and development of the affective domain?

4. When designing (or redesigning) a course, which elements are best offered online? In the classroom? Synchronously or asynchronously?

5. What research questions should be posed to advance the science of teaching and learning in the online learning community?

6. What strategies can be used to prevent academic dishonesty in online courses? What are the cost and benefit considerations of these strategies?

REFERENCES

Alexander, B. (2004). Going nomadic: Mobile learning in higher education. *Educause, 39*(5), 29–35.

Ali, N., Hodson-Carlton, K., & Ryan, M. (2004). Students' perception of online learning: Implications for teaching. *Nurse Educator, 29*(3), 111–115.

Ali, N., Hodson-Carlton, K., Ryan, M., Flowers, J., Rose, M. A., & Wayda, V. (2005). Online education: Needs assessment for faculty development. *The Journal of Continuing Education in Nursing, 36*(1), 32–38.

Allen, I. E., & Seaman, J. (2010). *Learning on demand: Online education in the United States, 2009.* Newburyport, MA: Babson Survey Research Group and The Sloan Consortium. Retrieved from http://sloanconsortium.org/publications/survey/pdf/learningondemand.pdf

Anderson, K. & Avery, M. (2008). Faculty teaching time: A comparison of web-based and face-to-face graduate nursing courses. *International Journal of Nursing Education Scholarship, Vol. 5*: Iss. 1, Article 2. Available at: http://www.bepress.com/ijnes/vol5/iss1/art2

Babenko-Mould, Y., Andrusyszyn, M., & Goldenberg, D. (2004). Effects of computer-based clinical conferencing on nursing students' self-efficacy. *Journal of Nursing Education, 43*(4), 149–155.

Baldwin, K., & Burns, P. (2004). Development and implementation of an online CNS program. *Clinical Nurse Specialist, 18*(5), 248–254.

Bata-Jones, B., & Avery, M. (2004). Teaching pharmacology to graduate nursing students: Evaluation and comparison of web-based and face-to-face methods. *Journal of Nursing Education, 43*(4), 185–189.

Beitz, J., & Snarponis, J. (2006). Strategies for online teaching and learning: Lessons learned. *Nurse Educator, 31*(1), 20–25.

Benner, P., Sutphen, M., Leonard, V., & Day, L. (2010). *Educating nurses.* San Francisco, CA: Jossey-Bass.

Billings, D. (2000). A framework for assessing outcomes and practices in web-based courses in nursing. *Journal of Nursing Education, 39*(2), 60–67.

Billings, D. (2002). Internal marketing. In D. Billings (Ed.), *Conversations in e-learning* (pp. 41–44). Pensacola, FL: Pohl.

Billings, D. (2009). Wikis and blogs: Consider the possibilities for continuing nursing education. *Journal of Continuing Education in Nursing, 40*(12), 534–535.

Billings, D., Connors, H., & Skiba, D. (2001). Benchmarking best practices in web-based nursing courses. *Advances in Nursing Science, 23*(3), 41–52.

Billings, D., Jeffries, P., Daniels, D., Rowles, C., Stone, C., & Stephenson, E. (2006). Developing and using online courses to prepare nurses for employment in critical care. *Journal for Nurses in Staff Development, 22*(2), 1–6.

Billings, D., Skiba, D., & Connors, H. (2005). Best practices in web-based courses: Generational differences across undergraduate and graduate nursing students. *Journal of Professional Nursing, 21*(2), 126–133.

Blood-Siegfried, J., Short, N., Rapp, C., Hill, E., Talbert, S., Skinner, J., . . . Goodwin, L. (2008). A rubric for improving the quality of online courses. *International Journal of Nursing Education Scholarship, 5*(1), 1–13.

Bloom, K. C., & Trice, L. B. (1997). The efficacy of individualized computerized testing in nursing education. *Computers in Nursing, 15*(2), 82–88.

Bolan, C. (2003). Incorporating experiential learning theory into the instructional design of online courses. *Nurse Educator, 28*(1), 10–14.

Bonk, C. (2010). *The world is open: How web technology is revolutionizing education.* San Francisco, CA: Jossey-Bass.

Bonk, C., & Graham, C. (2005). *The handbook of blended learning: Global perspectives, local designs.* Indianapolis, IN: Jossey-Bass.

Bonnel, W. (2008). Improving feedback to students in online courses. *Nursing Education Perspectives, 29*(5), 290–294.

Bristol, T. (2010). Twitter: Consider the possibilities for continuing education in nursing. *Journal of Continuing Education in Nursing, 41*(5), 199–200.

Broome, M., Halstead, J., Pesut, D., Rawl, S., & Boland, D. (2011). Evaluating the outcomes of a distance accessible PhD program. *Journal of Professional Nursing, 27*(2), 69–77.

Brownrigg, V. (2005). *Assessment of web-based learning in nursing: The role of social presence.* (Unpublished dissertation). University of Colorado Health Sciences Center, Denver, CO.

Buckley, K. M. (2003). Evaluation of classroom-based, web-enhanced, and web-based distance learning nutrition courses for undergraduate nursing. *Journal of Nursing Education, 42*(8), 367–369.

Burruss, N., Billings, D., Brownrigg, V., Skiba, D., & Connors, H. (2009). Class size as related to the use of technology, educational practices, and outcomes in web-based nursing courses. *Journal of Professional Nursing, 25*(1), 33–41.

Carruth, A. K., Broussard, P. C., Waldmeier, V. P., Gauthier, D. M., & Mixon, G. (2010). Graduate nursing online orientation course: Transitioning for success. *Journal of Nursing Education, 49*(12), 687–690.

Chao, T., Saj, T., & Tessier, F. (2006). Establish a quality review for online courses. *Educause Quarterly, 29*(3), 32–39.

Chickering, A., & Ehrmann, S. (1996). *Implementing the seven principles: Technology as a lever.* Retrieved from http://www.tltgroup.org/programs/seven.html

Chickering A., & Gamson, Z. (1987). *Seven principles of good practice in undergraduate education.* Racine, WI: Johnson Foundation.

Cobb, K., Billings, D., Mays, R., & Canty-Mitchell, J. (2001). Peer review of web-based courses in nursing. *Nurse Educator, 26*(6), 274–279.

Colwell, J., & Jenks, C. (2006). *The upper limit: The issues for faculty in setting class size in online courses.* Retrieved from http://www.ipfw.edu/

Coose, C. S. (2010). Distance nursing education in Alaska: A longitudinal study. *Nursing Education Perspectives, 31*(2), 93–96.

Daroszewski, E. B., Kinser, A., & Lloyd, S. (2004a). Online, directed journaling in community health advanced practice nursing clinical education. *Journal of Nursing Education, 43*(4), 175–180.

Daroszewski, E. B., Kinser, A., & Lloyd, S. (2004b). Socratic method and the Internet: Using tiered discussion to facilitate understanding in a graduate nursing theory course. *Nurse Educator, 29*(5), 189–191.

DeBourgh, G. A. (2001). Using web technology in a clinical nursing course. *Nurse Educator, 26*(5), 227–233.

DeBourgh, G. A. (2003). Predictors of student satisfaction in distance-delivered graduate nursing courses: What matters most? *Journal of Professional Nursing, 19*(3), 149–163.

Dell, D. (2002). Learning management systems. In D. Billings (Ed.), *Conversations in e-learning* (pp. 57–62). Pensacola, FL: Pohl.

Diekelmann, N., & Mendias, E. (2005). Being a supportive presence in online courses: Attending to students' online presence with each other. *Journal of Nursing Education, 44*(9), 393–395.

Edwards, N., Hugo, K., Cragg, B., & Peterson, J. (1999). The integration of problem-based learning strategies in distance education. *Nurse Educator, 24*(1), 36–41.

Halstead, J. A. (2002). How will my role change when I teach on the Web? In D. Billings (Ed.), *Conversations in e-learning* (pp. 105–112). Pensacola, FL: Pohl.

Halstead, J. A., & Coudret, N. A. (2000). Implementing web-based instruction in a school of nursing: Implications for faculty and students. *Journal of Professional Nursing, 16*(5), 273–281.

Hart, L., & Morgan, L. (2009). Strategies for online test security. *Nurse Educator, 34*(6), 249–253.

Hart, L., & Morgan, L. (2010). Academic integrity in an online registered nurse to baccalaureate in nursing program. *The Journal of Continuing Education in Nursing, 41*(11), 498–505.

Hollingsworth, C. (2002a). Layout, fonts, colors, graphics. In D. Billings (Ed.), *Conversations in e-learning* (pp. 141–154). Pensacola, FL: Pohl.

Hollingsworth, C. (2002b). Storyboards and course plans. In D. Billings (Ed.), *Conversations in e-learning* (pp. 137–140). Pensacola, FL: Pohl.

Hunter, J., & Krantz, S. (2010). Constructivism in cultural competence. *Journal of Nursing Education, 49*(4), 207–214.

Institute for Higher Education Policy. (2000). *Quality on the line: Benchmarks for success in Internet-based distance education.* Washington, DC: Author. Retrieved from http://www.ihep.org/assests/files/publications/m-r/QualityOnTheLine.pdf

Jafari, A., McGee, P., & Carmean, C. (2006). Managing courses, defining learning. *Educause, 41*(4), 50–70.

Johnston, J. (2008). Effectiveness of online instruction in the radiologic sciences. *Radiologic Technology, 79*(6), 497–506.

Kirkpatrick, J. (2002). Principles of good practice in e-learning. In D. Billings (Ed.), *Conversations in e-learning* (pp. 171–176). Pensacola, FL: Pohl.

Lahaie, U. (2007a). Strategies for creating social presence online. *Nurse Educator, 32*(3), 100–101.

Lahaie, U. (2007b). Web-based instruction: Getting faculty onboard. *Journal of Professional Nursing, 23*(6), 335–342.

Lashley, M. (2005). Teaching health assessment in the virtual classroom. *Journal of Nursing Education, 44*(8), 348–350.

Leasure, A. R., Davis, L., & Thievon, S. (2000). Comparison of student outcomes and preferences in a traditional vs. World Wide Web–based baccalaureate nursing research course. *Journal of Nursing Education, 39*(4), 149–154.

Leners, D., Wilson, V., & Sitzman, K. (2007). Twenty-first century doctoral education: Online with a focus on nursing education, *Nursing Education Perspectives, 28*(6), 332–336.

Leners, D. W., & Sitzman, K. (2006). Graduate student perceptions: Feeling the passion of caring online. *Nursing Education Perspectives, 27*(6), 315–319.

Little, B. (2009). Quality assurance for online nursing courses. *Journal of Nursing Education, 48*(7), 381–387.

Luke, R., Solomon, P., Baptiste, S., Hall, P., Orchard, C., Ruknolm, E., & Carter, L. (2009). Online interprofessional health sciences education: From theory to practice. *Journal of Continuing Education in the Health Professions, 29*(3), 161–167.

Mancuso-Murphy, J. (2007). Distance education in nursing: An integrated review of online nursing students' experiences with technology-delivered instruction. *Journal of Nursing Education, 46*(6), 252–260.

Mastrian, G., & McGonigle, D. (1999). Using technology-based assignments to promote critical thinking. *Nurse Educator, 24*(1), 45–47.

Mills, A. C. (2007). Evaluation of online and on-site options for master's degree and postmaster's certificate programs. *Nurse Educator, 32*(2), 73–77.

Mills, M., Fisher, C., & Stair, N. (2001). Web-based courses: More than curriculum. *Nursing and Health Care Perspectives, 22*(5), 235–239.

Mizra, N., & Staples, E. (2010). Webcam as a new invigilation methods: Students' comfort and potential for cheating. *Journal of Nursing Education, 49*(2), 116–119.

Moore, J. (2005). *The Sloan quality framework and the five pillars.* Newburyport, MA: The Sloan Consortium. Retrieved from http://sloanconsortium.org/

Nelson, R. (2007). Student support services for distance education students in nursing programs. *Annual Review of Nursing Education,* 183–205.

Nelson, R., Meyers, L., Rizzolo, M. A., Rutar, P., Proto, M., & Newbold, S. (2006). The evolution of educational information systems and nurse faculty roles. *Nursing Education Perspectives, 27*(5), 247–253.

Nesler, M., Hanner, M. B., Melburg, V., & McGowan, S. (2001). Professional socialization of baccalaureate nursing students: Can students in distance nursing programs become socialized? *Journal of Nursing Education, 40*(7), 293–302.

O'Neil, C., Fisher, C., & Newbold, S. (2004). *Developing an online course: Best practices for nurse educators.* New York, NY: Springer.

Palloff, R., & Pratt, K. (1999). *Building learning communities in cyberspace: Effective strategies for the on-line classroom.* San Francisco, CA: Jossey-Bass.

Palloff, R., & Pratt, K. (2003). *The virtual student: A profile and guide to working with online learners.* San Francisco, CA: Jossey-Bass.

Parker, E., & Howland, L. (2006). Strategies to manage the time demands of online teaching. *Nurse Educator, 31*(6), 270–274.

Patillo, R. E. (2007). Decreasing transactional distance in a web-based course. *Nurse Educator, 32*(3), 109–112.

Phillips, J. (2005). Strategies for active learning in online continuing education. *Journal of Continuing Education in Nursing, 36*(2), 77–83.

Pullen, D. (2006). An evaluative case study of online learning for healthcare professionals. *Journal of Continuing Education in Nursing, 37*(5), 225–232.

Reising, D. (2002). Online testing. In D. Billings (Ed.), *Conversations in e-learning* (pp. 213–220). Pensacola, FL: Pohl.

Rhoads, J., & White, C. (2008). Copyright law and distance nursing education. *Nurse Educator, 33*(1), 39–44.

Richard, P., Mercer, Z., & Bray, C. (2005). Transitioning a classroom-based RN-BSN program to the Web. *Nurse Educator, 30*(5), 208–211.

Rossignol, M., & Scollin, P. (2001). Piloting use of computerized practice tests. *Computers in Nursing, 18*(2), 72–86.

Ryan, M., Hodson-Carlton, K., & Ali, N. (2004). Reflections on the role of faculty in distance learning and changing pedagogies. *Nursing Education Perspectives, 25*(2), 73–80.

Ryan, M., Hodson-Carlton, K., & Ali, N. (2005). A model for faculty teaching online: Confirmation of a dimensional matrix. *Journal of Nursing Education, 44*(8), 357–365.

Shovein, J., Huston, C., Fox, S., & Damazo, B. (2005). Challenging traditional teaching and learning paradigms: Online learning and emancipatory teaching. *Nursing Education Perspectives, 26*(6), 340–343.

Sitzman, K. (2010). Student-preferred caring behaviors for online nursing education. *Nursing Education Perspectives, 31*(3), 171–176.

Sitzman, K., & Leners, D. W. (2006). Student perceptions of caring in online baccalaureate education. *Nursing Education Perspectives, 27*(5), 254–259.

Skiba, D. J. (2008). Nursing education 2.0: Twitter & tweets. Can you post a nugget of knowledge in 140 characters or less? *Nursing Education Perspectives, 29*(2), 110–112.

Skiba, D. J. (2010). Nursing education 2.0: Social networking and the WOTY. *Nursing Education Perspectives, 31*(1), 44–46.

Sternberger, C. (2002). Embedding a pedagogical model in the design of an online course. *Nurse Educator, 27*(4), 170–173.

Stewart, S., Pope, D., & Hansen, T. S. (2010). Clinical preceptors enhance an online accelerated bachelor's degree to BSN program. *Nurse Educator, 35*(1), 37–40.

Suen, L. (2005). Teaching epidemiology using WebCT: Application of the seven principles of good practice. *Journal of Nursing Education, 44*(3), 143–146.

VandeVusee, L., & Hanson, L. (2000). Evaluation of online course discussions. *Computers in Nursing, 18*(4), 181–188.

Vinten, S., & Partridge, R. (2002). E-learning and the clinical practicum. In D. Billings (Ed.), *Conversations in e-learning* (pp. 187–196). Pensacola, FL: Pohl.

Wills, C., & Stommel, M. (2002). Graduate nursing students' precourse and postcourse perceptions and preferences concerning completely web-based courses. *Journal of Nursing Education, 41*(5), 193–201.

Wink, D. (2009). Sources of fully developed course materials on the Web. *Nurse Educator, 34*(4), 143–145.

Zsohar, H., & Smith, J. (2008). Transition from the classroom to the Web: Successful strategies for teaching online. *Nursing Education Perspective, 29*(1), 23–28.

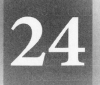

24 The Evaluation Process: An Overview

Mary P. Bourke, PhD, RN, MSN

Barbara A. Ihrke, PhD, RN

Nursing faculty are responsible for evaluating student learning, course, curriculum, and program outcomes as well as their own teaching practices. They are accountable to students, peers, administrators, employers, and society for the effectiveness of the nursing program. The purpose of this chapter is to present an overview of the process by which nursing faculty can evaluate instructional and program outcomes and report results to stakeholders. Terminology is often interchangeable between evaluation of classroom instruction and program evaluation. This chapter is a link to subsequent and previous chapters that cover specific evaluation activities and strategies. The chapter delineates a step-by-step evaluation process including the use of models; selection of instruments; data collection procedures; and the means to interpret, report, and use findings. Results can be used to make decisions about improvement in student learning; faculty performance; and course, curriculum, and program quality.

Definition of Terms

The many terms used to describe evaluation and evaluation activities are often used interchangeably. The following definitions are used throughout this chapter.

Evaluation

Evaluation is a means of appraising data or placing a value on data gathered through one or more measurements. Evaluation also involves rendering judgment by pointing out strengths and weaknesses of different features or dimensions. Evaluation is the "implementation form

for accountability as well as one of the basic ways of assuring quality" (Kai, 2009, p. 44). Rossi, Lipsey, and Freeman (2004) describe evaluation as judging a performance based on selected outcomes and standards. In education, evaluation assesses data collected through various methods to measure the outcome of the teaching–learning process.

Grading

Grading, often confused with evaluation, involves quantifying data and assigning value. Grades serve two purposes. Grades notify students of their achievement as it related to them and others and informs the public of student performance (Shoemaker & DeVos, 1999). Grading represents the achievement of the student as assessed by the faculty or grader.

Assessment

Assessment, in the broadest view, refers to processes that provide information about students, faculty, curricula, programs, and institutions to various stakeholders. More specifically, assessment refers to measures of student abilities and changes in knowledge, skills, and attitudes during and after participation in courses and programs (Angelo & Cross, 1993; Davis, 1993; Gates et al., 2002). Assessment data can be obtained to place students in courses, to provide information about learning needs (see Chapter 2), and to determine achievement in individual courses and programs (see Chapters 16 and 25 to 28). Findings are used to improve student learning and teaching (see Chapter 16) and to improve courses and programs.

Curriculum Evaluation

Curriculum evaluation is the process of determining the outcomes of student learning as a result of participation in a program or plan of learning. Curriculum evaluation involves establishing outcomes and verifying the extent to which these have been achieved (see Chapter 28).

Program Evaluation

Educational program evaluation or program review "can be defined as a systematic operation of varying complexity involving data collection, observations and analyses, and culminating in a value judgement" (Mizikaci, 2006, p. 41). Program reviews are typically conducted by the faculty as a self-study (see Chapter 28) and are undertaken to respond to accreditation reviews by state, education, and professional accrediting bodies (see Chapter 29).

Accreditation

Accreditation is "a voluntary, peer review process that has been a hallmark of quality in American higher education and professional education for decades" (Grumet, 2002, p. 114). This process serves as a mechanism to ensure the quality of educational programs. Accreditation signifies that an institution, school, or program has defined appropriate outcomes, maintains conditions in which they can be met, and is producing acceptable outcomes (Millard, 1994). According to Alstete (2004), accreditation can be viewed as "a positive, active learning exercise" (p. 3). Accreditation occurs following a period of self-study, evaluation, and periodic review and is primarily focused on the mission of the institution and on student outcomes.

Schools of nursing may be accredited by state and regional agencies as well as national nursing organizations. Historically and currently there are two organizations of interest in accrediting nursing education programs: the National League for Nursing Accrediting Commission and the Commission on Collegiate Nursing Education. Effective accreditation programs must be simple, relevant, and cost effective. Regardless of the agency or organization providing accreditation services, nursing faculty must be aware of the standards and participate in the process of their evaluation and review. See Chapter 29 for further information about accreditation of nursing programs.

Philosophical Approaches to Evaluation

A philosophy of evaluation involves the evaluator's beliefs about evaluation. The philosophy will influence how evaluations are conducted, when evaluations are conducted, what methods are used, and how results are interpreted. A philosophy is reflected in attitudes and behavior.

In nursing education, evaluations or judgments are made about performance (students), program effectiveness (a nursing curriculum or program), instructional media (a textbook, a computer-assisted instruction program), or instruction (course, faculty). Evaluation activities in nursing education are conducted from various perspectives, and these perspectives influence outcomes. Therefore evaluators should be aware of the perspective or orientation as they relate it to the evaluation process.

Several philosophical perspectives tend to influence evaluation. Educators who rely on goals, objectives, and outcomes to guide program, course, or lesson development will likely have an objectives approach to evaluation. The merits of the activity or program are largely indicated by the success of students meeting those objectives. A service orientation toward evaluation emphasizes the learning by students and includes self-evaluation, thus assisting educators to make decisions about learners and the teaching–learning process. Although all evaluation involves judgment, the evaluator with a judgment perspective will focus on establishing the worth or merit of the employee, student, product, or program. Others have a research orientation to evaluation and emphasize precision in measurement and statistical analysis to gain a general understanding of why students and programs do or do not succeed. The focus in this perspective is on tools, methods, and designs as they relate to validity and reliability of instruments. Yet another orientation is the constructivist view, which emphasizes the values of the stakeholders and builds consensus about what needs to be changed. Although faculty, in their role as evaluators, use a combination of these perspectives, one is likely dominant, and faculty should be aware of the perspective they bring to the evaluation process because their philosophical orientation toward evaluation will guide the evaluation process and influence outcomes.

The Evaluation Process

Evaluation is a process that involves the following systematic series of actions:

1. Identifying the purpose of the evaluation
2. Identifying a time frame
3. Determining when to evaluate
4. Selecting the evaluator
5. Choosing an evaluation design, framework, or model
6. Selecting an evaluation instrument
7. Collecting data
8. Interpreting data
9. Reporting the findings
10. Using the findings
11. Considering the costs of evaluation

The steps can be modified depending on the purpose of the evaluation, what is being evaluated (e.g., students, instruction, program, or system), and the complexity of the units being evaluated.

Identifying the Purpose of the Evaluation

As in the research process, the first step in the evaluation process is to pose various questions that can be answered by evaluation. These questions may be broad and encompassing, as in program evaluation, or focused and specific, as in classroom assessment (Box 24-1). Regardless of the scope of the evaluation, the purpose or reason for conducting an evaluation should be clear to all involved.

BOX 24-1 Purposes of Evaluation

- To facilitate learning—or change behavior of an employee or student
- To diagnose problems—to find learning deficits, ineffective teaching practices, curriculum defects, and so on
- To make decisions—to assign grades, to determine merit raises, to offer promotion or tenure
- To improve products—to revise a textbook, to add content to an independent study module
- To judge effectiveness—to determine whether goals or standards are being met
- To judge cost effectiveness—to determine whether a program is self-supporting

---

Identifying a Time Frame

The next step in the evaluation process is to consider when evaluation should occur. Time frames for evaluation can be described as formative or summative.

Formative Evaluation

Formative evaluation (or assessment) refers to evaluation taking place during the program or learning activity (Kapborg & Fischbein, 2002). Formative evaluation is conducted while the event to be evaluated is occurring and focuses on identifying progress toward purposes, objectives, or outcomes to improve the activities, course, curriculum, program, or teaching and student learning. Formative evaluation emphasizes the parts instead of the entirety. The aim of formative evaluation "is to monitor learning progress and to provide corrective prescriptions to improve learning" (Gronlund & Waugh, 2009, p. 8).

One advantage of formative evaluation is that the events are recent, thus guarding accuracy and preventing distortion by time. Another major advantage of formative evaluation is that the results can be used to improve student performance, program of instruction, or learning outcome before the program or course has concluded (Gronlund & Waugh, 2009; Sims, 1992). Disadvantages of formative evaluation include making judgments before the activity (classroom or clinical performance, nursing program) is completed and not being able to see the results before judgments are made. Formative evaluation can also be intrusive or interrupt the flow of outcomes. There is also a chance for a false sense of security when formative evaluation is positive and the results are not as positive as predicted earlier. There are many techniques available for formative evaluation of the classroom and program. For example, in the classroom student learning can be measured at a "point in time" using the one-minute paper method. Students are asked to write about the most important points discussed in class and what concepts need further clarification. This technique provides valuable insight into the teaching–learning process. The instructor has an opportunity to clarify information during the next class. For formative evaluation of a program, many schools of nursing use national standardized testing systems such as ATI (Assessment Technologies Institute). Each semester students take a test that identifies the student's competencies and their placement nationally. This helps to determine student progression through key concepts within the curriculum. Weaknesses within the curriculum can be identified using content-specific testing as the cohorts progress through the nursing program. Thus formative evaluation provides critical data for ongoing changes necessary to improve student outcomes.

Summative Evaluation

Summative evaluation (or assessment), on the other hand, refers to data collected at the end of the activity, instruction, course, or program (Grondlund & Waugh, 2009; Kapborg & Fischbein, 2002, Story et al., 2010). The focus is on the whole event and emphasizes what is or was and the extent to which objectives and outcomes were met for the purposes of accountability, resource allocation, assignment of grades (students) or merit pay or promotion (faculty), and certification (Davis, 1994). Summative evaluation therefore is most useful at the end of a learning module or course and for program or course revision. Summative evaluation of learning outcomes in a course usually results in assignment of a final grade.

The advantages of performing an evaluation at the end of the activity are that all work has been completed and the findings of the evaluation show results. The major disadvantage of summative evaluation is that nothing can be done to alter the results.

Determining When to Evaluate

The evaluator must also weigh each evaluation event and determine when evaluation is most appropriate. Typically both formative and summative evaluations are appropriate and lend respective strengths to the evaluation plan.

In determining when to evaluate, the evaluator must also consider the frequency of evaluation. Evaluation can be time consuming, but frequent evaluation is necessary in many situations. Frequent evaluations are important when the learning process is complex and unfamiliar and when it is considered helpful to anticipate potential problems if the risk of failure is high. Finally, important decisions require frequent evaluations (Box 24-2).

> **BOX 24-2** Situations in Which Frequent Evaluation Is Useful
>
> - Learning is complex
> - Trends are emerging
> - Problems have been identified
> - Problems are anticipated
> - There is a high risk of failure
> - Serious consequences would result from poor performance
> - Immediately after major changes in curriculum or requirements of a program

---

Selecting the Evaluator

An important element in the evaluation process is the evaluator. Selection of an evaluator involves deciding who should be involved in the evaluation process and whether the evaluator should be chosen from the "inside" (internal evaluator) or from the "outside" (external evaluator). Both have merits.

Internal Evaluators

Internal evaluators are those directly involved with the learning, course, or program to be evaluated, such as the students, faculty, or nursing staff. Many individuals (stakeholders) have a vested interest in the evaluation process and could be selected to participate. There are advantages and disadvantages associated with internal evaluators, and often several evaluators are helpful to obtain the most accurate data.

Advantages of using internal evaluators include their familiarity with the context of the evaluation, experience with the standards, cost effectiveness, and potential for less obtrusive evaluation. Additionally, the findings of evaluation can be acted on quickly because the results are known immediately. *Disadvantages* of using internal evaluators include bias, control of evaluation, and reluctance to share controversial findings. When internal evaluators are chosen and employed, it is important to note their position in the organization and responsibility and reporting lines.

External Evaluators

External evaluators are those not directly involved in the events being evaluated. They are often employed as consultants. State, regional, and national accrediting bodies are other examples of external evaluators. The *advantage* of using external evaluators is that they do not have a bias, are not involved in organizational politics, may be very experienced in a particular type of evaluation, and do not have a stake in the results. *Disadvantages* of using external evaluators include expense, unfamiliarity with the context, barriers of time, and potential travel constraints. Because evaluators are so critical to the evaluation process, faculty should select evaluators carefully. Box 24-3 lists questions to ask when selecting an evaluator.

Choosing an Evaluation Design, Framework, or Model

This step of the evaluation process involves selecting or developing an evaluation model. An evaluation model represents the ways the variables, items, or events to be evaluated are arranged, observed, or manipulated to answer the evaluation question. A model serves to clarify the relationship of the variables to be evaluated and provides a systematic plan or framework for the evaluation.

Evaluation models for nursing education may be found in the nursing literature or may be developed by nurse educators for a specific use. Although evaluation models have been adapted from those used in education (Guba & Lincoln, 1989; Madaus, Scriven, & Stufflebeam, 1988; Scriven, 1972; Stake, 1967) and business, nursing education evaluation models reflect closely the aspects of nursing education and practice that are being evaluated (Billings, Connors, & Skiba, 2001; Germain, Deatrick, Hagopian, & Whitney, 1994; Kapborg & Fischbein, 2002).

BOX 24-3 **Questions to Ask When Selecting an Evaluator**

1. What is the evaluator's philosophical orientation?
2. What is the evaluator's experience?
3. What methods or instruments does the evaluator use? Have experience with?
4. What is the evaluator's style?
5. Is the evaluator responsive to the client?
6. Does the evaluator work well with others?
7. Is the evaluator supportive versus critical?
8. What is the evaluator's orientation to evaluation?

Using an evaluation model has several advantages. A model makes variables explicit and often reflects a priority about which variables should be evaluated first or most often. A model also gives structure that is visible to all concerned; the relationships of parts are evident. Using an evaluation model helps focus evaluation. It keeps the evaluation efforts on target: those elements that are to be evaluated are included; those not to be evaluated are excluded. Finally, a model can be tested and validated.

A model should be selected according to the demands of the evaluation question, the context, and the needs of the stakeholders. Several models are used in nursing evaluation activities; they are described briefly here. For detailed information and an example of the use of one model, see Chapter 28.

Theory-Driven Model

Chen supports the use of a theory-driven model during evaluation and provides "information on not only the performance or merit of a program but on how and why the program achieves such a result" (Chen, 2004, p. 415). According to Rosas (2005), "a critical requirement of theory-driven evaluation is the development and articulation of a clear theory" (p. 390). Thus the evaluation process flows from a theory-based evaluation of program curriculums or instructional methods. The theory will direct the evaluation process from identifying variables to be measured to the final report (Stufflebeam, 2001). Various theories or models provide the structure for the evaluation processes. Theories can be grounded in the social sciences, in nursing, or in business.

Using Logic Models

McLaughlin and Jordan (as cited in Wholey, Hatry, & Newcomer, 2004) recommend that, before an evaluation is conducted, it is helpful to use a "logic model" approach as an advance organizer. The logic model is a tool that is useful for conceptualizing, planning, and communicating with others about their program. McLaughlin and Jordan further describe one of the first steps in the model as the development of a flowchart that clarifies and summarizes key elements of a program such as resources and other program inputs, program activities, and the intermediate outcomes as well as the end outcomes that the program strives to achieve. It is also capable of showing assumed cause-and-effect linkages among elements in the model. Sanders and Sullins (2006) explain that in order to clarify a program, the logic model describes inputs (resources—fiscal and human—needed to run the program as well as equipment, books, materials), activities (what you are doing), outputs (student demographics, contact hours, assignments, tests), initial outcomes (change in students from activities), intermediate outcomes (longer-term student outcomes), and finally ultimate outcomes (vision for students who have completed the program). This model is extremely helpful when designing a program evaluation.

Decision-Oriented Models: CIPP

The concepts of the CIPP model (context, input, process, and product) facilitate delineating, obtaining, and providing useful information for judging decision alternatives (Stufflebeam, 1971; Stufflebeam & Webster, 1994). *Context* evaluation identifies the target population and assesses its needs. For example, the target population of first-year college students is identified and, with surveys, interviews, and focus groups, their needs are assessed. *Input* evaluation identifies and assesses system capabilities, alternative program strategies, and procedural designs for implementing the strategies. In this case, a college would identify and assess its ability or capacity to start a weekend college program. A plan of action would be designed to implement the new program. *Process* evaluation detects defects in the design or implementation of the procedure. *Product* evaluation is a collection of descriptions and analyses of outcomes and correlates them to the objectives, context, input, and process information, resulting in the interpretation of results.

The CIPP model measures the weaknesses and strengths of a program, identifies the needs of the target population, identifies options, and provides evidence of beneficial results or lack thereof. In this model, evaluation is performed in the service of decision making; for this reason it should provide information useful to decision makers. Evaluation is also a cyclic, continuing process and therefore must be implemented through a systematic program.

Singh (2004) stated that there were "4 key factors in successfully conducting a program evaluation that is based on the CIPP model" (p. 2). The key factors are (1) "create an evaluation matrix," (2) establish a group to direct the evaluation, (3) "determine who will conduct the evaluation," and (4) make certain that the evaluators "understand and adhere to the program evaluation standards of utility, feasibility, propriety, and accuracy" (p. 2). The article included several useful tables of questions, data sources, and collection methodologies, thus providing clarity and a systematic design for the use of CIPP for evaluation of nursing programs.

Client-Centered (or Responsive Evaluation) Models

Stake's (1967) countenance model focuses on the goals and observed effects of the program being evaluated in terms of antecedents, transactions, and outcomes (Stufflebeam & Webster, 1994). *Antecedents* are conditions that exist that may affect the outcome; for example, students with prior college experience will affect the outcome of freshmen scores. *Transactions* are all educational experiences and interactions, and *outcomes* are the abilities, achievements, attitudes, and aspirations of students that result from the educational experience. The purpose of this model is to promote an understanding of activities in a given setting. Case studies and responsive evaluations (Stake, 1967) elicit information about the program from those involved in this action-research approach to educational evaluation. In this model, evaluators "interact continuously with, and respond to, the evaluative needs of the various clients, as well as other stakeholders" (Stufflebeam, 2001, p. 63).

The Cybernetic Model by Veney and Kaluzny (1991; as cited in Jones & Beck, 1996) is a problem-oriented model focused on immediate feedback within a system. The three phases include:

- *Phase one: Needs assessment.* What are the desired outputs or goals for the program? What is the nature of any problems and what are the expected outcomes for resolution? Determine program strategies and specify goal criteria.
- *Phase two: Implementation.* Is the program progressing as expected?
- *Phase three: Results assessment.* Were the program objectives met? Are program outputs sufficient to justify costs? What is the long-term impact on improvement in health and quality of life?

Feedback results are used to make changes to the inputs, outputs, processes, or desired goals.

Assessment Models

Assessment models focus on the outcomes of general and professional education. Assessment models tend to be locally developed and locally implemented, and the results are used by the participants for course, curriculum, and program improvement. Assessment begins with educational values; works best when the program has clear purposes; and makes a difference when it illuminates questions of concern to the stakeholders, is ongoing, and meets responsibilities to students and the public (American Association of Higher Education Assessment Forum, 1994).

Naturalistic, Constructivist, or Fourth-Generation Evaluation Models

Fourth-generation evaluation is a "sociopolitical process that is simultaneously diagnostic, change-oriented, and educative for all the parties involved" (Lincoln & Guba, 1985, p. 141). Fourth-generation evaluation takes into account the values, concerns, and issues of the stakeholders involved in the evaluation (students, faculty, clients, and administrators). The result is a construction of and consensus about needed improvements and changes (Clendon, 2003). Both the evaluator and the stakeholders are responsible for change.

Fourth-generation evaluation incorporates techniques of evaluator observation, interviews, and participant evaluations to elicit views, meanings, and understanding of the stakeholders. As a result, the evaluation becomes not the opinion or judgment of the evaluator but the working toward meaning, understanding, and consensus of all involved in the process. This responsive evaluation informs and empowers the stakeholders for reflection and change. Haleem et al. (2010) determined that a constructivist evaluation approach improved their NCLEX-RN pass rate by 40%. They created a working retreat that involved all faculty in the evaluation process. The goal was to evaluate their entire nursing program and then work on evidence-based solutions to identified problems and thus improve program outcomes. As a group, they evaluated courses, objectives, instruction, curriculum, NCLEX scores, credit loads, courses, sequencing of content, overlap in content, et cetera. The entire process led to an informed, involved faculty. As a result, faculty were stakeholders in the evaluation process and thus collaborators in change. Lessons learned were expressed as "take the time to evaluate the program in a meaningful way, work as a team, and listen to other faculty and the students. These lessons made the difference in promoting student success" (p. 121).

Specific changes that resulted in improved scores involved a multifaceted approach. Changes instituted by Haleem et al. (2010) to improve student learning included the following:

1. Ninety percent of the course grade for each clinical course was based on objective testing.
2. Implementing application and analysis-level test items only for nursing exams.
3. Each clinical course was assigned homework to include case studies.
4. All students are required to complete 700 NCLEX-RN practice questions.
5. A workshop was developed that focused on a "good thinking" approach to questions.
6. Comprehensive standardized examinations to be used in each clinical course and at the end of the program. The results are computed as 10% of the student's grade.
7. Students are required to take an NCLEX-RN review course prior to the NCLEX-RN exam.
8. A new course entitled Boot Camp was developed: a 10-week course meeting 16 hours per week and focusing on content reviews, testing, and remediation. A minimum of 3000 review questions are required for each student.
9. Students are allowed to repeat only one nursing course. If a student receives a C in two nursing or cognate courses, he or she is dismissed from the program.

Quality Assurance Models: Total Quality Management and Continuous Quality Improvement

Adapted from business and nursing services, quality assurance models can be used to guide evaluation and improve educational programs and nursing programs. Total quality management (TQM) and continuous quality improvement (CQI) are structured approaches that examine organizational processes as a way of understanding their contributions to outcomes. Organization-wide participation is focused on meeting the customer's needs and continuously improving the processes that contribute to an effective organization and organizational outcomes (Clark & Rice, 1994). The process involves all stakeholders and uses team knowledge to improve decision making. Benchmarking is used in the "pursuit of continuous quality improvement" (Murphy, 1995, p. 45). Benchmarking "involves determining optimal performance in any specific area and detailing how that level of performance can best be achieved" (Chambliss, 2003, p. 3). The faculty develop benchmarks for levels of student achievement and measure outcomes based on the benchmarks.

Accreditation Model: Evidence-Based Evaluation

Accreditation in higher education is the result of an educational review process. Colleges and universities are accredited by one of 19 recognized institutional accrediting organizations. Programs are accredited by one of approximately 60 recognized programmatic accrediting organizations. Accrediting organizations that are "recognized" have been reviewed for quality by the Council for Higher Education Accreditation or the United States Department of Education (Council for Higher Education Accreditation, 2006).

Nursing programs are accredited by two main organizations: Commission on Collegiate Nursing Education (CCNE) and National League for Nursing Accrediting Commission (NLNAC). Nursing program accreditation is based on evidence collected during an extensive self-evaluation. One of CCNE's principles is to "Focus on stimulating and supporting continuous quality improvement in nursing education programs and their outcomes" (CCNE Accreditation: A Value-Based Initiative, www.aacn.nche.edu). One benefit of accreditation according to NLNAC is that it "fosters on-going, self-examination, re-evaluation, and focus on the future" (Benefits of Accreditation, www.nlnac.org).

Successful accreditation indicates that a nursing program has clear and appropriate educational objectives and is working to achieve these objectives; consequently, the accreditation model could be considered an evidence-based evaluation model.

Benchmarking

Benchmarking has been widely used in the business arena, including health care, but has been used less often in educational settings. Benchmarking refers to the measurement and comparison of selected criteria with previously recognized ideal criteria. Licensing examination pass rates of nursing programs are compared, hence permitting evaluation of a program according to national standards. The number of students passing the licensing examination is an indication that an overall program has been successful in the teaching–learning process. Benchmarking or "best practices" is "a process improvement technique that provides factual data that allows institutions to compare performance on specific variables in order to achieve best-of-performance" (Billings et al., 2001, p. 42). Palomba and Banta (1999) define benchmarking as "the process of identifying and learning from institutions that are recognized for their outstanding practices" (p. 333). Gates et al. (2002) refer to benchmarking as the "comparison to leading-edge peers" (p. 98), thus relying "on the comparison of performance with that of external peers" (p. 143). Others have interchanged goals and objectives with the term *benchmarks* (Lignugaris-Kraft, Marchand-Martella, & Martella, 2001).

Welsh and Metcalf (2003) refer to performance benchmarking as a method of evaluating institutional effectiveness. Although most definitions indicate evaluation at an institutional level, benchmarking can also be used at the divisional or college level. Nursing programs evaluate themselves in comparison with nursing programs that are recognized for outstanding practices. Individual courses are judged against courses developed by "leading-edge peers" who are specialists in content and teaching–learning practices. Although few researchers have used benchmarking as an approach to assessment of the teaching–learning process (Parry & Dunn, 2000), it is a valid assessment model.

Billings et al. (2001) measured performance indicators in web-based nursing courses, and the mean of each indicator was "reported as the benchmark" (p. 46). According to Billings et al. (2001), one begins the process of assessment by defining the benchmarks to be used. Consequently, benchmarks depend on the evaluation purpose and can be defined for institutions, programs within institutions, or individual student performance.

Models for Evaluating Online Learning Environments

With increasing use of online courses and programs, educators must also use models for evaluating the unique aspects of these learning environments. Many online courses are compared with their classroom counterparts, and claims of increased critical thinking, comprehension, and academic success are made. However, when one examines the research closely, the evaluations are often incomplete or inadequate. Without a model or framework to be used as a guide for the school, faculty, or administration, a one-dimensional evaluation may result.

Evaluation models for online learning must account for the use of the technology, student support, faculty development, and effective use of principles of teaching and learning, as well as program outcomes. Formative evaluation is particularly important in the initiation of online courses and programs and typically includes usability testing and peer review of the courses (see Chapter 23).

Commercial Testing Systems Used in Program Evaluation

As a form of program evaluation, many schools of nursing are turning to commercial testing systems. These products provide a means for formative evaluation as well as end-of-program testing and remediation. Tests are given at the end of courses to measure student retention of content against their classmates and the wider cohort of peers in other nursing programs. The use of commercial testing programs has also been spurred by the schools of nursing's perceived risk of not producing the NCLEX-RN test results required by state boards of nursing and accreditation bodies. Here, the end-of-program comprehensive exam evaluates students' readiness to take the licensing exam, provides information about those students who may need additional preparation, and in some instances has been used to determine progression and graduation.

Although helpful in identifying a particular student's strengths, weaknesses, and type of remediation needed, the commercially available tests have limited value in predicting success on licensing exams, particularly for low-achieving students (Spurlock, 2006). Spurlock and Hunt (2008), Yvonne (2006), and Spurlock (2006) examined the use of the HESI test as a means to determine progression to graduation and found that there is little empirical evidence that a required exit examination competency can improve NCLEX-RN pass rates. They caution schools of nursing not to use a single test score to determine progression and graduation. Further, the National League for Nursing (2010) recommends that commercial tests used for progression and graduation be reviewed for validity, reliability, and cultural bias. Furthermore, they recommend that schools of nursing use a variety of tests and data points to make decisions about students' attainment of learning outcomes.

Selecting an Evaluation Instrument

After a model has been selected, and the variables to be evaluated and their relationship to each other have been identified, the evaluator then selects evaluation instruments that can be used most easily to obtain the necessary data. The selection of evaluation instruments is determined by the evaluation question and the evaluation model. Many instruments are available for measurement and can be found by doing a literature review. To use a published instrument you must contact the publisher and obtain permission. If one that is appropriate for your needs is not available, then an instrument can be developed using Construct Modeling. Wilson (2005) describes Construct Modeling as a framework used to understand how an instrument is constructed and how it works. There are four building blocks used in the instrument development process.

1) The Construct Map: A precise concept, a one-dimensional latent variable. It distinguishes the dimensions within the construct we are trying to measure.
2) The Item Designs: The theoretical concept must be manifested in a form that can be used for measurement. Items are written for the instrument that are guided by the construct map.
3) The Outcome Space: Refers to the response categories for each item. For example, the Likert-type scale has the following levels: strongly disagree, disagree, neutral, agree, and strongly agree. This functions as ordered levels for the respondent to use as a guide for responses.
4) The Measurement Model: This is a statistical model that will help the instrument developer to understand and evaluate the scores that come from the item responses and hence tell us about the construct, and it must also guide the use of the results in practical applications. (Wilson, 2005, p. 17)

Types of Instruments

Many evaluation instruments can be used or adapted to elicit information about nursing education activities. Commonly used instruments are discussed briefly here. Actual examples of evaluation instruments are provided in related chapters.

Questionnaire

A *questionnaire* is a method in which a person answers questions in writing on a form. The questionnaire is usually self-administered. The person reads the question and then responds as instructed. Questionnaires are cost effective but often lack substance. Questions must be clear, concise, and simple (Polit & Beck, 2006). This type of instrument is often used to measure qualitative variables, such as feelings and attitudes. Questionnaires could be used to measure a student's level of confidence in the clinical setting or to determine students' satisfaction with the nursing program after graduation.

Interview

An *interview* involves direct contact with individuals participating in the evaluation. Exit interviews, for example, are often conducted as a faculty member leaves the school of nursing or as students graduate. Interviews can be used to elicit both qualitative and quantitative data. Interviews can be conducted with an individual or in focus groups. Students or external evaluators may be assigned to collect the data. The interview should be scheduled at a time that is convenient for both the interviewer and the participant.

The interviewer should provide a quiet private room or office to allow the participant to speak in privacy. A participant may open up more if he or she feels that the conversation will be private and confidential. An objective outline should be created and followed during the interview, and notes should be kept in a file. Great care must be taken to avoid personalizing the information. One negative aspect of interviews is that they are time intensive (Polit & Beck, 2006). Sanders and Sullins (2006) define the guidelines for interviews as follows:

Keep the language pitched to the level of the respondent.
Clearly explain the purpose of the interview, who has access to the recordings or transcripts, and how it will be kept confidential.
Encourage honesty, but let people know they can refuse to answer a question if they choose.
Establish rapport by asking easy, impersonal questions first.
Avoid long questions.

Avoid ambiguous wording.
Avoid leading questions.
Limit questions to a single idea.
Do not assume too much knowledge. (p. 31)

Observation

Observation is the direct visualization of performance of a task or behavior. Observation or performance appraisal is useful for evaluation of clinical performance, skill competence, and development of attitudes and values. Observation allows for immediate feedback and opportunity for remediation. Difficulties often arise in scheduling observation; when there are no objective criteria for observation, observations are biased opinions that skew results. The student, knowing he or she is being observed, will often inadvertently distort accuracy of data collected because of anxiety. In addition, distortion of one problem observed can affect results of future observed outcomes. To avoid obtaining inaccurate results, the observer must have an objective tool that can be used to collect information accurately and without bias.

If the student is aware of objective criteria before evaluation, he or she has a clear understanding of expected behavior. Prior preparation will decrease anxiety among students, enabling a fair assessment. Faculty may provide a list of skills to be observed and the criteria for competence to the student. The student has a responsibility to prepare for the observation according to the criteria specified. This will give the student a sense of control over his or her educational experience and evaluation, hence decreasing anxiety.

Rating Scale

A *rating scale* is used to measure an abstract concept on a descriptive continuum. The rating scale is designed to increase objectivity in the evaluation process. Rating scales work well with norm-referenced evaluation, although they are not the best tools to use for this type of evaluation. Grades can easily be assigned to the ratings.

Checklist

A *checklist* is two-dimensional in that the expected behavior or competence is listed on one side and the degree to which this behavior meets the level of expectation is listed on the other side. With a detailed checklist of items and well-defined criteria being measured, the evaluator can easily identify expected behavior or acceptable competence. This type of instrument is useful for formative and summative evaluations. A checklist can be used to evaluate a student's performance of clinical procedures. The steps to be followed can be placed in sequential order and the observer can then check off each action that is taken or not taken.

Attitude Scale

An *attitude scale* measures how the participant (usually a student) feels about a subject at the moment when he or she answers the question. Several popular types of attitude scales are used in nursing education evaluation.

The most popular is the Likert scale. In a Likert scale, several items in the form of statements (10 to 15 recommended) are used to express an opinion on a particular issue. Each item represents a construct of that issue; for example, a particular item may express an opinion about Latino students in nursing when the theme of the survey is diversity. Participants are asked to indicate the degree to which they agree or disagree. Equal numbers of positively and negatively worded items should be used to prevent bias in the responses.

Semantic differential is another scale used to measure attitude. Bipolar scales are used to measure the reaction of the participant. Each item on the scale is followed by bipolar adjectives such as good–bad, active–passive, or positive–negative. The number of intervals between each adjective is usually odd so that the middle interval is neutral. A list of five to seven intervals is adequate. Analysis is performed by adding values for each item, which is similar to what is done with the Likert scale (Polit & Beck, 2006).

For analysis of Likert scale data and semantic differential scale data, it is recommended to refrain from treating the data as interval data and to use the Rasch model for analysis. By applying the Rasch model, a more appropriate analysis of the tool and data are accomplished. Typically, Likert data are treated as interval data, although the individual responses are scaled as ordinal. Interval data are assumed. As Bond and Fox (2001) illustrate:

> Five endorsements of the coding of a Likert type scale by a respondent (SD D N A SA) results in a satisfaction score of 25, five times the amount of satisfaction indicated by the respondent who endorses the five SD categories ($5 \times 1 = 5$), or

almost exactly twice the satisfaction of someone who endorses two N's and three SD's ($2 \times 3 \times 2 = 12$). Whenever scores are added in this manner, the ratio, or at least the interval nature of the data, is being presumed. That is, the relative value of each response category across all items is treated as being the same, and the unit increases across the rating scale are given equal value . . . the data are subsequently analyzed in a rigidly prescriptive and inappropriate statistical way. (p. 67)

The Rasch model treats Likert scale data mathematically more justifiably than the ordered sequence of 1 to 5 "then add them up" approach. Rasch recognizes coding as ordered categories only, in which values of each category are higher than for the previous category but by an unspecified amount. Likert-type scale data need to be regarded as ordinal data, whereas the Rasch model transforms the counts of items into interval scales based on empirical evidence as opposed to an assumption. The empirical evidence is calculated using log transformations of raw data odds and abstraction is accomplished through probabilistic equations.

The Rasch model is "the only model that provides the necessary objectivity for the construction of a scale that is separable from the distribution of the attribute in the persons it measures" (Bond & Fox, 2001, p. 7). The conceptual understanding of the Rasch model is best described as a model created within item response theory. *Item response theory*, as explained by Rudner (2001), uses test scores and specific test item scores based on assumptions concerning the mathematical relationship between abilities or attitudes and item responses. The Rasch model has the ability, through several diagnostic procedures, to diagnose the tool's ability to measure accurately the author's and respondent's intentions. The design of a rating scale has a tremendous influence on the quality of responses provided by the respondents. Diagnostic ability provides a powerful tool for designing, analyzing, and revising attitude scales.

Self-Report, Journal, or Diary

A *self-report*, *journal*, or *diary* is a student's written narrative of his or her critical reflections, thoughts, fears, goals progress, improvements needed, and tasks completed. These reports can involve a one-time assignment or a continuous record over a semester of clinical experience or even a curriculum. A spiral notebook is a useful tool for keeping a progressive record together. The notebook can be evaluated on a daily, weekly, or semester basis. The more frequent the evaluation, the more effective this tool will be in the evaluation process.

The diary or journal is valuable in a long-term analysis of the student's progress. The value of this tool is directly correlated with the planning and construction of its intended purpose and how it is used. Diaries or journals require student compliance and may involve considerable time to grade.

Anecdotal Notes

Anecdotal notes are the instructor's notations or comments on student performance or behavior during clinical experience. The value of these notes will be directly related to the objectives to be measured. Planning and identification of what is to be noted will prevent negative bias or lack of constructive value. Anecdotal notes are a valuable tool when accumulated and then used for a summative evaluation of the student's performance. This continual assessment allows the student to be judged fairly, especially in cases in which the student may have performed unsatisfactorily during one clinical learning experience; as a consequence, continual assessment prevents the possibility that one event will cloud the entire clinical experience.

Selection and Development of Evaluation Instruments

The evaluator should give careful consideration to selection (or development) of an evaluation instrument. Several guidelines can be used for selecting evaluation instruments. The instrument should have the following characteristics:
1. Appropriate for what is being evaluated
2. Appropriate for the domain being evaluated
3. Comprehensive: inclusive of all variables in the evaluation model
4. Easy to use: understandable to the evaluator and user
5. Cost effective
6. Time efficient
7. Valid and reliable

When evaluation tools or instruments are not available, faculty can develop their own. However, the cost of development can be significant in terms of time. Schools of nursing tend to have instruments developed that can be used as a starting point for evaluation activities.

Although there are many advantages to use of existing instruments, Polit and Beck (2006) point out that the potential for serious problems must be understood before any instrument is used. First, the selection of an inappropriate or technically inadequate instrument will lead to inadequate measurement of desired data. The instrument must meet minimum standards of validity, reliability, and interpretability. Second, the instrument or tool must be valid. Third, faculty must consider that the use of some existing instruments, such as examinations, increases the chance of material not being taught or learned according to the objectives but according to material being tested or observed. An evaluation of the instrument, with these criteria, will increase success in measuring accurately what is intended to be evaluated.

Reliability and Validity of Evaluation Instruments Used in Nursing Education

When any instrument is used, its validity and reliability for evaluation should be ensured. Special procedures can be used to determine reliability and validity of instruments used for clinical evaluation, program evaluation, and examinations given to measure classroom achievement. Specific procedures are discussed in appropriate chapters of this book. A general overview of the concepts of validity and reliability are provided here.

Validity

Measurement validity verifies that faculty are in fact collecting and analyzing results they intend to measure. Measurement validity, particularly in the area of educational assessment and evaluation, has attributes of relevance, accuracy, and utility (Prus & Johnson, 1994; Wholey et al., 2004). *Relevance* of an instrument is achieved when the instrument measures the educational objective as directly as possible. The instrument is *accurate* if it is measuring the educational objective precisely. The instrument has *utility* if it provides formative and summative results that have implications for evaluation and improvement. As a result, valid evaluation instruments have relevance for the local program or curriculum and can provide meaningful results that indicate directions for change (Prus & Johnson, 1994).

Although there are several types of validity, measurement validity is now viewed as a single concept (Goodwin, 1997; Wholey et al., 2004). Content-related evidence, criterion-related evidence, and construct-related evidence are considered categories of validity. For interpretation, evidence from all categories is ideal. The validity of an instrument can best be determined when faculty understand the nature of the content and specifications in the evaluation design, the relationship of the instrument to the significant criterion, and the constructs or psychological characteristics being measured by the instrument (Gronlund, 1993).

Content-related evidence refers to the extent to which the instrument is representative of the larger domain of the behavior being measured. Content-related evidence is particularly important to establish for clinical evaluation instruments and classroom tests. For example, with classroom tests, the following question is raised: "Does the sample of test questions represent all content described in the course?" In clinical evaluation, the question posed is: "Does the instrument measure attitudes, behaviors, and skills representative of the domain of being a nurse?"

Criterion-related evidence refers to the relationship of a score on one measure (test, clinical performance appraisal) to other external measures. There are two ways to establish criterion-related evidence: concurrent and predictive. *Concurrent evidence* is the correlation of one score with another measure that occurs at the same time. The most common example of concurrent validity is correlation of clinical course grades with didactic course grades. Concurrent validity of the instrument is said to occur, for example, when there is a high correlation between clinical evaluation and examination scores in a class of students. *Predictive study*, on the other hand, is a correlation with measures obtained after completion of an event or intervention, such as a course or lesson. For example, there may be predictive validity between course grades and licensing examination or certification examination scores.

Criterion-related evidence is used to relate the outcomes of one instrument to the outcomes of another. In this sense, it is used to predict success or establish the predictability of one measure with another one. Criterion-related evidence is established by using correlation measures. One example is the correlation between grade point average and scores on licensing or credentialing examinations. When there is a high positive correlation between the grade point average and the examination score, there is said to be criterion-related evidence.

Construct-related evidence is a relationship of one measure (e.g., examination) to other learner variables such as learning style, IQ, clinical competence, or job experience. Construct-related evidence is used to infer the relationship of a test instrument and student traits or qualities to identify what factors might be influencing performance. Examples include the relationship of IQ scores, Scholastic Aptitude Test (SAT) scores, and other test scores or working for pay as a student nurse and clinical performance.

Reliability

Reliability is the extent to which an instrument (self-report examination, observation schedule, or checklist) is dependable, precise, predictable, and consistent. Pedhazur and Schmelkin (1991) refer to reliability as the degree to which test scores are free from errors of measurement. Reliability answers the question: "Will the same instrument yield the same results with different groups of students or when used by different raters?" According to Newby (1992), "Reliability in testing refers to the idea that tests should be consistent in the way that they measure performance" (p. 253).

Several types of reliability—stability reliability, equivalence reliability, and internal consistency reliability—are relevant to evaluation instruments and achievement examinations. *Stability reliability* of an instrument is the perceived consistency of the instrument over time. An assumption of stability in results is assumed. *Equivalence reliability* entails the degree to which two different forms of an instrument can be used to obtain the same results. For example, when two forms of a test are used, both tests should have the same number of items and the same level of difficulty. The test is given to the group at the same time as the equivalent test is given or the equivalent test is administered at a later date. *Internal consistency reliability* is associated with the extent to which all items on an instrument measure the same variable and with the homogeneity of the items. This reliability is considered only when the instrument is being used to measure a single concept or construct at a time. Because the validity of findings is threatened when an instrument is unreliable, faculty should use measures to ensure instrument reliability.

Collecting Data

The next step of the evaluation process is use of the evaluation instrument to gather data. Although the instrument will determine to some extent what data are collected and how, several other factors should be considered at this time. These include the data collector, the data sources, amount of data, timing of data collection, and informal versus formal data collection.

Data Collector

Consideration must be given to who is collecting the data. In some instances, the data are gathered by the evaluator, for example, the faculty member evaluating clinical performance of the students. In other situations, students or research assistants may administer instruments. If the data collectors are not familiar with the data-collecting procedures, they should be oriented to the task. Interrater reliability must be ensured when more than one person is collecting data.

Data Source

Before evaluation, the evaluator must identify sources from which the data will be collected. Will the data be observed (as in clinical evaluation), archival (as when grade point average is obtained from student records), or reported (as obtained from a longitudinal questionnaire of graduates)? At this time in the evaluation process, it is important to determine whether it is possible to have access to records, particularly if permission must be obtained from the participants.

Amount of Data

The amount of data to be collected must also be determined and specified. All data may be collected or a sample may be sufficient, but a decision must be made. For example, in clinical evaluation or classroom testing it is impossible to collect data about each instance of clinical performance or knowledge gained from the classroom experience. In this instance, a sampling procedure is used and guided by the clinical evaluation protocol, blueprint, or plan for the classroom test. It is important to note that the sampling plan must be established at this stage of the evaluation process.

Timing of Data Collection

When is the best time to collect the data? An understanding of the context of evaluation is helpful here. Should the data be collected at the beginning, middle, or end of the activity being evaluated? When gathering data from students, it is important to allow adequate time and to gather data when students are able to give unbiased responses. (For example, course evaluation data collected immediately after test results have been given may not yield the most reflective responses.)

Formal versus Informal Data Collection

Decisions about use of formal and informal data must also be made. Data can be obtained in a formal manner, such as by using a structured evaluation tool. Data can also be collected with informal methods, such as in the form of spontaneous comments made by students. The evaluator must decide whether both formal and informal data will be used in the plan.

Interpreting Data

This step of the evaluation process involves translating data to answer the evaluation questions established at the beginning of the evaluation process. This involves putting the data in usable form, organizing data for analysis, and interpreting the data against preestablished criteria. When data are interpreted, the context, frame of reference, objectivity, and legal and ethical issues must also be considered.

Frame of Reference

Frame of reference refers to the reference point used for interpretation of data. Two frames of reference are discussed here, norm-referenced interpretation and criterion-referenced interpretation.

Norm-Referenced Interpretation

Norm-referenced interpretation refers to interpreting data in terms of the norms of a group of individuals who are being evaluated. The scores of the group form a basis for comparing each individual with the others. In norm-referenced evaluation, there will always be an individual who has achieved at the highest level, as well as one who has achieved at the lowest level.

Norm-referenced interpretation permits evaluators to compare achievement of students in several ways. Students in the same group can be compared and ranked. Students can be compared with students in another group or class section or with national group norms, as in the case of licensing examinations or nursing specialty certification examinations. As a consequence, an *advantage* of norm-referenced interpretation is the ability to make comparisons within groups or with external groups and to use the data for predictive purposes, such as admission criteria. A *disadvantage* of norm-referenced interpretation is the focus on comparison, which may foster a sense of competitiveness among students.

Criterion-Referenced Interpretation

In *criterion-referenced interpretation*, on the other hand, results are judged against preestablished criteria and reflect the degree of criteria attainment. Criterion-referenced interpretation is typically used in competence-based learning models in which the goal is to assist the learner to achieve competence in or mastery of specified learning outcomes. Because students are compared with the outcomes and not each other, all students can achieve competence.

The *advantages* of criterion-referenced interpretation include the following: emphasis on mastery and the potential for all learners to achieve increased learner motivation, sharing and collaboration among students, and ability to give clear progress reports to learners. *Disadvantages* of criterion-referenced interpretation include the inability to compare students with each other or with other groups.

Issues of Objectivity and Subjectivity

The issues of objectivity and subjectivity in evaluation always arise when data are interpreted. Different evaluators can look at the same data yet render different judgments. The differences may be a result of evaluator bias or degrees of difference in objectivity. Studies of performance appraisals in work settings have shown the effects of recency—interpreting findings when other favorable findings have preceded the evaluation (Polit & Beck, 2006). In some ways, faculty need to accept that there is a certain amount of subjectivity in evaluation; after all, this is "evaluation" and not "measurement." However, faculty should recognize subjectivity and the role it may play in interpretation of findings.

Legal Considerations

There may be *legal aspects* involved in interpretation of findings. Legal consideration is particularly important in the area of student rights. How will the results of evaluations be shared? What data about students can be collected? Does evaluation involve protection of human subjects? Will there be moral or ethical dilemmas in reporting the data? Who is affected by evaluations? How will they respond to the results? What impact will evaluation have on a student, a program, or a curriculum? Accordingly, the evaluator and the audience must be aware of the context of evaluation because these elements can influence how the evaluation is conducted, how results are reported, what will change as a result of the evaluation, and how due process will be handled. See Chapter 3 for additional discussion of legal aspects of evaluating students' academic and clinical performance.

Reporting the Findings

In this step of the evaluation process, the results of evaluation are communicated to appropriate persons. Factors to consider when findings are reported include when, how, and to whom the findings will be provided.

Who Receives the Findings

The evaluator must know to whom the data should be reported. Typically, both the persons and group being evaluated and those requesting evaluation receive evaluation reports. Issues of reporting and confidentiality should be established at the outset of evaluation. Confidentiality of the report must be maintained. Only those persons designated to receive the report should do so. The evaluator should then destroy unneeded background information after the report is completed.

In reporting findings, it is also important to consider the recipient of the report. What will the recipient want and need to know? For example, students receiving a test grade are usually prepared only to understand the grade, not the complex methods that were used to determine the grade or the item analysis statistics. Preparing the recipient for the evaluation report may also be helpful if the recipient does not have adequate background information to receive the report.

When to Report Findings

The timing of the report is also crucial. There tends to be a readiness to know the results of evaluation, and if the report of results is delayed, the recipients may lose interest. For example, students prefer having immediate results and can have increased anxiety or lose interest if results are delayed. The timing of the report may also be based on when information is needed, for example, at the end of the semester when grades are to be reported to the registrar.

How to Report Findings

Evaluation reports can take many forms. They may be written or oral, formal or informal. An example of an informal evaluation is talking with the student about his or her performance in a clinical experience, without a structured evaluation. This type of evaluation is far from ideal and leaves the student and the instructor without objective criteria and a sense of fairness. In the event that the student should fail the course, the instructor is not able to defend the decision. In a formal report, statistical analysis of the data will be accessible along with the findings. Specific methods of reporting findings to students, faculty, administrators, and external audiences are discussed in subsequent chapters.

Using the Findings

Evaluation is a mutual effort between the evaluator and the individual, group, or program being evaluated. Although using the findings is the last, and often forgotten, step of the evaluation process, both parties have obligations to use the findings as explained by Sanders and Sullins (2006). It is a waste of valuable resources to conduct an evaluation without follow-up. Target the evaluation results toward uses that will provide the most impact on the program. Barrett-Barrick (1993) states that the use of evaluation findings requires purposeful, strategic planning. Four perspective strategies are purpose, people, planning, and packaging. The *purpose* of the evaluation must be identified by faculty and administration. Types of evaluation used in nursing programs include accreditation, criterion-referenced evaluation, decision-focused evaluation, external evaluation, formative evaluation, internal evaluation, outcome evaluation, process evaluation, and summative evaluation. For an evaluation to be successful, the *people* involved in the evaluation should be included in the process. The main strategy in promoting evaluation is *planning* the activities and disseminating the evaluation information. *Packaging* the evaluation report to meet the needs of those who will use the report is a priority. The report should be in a format that is easily understood, and graphs and other visual aids should be used as needed.

Evaluation results can be used in a variety of ways. Common uses in nursing are to assign grades; revise instruction, courses, curricula, or programs; and demonstrate program effectiveness.

Several ways to improve the use of evaluation efforts are as follows:

1. Encourage persons involved in results to be involved in designing the evaluation plan.
2. Involve all concerned in the evaluation process. For example, students can do self-evaluation; faculty can do peer review.
3. Report findings in a timely manner.
4. Make recommendations that are realistic and can be used. For example, when reporting results of a test to a student, the evaluator (teacher) can make recommendations as to how to study for the next test to improve scores. In this way, the report of the results can be useful to the student.
5. Build in time for sharing results. This can be done by having an examination review, an evaluation conference, or a curriculum evaluation workshop.
6. Encourage the recipient to generate alternatives to behavior. For example, the student can make his or her own suggestions about improving test scores. Faculty and staff can establish goals and objectives for course change.
7. Establish trust and be cautious with sensitive findings.
8. Place findings in context. Explain to the recipients what the findings mean and how they can use the results in their own setting.

Considering the Costs of Evaluation

Evaluation can be costly throughout the entire process, and therefore the evaluator and audience must be assured that the cost will match the benefit.

Answers to the following cost-related questions need to be determined at the outset:

- What fees (or faculty time) are associated with evaluation?
- How much time will the evaluator spend in developing tools, administering tools, interpreting data, and reporting results?
- Will undue time be spent on the part of those being evaluated in filling out evaluation tools?
- Will complex evaluation methods involving lengthy evaluation tools or computer time for data analysis contribute to the outcome?
- Will the results of evaluation require changes?
- Will the student fail the course and need to repeat it?
- Will the curriculum require massive revision?

SUMMARY

Evaluation is a means of appraising data or placing a value on data gathered through one or more measurements. The evaluation process involves a systematic series of actions including identification of a clear purpose, the time frame, and the evaluator. Models or frameworks can be used to guide the process, choice of instruments, data collection methods, and reporting procedures. Would a builder construct a house without plans? The same principle applies in evaluation. The framework establishes the guide to the construction of purposeful evaluation. Researching and developing the framework are the most valuable first steps. Selection of the appropriate instruments is integral to success. The instruments should be appropriate for what is being evaluated, easy to use, cost effective, time efficient, valid, and reliable. Results must be interpreted and reported accurately. Finally, after analysis, the findings must be used. To design and implement an evaluation plan and then ignore the results would defeat the purpose of evaluation. It would be analogous to leaving a newly constructed house empty. Box 24-4 presents several websites that provide useful information about the evaluation process.

BOX 24-4 Internet Resources Related to Evaluation

- **www.scup.org/** Society for College and University Planning.
- **http://nces.ed.gov/ipeds/** Integrated Postsecondary Education Data System (IPEDS).
- **http://nces.ed.gov/** "The National Center for Education Statistics (NCES), located within the U.S. Department of Education and the Institute of Education Sciences, is the primary federal entity for collecting and analyzing data related to education."
- **http://nces.ed.gov/NPEC/** "NPEC's mission is to promote the quality, comparability and utility of postsecondary data and information that support policy development at the federal, state, and institution levels."
- **http://eric.ed.gov/** "The Education Resources Information Center (ERIC), sponsored by the Institute of Education Sciences (IES) of the U.S."
- **www.chea.org/Research/crossroads.asp** *Accreditation at a Crossroads*.
- **www.chea.org/Events/Usefulness/98May/98_05Ewell.asp** *Examining a Brave New World: How Accreditation Might Be Different*.
- **www.chea.org/pdf/HED_Apr1998.pdf#search="Distance learning"** *Distance Learning in Higher Education*.
- **www.chea.org/degreemills/default.htm** *The Fundamentals of Accreditation*.
- **www.ion.illinois.edu/resources/tutorials/pedagogy/index.asp** Instructional Strategies for Online Courses.
- **www.umass.edu/oapa/oapa/publications/online_handbooks/program_based.pdf** *PROGRAM-Based Review and Assessment: Tools and Techniques for Program Improvement*.
- **www.managementhelp.org/evaluatn/fnl_eval.htm** Basic Guide to Program Evaluation.
- **http://paws.wcu.edu/gjones/as.assessment_wcu.html** Assessment and evaluation topics.

REFLECTING ON THE EVIDENCE

1. A national nursing accrediting body has notified you that your program is due for reaccreditation in 3 years. What steps must you take to be prepared for the accreditation team? Develop a plan of action to evaluate and document student and program outcomes, and organize the documents obtained.

   a. Based on the best evidence, choose an evaluation model and evaluation tools, develop a method to track outcome evidence, and develop a plan to delegate certain evaluation components.

   b. Develop a timeline and action plan.

   c. Discuss your timeline, action plan, and impact of accreditation with at least two other students.

   d. What are the evaluation obstacles facing your nursing program and what plan do you have to overcome these obstacles?

2. You have been assigned by your program chair to design the evaluation process for your school of nursing. The school of nursing is a baccalaureate program with 160 students, 12 full-time faculty, and 20 adjunct faculty. Your curriculum has not been revised for 10 years and your NCLEX pass rate has averaged 70% for 6 years. What model would you choose for evaluation and why?

3. After you have chosen a model in question 2, design a framework to collect data. Address the evaluation process and stakeholders. Also, create a theoretical budget for the evaluation process.

4. Your school of nursing has decided to hire an outside evaluator to evaluate the master's degree (NP) program. What criteria would you use to hire an outside evaluator? Who will interact with the evaluator? What documents will he or she need to access? What possible outcomes might occur after an evaluation of this sort? Why might an "outside" evaluator be necessary instead of an "inside" evaluator?

REFERENCES

Alstete, J. W. (2004). *Accreditation matters: Achieving academic recognition and renewal.* ASHE-ERIC Higher Education Report, *30*(4). San Francisco, CA: Wiley Periodicals.

American Association of Higher Education Assessment Forum, The. (1994). Principles of good practice for assessing student learning. In J. S. Stark & A. Thomas (Eds.), *Assessment and program evaluation* (pp. 769–772). Needham Heights, MA: Simon & Schuster.

Angelo, T., & Cross, P. (1993). *Classroom assessment techniques: A handbook for college teachers.* San Francisco, CA: Jossey-Bass.

Barrett-Barrick, C. (1993). Promoting the use of program evaluation findings. *Nurse Educator, 18*(1), 10–12.

Billings, D. M., Connors, H. R., & Skiba, D. J. (2001). Benchmarking best practices in web-based nursing courses. *Advances in Nursing Science, 23*(3), 41–52.

Bond, T., & Fox, C. (2001). *Applying the Rasch model: Fundamental measurement in the human sciences.* Mahwah, NJ: Lawrence Erlbaum.

Chambliss, C. (2003). *Making departments distinctive: The continuous quality improvement (CQI) mindset.* ERIC Document Reproduction Service No. ED479751. Retrieved from EBSCOHost ERIC database.

Chen, H.-T. (2004, October 21). Theory-driven evaluation. Retrieved from http://www.mywire.com/a/Evaluation/TheoryDriven-Evaluation/17671523/

Clark, A. T., & Rice, D. R. (1994). TQM and assessment: The North Dakota experience. In J. S. Stark & A. Thomas (Eds.), *Assessment and program evaluation* (pp. 797–802). Needham Heights, MA: Simon & Schuster.

Clendon, J. M. (2003). Nurse-managed clinics: Issues in evaluation. *Journal of Advanced Nursing, 44*(6), 558–565.

Council for Higher Education Accreditation. (2006). *Informing the public about accreditation.* Retrieved from http://www.chea.org/public_info/index.asp

Davis, B. G. (1994). Demystifying assessment: Learning from the field of evaluation. In J. S. Stark & A. Thomas (Eds.), *Assessment and program evaluation* (pp. 45–58). Needham Heights, MA: Simon & Schuster.

Davis, J. R. (1993). *Better teaching, more learning: Strategies for success in postsecondary settings.* Phoenix, AZ: Oryx Press.

Gates, S. M., Augustine, C. H., Benjamin, R., Bikson, T. K., Kaganoff, T., Levy, D. G., . . . Zimmer, R.W. (2002). *Ensuring quality and productivity in higher education.* San Francisco, CA: Jossey-Bass.

Germain, C. P., Deatrick, J. A., Hagopian, G. A., & Whitney, F. W. (1994). Evaluation of a PhD program: Paving the way. *Nursing Outlook, 42*(3), 117–122.

Goodwin, L. D. (1997). Changing concepts of measurement validity. *Journal of Nursing Education, 36*(3), 102–107.

Gronlund, N. E. (1993). *How to make achievement tests and assessments* (5th ed.). Boston, MA: Allyn & Bacon.

Gronlund, N. E., & Waugh, C. K. (2009). *Assessment of student learning* (9th ed.). Columbus, OH: Pearson.

Grumet, B. R. (2002). Demystifying accreditation: How NLNAC is making the process relevant for today's educators. *Nursing Education Perspectives, 23*(3), 114–117.

Guba, E. G., & Lincoln, Y. S. (1989). *Fourth generation evaluation.* Newburg Park, CA: Sage.

Haleem, D., Evanina, K., Gallagher, R., Golden, M., Healy-Karabell, K., & Manetti, W. (2010). Program evaluation: How faculty addressed concerns about the nursing program. *Nurse Educator, 35*(3), 118–121.

Jones, R., & Beck, S. (1996). *Decision making in nursing.* Albany, NY: Delmar.

Kai, J. (2009). A critical analysis of accountability in higher education: Its relevance to evaluation of higher education. *Chinese Education and Society, 42*(2), 39–51.

Kapborg, I., & Fischbein, S. (2002). Using a model to evaluate nursing education and professional practice. *Nursing and Health Sciences, 4*(1–2), 25–31.

Lignugaris-Kraft, B., Marchand-Martella, N., & Martella, R. C. (2001). Writing better goals and short-term objectives or benchmarks. *Teaching Exceptional Children, 34*(1), 52–58.

Lincoln, Y. S., & Guba, E. G. (1985). *Naturalistic inquiry.* Beverly Hills, CA: Sage.

Madaus, G., Scriven, M., & Stufflebeam, D. (1988). *Evaluation models.* Boston, MA: Kluwer-Nijhoff.

Millard, R. M. (1994). Accreditation. In J. S. Stark & A. Thomas (Eds.), *Assessment and program evaluation* (pp. 151–164). Needham Heights, MA: Simon & Schuster.

Mizikaci, F. (2006). A systems approach to program evaluation model for quality in higher education. *Quality Assurance in Education, 14*(1), 37–53.

Murphy, P. S. (1995). Benchmarking academic research output in Australia. *Assessment & Evaluation in Higher Education, 20*(1), 45–58.

National League for Nursing. (2010). Reflection and dialogue, high stakes testing. Retrieved from https://www.nln.org/aboutnln/reflection_dialogue/refl_dial_7.htm

Newby, A. C. (1992). *Training evaluation handbook.* San Diego, CA: Pfeiffer.

Palomba, C. A., & Banta, T. W. (1999). *Assessment essentials: Planning, implementing, and improving assessment in higher education.* San Francisco, CA: Jossey-Bass.

Parry, S., & Dunn, L. (2000). Benchmarking as a meaning approach to learning in online settings. *Studies in Continuing Education, 22*(2), 221–234.

Pedhazur, E., & Schmelkin, L. (1991). *Measurement, design, and analysis: An integrated approach.* Hillside, NJ: Lawrence Erlbaum.

Polit, D. F., & Beck, C. T. (2006). *Essentials of nursing research: Methods, appraisal, and utilization.* Philadelphia, PA: Lippincott Williams & Wilkins.

Prus, J., & Johnson, R. (1994). A critical review of student assessment options. In J. S. Stark & A. Thomas (Eds.), *Assessment and program evaluation* (pp. 603–618). Needham Heights, MA: Simon & Schuster.

Rosas, S. R. (2005). Concept mapping as a technique for program theory development. *American Journal of Evaluation, 26*(3), 339–401.

Rossi, P. H., Lipsey, M. W., & Freeman, H. E. (2004). *Evaluation: A systematic approach* (7th ed.). Thousand Oaks, CA: Sage.

Rudner, L. M. (2001). Item response theory. Retrieved from http://echo.edres.org:8080/irt/

Sanders, J. R., & Sullins, C. D. (2006). *Evaluating school programs.* Thousand Oaks, CA: Corwin Press.

Scriven, M. (1972). Pros and cons about goal-free evaluation. *Evaluation Comment, 3*(4), 1–4.

Shoemaker, J. K., & DeVos, M. (1999). Are we a gift shop? A perspective on grade inflation. *Journal of Nursing Education, 38*(9), 394–398.

Sims, S. J. (1992). *Student outcomes assessment: A historical review and guide to program development.* New York, NY: Greenwood Press.

Singh, M. D. (2004). Evaluation framework for nursing education programs: Application of the CIPP model. *International Journal of Nursing Education Scholarship, 1*(1), 1–16. doi:10.2202/1548-923X.1023

Spurlock, D. (2006). Do no harm: Progression policies and high-stakes testing in nursing education. *The Journal of Nursing Education, 45*(8), 297–302.

Spurlock, D., & Hunt, L. (2008). A study of the usefulness of the HESI exit exam in predicting NCLEX-RN failure. *Journal of Nursing Education, 47*(4), 157–166.

Stake, R. (1967). The countenance of educational evaluation. *Teachers College Record, 68*(7), 523–540.

Story, L., Butts, J. B., Bishop, S. B., Green, L., Johnson, K., & Mattison, H. (2010). Innovative strategies for nursing education program evaluation. *Journal of Nursing Education, 49*(6), 351–354.

Stufflebeam, D. L. (Ed.). (1971). *Educational evaluation and decision-making.* Itasia, IL: Peacock.

Stufflebeam, D. L. (2001). *Evaluation models.* San Francisco, CA: Jossey-Bass.

Stufflebeam, D. L., & Webster, W. J. (1994). An analysis of alternative approaches to evaluation. In J. S. Stark & A. Thomas (Eds.), *Assessment and program evaluation* (pp. 331–348). Needham Heights, MA: Simon & Schuster.

Welsh J. F., & Metcalf, J. (2003). Cultivating faculty support for institutional effectiveness activities: Benchmarking best practices. *Assessment & Evaluation in Higher Education, 28*(1), 33–45.

Wholey, J. S., Hatry, H. P., & Newcomer, K. E. (2004). *Handbook of practical program evaluation.* San Francisco, CA: Jossey-Bass.

Wilson, M. (2005). *Constructing measures: An item response modeling approach.* Mahwah, NJ: Lawrence Erlbaum Associates, Inc.

Yvonne, M. (2006). Commentary from the perspective of an expert in psychometrics. *Journal of Nursing Education, 45*(8), 309–310.

Strategies for Assessing and Evaluating Learning Outcomes

Jane M. Kirkpatrick, PhD, RN

Diann A. DeWitt, PhD, RN , CNE

This chapter is dedicated to our outstanding colleague and friend Dr. Lillian Yeager, who died in May 2006. Dr. Yeager was appointed Dean for the School of Nursing at Indiana University Southeast in 2002 following approximately 30 years as an exceptional educator there. It was our pleasure to collaborate with such an outstanding nurse educator and administrator. Lillian had a keen sense of humor and zest for life, both of which aided in her valiant efforts to live life fully in her fight with cancer. She is greatly missed and will long be remembered by many. Thanks for inspiring us, Lillian!

The purpose of this chapter is to discuss the uses, advantages, disadvantages, and issues related to a variety of strategies that faculty can use to assess and evaluate student learning. The Carnegie Foundation's report on nursing education (Benner, Sutphen, Leonard, & Day, 2009) calls for stronger integration of both clinical and classroom instruction and "radical transformation" in how nursing education is provided. Just as teaching methods are expanding to ensure that graduates achieve desired outcomes as identified by the American Association of Colleges of Nursing (AACN) essentials (2008) and National League for Nursing (NLN) competencies (2010), we must also expand our assessment and evaluation strategies to determine if these competencies are attained. Competency in clinical judgment, critical thinking, and best nursing practices may need multiple measures to be evaluated accurately. As educators expand teaching methods and seek to assess deep learning and critical thinking, we can explore ways that our active learning teaching strategies can be transformed to assess the desired learning outcomes. The chapter includes practical information on a variety of outcome assessment strategies. Included are ways to select strategies, improve validity and reliability of the assessment strategies, and increase the effectiveness of their use.

Assessment and Evaluation

Just what is the difference between assessment and evaluation? In many instances it seems that these two terms are interchangeable. Assessment basically means obtaining information for a specific purpose. The information collected may be quantitative or qualitative depending on how it will be used (Brookhart, 2005). The main purpose of assessment is understanding and improving student learning (T. A. Angelo, personal communication, November 7, 2006). "It involves making our expectations explicit and public; setting appropriate criteria and high standards for learning quality; systematically gathering, analyzing, and interpreting evidence to determine how well performance matches those expectations and standards; and using the resulting information to document, explain, and improve performance" (Angelo, 1995, pp. 7–9). This definition of assessment is quite similar to formative evaluation, a process of determining progress with the goal of making improvements.

Evaluation is a term that is more commonly associated with summative evaluation, which takes assessment to the next level of judging the value and quality of performance at a defined end point. Summative evaluation suggests that a decision may be made. In clinical disciplines, faculty must evaluate student attainment of course outcomes and defined program competencies.

Selecting Strategies

The strategies discussed in this chapter provide faculty with a variety of techniques to use to assess and evaluate student learning outcomes. Several of the strategies discussed may be more familiar as teaching strategies. The idea of adapting a teaching strategy as an assessment or assessment tool allows students to practice the same process by which they will ultimately be evaluated.

The major reasons for faculty to consider new assessment and evaluation strategies are so they can better (1) assess and evaluate all domains of learning, (2) assess higher levels of the cognitive domain (e.g., analysis, synthesis), (3) assess critical thinking, and (4) prepare students for licensing or certification examinations. By providing a more authentic assessment wherein the student is asked to perform or demonstrate the learning in a way that is as closely related to the ultimate performance required in the real world, the faculty will have richer and deeper evidence of student progress.

In selecting strategies, the philosophy of the faculty regarding accountability and responsibility for learning must be considered. Many of the strategies discussed are compatible with active teaching techniques. Critical reflections, short essays, and guided writing assignments encourage students to interact with the material in a different way than if they were learning the material for a multiple-choice test. The major challenges of using these strategies include (1) the time it takes to use the strategy and (2) difficulty in establishing validity and reliability of data-gathering instruments and methods. To avoid some of the pitfalls associated with these strategies, faculty should do the following:

1. Clearly delineate the *purpose* of the assessment and evaluation.
2. Consider the *setting* in which the learning and assessment and evaluation will take place.
3. Choose the best assessment and evaluation *strategy* for the purpose.
4. Determine the *procedure* for the strategy selected.
5. Establish *validity* and *reliability* of the strategy.
6. Assess and evaluate the overall *effectiveness* of the process.

Purpose

The purpose of assessment and evaluation is to ascertain that students have achieved their potential and have acquired the knowledge, skills, and abilities set forth in courses and curricula. The instructional goals and course objectives will indicate the type of behavior (cognitive, affective, or psychomotor) to be assessed. The learning experiences must

have relevance to the students and be valued in the grading system. Finally, the grading criteria should be shared with the students before the assessment occurs.

The timing of the assessment relates closely to the purpose. Assessment or formative evaluation is much like feedback for the purpose of recognizing progress. This type of evaluation would be appropriate throughout the class term. Summative evaluation suggests that a decision may be made. This might be a grade or a decision for passing or failing a course.

Setting

Another critical factor to consider is the setting in which the instruction and assessment will occur. Most faculty are comfortable with assessment and evaluation in traditional classroom settings, but more than half of all nursing schools are now using some form of computer-based learning support. For some, technology provides an adjunct or support to the nursing course. For others, the entire course is web-based and delivered online.

When considering how to implement assessment and evaluation strategies in an electronic environment, faculties need to address how the technology supports the assessment purpose. Most of the strategies discussed in this chapter can be used in an online community. For example, a threaded discussion can be used for critiquing or even as a forum for verbal questioning. Concept maps can be developed in an electronic format. Students or faculty can maintain an electronic portfolio representative of student work throughout the course.

Choice of Strategy

When choosing the best strategy for the purpose, faculty must weigh the advantages and disadvantages of each strategy. Faculty should also consider time for preparation, implementation, and grading. Other issues, such as cost, may also be a determining factor. Faculty must decide how often to assess, who will assess, and how the students will be prepared for the assessment and evaluation technique. When selecting an assessment method, students should have ample opportunity to practice the technique on which they will be tested.

Procedures

Although procedures for using assessment strategies vary, any procedure selected must be well planned. The strategy should be pilot-tested before it is fully implemented. This process should help prevent unexpected difficulties and allow for refinement and quality improvements prior to full-scale implementation. It is also important to delineate the responsibilities associated with the methods used. For example, in the case of portfolio assessment, a decision must be made about whether students or faculty will collect and keep the work. Another area of concern is the environment in which the assessment will take place. Because of the anxiety and stress associated with the process of being evaluated, faculty must attempt to provide an atmosphere conducive to the process. Humor, when used appropriately, may help place students at ease.

Validity and Reliability

The issues of validity and reliability are critical, especially when the purpose is for summative assessment and evaluation. The terms *validity* and *reliability* are defined and described in Chapter 24. For the purposes of this chapter, specific examples are given to clarify establishment of validity and reliability in nonmultiple-choice assessment methods.

In determining validity, faculty must ask whether the assessment technique is appropriate to the purpose and whether it provides useful and meaningful data (Linn & Gronlund, 2005). Faculty must consider the fit of the assessment strategy with the identified objectives. In other words, does the strategy measure what it is supposed to measure? For instance, if the objective for an assignment is for the student to demonstrate skill in written communication, evaluating student performance through oral questioning will not provide valid data. Similarly, at the nursing department level, faculty should coordinate assessment and evaluation strategies with nursing program outcomes such as critical thinking and communication. It is a challenge to develop sound criteria for assessment that accurately reflect the specified outcomes, objectives, and content. To establish *face validity*, faculty must seek input from colleagues by asking questions such as "Do these criteria appear to measure what my objectives are?" In addition, obtaining the opinion of other content experts can assist in determining whether there is adequate sampling of the content (*content validity*). Whereas these types of validity (e.g., face, content) constitute the traditional approach to establishing validity, Gronlund (2006) asserts that this view is being replaced by validity as a unitary concept, based on several different categories of evidence (e.g., face-related evidence, content-related evidence). The evidence available to establish validity determines whether validity is considered low, medium, or high.

Once assessment and evaluation criteria or rubrics are developed, it is essential to establish their reliability. The most commonly used method for establishing reliability in this situation is when two or more instructors independently rate student performance using the agreed upon criteria or rubric for sample work. Then the ratings are correlated to establish *interrater reliability*. Interrater reliability is expressed as a percentage of agreement between scores. An example of using criteria to establish interrater reliability is provided in Box 25-1.

A multiplicity of assessment strategies can provide a more complete picture of the student's abilities and therefore contribute to the trustworthiness of the process. It is a serious limitation to rely on a single technique. Each assessment technique

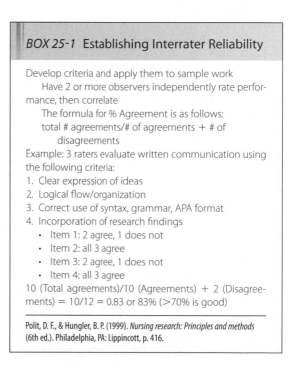

BOX 25-1 Establishing Interrater Reliability

Develop criteria and apply them to sample work
 Have 2 or more observers independently rate performance, then correlate
 The formula for % Agreement is as follows:
 total # agreements/# of agreements + # of
  disagreements
Example: 3 raters evaluate written communication using the following criteria:
1. Clear expression of ideas
2. Logical flow/organization
3. Correct use of syntax, grammar, APA format
4. Incorporation of research findings
 • Item 1: 2 agree, 1 does not
 • Item 2: all 3 agree
 • Item 3: 2 agree, 1 does not
 • Item 4: all 3 agree
10 (Total agreements)/10 (Agreements) + 2 (Disagreements) = 10/12 = 0.83 or 83% (>70% is good)

Polit, D. F., & Hungler, B. P. (1999). *Nursing research: Principles and methods* (6th ed.). Philadelphia, PA: Lippincott, p. 416.

has limitations and issues that can influence the reliability, validity, and appropriateness of the technique for given student populations. Using multiple assessment techniques provides a more robust and accurate framework for making evaluative decisions.

Effectiveness

After the assessment strategy is implemented, it is essential to determine its overall effectiveness. Issues related to the implementation of the assessment strategy should be examined as well. Some questions faculty should ask include the following: Was the strategy an effective use of resources (e.g., student and faculty time and financial resources)? Were there adequate data to determine if the learning outcome was met? Are there any problems with the implementation of the technique? What revisions are necessary? Would the faculty consider this strategy to be a good choice for future use?

Matching the Assessment Strategy to the Domain of Learning

Educators must also be mindful of the domain of learning being assessed or evaluated (see Chapter 13). Cognitive learning is typically assessed with strategies requiring the students to write, submit portfolios, or complete tests (see Chapter 11). Assessment in the psychomotor domain typically involves simulations and simulated patients and ultimately occurs in clinical practice (see Chapters 19 and 20). Assessment in the affective domain is particularly important in nursing and is discussed further here.

The taxonomy of affective assessment and evaluation as applied to nursing (Krathwohl, Bloom, & Mases, 1964) lists five behavioral categories: (1) receiving, (2) responding, (3) valuing, (4) organization of values, and (5) characterization by a value or value complex. The beginning student may be at the receiving level, able to hear and recognize the values. As the student progresses, more sophisticated affective growth would demonstrate the ability to respond to or communicate about the particular value or issue. At the next level, the student embraces the value. Ultimately, the student would act on the value. Once actions are consistent, the highest levels of the affective domain would be realized.

Examples of areas in which nursing students encounter the affective domain include socialization to the roles of the nurse, caring for patients who are dying, meeting spirituality needs, working with sexuality concerns, and becoming culturally competent.

For example, students are expected to increase their level of cultural competence throughout the curriculum. At the beginning level students may be expected to become self-aware using exploration of their own cultural and health care practices as well as values. A mid-program outcome could focus on student awareness of the cultural orientation of the patients under their care. At graduation the expected outcomes would be to act in a culturally competent manner when providing care to all patients and demonstrate the ability to advocate for an individual patient's unique needs.

Multiple strategies could be used for assessment of these outcomes, including written papers identifying the student's own cultural background, a critical review of an interaction in caregiving with a patient of another culture, or perhaps the use of media (e.g., video recording, web page development, or even a collage) to demonstrate key concepts and values held by a given culture. The assessment and evaluation strategy would be designed to assess evidence of self-awareness, recognition of the values and conflicts in areas in which judgments must be made, and mechanisms for advocacy.

Development of the affective domain is progressive and can be tied to critical thinking. Because of the progressive nature of development, formative assessment and evaluation across the curriculum may be most appropriate, with a summative assessment and evaluation at the time of graduation. Many of the assessment methods listed in this chapter can be adapted to evaluate the affective domain.

Communicating Grading Expectations

When assessment strategies are used to collect data for grading purposes, it is imperative that the grading requirements be communicated to the students. Information about grading criteria is typically provided to students in the course syllabus. Other methods such as checklists, guidelines, or grading scales can be used as well. See Box 25-2 for an example of a writing assignment with grading rubric.

Rubrics are another way to inform students about grading expectations. According to Stevens and Levi (2005), rubrics are rating scales used to assess performance. The two types of rubrics are *holistic* and *analytic*. The holistic approach is based

BOX 25-2 Sample Writing Assignment with Grading Rubric

COURTESY OF COLORADO CHRISTIAN UNIVERSITY

COLLEGE OF ADULT AND GRADUATE STUDIES

Division of Nursing and Sciences
NUR 400A Transitions in Nursing: Career Advancement
Scholarly Paper Assignment
Please select a nursing topic of interest to you for this scholarly paper assignment. The purpose of this paper is, in part, to assess your ability to think critically and communicate clearly as you begin the RN-BSN program.

The paper is to be 6–8 pages in length and follow APA format. Please refer to *CAGS Guidelines for APA Style* in Doc Sharing for additional information. A minimum of three (3) professional journal articles (less than five years old) should be used. All scholarly papers should have an introduction that includes a thesis statement, the body of the paper and a conclusion or summary.

Make sure the paper includes the following:
• A title page
• Body of the paper
  • Introduction (including thesis statement or focus for the paper)
  • At least one direct quote from a credible information source (such as a nursing article)
  • At least one in-text citation of an information source (from a different source than the one you obtained the quote from). This should not be a direct quote. It should be a reference to an idea or concept presented by the author.
  • Conclusion (summary of main points)
• A reference page
Please refer to the **NUR 400A Grading Rubric for Scholarly Paper** (in Doc Sharing) for specific grading criteria.

NUR 400A GRADING RUBRIC FOR SCHOLARLY PAPER

Critical Thinking and Written Communication

Objectives	Below Expectations <75%	Meets Expectations 75–90%	Exceeds Expectations 90–100%	Points
Organization (introduction and conclusion as well as transitions) The student will provide an introduction (including a clear thesis statement) and conclusion as well as use transitions to provide a logical flow.	Missing the introduction (with a thesis statement), the conclusion, or both. AND Transitions not used or transitions are inconsistent which provides some confusion to the reader.	Adequate introduction clearly focuses the paper and includes a thesis statement. Plausible conclusion summarizes paper. AND Transitions are ordinary (get the job done but in a routine fashion) but purposefully connect content providing logical flow.	Insightful, original introduction (including the-sis statement) clearly focuses the paper. Convincing conclusion summarizes paper. AND Transitions are original and purposefully connect content providing strong logical flow.	___ of 20
Development and Evidence (Analysis and Development) The student will analyze and develop content in a logical progression.	Content analysis and de-velopment are general or vague but presented in a somewhat logical progression or no logi-cal progression at all.	Content analysis and development are adequate and pre-sented in a logical progression.	Content analysis and development are insightful and pre-sented in logical progression.	___ of 20

Continued

BOX 25-2 Sample Writing Assignment with Grading Rubric—cont'd

Critical Thinking and Written Communication

Objectives	Below Expectations <75%	Meets Expectations 75–90%	Exceeds Expectations 90–100%	Points
Development and Evidence (Support) The student will support thesis, main points, and/or claims with appropriate evidence.	The topic statement, main points, announcement and/or claims are not supported or are supported with general or vague (reader gains few insights) personal examples and obvious textual sources.	The thesis, main points, and/or claims are supported with relevant personal examples (reader gains some insight), textual sources, and appropriate external sources.	The thesis, main points, and/or claims are supported with relevant personal examples (reader gains insight), textual sources, and scholarly academic sources.	___ of 20
Structure and Usage (Language) The student will use effective academic language, variety in sentence structure, and active voice.	Conversational word choice; some variety in sentence structure; active and passive voice are used or passive voice is primarily used.	Academic word choice; variety in sentence structure; active voice is primarily used.	Strong effective academic word choice; variety in sentence structure; active voice is primarily used.	___ of 20
Structure and Usage (Conventions— Mechanics & APA) The student will use writing mechanics properly (spelling; capitalization; punctuation; pronoun references; subject–verb agreement; consistent verb tense). The student will use APA format correctly.	The paper contains numerous (7+) mechanical errors and the errors seriously distract from the writer's purpose. AND APA format errors are numerous (7+).	The paper contains a few (4–6) mechanical errors but the errors do not distract from the writer's purpose. AND There are a few (4–6) APA format errors.	Mechanical errors are rare (0–3) and the errors do not distract from the writer's purpose. AND APA format errors are rare (0–3).	___of 20
			Total Points	/100

on global scoring, often with descriptive information for each area based on a numerical scoring system, whereas analytic scoring involves examining each significant characteristic of the written work or portfolio. For example, in assessment of writing, the organization, ideas, and style may be judged individually according to analytic scoring (Linn & Gronlund, 2005). The global method seems more suitable for summative assessment, whereas the analytic method is useful in providing specific feedback to students for the purpose of performance improvement.

Regardless of the type, rubrics are composed of four parts: (1) a task description (the assignment), (2) a scale, (3) the dimensions of the assignment, and (4) descriptions of each performance level (Stevens & Levi, 2005). The first portion of a rubric contains a clear description of the assignment and should be matched to the learning outcomes of the course. The next part of the rubric is a scale to describe levels of performance. Such a scale may include levels such as "excellent," "competent," and "needs work." The dimensions of the assignment are the third part of rubric development, where the task is broken down into components. Last, differentiated descriptions of each performance level are explicitly identified. Rubrics thus provide clarity of expectations to assist students in the successful completion of assignments as well as making grading of these assignments more objective for the faculty. See Box 25-3 for an example of grading rubrics.

BOX 25-3 Examples of Grading Rubrics

"A" GRADE

The final course *synthesis paper* clearly defines a researchable problem; the search strategy provides sufficient relevant data for understanding the problem; the coding sheet is focused and guides the analysis of the data; issues of reliability and validity are identified; the literature is synthesized, rather than reviewed or summarized; the paper concludes with recommendations based on the research synthesis. The paper is written using the IUSON writing guidelines.

Participation in discussions and learning activities integrates course concepts and reflects critical thinking about research synthesis. Participation is thoughtful, respectful, informed, and substantiated. Peer review of the synthesis paper reflects the reviewers' understanding of the synthesis process, provides practical suggestions, and is presented in a collegial manner.

Dissemination of the findings of the research synthesis includes a written *plan for publication* and an oral *presentation* to faculty and classmates. The plan for publication includes thoughtful selection of a journal; draft of a query or cover letter; and, if the paper needs revisions to suit publication guidelines, a statement about revisions needed that matches the journal publication guidelines. The professional presentation is well organized, supported by visual aids (e.g., Power-Point slides), and uses professional communication style to suit the audience.

"B" GRADE

The final *synthesis paper* clearly defines a researchable problem; the search strategy yields mostly relevant data for understanding the problem; the coding sheet lacks one or more important data and/or does not reflect the scope of the problem statement; issues of reliability and validity are unclear; the review of literature is primarily synthesis with minimal summary; the paper concludes with mostly appropriate recommendations. The paper is free of major errors in grammar or style.

Participation in discussions and learning activities usually integrates course concepts and reflects critical thinking about research synthesis. Participation is helpful but may not contribute substantially to the focus of the course. Peer review of the synthesis paper does not include relevant aspects of the peer review checklists or overlooks areas in which feedback is needed.

Dissemination of the findings of the research synthesis includes a written *plan for publication* and an oral *presentation* to faculty and classmates. The plan for publication includes appropriate selection of a journal; the drafts of the query or cover letter are generally appropriate to the situation; general revisions are noted but do not consider manuscript guidelines of the journal. The professional presentation is fairly well organized; the visual aids (e.g., PowerPoint slides) enhance the presentation; the presentation is delivered with consideration for the audience.

"C" GRADE

The final *synthesis paper* has an ill-defined problem; the search strategy yields irrelevant or tangential data for understanding the problem; the coding sheet is not well focused or neglects key variables or includes irrelevant variables; issues of reliability and validity are not identified or are ignored; the review is more summary than synthesis; the paper does not include recommendations or includes recommendations that are not drawn from the data. There are substantial errors in grammar and/or writing style.

Participation in discussions occurs on an irregular basis and is not grounded in course concepts, comments do not reflect critical thinking, and there are breaches of course norms and etiquette. Peer review of the synthesis paper does not provide substantive or helpful feedback to classmates; significant aspects of the peer review checklist are ignored.

Dissemination of the findings of the research synthesis includes a written *plan for publication* and an oral *presentation* to faculty and classmates. There is no plan for publication or the journal selected is not appropriate for the content of the paper; the drafts of the query or cover letters are not clearly written and do not capture attention of the reader; there is not clear understanding of the revisions needed of the paper for the style requirements for the selected journal. The professional presentation is not well organized; visual aids (e.g., PowerPoint slides) or the visuals do not clarify or highlight key points of the presentation; the presentation exceeds time limits and/or is not suited to the audience. The presenter is unable to answer audience questions, if any, about the material.

Courtesy of Indiana University School of Nursing.
IUSON, Indiana University School of Nursing.

Strategies for Assessing and Evaluating Learning Outcomes

Nursing faculty can use a variety of strategies to assess and evaluate student learning. This section identifies several strategies known to be effective in nursing. Table 25-1 provides an overview of these strategies.

Portfolios

Description and Uses

Portfolios are simply collections of student work. The medium most widely used for pen-and-paper portfolios is some type of binder to contain the data. Recently, electronic portfolios are more prevalent (see Internet Resources Related to Chapter

---

TABLE 25-1 Overview of Assessment and Evaluation Strategies

Technique	Domain and Assessment Purpose	Possible Applications	Advantages	Disadvantages	Issues
Portfolio (paper and electronic)	High-level cognitive Affective Psychomotor (if video) Formative Summative	Placement in program of study For evidence of progress Outcome measure for individual or program Marketing tool for job placement	Broad sample of student work Documents progress Identifies student strengths and weaknesses Critical thinking with student reflection If electronic portfolio, is easier to make updates and convenient for online programs	Time for collection and grading Need storage space Not direct observation Limited reliability Additional expenses with electronic portfolios Time needed for learning	Ownership Responsibility for collection Nonselective versus selective portfolio Are you evaluating process or product? Deciding on the format for organizing the portfolio
Role play	Cognitive Affective Psychomotor Formative	Formative feedback for psychomotor skills, communication techniques, problem-solving skills	Active participation of student Stimulates creativity Variables can be controlled Can repeat Provides practice in peer review skills	Immediate feedback may not be possible Self-consciousness of participant	Takes time to build comfort with technique Need familiarity with material
Reflection	High-level cognitive Affective Formative Summative (for trending)	Self-assessment Integration of learning can be demonstrated Appropriate for evaluating the higher-level cognitive skills; critical thinking can be assessed	Active student involvement Encourages students to form connections within and between content Assists students to practice self-assessment based on criteria Encourages recognition of learning in students' life experience	Time consuming for both students and faculty Student frustration with lack of clarity of assignment	Grading criteria can be developed jointly Requires a high degree of trust Students will need orientation to this process May want to consider anonymous grading

TABLE 25-1 Overview of Assessment and Evaluation Strategies—cont'd

Technique	Domain and Assessment Purpose	Possible Applications	Advantages	Disadvantages	Issues
Paper	High levels of cognitive and affective domains Formative Summative	Critical thinking skills Writing skills Develop arguments Synthesis of ideas	More in-depth information in area of interest A public work to be assessed Writing is the scholarly model for self-expression	Time for both faculty and student Subjectivity in grading Limited sample of ability	Reliability Grading criteria
Essays	High levels of cognitive and affective domains Formative Summative	Critical thinking skills Free-form Demonstrate problem-solving abilities, decision making, and rationale Analysis	Shorter than a paper Assess recall and synthesis at one moment rather than at several times Creativity Easy to construct and administer	Less sample of content and ability Time to write and time to grade	Reliability Grading criteria Clarity of questions Use a test plan to better cover content
Oral (verbal) questioning	All ranges of cognitive domain Affective Formative Summative	Evidence of thinking process with "why" questions Evidence of verbal skills Defense: determines content mastery and evidence of synthesis	Quick to prepare Inexpensive Opportunity for student to receive immediate corrective feedback Works well for nonlinear ideas	Perceived by students as threatening Bias of evaluator	Must determine the difference between questions for teaching versus assessment Criteria for assessment should be established before use Can be subjective
Concept mapping	All ranges of cognitive domain Affective Formative	Concepts expressed in a visual way Shows relationships between and among topics	Works well for students who are highly visual in their orientation Computer-based tools available for electronic submissions	Artistic students may have an advantage Can be frustrating to concrete thinkers	Reliability Grading criteria must be defined Allow for student creativity
Audio and video recording	All ranges of cognitive domain Affective Video gives evidence of psychomotor domain Formative Summative	Verbal skills Interviews Group discussion Video captures nonverbal performance	Provides evidence when presence of faculty may be intrusive or when faculty are unable to be present Relatively inexpensive Less intrusive than video camera Is a permanent record Evidence can be replayed Works for self-assessment	Limited by mode of recording May be difficult to get quality recording of each group member Requires time to listen Expense and maintenance of equipment	Requires consent Student should be aware of how the recording will be used Must determine whether entire tape or a sampling of the tape will be assessed Confidentiality of patient data is critical

Continued

TABLE 25-1 Overview of Assessment and Evaluation Strategies—cont'd

Technique	Domain and Assessment Purpose	Possible Applications	Advantages	Disadvantages	Issues
Patient simulation	Psychomotor High-level cognitive Affective	Safe practice environment for psychomotor skills Preparation for clinical	Active involvement of students and faculty Team interaction	Expensive Specially trained personnel, including faculty Small numbers of active students per scenario	Integration into the curriculum Selection of scenarios Opportunity to practice prior to evaluation Equipment maintenance Faculty education and training Personnel needs Efficient scheduling of students
Service learning	Higher levels of cognitive domain Affective Formative Summative	Evidence of complex communication and problem-solving skills Teamwork, if group project	Authentic learning and assessment Impact on student, preceptor, and community Student exposure to diverse or underserved populations	Time to coordinate with students, agency personnel Risk that expectations of students and agency for scope of project are not alike	Assessment should include outcomes for student learning, preceptor and agency satisfaction, and impact on targeted community

Content) and a variety of resources are available to facilitate their use. Regardless of the format, portfolios are used to obtain a broader sample of student performance (Gordon, 2003; Linn & Gronlund, 2000). Although portfolios have been used in other disciplines (e.g., art) for decades, they have more recently become commonplace in education and nursing education.

Portfolios are used for a variety of purposes. They can be used (1) as proof of achievement in a class, (2) as an outcome or assessment measure of a program, (3) as a marketing tool for job placement, or (4) for student placement in a program of study.

The purpose of the portfolio needs to be clearly established before work is collected for inclusion. The use of portfolios for student *assessment* in the classroom provides evidence of student progress within the course in addition to specific feedback to aid their learning. Student work (either all or selected assignments) may be collected from the beginning to the end of the course. Assessment of student work may occur during the course

(formative) or at the end of the course (summative). It is important that clearly established criteria be identified for the assessment and evaluation of the portfolio. These criteria need to be shared with students at the beginning of the course.

Students may be required to write a paper (or papers) in which they *critique* their *progress* during the course. When clearly delineated criteria are used, this exercise could assist students in development of self-assessment skills to more effectively prepare them for real-world practice.

Portfolios used as an *outcome measure of a program* can include selections of student work acquired throughout the curriculum. Samples of these portfolios can be used to assess student progress in an area such as writing skills to provide feedback about the effectiveness of the program. Karlowicz (2000) and Robertson et al. (2010) describe the benefits and limitations of portfolios in program assessment and evaluation and share their experiences in using this approach for program assessment.

Although art students have used portfolios of their work when seeking *employment* and further study, this approach is not widespread in nursing. Some BSN completion programs use student portfolios to validate prior learning and experience and some employers, such as academic institutions, wish to see samples of published research that could be compiled as a portfolio or dossier.

Portfolios are often used in nursing programs for *advanced placement* of students. In this process, students compile objective evidence that they have acquired certain content and skills through prior learning, practice experience, or both. Through the use of portfolios, students may demonstrate attainment of learning objectives or competencies required of a specific nursing course within a program of study. Guidelines for compiling and evaluating such portfolios must be clearly delineated. Examples of documentation that may be included in this type of portfolio include (but are not limited to) a résumé, performance evaluation, course syllabi or outlines, and evidence of professional activity.

Similar to student portfolios are those used by *faculty*; faculty may use portfolios when they are seeking *promotion* or showing evidence in performance evaluations. Guidelines for construction of such portfolios usually include evidence and assessment of teaching, scholarship, and service, although specific requirements differ among institutions.

Advantages

Portfolios provide a broad sample of student work and can show evidence of progress or accomplishment. Identification of student strengths and weaknesses allows students to make improvements. Student reflection on the work in a portfolio can stimulate critical thinking. Using portfolios for advanced placement in programs enables students to receive credit for previous experience and reduces repetition of content. In addition, once an electronic portfolio is assembled, it is easier to make changes as well as more convenient for online programs.

Disadvantages

Although collection of the portfolio papers is not time consuming, the main disadvantage associated with portfolios is the time needed to provide feedback and grades. In addition, it is challenging and takes time to determine validity and reliability for the established grading criteria or rubrics. As indicated earlier, it is beneficial for faculty to collaborate with one another, which also requires that valued commodity: time. If electronic portfolios are used, additional expenses may be incurred as well as increased time to learn the format used to organize the portfolio.

Issues

Major issues related to student portfolios are ownership of the portfolio, responsibility for collection, fair grading, use of nonselective versus selective portfolios, and the format used to organize the portfolio. The format used to organize portfolios needs to be decided. Both paper and electronic formats are used, although electronic ones are gaining in popularity. When a portfolio is used for classroom or program assessment, the faculty must decide the purpose of the portfolio (e.g., to assess writing skill or critical thinking), which works will be collected, who is responsible for maintaining the portfolio, what criteria will be used to assess the collection, the scoring method, and when feedback will be given to students. Scoring is another issue surrounding portfolio use.

Nonselective portfolios are collections of all student work for a specified period. The focus of these is formative assessment and evaluation of student progress. A compilation of certain completed works of students is called a *selective portfolio*. A selective portfolio often contains works that are the best efforts of the student and are usually part of a summative assessment and evaluation (Courts & McInerney, 1993).

When a portfolio is used for program assessment and evaluation purposes, faculty buy-in and adequate faculty development are key (Robertson et al., 2010). These authors emphasize the implications for organizational culture change, the need to clarify faculty role expectations for development and participation in the portfolio review process, institution of reward structures to recognize faculty service provided, and development of tools that adequately reflect the program outcomes that are necessary for successful implementation of the portfolio for program assessment.

Reflection

Description and Uses

The development of self-assessment skills via the mechanism of reflection is an essential component of professional development (Benner, Sutphen,

Leonard, & Day, 2009; Branch, 2010; Mann, Gordon, & MacLeod, 2009). Learning to evaluate self is a component of lifelong learning (Boud & Falchikov, 2006).

Epstein, Siegel, and Silberman (2008) suggest that self-monitoring of clinical practice (paying attention to clinical actions while in the moment, purposely examining the impact of one's actions, and using these insights to improve future thinking and practice) should be cultivated. Their hope is that building student skills in self-monitoring will create a more thoughtful, self-aware, and reflective practitioner who will ultimately contribute to improved quality of care. However, in their systematic review Mann et al. (2009) were unable to locate studies measuring change in clinical practice as an indirect or direct result of reflection.

Reflections allow faculty to view the student's ability to fully consider a question, an experience, or a thesis. Depending on the desired learning outcome, the reflection may be focused on preexperience exploration of values, reactions to a clinical experience, or a self-assessment of professional development (Billings, 2006). Reflection may be implemented through a variety of techniques: short (one- to two-page) papers, progressive journaling, as well as questioning and discussion with individuals or in groups.

A reflective approach to assessment is based on an educational connoisseurship model in which students become connoisseur critics. According to Eisner (1985), a connoisseur is able to appreciate and distinguish the important from the trivial. Although students may not have enough experience to be true connoisseurs, the faculty member can act as a role model and coach students to develop these skills. Bevis and Watson (1989), in a modification of Eisner's work, identified six levels of critiquing: looking, seeing, perceiving and intuiting, rendering, interpreting meaning, and judging. These steps include identifying an event, viewing it with a focus, interpreting the event on a personal level (complete with value clarification), and discerning the significance of the event. Assessment criteria can be built around these steps.

Reflections allow faculty to assess the students' level of understanding, guide students in the development of mental models, and help students expand critical thinking skills (Atchison et al., 2006). Reflective journaling can be used prior to class to assist students prepare for the class, and then followed by taking notes during class; after the class the students can write a reflection to summarize what they have learned.

Providing feedback to student reflections requires thoughtful responses by faculty. Seven components for responding to writing identified by Beach and Marshall (1991) are described in Box 25-4. Effective assessment and evaluation includes feedback about the student's efforts, individualized and clearly expressed comments that focus on the work and not on the student as an individual, and concern for the student's learning. Faculty comments should focus on the learning to be obtained from the assignment.

Advantages

As an assessment strategy, reflection provides an opportunity to examine critical thinking and values awareness. Practice in critical reflection increases student self-awareness. The process of completing reflection on experiential learning serves to reinforce the expected standards and can contribute to deep learning (Dummer, Cook, Parker, Barrett, & Hull, 2008). Sequential reflections provide evidence of learning over time.

BOX 25-4 Seven Components for Responding to Writing

1. **Praising**: providing positive reinforcement for students
2. **Describing**: providing "reader-based" feedback about one's own reactions and perceptions of the students' responses that imply judgments of those responses
3. **Diagnosing**: determining the students' own unique knowledge, attitudes, abilities, and needs
4. **Judging**: evaluating the sufficiency, level, depth, completeness, validity, and insightfulness of a student's responses
5. **Predicting and reviewing growth**: predicting potential directions for improving student's responses according to specific criteria and reviewing progress from previous responses
6. **Record keeping**: keeping a record to chart changes across time in student's performance
7. **Recognizing/praising growth**: giving students recognition and praise for demonstrating growth

Excerpt from *Teaching literature in the secondary school* (pp. 211–212), by Richard W. Beach and James D. Marshall. Copyright by Harcourt Brace & Company, 1991. Reprinted by permission of the publisher.

Disadvantages

The use of reflection and critical self-reflection for assessment and evaluation requires the time of both students and faculty. Students may experience initial frustration if the scope of the assignment is not well defined and the skills required for critiquing are not practiced. The process used to grade the critique must be clearly defined. Goldenberg (1994) suggests that the faculty and students work together to determine the necessary criteria. This puts the student and faculty in more collaborative roles, which may be new to both students and faculty.

Issues

Students must be oriented on the elements that are essential to a high-quality reflection, just as they are oriented to more traditional approaches of assessment. The authors' initial experience with reflection found that students spent the majority of a written reflection assignment describing the event or incident and providing minimal analysis. If the purpose of the reflection activity is to provide evidence of analysis and application, the assignment needs to be structured for this. A three-part journal framework can accomplish this goal. The first section is for description of the event, the second section requests that the student demonstrate an understanding of the concepts by applying the content from the course to the experience, and the third section asks the student to apply the understanding gained from the analysis to a future professional experience.

Time involved for both students and faculty is an issue. Writing thoughtful reflections requires a time commitment on the part of students. Those who procrastinate may not obtain the benefits of the exercise. For faculty, reading and responding can be a lengthy process. For example, if reflections are assigned in the framework of a sequential journal, faculty must decide whether they are going to read each entry for assessment purposes or take a sample.

The purpose of the assignment must be clearly established for its full benefits to be realized. Establishing grading criteria before students complete the assignment will convey outcome expectations. Faculty feedback should also be of a critically reflective nature and may be most effective as a formative assessment and evaluation. The use of anonymity could be appropriate for grading this kind of assignment, because it can enhance objectivity on the part of the evaluator and minimize student fears that can inhibit honesty and creativity.

In critical reflection, the relationship of the student and faculty changes to shared power in the learning environment. The faculty–student relationship becomes more collegial, and a high level of mutual trust and desire to grow is essential. It is also imperative that the philosophy of the school and faculty support the practice of critical reflection. Students should also know who will view their reflections. If peers will view the reflections (e.g., via threaded discussions) the amount of self-disclosure students choose to provide may be affected. Confidentiality for the student reflection is an important consideration. If the reflection assignments are kept in an electronic format, password protection adds security.

Papers and Essays

Description and Uses

Papers and assigned essays or essay questions on examinations can be used to demonstrate organizational skills, critical thinking, and written communication while encouraging creativity. Papers are written reports, whereas essays are free-form responses to open-ended questions. Students are encouraged to be creative in responding to essay questions. Both papers and essays can measure the affective domain as well as higher levels of the cognitive domain.

Advantages

In-depth information can be obtained through the writing of papers. This helps students clarify their own thinking about topics and learn to write better. Papers are a public work and can be assessed by others in the profession. Writing papers requires students to integrate their ideas with those found in other sources. Similarly, essays are useful for evaluating higher-level cognitive skills such as analysis and synthesis.

Using essay questions in a testing environment has the advantage that essay questions are easier to construct than multiple-choice examination questions. It is important to make the essay question clearly understood and focused; providing the grading criteria to students will help them allocate their response time more effectively during the testing session (Davis, 2009). Essay tests can demonstrate the ability of the student to synthesize material they have learned and convey their ideas clearly without the benefit of resources.

Disadvantages

The major disadvantage of papers for both students and faculty is the amount of time involved in writing and grading. Faculty can become distracted from the content of the paper when a student exhibits poor writing skills. Providing constructive comments can be accomplished through facilitative comments by posting questions versus being authoritative. Davis (2009) suggests using a question—"What do you hope your reader will understand your thesis to be?"—as compared to a directive statement—"State your thesis more clearly" (p. 328). Faculty should also avoid the temptation to rewrite papers while they are grading. An essay test may involve less sampling of the content than a multiple-choice examination.

Issues

Reliability in grading papers is an issue. Reliability can be increased by having more than one person grade the paper and by having clearly established grading criteria. This is especially important for papers that receive low or failing grades. Anonymous grading can increase the objectivity of the grader. Faculty should determine the purpose of the paper. For example, if the purpose is to demonstrate critical thinking and creativity, the format of the paper may have less value in the total grade of the paper. If the purpose is for the student to practice writing a scholarly paper, the format score may be emphasized.

Writing a clear and focused essay question can be a challenge for faculty. The question needs to be stated in such a way that the scope is clear to the students. It is also important to follow a test plan when essay tests are constructed so that the content is adequately sampled. Before grading an essay examination, faculty must establish clear grading criteria. When more than one person is grading, interrater reliability needs to be established. Time required to answer the essay should be determined. Davis (2009) suggests providing approximately twice the amount of time for students to provide their answers in a testing environment as it takes for the faculty member to write out the answer to the essay.

Concept Mapping

Description and Uses

Concept, mind, and nursing process mapping are all descriptive terms applied to a technique in which students express concepts and their relationships in a visual format. This strategy provides a visual means for students to demonstrate their ability to think critically, organize information, understand complex relationships, and integrate theoretical knowledge into practice (Caputi, 2010; Hill, 2006; King & Shell, 2002; Novak & Cañas, 2008; Schuster, 2008; Sutton & Koehler, 2010). Concept mapping is frequently used as an alternative to traditional nursing care plans as a method for students to demonstrate their understanding of the underpinnings that guide the delivery of nursing care. Multiple problems can be incorporated into a patient-oriented concept map, allowing students to demonstrate the interrelationship of the problems to patient care. Examples of concept mapping are provided in Figures 25-1 and 25-2.

Several concepts to be mapped can be provided by the faculty or generated by the students; the structure can be defined or left open to student creativity. A number of computer-based programs are available for constructing concept maps. Each piece of the concept map can be hyperlinked to a resource. This application of concept mapping is called a *concept resource map*.

When concept mapping is chosen for assessment and evaluation, the purpose of the assignment will drive the assessment criteria. For example, assessment and evaluation criteria may include such things as a content analysis (the number of items included), the clarity of the organizational structure, accuracy of relationships, and categorization of content. It is possible to have students self-assess or peer assess concept maps as a way of building the professional skills of self-assessment and peer assessment.

Advantages

Concept mapping is a technique that requires students to demonstrate cognitive synthesis skills with a minimum of writing. Mapping also allows faculty to gain insight into the way students assimilate new information and how students are connecting the material. Mapping also lends itself well to formative assessment and evaluation, especially in determining the way students view relationships. Having students explain the concept map can add clarity to

Example of a Concept Map for Synthesizing Course Concepts in a Graduate Course in Computer Technologies for Nurse Educators

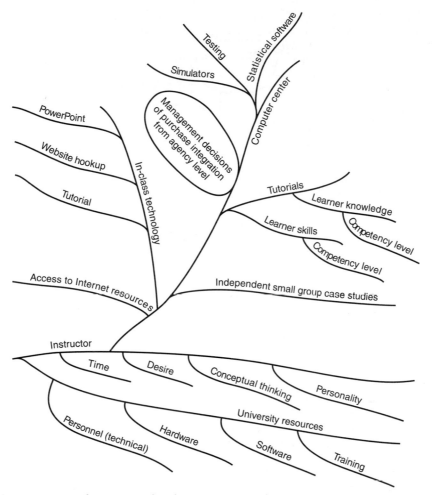

Figure 25-1 Concept map used to assess and evaluate attainment of major course concepts. (Courtesy Mary Beth Riner, Indiana University School of Nursing.)

their understanding of the relationships expressed by the lines on the map.

Disadvantages

The concept map may be large and difficult to follow. It may be more challenging to interpret the student's intent because only key words and phrases are used. It is possible that the artistic ability and overall appearance of the map, much like handwriting,

could influence faculty. Special software is required to create concept maps in an electronic environment. Time involved in reading and responding to concept maps can be lengthy.

Issues

The faculty must teach students how to successfully create a map before using it as an assessment strategy. If faculty model the mapping strategy for

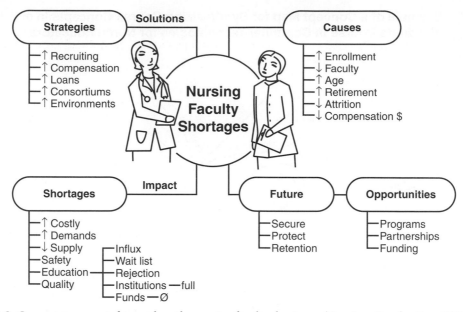

Figure 25-2 Concept map created to analyze the nursing faculty shortages. (Courtesy Carolyn Low, RN to BSN student, Colorado Christian University.)

in-class learning experiences, the students will have a greater familiarity with the process. Special software can improve the capabilities of concept mapping in an electronic environment. Software to support concept mapping can add a learning curve for students. Regardless of the method used to construct the map, a limitation of mapping is the lack of rationale presented for the relationship of ideas. One way of addressing this limitation would be to use the map as the focus for a faculty–student conference.

The assessment of the exercise can easily become subjective unless clear criteria for grading are established. These criteria should be defined for the students before submission of their work. Faculty need to establish the validity and reliability of their assessment tools for this strategy.

Oral Questioning

Description and Uses

In the quest to assess the student's ability to think critically, faculty can use questions. These questions should allow the student to demonstrate knowledge, skills, and values. Questions can be designed to elicit assessment at all levels of the cognitive domain and evidence of critical thinking. Questions may solicit only factual information or ask for comparisons, priorities, and rationales. Students can be asked to elaborate and justify their responses. Questioning as an assessment technique can be sequenced to move the student from a basic level (factual information) to a higher cognitive level (clarifying relationships).

Oral questioning has been a tradition for the defense of the dissertation and thesis at the graduate level. In this process, the student must demonstrate a working knowledge of the discipline and the ability to express arguments orally. Students in undergraduate nursing programs may experience oral questioning during their clinical experiences. Box 25-5 provides examples (adapted from Hansen, 1994, and King, 1994) of questions that assess the cognitive domain as defined in Bloom's taxonomy (Krathwohl, 2002).

Advantages

Oral questioning is inexpensive, requires no special equipment, and can be quickly developed by faculty. It is possible to give immediate feedback to the student.

BOX 25-5 Examples of Questions to Assess the Cognitive Domain

REMEMBER

Define _____.
List the five principles for _____.
Based on your assignment, what do you recall about _____?

UNDERSTAND

Explain the meaning of _____.
Tell me in your own words what is meant by _____.
Which of the examples demonstrates _____?

APPLY

What is a new example of _____?
How could _____ be used to _____?
Show how this information could be graphed.

ANALYZE

What are the implications of _____?
What is the meaning of _____?
What are the key components of _____?

EVALUATE

Explain the effectiveness of this approach.
Which solution would you choose? Justify your opinion.
What are the consequences of _____?

CREATE

What are some possible solutions to the problem of _____?
From this information, create your own model of _____.
Suppose you could _____. How would you approach _____?

Adapted from Hansen, C. (1994). Questioning techniques for the active classroom, and King, A. Inquiry as a tool in critical thinking. In D. F. Halpern (Ed.), *Changing college classrooms: New teaching and learning strategies for an increasingly complex world* (pp. 13–38, 93–106). San Francisco, CA: Jossey-Bass. Cognitive taxonomy dimensions based on Krathwohl, D. (2002). A revision of Bloom's taxonomy: An overview. *Theory into Practice, 41*(4), 212–218.

Disadvantages

Students may feel stressed by the experience. Unless the session is recorded, there is no permanent record of it. The evaluator may be biased by a variety of factors during the assessment. For example, if the student performs well at the beginning of the session and the performance deteriorates as the session progresses, the earlier performance may be biased by what occurred subsequently. It is imperative that the criteria for assessment be fully developed before the questioning session.

Issues

Using questions for assessment and evaluation must be distinguished from using questions to encourage active student learning. Avoid leading or loaded questions. Give students a minute to write down an answer. This can minimize the stressful impact of a questioning session. It is important for faculty to avoid interrupting the student as an answer is being given. The criteria for assessment must be established before the session with the student. Because of the lack of a permanent record of the interaction, risk of subjectivity is greater in assessment.

Audio and Video Recording

Description and Uses

Audio recording can be used to demonstrate communication skills, group process, and interviewing skills. Audio recording allows the evaluator to focus on verbal communication without other distracters. Video recording captures a more complete essence of the competencies being evaluated.

Using a video camera to record student performance can be a means of evaluating several performance parameters. Video of student performance is useful for evaluating communication skills because it picks up the student's actual words and inflections as well as body language. The live-action feature of the video recording provides evidence of the sequencing of student actions in hands-on skill performance. This method works well for skill validation and is very useful in debriefing after simulations. Graf (1993) has found that grading takes less time when the video return demonstration, rather than the traditional method of skill demonstration, was used. Rinne (1994) used videotaping and computers to allow students to record their performance and play it back on a split computer screen. On half of the screen is the student's work and on the other half is the expert performance; students can critique their performance side by side with that of the expert. Basic video recording equipment has become fairly inexpensive.

Advantages

Obtaining audio recording equipment is relatively inexpensive. Most digital cameras and many cell phones have video recording capabilities and are fairly inexpensive. In the case of audio recording, the presence of the microphone may be less threatening to the student than use of a video camera or direct faculty observation. Video recording works well for demonstration of mastery, particularly with psychomotor skills. These techniques allow students to practice and record their skills in private; listen to, view, and critique their own performance; and even re-record the procedure until they are satisfied with the performance prior to submitting for a grade.

This technique affords flexibility in scheduling for both students and faculty. Faculty can conduct a secondary analysis of the recording if necessary. With both audio and video recording, faculty can assess student performance with patients without being intrusive in the dynamic of the student–patient relationship.

Disadvantages

It can be difficult to distinguish individual voices in a group of participants when listening to an audio recording. One suggestion is to have each group member state his or her name at the beginning of the recording so that voices can be identified. In addition, communication has both verbal and nonverbal components. Thus, one limitation of audio recording as a strategy is that only the verbal components of the skill can be assessed.

A certain level of competence is required in knowing how to position video equipment correctly to secure quality visual and audio recording. The skill of the cameraperson and the camera angle can affect the quality of the recording. It may be necessary to use small microphones to adequately secure the audio components. More expensive options are commonly found in high-fidelity simulation rooms where video cameras may be mounted in multiple sites throughout the room and inputs from each camera are synchronized in a control room. Extra tech personnel are usually needed to maintain the equipment. If patients are involved, their consent is required. Requirements of the Health Insurance Portability and Accountability Act of 1996 (HIPAA) privacy rules are of concern whenever there is digital data from patients; therefore protocols should be in place to maintain security. Students should be educated about the uses of the recordings, especially the issues surrounding confidentiality of the materials, and sign agreements indicating their understanding.

The experience of being recorded can cause stress to some students who may feel self-conscious about being "on camera." In some cases, the stress level may be lower than that experienced with direct observation by the faculty member. If patients are also being videotaped, explanations of expectations should be given before the recording begins. Evaluators need good observational skills.

Issues

The protocol for scoring must be determined before this assessment technique is instituted. Students need an opportunity to practice with the technique before it is used in the assignment of a grade. A decision needs to be made about whether the entire recording or a sampling will be assessed. Confidentiality is an issue, as well as the need to obtain consent from all individuals who are included in the recording. HIPAA guidelines are required for digital patient data.

Role Play

Description and Uses

In role play, the learner portrays a specific individual and is generally given much freedom to act out that role spontaneously. Role play is particularly appropriate for objectives related to developing interpersonal relationships with patients, peers, and other health care providers (Oermann & Gaberson, 2009). The role-playing process provides a live sample of human behavior that serves as a vehicle for students to (1) explore feelings; (2) gain insight into their abilities, values, and perceptions; (3) develop their problem-solving skills and attitudes; and (4) explore subject matter in different ways.

The time for role play can vary according to the time available and the complexity of the role-play situation. The student is informed of the concept or role to be performed and given time to be creative in its presentation. The content, and not the performance ability, should be assessed. The content and process can be assessed for use of communication techniques. Role reversal is used in situations in which the purpose is to change attitudes. This facilitates an understanding of opposing beliefs. On termination of the role play, the student observers analyze what occurred, what feelings were generated, what insights were gained, why things happened as they did, and how the situation is related to reality.

Advantages

Situations can be structured or prepared as open-ended responses. After students critique the role play, the process can be repeated. Role play affords the opportunity for students to practice peer review. This technique actively involves the students and fosters creativity.

Disadvantages

Role play can be awkward for the faculty and student if it is not practiced before the time of assessment. Immediate feedback is difficult to provide if many groups are performing at the same time.

Issues

Role play as a teaching mode before its use in assessment assists students and faculty to become familiar with the technique and material. All that could happen cannot be anticipated. Students need to be informed in advance about the use of this technique for assessment. It may take time and experience to build comfort with this technique.

Patient Simulation

Description and Uses

Simulation is the creation of a representation or model of a real-life situation (adapted from http://sb.thefreedictionary.com/simulate). In nursing, simulations are used to provide a safe practice environment for both student learning and evaluation (Garrett, MacPhee, & Jackson, 2010; Jeffries, 2007; Nehring, 2010). According to Nehring (2010), the continuum of simulation ranges from role playing to high-fidelity simulation. High-fidelity patient simulations use the most up-to-date manikins and computer-driven equipment to closely replicate real-life situations. Faced with limited clinical resources, high-fidelity simulations are being widely adopted in nursing education programs. Nursing research related to the use of simulations as a teaching strategy is increasing; however, there is a paucity of research regarding evaluation of student competencies through the use of simulation (Garrett et al., 2010; Nehring, 2010). Eight of 22 nursing education research studies on simulation reviewed by Nehring evaluated the competence of skill performance as a result of high-fidelity simulation. These studies found that skill performance improved with the use of simulation; however,

limitations of the studies preclude generalization. Reed (2010) proposed the use of Scriven's Key Evaluation Checklist to assist nurse educators to plan, design, implement, assess, and evaluate simulation. More comprehensive information regarding use of simulations in nursing education is found in Chapter 20.

Advantages

High-fidelity simulation provides a safe environment to evaluate skills that are essential for quality nursing practice. Low-fidelity simulations can allow the opportunity for students to practice psychomotor skills in a more authentic environment. For example, instead of setting up individual stations where students validate their ability to perform procedures, a more authentic simulation would be with new orders on a given patient that required performance of the skills in the context of patient care. The combination of video recording with simulation provides opportunities for debriefing with students.

In addition to evaluating individual skill performance and demonstration of higher-order thinking skills, simulations allow for assessment of team interaction. High-fidelity simulations have been used with students of various disciplines to improve communication across disciplines. Students and faculty alike find the simulated patient care environment interesting and stimulating.

Disadvantages

The main disadvantage of using high-fidelity simulations is the expense involved. While equipment cost is decreasing, it remains rather high for the initial purchase. Along with the initial costs are maintenance fees and the need for specially trained personnel who maintain and operate the equipment. Other less obvious costs include space for the simulators, a central control room (for large simulation units), and additional video recording equipment and digital storage space for the recordings. Time for faculty development, scenario development, and staffing of the simulation lab also contributes to the total cost. Another disadvantage is that simulations can accommodate only a small number of active participants at a given time.

Issues

Major issues related to high-fidelity patient simulation include, but are not limited to, integration of simulations into the curriculum, selection of scenarios, opportunity for practice prior to evaluation, maintenance of equipment, faculty education and training, personnel needs, and efficient scheduling of students.

Faculty must determine the best way to *integrate simulations into the curriculum*. It is a sound educational principle that the curriculum develop from simple to complex and simulations are no exception. Faculty need to decide which courses will include simulation. Will it be used as a teaching strategy and an evaluation method? What is the timing in the course? Will an evaluation of student competence be used prior to clinical?

Faculty may choose from an increasing number of high-fidelity simulations available for purchase or decide to construct their own. Therefore *selection of scenarios* is another issue related to the use of simulations for evaluation. The format of the scenario for evaluation should match the format used for practice. There is a need for ample *opportunity for student practice prior to being evaluated*. This assists the students to become more comfortable with the simulated environment before they receive a grade (even if that grade is satisfactory or unsatisfactory).

Maintenance of equipment is another issue related to use of high-fidelity patient simulations. The simulators must be programmed for their environment as well as regularly maintained by technicians who are well versed in their operation.

Faculty training related to simulation must include, but is not limited to, establishing correlation of simulations with learning outcomes, building simulations from simple to complex, how to conduct the simulation, and the methods used for evaluation of simulations. Consistent evaluation of students is also important; therefore measures for creating reliability and validity of simulation evaluations are indispensable.

Additional *personnel needs* must be considered as well. Not only is a technician needed for the daily operations and maintenance of the simulators, but faculty committed to simulations is needed.

How to *efficiently schedule students* must be addressed, as simulations accommodate only a small number of active participants. It is necessary to work out the mechanics of scheduling students whether simulations are used as a teaching or evaluation strategy. If collaborative partnerships have been developed between practice and academia for shared simulation equipment and space, then scheduling issues may be more complicated.

Service Learning

Description and Uses

Many college campuses have embraced service learning either as the framework for a course or as a component within a course. According to the Corporation for National and Community Service, two essential elements must be in place for an experience to be considered service learning. First, the service activities must meet needs that the community identifies as important. Second, the educational experience must be structured in such a way that critical thinking is enhanced and students reflect to better understand course content and the role their service learning plays as a value to the community (Billig & Eyler, 2003; Kirkpatrick & Braswell, 2010). A service-learning project can take multiple forms. It can be designed as an individual project where one student works on a project that meets a need for an agency (e.g., developing an in-service for a nursing unit on a given topic) or it may be a group project wherein several students work together (e.g., develop and carry out a health fair for senior citizens at a community center). The ability to effectively work as a member of a team is a common outcome associated with service learning. Using formative assessment strategies such as an appreciative inquiry reflection (Keefe & Pesut, 2004) at the midpoint of the project can be useful in addressing challenges with the group. Timing of this assessment midway through the project allows readjustments in group processes and helps with self-awareness. Typically a final group presentation or report would be completed.

Advantages

A service-learning project has relevance for the students because the learning experience is authentic and based in a real-world situation. It also is meaningful to those who benefit from the projects these students complete. Setting the learning in the context of reality exposes students to situations they may encounter upon graduation and allows them the opportunity to find their way while still having the support of faculty. There can be very positive visibility for the school when contributions provided by the service-learning projects meet needs of the community. Service-learning projects may provide students the opportunity to better understand the social issues associated with meeting health care needs for the underserved (Bentley & Ellison, 2005).

Disadvantages

Time for faculty to manage service-learning projects can be viewed as a disadvantage because out-of-class time is required to meet with the agencies, arrange the experiences, and follow up regularly with students and agencies. Assuring that the expectations of the agency are in concert with the expectations of the faculty for the learning requirements requires extra effort. Faculty may need to help students clarify and resolve conflicts with agencies and within groups. There is also a risk that the student group may fall short of the expectation of the agency and that the reputation of the school could be jeopardized in the community.

Issues

The ultimate question becomes how to assess the learning that takes place. Again, the faculty must focus on the desired learning outcomes. A multidimensional assessment, including both product and process, is appropriate (Peterson, 2005). For example, if the primary purpose is to help students learn to work in teams, evaluating process using techniques that demonstrate growth in self-awareness, communication, and conflict resolution are appropriate. A variety of assessment strategies may be used. It is fairly common to have reflections or papers as a means to consider the outcomes. Group work or teamwork can be triangulated by looking at individual and group reports as well as observation by the faculty and the agency staff. In some cases, students may be asked to provide peer review. The assessment should also evaluate the measurable impact of the experience on the student as well as the impact on the agency, the preceptor, and the community served (Atchison et al., 2006). The students can be mentored by the faculty to help develop the assessment tools used for the service-learning project (La Lopa, 2005).

SUMMARY

There are many strategies to effectively assess learning outcomes in both the classroom and the clinical setting. Using more than one strategy will more fully demonstrate student outcome achievement. When using a nontraditional assessment strategy, the students should have the opportunity to practice before the activity is used for grading. The strategies addressed in this chapter include portfolios, reflections, papers, essays and essay tests, concept mapping, oral questioning, audio and video recordings, simulations, role play, and service learning. To select the best assessment strategy, faculty members must consider the purpose and setting of the assessment; the time required for preparation, implementation, and grading; the cost; and the advantages and disadvantages of each strategy. Although it requires time, energy, and persistence to plan assessment of student achievement of outcomes, the effort will ultimately benefit students and the patients they are preparing to serve.

Faculty who implement alternative assessment strategies will continue to increase the evidence base for best practices and contribute to the scholarship of teaching. The findings from assessment strategies can be used for a variety of purposes. The most obvious is to provide feedback to the learner and to revise instruction and learning activities. Evidence of critical thinking and therapeutic communication are a part of the systematic program assessment plan. In addition, assessment data are helpful for the individual faculty as evidence of teaching excellence. As nursing education meets current challenges, the refinement of assessment strategies will continue to expand in tandem with the development of teaching strategies, thereby contributing to the ever-increasing quality of education for nurses of the future.

REFLECTING ON THE EVIDENCE

1. Select a course or program outcome and determine an assessment and evaluation strategy for that outcome by applying the six steps discussed in the chapter.

2. Compare and contrast two different assessment and evaluation strategies and discuss their application in the classroom or clinical setting.

3. Identify ways to enhance the reliability and validity of assessment and evaluation strategies presented in the chapter. Construct a grading rubric for an assessment and evaluation strategy to be used to assess learning outcomes in a course.

Internet Resources Related to Chapter Content

ELECTRONIC PORTFOLIO WEB RESOURCES

http://bearlink.berkeley.edu/ePortfolio/ page48.html
http://ddp.alverno.edu/

CONCEPT MAPPING WEB RESOURCES

http://cord.org/txcollabnursing/onsite_ conceptmap.htm
http://hsc.unm.edu/consg/critical/concept_map. shtml

http://www.socialresearchmethods.net/ mapping/mapping.htm
http://cmap.ihmc.us/

SERVICE LEARNING WEB RESOURCES

http://www.compact.org/initiatives/ service-learning/
http://www.compact.org/disciplines/reflection/ structuring/
http://www.ohiocampuscompact.org/cffm/ custom/File/Recommended%20Reading%20 Jan%2009.pdf

REFERENCES

American Association of Colleges of Nursing (2008). Essentials of Baccalaureate Education. http://www.aacn.nche.edu/publications/positions/index.htmngelo, T. A. (1995). Reassessing (and defining) assessment. *The AAHE Bulletin, 48*(2), 7–9.

Atchison, C., Boatright, D., Merrigan, D., Quill, B., Whittaker, C., Vickery, A., & Aglipay, G. (2006). Demonstrating excellence in practice-based teaching for public health. *Journal of Public Health Management and Practice, 12*(1), 15–21.

Beach, R., & Marshall, J. (1991). *Teaching literature in the secondary school.* San Diego, CA: Harcourt.

Benner, P., Sutphen, M., Leonard, V., & Day, L. (2009). *Educating nurses: A call for radical transformation.* San Francisco, CA: Jossey-Bass.

Bentley, R., & Ellison, K. (2005). Impact of a service-learning project on nursing students. *Nursing Education Perspectives, 26*(5), 287–290.

Bevis, E. O., & Watson, J. (1989). *Toward a caring curriculum: A new pedagogy for nursing.* New York, NY: National League for Nursing.

Billig, S., & Eyler, J. (2003). *Deconstructing service-learning: Research exploring context, participation, and impacts.* Greenwich, CT: Information Age.

Billings, D. (2006). Journaling: A strategy for developing reflective practitioners. *Journal of Continuing Education in Nursing, 37*(3), 104–105.

Boud, D., & Falchikov, N. (2006). Aligning assessment with long-term learning. *Assessment and Evaluation in Higher Education, 31*(4), 399–413.

Branch, W. T. (2010). The road to professionalism: Reflective practice and reflective learning. *Patient Education and Counseling, 80*(3), 327–332.

Brookhart, S. M. (2005). Assessment theory for college classrooms. In M. V. Achacoso & M. D. Svinicki (Eds.), *Alternative strategies for evaluating student learning* (pp. 5–14). San Francisco, CA: Jossey-Bass.

Caputi, L. (2010). Using concept maps to foster critical thinking. In L. Caputi (Ed.), *Teaching nursing: The art and science* (2nd ed., Vol. 2, pp. 454–477). Glen Ellyn, IL: College of DuPage Press.

Courts, P. L., & McInerney, K. H. (1993). *Assessment in higher education: Politics, pedagogy, and portfolios.* Westport, CT: Praeger.

Davis, B. G. (2009). *Tools for teaching* (2nd ed.). San Francisco, CA: Jossey-Bass.

Dummer, T., Cook, I., Parker, S., Barrett, G., & Hull, A. (2008). Promoting and assessing "deep learning" in geography fieldwork: An evaluation of reflective field diaries. *Journal of Geography in Higher Education, 32*(3), 459–479.

Eisner, E. (1985). *The educational imagination* (2nd ed.). New York, NY: Macmillan.

Epstein, R., Siegel, D., & Silberman, J. (2008). Self-monitoring in clinical practice: A challenge for medical educators. *Journal of Continuing Education in the Health Professions, 28*(1), 513.

Garrett, B., MacPhee, M., & Jackson, C. (2010). High-fidelity patient simulation: Considerations for effective learning. *Nursing Education Perspectives, 31*(5), 309–313.

Goldenberg, D. (1994). Critiquing as a method of evaluation in the classroom. *Nurse Educator, 19*(4), 18–22.

Gordon, J. (2003). Assessing students' personal and professional development using portfolios and interviews. *Medical Education, 37*(4), 335–340.

Graf, M. A. (1993). Videotaping return demonstration. *Nurse Educator, 18*(4), 29.

Gronlund, N. E. (2006). *Assessment of student achievement* (8th ed.). Boston, MA: Allyn & Bacon.

Hansen, C. (1994). Questioning techniques for the active classroom. In D. F. Halpern (Ed.), *Changing college classrooms: New teaching and learning strategies for an increasingly complex world* (pp. 93–106). San Francisco, CA: Jossey-Bass.

Hill, C. (2006). Integrating clinical experiences into the concept mapping process. *Nurse Educator, 31*(1), 36–39.

Jeffries, P. (2007). *Simulation in nursing education: From conceptualization to evaluation.* New York, NY: National League for Nursing.

Jeffries, P., & McNelis, A. (2010). Evaluation. In W. M. Nehring & F. R. Lashley (Eds.), *High-fidelity patient simulation in nursing education* (pp. 405–424). Sudbury, MA: Jones & Bartlett.

Karlowicz, K. A. (2000). The value of student portfolios to evaluate undergraduate nursing programs. *Nurse Educator, 25*(2), 82–87.

Keefe, M.R. & Pesut, D. (2004). Appreciative inquiry and leadership transitions. *Journal of Professional Nursing. 20*(2), 103–109.

King, A. (1994). Inquiry as a tool in critical thinking. In D. F. Halpern (Ed.), *Changing college classrooms: New teaching and learning strategies for an increasingly complex world* (pp. 13–38). San Francisco, CA: Jossey-Bass.

King, M., & Shell, R. (2002). Teaching and evaluating critical thinking with concept maps. *Nurse Educator, 27*(5), 214–216.

Kirkpatrick, J., & Braswell, M. (2010). Service-learning. In L. Caputi (Ed.), *Teaching nursing: The art and science* (2nd ed., *Vol. 2*, pp. 879–899). Glen Ellyn, IL: College of DuPage Press.

Krathwohl, D. (2002). A revision of Bloom's taxonomy: An overview. *Theory into Practice, 41*(4), 212–218.

Krathwohl, D. R., Bloom, B. S., & Mases, B. (1964). *Taxonomy of educational objectives. Handbook II, affective domain.* New York, NY: David McKay.

La Lopa, J. M. (2005). Developing a student-based assessment tool for authentic assessment. In M. V. Achacoso & M. D. Svinicki (Eds.), *Alternative strategies for evaluating student learning* (pp. 31–36). Hoboken, NJ: Wiley.

Linn, R., & Gronlund, N. (2005). *Measurement and assessment in teaching.* Upper Saddle River, NJ: Prentice-Hall.

Mann, K., Gordon, J., & MacLeod, A. (2009). Reflection and reflective practice in health professions: A systematic review. *Advances in Health Science Education, 14*(4), 595–621.

Nehring, W. (2010). A synthesis of theory and nursing research using high-fidelity patient simulation. In W. M. Nehring & F. R. Lashley (Eds.), *High-fidelity patient simulation in nursing education* (pp. 27–56). Sudbury, MA: Jones & Bartlett.

National League for Nursing. Competencies. http://www. Nln. org/facultydevelopment/competencies/index.htm

Novak, J. D., & Cañas, A. (2008). *The theory underlying concept maps and how to construct and use them* (Technical Report IHMC Cmaptools 2006. 01 Rev 2008. 01). Pensacola, FL: Florida Institute for Human and Machine Cognition. Retrieved from http://cmap.ihmc.us/

Oermann, M., & Gaberson, K. (2009). *Evaluation and testing in nursing education* (3rd ed.). New York, NY: Springer.

Peterson, T. (2005). Assessing performance in problem-based service-learning projects. In M. V. Achacoso & M. D. Svinicki (Eds.), *Alternative strategies for evaluating student learning* (pp. 55–63). San Francisco, CA: Jossey-Bass.

Reed, S. J. (2010). Designing a simulation for student evaluation using Scriven's key evaluation checklist. *Clinical Simulation in Nursing, 6*(2), 41–44.

Rinne, C. (1994). The SKILLS system: A new interactive video technology. *THE Journal, 21*(8), 81–82.

Robertson, J., Rossetti, J., Peters, B., Coyner, S., Koren, M., Hertz, J., & Elder, S. (2010). Portfolio assessment: One school of nursing's experience. In L. Caputi (Ed.), *Teaching nursing: The art and science* (2nd ed., Vol. 2, pp. 525–558). Glen Ellyn, IL: College of DuPage Press.

Schuster, P. (2008). *Concept mapping: A critical thinking approach to care planning* (2nd ed.). Philadelphia, PA: F. A. Davis.

Stevens, D. D., & Levi, A. J. (2005). *Introduction to rubrics: An assessment tool to save grading time, convey effective feedback and promote students learning.* Sterling, VA: Stylus.

Sutton, S., & Koehler, C. (2010). Nursing process mapping. In M. Bradshaw & A. Lowenstein (Eds.), *Innovative teaching strategies in nursing and related health professions* (5th ed., pp. 423–436). Boston, MA: Jones & Bartlett.

Developing and Using Classroom Tests

Prudence Twigg, PhD(c), APRN-BC

Using teacher-made tests is one more strategy that nurse educators can use to assess outcomes of learning in didactic and clinical courses. Although developing classroom tests seems like a relatively straightforward task, it is a very involved process. The purpose of this chapter is to offer a step-by-step approach to planning, developing, administering, analyzing, and revising classroom tests.

Planning the Test

Developing a test that is valid (representative) and reliable (consistent) requires much thought and planning. The following section describes how to develop a test. This section covers the purpose of the test, criterion-referenced versus norm-referenced tests, development of a table of specifications, and how to improve the reliability and validity of a test.

Purpose of the Test

The first question that must be addressed is: "What purpose will the test serve?" If the test is to be given before instruction, it may be used to determine *readiness* (the grasp of prerequisite skills needed to be successful) or *placement* (the level of mastery of instructional objectives). During instruction, the test may be used as a *formative* evaluation of learning or as a diagnostic tool to identify learning problems. With the wide availability of test banks, such as those that accompany textbooks, and the ease of creating tests in a test-authoring component of a

learning management system, faculty can also use tests as a way for students to *practice* and *assess* their own learning. As measures of learning outcomes, tests provide *summative evaluation* of learning on which progression and *grading* decisions may be based. See Table 26-1 for a summary of test measures based on timing of administration.

Tests may serve a variety of additional functions. For example, testing may provide the structure (e.g., deadlines) that some students need to direct their learning activities or faculty may use testing as one means of evaluating teaching effectiveness by measuring the outcomes of student learning. Faculty may also use posttest reviews as a learning opportunity for students to discuss rationales for answers (Morrison & Free, 2001) and gain insight into their own strengths and weaknesses (Flannelly, 2001).

Types of Tests

Criterion-Referenced Tests

Criterion-referenced tests are those that are constructed and interpreted according to a specific set of learning outcomes (McDonald, 2008). This type of test is useful for measuring mastery of subject matter. An absolute standard of performance is set for grading purposes.

Norm-Referenced Tests

Norm-referenced tests are those that are constructed and interpreted to provide a relative ranking of students (McDonald, 2008). Norm-referenced tests are based on measurement of content according to a table of specifications (test map, test plan, test blueprint). This type of test is useful for measuring differential performance among students. A relative standard of performance is used for grading purposes.

The author acknowledges the work of Lori Rasmussen, MSN, RN, and Diana J. Speck, MSN, RN, in the previous edition(s) of the chapter.

TABLE 26-1 Test Measures Based on Timing of Administration

Timing	Type of Test	Measure
Before	Readiness	Prerequisite skills
	Placement	Previous learning
During	Formative	Learning progress
	Diagnostic	Learning problems
After	Summative	Terminal performance

TABLE 26-2 Bloom's Taxonomy with Action Verbs for the Cognitive Levels

Cognitive Level	Action Verbs
Knowledge	Define, identify, list
Comprehension	Describe, explain, summarize
Application	Apply, demonstrate, use
Analysis	Compare, contrast, differentiate
Synthesis	Construct, develop, formulate
Evaluation	Critique, evaluate, judge

TABLE 26-3 Anderson and Krathwohl's Taxonomy with Action Verbs for the Cognitive Processes

Cognitive Processes	Action Verbs
Remember	Retrieve, recognize, recall
Understand	Interpret, classify, summarize, infer, compare, explain, exemplify
Apply	Execute, implement
Analyze	Differentiate, organize, attribute
Evaluate	Check, critique
Create	Generate, plan, produce, reorganize

Both criterion- and norm-referenced tests may be used in nursing education. Criterion-referenced tests are frequently used to ensure safety in areas such as drug dosage calculation, in which the absolute standard of performance may be set as high as 100%, regardless of the performance of other students.

Table of Specifications

The purpose of developing a table of specifications (test map, test grid, test blueprint) is to ensure that the test serves its intended purpose by representatively sampling the intended learning outcomes and instructional content. The first step in developing a table of specifications is to define the specific learning outcomes to be measured. Specific learning outcomes, which are derived from more general instructional outcomes (e.g., course and unit objectives), specify tasks that students should be able to perform on completion of instruction (Miller, Linn, & Gronlund, 2009).

Bloom's taxonomy (1956) has been used as a guide for developing and leveling general instructional and specific learning outcomes (see Chapter 11 for details). Although the cognitive components of the affective and psychomotor domains can be evaluated with classroom tests, tests have most often been used to determine achievement of outcomes in the six levels of Bloom's cognitive domain (Table 26-2). Anderson and Krathwohl (2001) have revised Bloom's taxonomy, defining knowledge dimensions and cognitive processes. The knowledge dimensions are factual, conceptual, procedural, and metacognitive. The cognitive processes are remembering, understanding, applying, analyzing, evaluating, and creating (Table 26-3). Any of the six cognitive processes may be applied to the various dimensions of knowledge.

Additional attention is being given to those cognitive processing skills used by nurses, such as critical thinking, clinical judgment, and clinical decision making (Wendt & Harmes, 2009a). Test items should address these processes as well, and a mixture of cognitive processes should be evaluated at each stage of instruction, placing an increasing emphasis (or weight) on higher-level skills. This is vital because higher-level skills are more likely to result in retention and transfer of knowledge. In addition, this will assist in preparing students for the licensing and certification examinations that test primarily at the levels of application and analysis (National Council of State Boards of Nursing, 2010).

The second step in developing a table of specifications involves determining the instructional content to be evaluated and the weight to be assigned to each area. This can be accomplished by developing a content outline and using the amount of time spent teaching the material as an indicator for weighting (Table 26-4).

TABLE 26-4 Content Outline and Relative Teaching Time

	Content	Teaching Time (%)	No. of Items/Section*
I.	Antipsychotic agents	25	10
II.	Antianxiety agents	25	10
III.	Antidepressant agents	25	10
IV.	Antimanic agents	12.5	5
V.	Antiparkinson agents	12.5	5
Totals		100	40

*Percentage of teaching time × Total no. of items = No. of items/section.

weight, whereas all stages may be tested equally by the end of instruction. Tables 26-6 and 26-7 are examples of three-way tables of specifications.

Alternatively, or additionally, a table of specifications can be created by using the test plan of the current licensure examination (NCLEX-RN). The NCLEX-RN tests content in four categories of client needs as follows (National Council of State Boards of Nursing, 2010):
1. Safe, effective care environment
2. Health promotion and maintenance
3. Psychosocial integrity
4. Physiological integrity

In addition to the category of client needs, the NCLEX-RN integrates concepts and processes of nursing practice (nursing process, caring, communication and documentation, self-care, teaching and learning) throughout the questions. One possible disadvantage of using the NCLEX-RN test plan in a table of specifications for development of a classroom test is that the content of most nursing courses is not organized according to these categories.

Other Considerations in the Planning Stage

Selecting Item Types

Items may be *selection-type*, providing a set of responses from which to choose, or *supply-type*, or a constructed response type requiring the student to provide an answer. Common selection-type items include true–false, matching, ordered-response, and multiple-choice questions. Supply-type items include fill-in-the blank (usually requiring an absolute answer derived from a mathematical calculation),

Finally, a two-way grid is developed, with content areas being listed down the left side and learning outcomes being listed across the top of the grid (Table 26-5). Each cell is assigned a number of questions according to the weighting of content and cognitive processes of learning outcomes.

Some faculty prefer to use a three-way table of specifications. With a three-way grid, the five steps of the nursing process are listed on the left side, outcomes are listed across the top, and the number of items or specific content areas is listed within each cell. Weighting of the steps of the nursing process again depends on the level of instruction. For example, early in the instructional process, assessment and diagnosis might carry the most

TABLE 26-5 Two-Way Table of Specifications

Outcomes* (Content†)	Remember (20%)	Understand (40%)	Apply (40%)	Totals
Antipsychotic agents (25%)	2	4	4	10
Antianxiety agents (25%)	2	4	4	10
Antidepressant agents (25%)	2	4	4	10
Antimanic agents (12.5%)	1	2	2	5
Antiparkinson agents (12.5%)	1	2	2	5
Totals	8	16	16	40

* Arbitrarily determined by level of instruction.
† Percent determined by teaching time.

TABLE 26-6 Three-Way Table of Specifications: Number of Items per Cell

Outcomes*(Content†)	Remember (20%)	Understand (40%)	Apply (40%)	Totals
Assessment (40%)	6	6	4	16
Diagnosis (10%)	1	3	—	4
Planning (10%)	1	2	1	4
Intervention (20%)	—	2	6	8
Evaluation (20%)	—	3	5	8
Totals	8	16	16	40

* Arbitrarily determined by level of instruction.
† Percent determined by teaching time.

TABLE 26-7 Three-Way Table of Specifications: Content to Be Tested per Cell*

Outcomes*(Content†)	Remember (20%)	Understand (40%)	Apply (40%)	Totals
Assessment (40%)	P, A, A, D, D, M	P, P, A, D, M, PA	P, A, D, PA	16
Diagnosis (10%)	P	A, D, M	—	4
Planning (10%)	PA	A, D	P	4
Intervention (20%)	—	P, A	P, A, A, D, M, PA	8
Evaluation (20%)	—	P, PA, D	P, A, D, D, M	8
Totals	8	16	16	40

A, Antianxiety agents; D, antidepressant agents; M, antimanic agents; P, antipsychotic agents; PA, antiparkinson agents.
* No. of each type of content item determined by teaching time.
† Percent determined by teaching time.

short-answer, multiple-response, hotspot, and essay questions (Wendt & Kenny, 2009).

The primary reason for choosing one type of item over another can be determined by answering the question: "Which type of item most directly measures the intended learning outcome?" Both selection-type and supply-type questions can be developed for all levels of the cognitive domain (Su, Osisek, Montgomery, & Pellar, 2009) and to test critical thinking, problem solving, and clinical decision-making skills. Other factors may also influence the item-type selection. For example, a large class size may prohibit the use of supply-type items because of the time required for grading.

In addition to multiple-choice items with one correct answer, the NCLEX-RN uses alternative format questions, which include fill-in-the-blank questions, multiple-response questions, drag-and-drop or ordered-response questions, picture or graphic questions, as well as questions that use audio files; using video clips in test questions is under consideration (Wendt & Harmes, 2009a). Current information on the examination format can be obtained at the website for the National Council of State Boards of Nursing (www.ncsbn.org).

Selecting Item Difficulty

Item difficulty primarily depends on the purpose of the test. If it is a criterion-referenced test, difficulty should match the level of the learning that reflects the skills to be mastered. Norm-referenced tests involve eliminating easy items and using average-difficulty items to maximize the differences among students.

Determining Number of Items

Test reliability usually increases with the number of test items. However, the number of test items is limited by many practical constraints. For example, more selection-type items than supply-type items can be answered in a given period. Similarly, items that require higher-level thinking skills take more time to answer than those that require lower-level skills.

A general guide for planning is to allow 1 minute for each moderately difficult multiple-choice item. For a 60-minute class, a test with about 50 items is appropriate (McDonald, 2008).

Writing Test Items

Writing items for true–false, matching, interpretive, short-answer, multiple-choice, and alternative format tests requires time and skill. The definitions, advantages, disadvantages, guidelines for writing, and examples of each of these types of test items follow.

True–False Items

Definition

A true–false or binary choice question is a declarative sentence that the student must determine to be true or false (Oermann & Gaberson, 2009).

Advantages

1. Faculty can sample more information about a topic using this format.
2. The student can complete more of these items in a given period.
3. This type of item works well when there are only two alternatives.
4. Scoring is easy and objective.

Disadvantages

1. Students' scores are influenced by guessing. By chance alone, a student could get a score of 50% on a test.
2. This item type encourages memorization of text or lectures.
3. A true–false item presents two extremes that rarely match up with the real world.
4. Marking a question "false" does not mean the student knows what is really true.
5. It is difficult to write this item type at the higher levels of cognitive processes.

Guidelines for Writing True–False Items

1. Avoid the use of absolute terms such as "all" or "always," which indicate that the item is false. Likewise, qualifiers such as "sometimes" or "typically" indicate that the item is true.

2. State the item in a positive, declarative sentence, as simply as possible.
3. Avoid negative and double-negative statements.
4. Keep true and false statements equal in length.
5. Randomize the true and false items so the student will not detect a pattern.
6. Write each item so it is clearly true or clearly false.
7. Credit opinions to a source if understanding of beliefs is being measured.
8. Do not include two concepts in one statement.

Examples

Read the following statements and decide whether they are true or false. Circle T for true and F for false.
1. T F Oxytocin is released from the anterior pituitary gland.
2. T F Lochia rubra is a normal finding for the tenth postpartum day.

Matching Items

Definition

A matching item consists of two parallel lists of words that require the student to match according to certain associations between the two lists. One column consists of problems (premises); the other contains answers (responses) (Oermann & Gaberson, 2009).

Advantages

1. A matching item is compact so a great deal of information can be tested on a single page.
2. The items can be scored quickly and objectively.
3. Students can respond to a large number of these items because reading time is short.
4. Students are required to integrate knowledge to discover the relationship.

Disadvantages

1. These items can be difficult to write without including unintended clues.
2. Questions of this nature tend to be restricted to lower-level cognitive processes.
3. It is difficult to generate enough plausible responses.

Guidelines for Writing Matching Items

1. The items being matched should be homogeneous. Otherwise the student can quickly find the correct responses.
2. The entire set of matching items should be on a single page to eliminate page turning.

3. Use a larger or smaller set of responses and permit them to be used more than once or not at all.
4. Arrange items in a systematic order to make the selection process quicker.
5. State in the directions the basis of relationship for matching.
6. Place the stimulus column on the left with each item numbered and the response column on the right with each item lettered.

Example

Column A contains statements by the nurse. Column B is the type of communication. On the line to the left of the items in column A, write the letter of the item in column B that best matches. Responses in column B may be used once, more than once, or not at all.

Column A: Statements	Column B: Communication Type
_____ 1. "I'm here if you need me."	A. Checking perceptions
_____ 2. "What do you think about it?"	B. Defending
_____ 3. "I'm sure he knows that."	C. Exploring
_____ 4. "Tell me more about that."	D. Offering self
	E. Probing

Interpretive Items

Definition

An interpretive item requires a response based on introductory material such as a paragraph, table, chart, map, or picture (Miller, Linn, & Gronlund, 2009). The student must make a judgment about the material presented. These items are often used on nursing examinations to evaluate a student's ability to interpret laboratory data, electrocardiogram or fetal monitor strips, or other pictorial items. The questions of the NCLEX-RN examination use charts and graphic or pictorial items that may require interpretation.

Advantages

1. Use of interpretative items is a way to measure a student's ability to understand printed information.
2. More complex cognitive processes can be measured.
3. Scoring is easy and objective.

Disadvantages

1. It is difficult to construct effective items.
2. Items may contain unintended clues.
3. Interpretative items do not measure a student's ability to express ideas.

Guidelines for Writing Interpretive Items

1. Keep the printed information brief and readable.
2. Phrase the question so it can be answered in either short-answer or multiple-choice format.
3. Present introductory material before the question.
4. Keep elements of items on the same page.

Examples

Complete the following:
1. [insert labor graph]
   How long did the first stage of labor last?

   _____

   How long was the transition phase?

   _____

2. [insert laboratory data]
   For which laboratory value, in a patient about to go to surgery, should the nurse notify the physician?
   1. hematocrit
   2. hemoglobin
      platelets
   3. white blood cell count
3. [insert electrocardiogram strip]
   What arrhythmia does the patient have?

   _____

Chart and Exhibit Questions

Definition

These questions, another example of interpretive questions, assess the test-taker's ability to seek and use data presented on a client's chart. The data will be presented from one or more chart "tabs": prescriptions, history and physical, laboratory results, miscellaneous reports, imaging results, flow sheets, intake and output, medication administration record, progress notes, and vital signs. When the test is administered by computer, the test-taker will be required to search in a way that simulates search through a client's chart or computerized patient record. The current NCLEX-RN examination includes chart and exhibit questions (National Council of State Boards of Nursing, 2010).

Advantages

1. Tests the ability to consider which data are needed for client care.
2. Tests in higher levels of cognitive domain.
3. Requires test-takers to use data for clinical decision making.
4. Requires test-takers to interpret a set of data, for example, trend data on a vital signs record.
5. Simulates obtaining data from a client's chart; test-takers can be timed to ascertain whether they know what data to obtain and where on a chart to find it.

Disadvantages

1. Chart and exhibit questions are time consuming to develop.
2. Chart and exhibit questions may require duplicating chart forms to develop the test questions.

Example

A parent has brought a 4-month-old to the immunization clinic. The nurse is reviewing the immunization record on the progress notes (see below).

Progress Notes

11/1/2011 1-month well-child visit; administered HepB #1

12/3/2011 2-month well-child visit; administered DTaP #1, IPV #1

The parent asks the nurse which immunizations the baby will receive on this visit. The nurse should tell the parent that the infant will receive which of the following? (Select all that apply.)

1. DTaP #3
2. HepB #2
3. IPV #2
4. MMR #1
5. Varicella

Short-Answer and Fill-in-the-Blank Questions

Definition

The short-answer or fill-in-the-blank item requires the student to produce an answer (Miller, Linn, & Gronlund, 2009). The question can be answered in one or two words. This item type is used when the instructor wants the student to recall or calculate the answer (fill in the blank). The student could also be asked to visually represent the answer; for example, "Calculate a drug dosage, then mark the answer on a picture of a syringe." Fill-in-the blank questions are used on the licensing exam; the test-taker provides one answer that can be noted to be either correct or incorrect.

Advantages

1. This item type reduces guessing.
2. This item type works well for math problems because it requires the student to work out the answer.
3. A broad range of material can be tested.

Disadvantages

1. It is difficult to phrase the question so there is only one correct answer.
2. Scoring can be time consuming because the student may supply an answer the instructor had not considered.
3. The student's spelling can make it difficult to score.

Guidelines for Writing Short-Answer and Fill-in-the-Blank Items

1. Write completion items that can be answered with one word or number.
2. Phrase statements or questions so there is only one correct answer.
3. Avoid giving grammatical clues to the answer (e.g., use of *a* or *an*).
4. Keep the length of the blanks the same.
5. Do not take statements directly from the text or lecture; this encourages memorization.
6. If spelling is a problem, a list of words from which to choose can be provided.
7. For math problems, indicate how precise the answer should be; indicate if the answer should be "rounded" or if the answer should be presented in milliliters or ounces.

Examples

Supply the appropriate word to answer the question or complete the sentence.

1. Using the Apgar scoring system as a guide, fill in the blanks to complete the score for a newborn with the following characteristics:

Characteristic	Score
a. Active motion of extremities	_____
b. Crying, good respirations	_____

Characteristic	Score
c. Heart rate greater than 100	_____
d. Pink color, blue extremities	_____
e. Vigorous cry	_____
Total	_____

2. The nurse is to give morphine elixir, 4 mg, sublingually. The drug available is morphine, 20 mg/mL. How much should the nurse give? (Round to the nearest tenth.)

_____ mg

3. What is the antidote for warfarin (Coumadin)? _____

4. Which serum laboratory value is the best indicator of renal function? _____

Hotspot (Rollover) Questions

Definition

Hotspot questions ask the test-taker to locate a specific "spot" on a chart or figure. While the questions can be developed and administered in paper-and-pencil formats, they are more effectively developed for computer-administered examinations in which the test-taker can use the mouse to "roll over" the correct spot on the chart or figure. When these questions are administered by the computer, the test-taker uses the mouse to "roll over" the area that is the correct answer and, once located, to click on the mouse to identify the answer choice. The NCLEX-RN examination includes hotspot questions (National Council of State Boards of Nursing, 2010).

Advantages

1. Provides an easy way to test understanding and application of anatomical knowledge.
2. Offers an effective way to test understanding of physical assessment techniques.
3. Used to test procedures and nursing skills with correct or incorrect positioning.

Disadvantages

1. Most effective in computer applications where a mouse can be used to "roll over" to identify the "hotspot."
2. Hotspot questions may be more difficult to develop due to the need to have an illustration as a reference point.

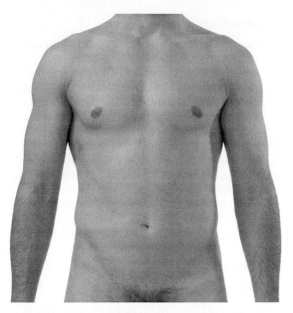

From Wilson, S. F., & Giddins, J. F. (2008). *Health assessment for nursing practice* (4th ed.). St. Louis, MO: Mosby.

Example

A client has not voided for 10 hours. Identify the anatomical area where the nurse should assess for bladder distension.

Drag-and-Drop and Ordered-Response Questions

Definition

These questions require the test-taker to place information in a specified order. For example, questions can be developed to ask the test-taker to put steps of a procedure in order or, given a set of clients, to determine priorities for nursing care. On the licensing examination, candidates will "drag" each response in the left column and "drop" it into the correct order in the right column (National Council of State Boards of Nursing, 2010).

Advantages

1. Evaluates test-takers' understanding of the order for steps of a procedure or how to set priorities for a client or groups of clients.
2. Relatively easy to develop.
3. When writing for paper-and-pencil tests, the order can be "scrambled" and the item writer can pose four or more possible sequences.

Disadvantages

1. May be confusing for test-takers to order all of the steps or priorities.
2. Steps, sequences, and priorities may be controversial or context-specific; thus the item needs to be structured such that experts will agree on the correct order, correct answer, and rationale.

Example

A client begins to have a seizure. The nurse should do which of the following in order from first to last?
1. Note the time.
2. Notify the physician.
3. Protect the client from injury.
4. Obtain a history of events prior to the seizure.

Graphic Items

Definition

Graphic items use photographs or illustrations in the question or in the answer options. The test-taker responds to details in the graphic to answer the question, or chooses the answer by selecting the correct answer from four different graphics.

Advantages

1. Tests assessment and evaluation skills.
2. Tests clinical decision making.

Disadvantages

1. Requires use of art; expense could be involved to obtain images of incorrect responses.
2. Time consuming to develop.

Example

The nurse is evaluating a client who has just been instructed on how to walk with crutches. The nurse should instruct the client (see figure) to:
1. Lean forward 30 degrees.
2. Pad the tops of the crutches.
3. Keep the arms on the rungs of the crutches as shown.
4. Lower the head to watch for objects on the floor.

Audio and Video Items

Definition

In audio and video items, an audio or video clip is used as a stimulus in a part of the question or answer. The student clicks on the icon that brings

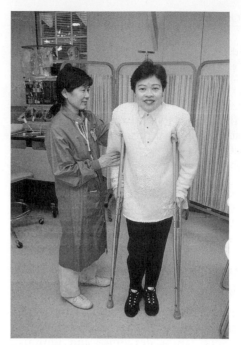

From Ignatavicius, D. D. (2009). *Medical-surgical nursing: Patient-centered collaborative care* (6th ed.). Philadelphia, PA: W. B. Saunders Company.

up the file. The NCLEX-RN exam currently uses audio item types and is exploring the use of video item types (Wendt & Harmes, 2009a, 2009b).

Advantages

1. Tests students' ability to identify sounds or respond to video information and make a clinical judgment based on information provided in the audio or video file.
2. Test questions can be written at higher levels of the cognitive domain and require students to synthesize data from the scenario and the data provided in the audio or video file.
3. Tests competencies that may be difficult to assess with other test item formats.

Disadvantages

1. Audio and video items can be administered only in a computer-managed environment that supports access to the audio and video files.
2. Finding access to no-cost or low-cost files may be difficult; purchase of files may be necessary as copyright protections must be observed.

Example

The nurse is assessing the breath sounds of a client who is hospitalized with bacterial pneumonia. Click here to listen to the breath sounds. [The sounds are course crackles.] The nurse should do which of the following first? [Note: The correct answer is dependent on the test-taker correctly identifying the breath sound and selecting the appropriate nursing action.]

1. Have the client to take a deep breath and cough to expectorate retained secretions.
2. Encourage the client to drink one glass of fluids every hour.
3. Check the blood levels of the antibiotic the client is receiving.
4. Tell the client the breath sounds are clear and to continue the deep-breathing exercises.

Multiple-Choice Items

Definition

A multiple-choice item consists of a *scenario*, which provides data about a client situation; a *stem*, which can be a question or an incomplete statement; and options (answers), one of which is correct and three of which are incorrect (distractors). Multiple-choice items, when carefully constructed, can measure critical thinking and higher levels of the cognitive domain (McDonald, 2008; Morrison & Free, 2001; Su et al., 2009).

Advantages

1. Multiple-choice items allow the faculty to sample a large amount of content in a single test.
2. Test items can be scored easily and objectively.
3. Scores on multiple-choice tests are less influenced by guessing than are scores on true–false tests.
4. These items are versatile because they can measure learning of several levels of cognitive processes.

Disadvantages

1. Writing good items with plausible distractors can be time consuming.
2. This item type takes more time for the student to read and understand.
3. These items may discriminate against the creative, verbal student.

4. Scores can be affected by students' reading ability and the instructor's writing style.
5. This item type can raise the score of the student who can recognize rather than produce the correct answer.
6. It is difficult to write multiple-choice items at the evaluation and creation levels.

Guidelines for Writing Multiple-Choice Items

Scenario

1. Present a single problem in the scenario.
2. Include relevant and irrelevant data to test students' ability to differentiate significant data.
3. Specify age, gender, ethnicity, or race only when essential to answering the question.
4. Do not use names for clients.

Stem

1. Poses the question; can be a complete or an incomplete sentence; can ask for priorities such as what the nurse should do should first.
2. Should be clear enough to answer without looking at the options.
3. Write the stem in a precise manner. If it is too complex, the student will spend too much time trying to decipher it.
4. State the stem in a positive rather than a negative manner. Highlight (underline, italicize, or use bold font for) key words such as *not, never, first,* and *next.*
5. Use action verbs that are consistent with the cognitive process being measured.

Answers and Options

1. Keep all options grammatically consistent with the stem to avoid giving clues to the correct option.
2. Arrange the options in either alphabetical or numerical order.
3. Keep the options the same length or have two short responses and two long responses.
4. Make all the options reasonable and homogenous.
5. Use only one best answer on which all authorities would agree.
6. Avoid the use of "all of the above" or "none of the above." Students can often guess the correct answer with only partial knowledge.

Examples

Remembering

Which of the following supplements for a woman of childbearing age will help prevent neural tube defects in the developing embryo?
1. calcium
2. folic acid
3. iron
4. vitamin C

Understanding

A 98-year-old woman lives in a nursing home. Based on activity theory, which of the following would probably be the most enjoyable for her?
1. completing a craft project on her own
2. reading a book in her room
3. visiting with friends
4. watching television

Applying

Patient teaching for enteric-coated drugs should include which statement by the nurse?
1. "Always take the medication whole."
2. "Avoid taking this medication with water."
3. "Lie down after taking this medication."
4. "This medication is likely to irritate your stomach."

Analyzing

A 78-year-old is admitted to the hospital because of severe diarrhea. The client is thirsty and skin turgor is poor. The blood pressure is 92/64 and pulse is 100. The serum sodium (Na^+) level is 165 mmol/L. The primary goal of nursing care for this client is to:
1. protect the skin from friction.
2. increase fluids.
3. prevent excoriation of the rectal area.
4. place the client on "falls alert."

Multiple-Response Items

Definition

A multiple-response item, like a multiple-choice item, has a stem and options; however, the options are written so that several of the responses are correct. Students should be instructed to choose all correct responses to receive credit for the question.

Advantages

1. Multiple-response items allow for several correct answers and require students to cluster correct responses.

2. There is less opportunity for choosing options by process of elimination than with standard multiple-choice items.
3. The use of multiple-response items avoids "all of the above" as an option.

Disadvantages

1. Multiple-response items require more options (usually five or six) and thus more distractors than standard multiple-choice items.
2. Scoring, particularly by computer, may be more difficult.

Guidelines for Writing Multiple-Response Items

For the stem, use the same general guidelines as for writing multiple-choice items. For the options, use the same general guidelines but include at least two correct responses and at least one incorrect response.

Examples

Remembering

The patient is taking digoxin (Lanoxin). For which of the following toxic effects of this drug should the nurse monitor? (Select all that apply.)
1. anorexia
2. dyspnea
3. hives
4. nausea
5. tachycardia
6. visual changes

Understanding

The patient is on a clear liquid diet. Which of the following foods and fluids are allowed? (Select all that apply.)
1. bouillon
2. gelatin
3. milk
4. orange juice
5. pudding
6. water

Applying

The nurse is the first to arrive on the scene of an auto accident and finds an unconscious man still in the driver's seat. The man's left femur is protruding through the skin. Which of the following actions should the nurse take? (Select all that apply.)
1. Assess airway, breathing, and circulation.
2. Call for emergency assistance.
3. Check for bleeding.

4. Move the left leg to align the bone.
5. Place a tourniquet high on the left thigh.
6. Remove the man from the car.

Evaluating

The nurse implements a medication safety teaching plan for the community-dwelling older adult. Which statements by the patient indicate that the teaching has been effective? (Select all that apply.)
1. "I will throw away any medications I am no longer using."
2. "I will have my prescriptions filled at different pharmacies to get the best price."
3. "I will tell my physician about any nonprescription medications I am taking."
4. "I will crush any medications that I have difficulty swallowing."
5. "I will take all of my medications with food to avoid stomach upset."
6. "I will report possible side effects of my medications to my physician."

Using Test Banks and Test-Authoring Systems

Faculty should attempt to create a large pool of questions from which the items for a specific test can be drawn. While time consuming to amass a large number of questions, the effort is rewarded by being able to administer different versions of the test or to generate a "makeup" test for students who were not able to take the test at a regularly scheduled time. Having the test items available in a word-processing file makes revision of the test easier. All test files should be secured in password-protected areas of a file server.

Many textbook publishers provide test items free of charge to faculty adopting their texts. Often these test items are written to test specific knowledge presented in the various chapters of the textbook, are written at lower levels of the cognitive domain, and do not test critical thinking or clinical judgment skills (Clifton & Schriner, 2010). If using these test items, faculty must review them for fit with their learning outcomes and test blueprints. Faculty can revise these questions to test at higher cognitive levels and to meet the needs of a particular course.

The task of creating test items can be simplified by using computerized test development software that typically is included as a component of a learning management system (see Chapter 23). This software can facilitate test development by creating a collection of test items (test bank) from which faculty can select appropriate questions according to the test blueprint. Alternate forms of tests can also be generated because the item pool can be large enough so that questions can be selected randomly. Some test-authoring software can be used for online testing in a computer classroom or on the Internet, thus simplifying the test administration process.

Editing Test Items

After test items have been developed, it is necessary to edit them and make any needed corrections. At this stage, peer review of the questions is helpful for refining the questions, ensuring accuracy and readability, reviewing the test items for fairness and cultural sensitivity (Wendt, Kenny, & Riley, 2009), and eliminating grammatical errors. This editing can be done in a question or checklist format. Questions to consider include the following:
1. Are items stated in a precise manner?
2. Do items match the table of specifications?
3. Is there one best answer for each item (except for multiple-response items)?
4. Does each item stand alone?
5. Are sentence construction and punctuation correct?
6. Have stereotyping, prejudices, and biases been eliminated?
7. Have "slang" or words with several meanings been eliminated?
8. Does the question eliminate gender bias, such as referring to the nurse as "she"?
9. Has the use of humor been avoided?
10. Has extraneous information been deleted?
11. Has a colleague reviewed the test?
12. Is the placement of correct options varied so there is no obvious pattern?

Potential Bias in Test Items

Students of equal ability should have an equal probability of correctly answering a test item. If systematic differences in responses to an item exist among members of particular groups, independent of total scores, then the item may be biased. Bosher (2003) classifies potential areas of bias in test items in four categories: testwise flaws, irrelevant difficulty, linguistic or structural bias, and cultural bias. Testwise flaws are those errors in items that provide cues to the correct answer within the item or test itself, thus potentially providing an unfair advantage to students with more test-taking experience or training and to native English speakers who can more easily recognize grammatical and other cues. Items with irrelevant difficulty may be missed for reasons related more to format (e.g., unclear stems, superfluous information, negative phrasing) than to content. Similarly, linguistic complexity, grammatical errors, and inconsistent word use may result in biased items. Finally, items that depend on culturally specific knowledge should not be used unless cultural practices per se are the domain of the question. The guidelines for writing items are designed to avoid bias.

Assembling and Administering a Test

Once the items are written and edited, they must be assembled into a test. This step includes arranging the items, writing test directions, reproducing the test, and administering the test (McDonald, 2008).

Arranging Items

Once items have been selected and edited, the next step is to decide how items will be arranged on the test. For the purposes of enhancing thought tracking, increasing student confidence, and preventing students from becoming anxious about early items, the following guidelines are suggested:
1. Group similar item types together (e.g., all true–false items).
2. Place items within each group in ascending order of difficulty.
3. Place item types in ascending order of difficulty (e.g., true–false items first, essay items last).
4. Begin the test with an easy question.

Writing Test Directions

Test directions should be self-explanatory and include the following information:
1. *Purpose of the test*: This may not need to be included if it has been addressed earlier in the instructional process.
2. *Time allotted to complete the test*: This information allows the students to pace themselves when responding to items.

3. *Basis for responding*: This provides the student with information necessary to choose the appropriate response (e.g., choose only one answer; matching options can be used more than once).
4. *Recording answers*: Answers may be recorded in a variety of ways to expedite grading (e.g., recording answers on a computer sheet using a No. 2 pencil, marking an X through the correct answer on a separate answer sheet for stencil grading, marking answers directly on the test booklet in the left column).
5. *Guessing*: Encouraging students to answer all questions prevents the inflation of scores of bolder students as a result of guessing.
6. *Value assigned to items*: This information allows the student to effectively plan the use of his or her time.

Example

Circle the one best answer. Because your score is the total number of correct answers, you should answer all questions. Each question is worth 2 points. You have 50 minutes to complete this 50-item test.

Reproducing the Test

The test should be easy to read and follow. The following guidelines are suggested:
1. Use standard font and type size; observe guidelines for page layout and use of white space.
2. Space items evenly.
3. Number items consecutively.
4. Keep an item's stem and options on the same page.
5. Place introductory material (e.g., graph or chart) before item (and make sure it reproduces clearly).
6. Keep matching lists on the same page.
7. Proofread the test after it is compiled but before it is duplicated.

Administering the Test and Maintaining Security during the Test

The physical environment should be conducive to the task. This includes adequate lighting, a comfortable temperature, sufficient workspace, and minimal interruptions. To reduce student anxiety, the faculty member should maintain a positive, nonthreatening attitude and avoid unnecessary conversation before and during the test. Faculty should avoid giving unintentional hints to individual students who ask for clarification of questions during the test.

In recent years, maintaining a secure test environment has become a challenge (DiBartolo & Walsh, 2010). Some suggestions for reducing cheating include the following:

1. Maintain test security (e.g., lock up copies of the test). Number tests and make sure all copies of tests are returned to the instructor before students leave the classroom.
2. Modify tests from one semester to another.
3. State the consequences of cheating early in the instructional process and inform students of academic honesty policies at the time of testing.
4. Require that book bags, cell phones, and items of clothing such as hats in which "cheat sheets" can be stored be brought to the front of the room.
5. Monitor students consistently throughout testing; depending on class size, additional proctors may be necessary.
6. Designate special seating arrangements (e.g., have an empty chair between students; have students sit in alphabetical order).
7. Use alternate versions of the test.
8. Use alternative answer forms (e.g., listing responses down the page, listing responses across the page).
9. Use secured and proctored computer testing centers.

See Chapter 23 for information about maintaining security for online tests.

Analyzing Test Results

Once the test has been administered and scored, faculty should review the results using concepts of measurement and data analysis. On the basis of these findings, faculty assign grades. Faculty at most schools of nursing have access to test scoring services that calculate test statistics and provide item analysis. Although there may be a fee associated with the service, the data provided by test scoring services are helpful, particularly for the first few times the test is used. Faculty should seek the assistance of these services and the consultation that can be obtained at testing centers.

Concepts of Measurement

Validity

According to the *Standards for Educational and Psychological Testing* (American Education Research Association, American Psychological Association, & National Council on Measurement in Education, 1999), the concept of validity refers to the appropriateness, meaningfulness, and usefulness of inferences made from test scores. Validity is the judgment made about a test's ability to measure what it is intended to measure. This judgment is based on three categories of evidence: content-related, criterion-related, and construct-related.

Content-related patterns of evidence should show that the test adequately samples relevant content (Popham, 1999). In nursing education, the relevant content is defined by nurse educators, the course, and the profession. Some examples of content-related evidence of validity are correspondence of the test content with the following:

1. The table of specifications
2. Professional judgments of peers
3. Core material as defined by professional organizations
4. Standards of care as defined by agencies and professional organizations

Criterion-related patterns of evidence should show that the test adequately measures performance, either concurrently or predictively (Popham, 1999). The performance must be compared with some criterion variable. Nurse educators may use performance on the licensing examination (NCLEX-RN or NCLEX-LPN) as the criterion variable (pass or fail).

Construct-related patterns of evidence should show a relationship between test performance and some "quality" to be measured (Popham, 1999). This is a broad category of evidence that must include specifics about the test (from the content and criterion categories) in addition to a description of the quality or construct being measured.

Some of the factors that may adversely affect test validity are unclear directions, inconsistent or inadequate sampling from the table of specifications, poorly written test items, and subjective scoring (McDonald, 2008). Careful preparation of the test can improve test validity.

Reliability

Reliability refers to the ability of a test to provide dependable and consistent scores. A judgment about reliability can be made based on the extent to which two similar measures agree. Reliability is a necessary but not sufficient condition for validity. However, reliability may be high even with no validity (Popham, 1999). Nurse educators look for evidence to judge tests as both reliable and valid.

According to Lyman (1997), among the factors that may adversely affect test reliability are insufficient length and insufficient group variability. For the purpose of increasing reliability, a minimum test length of 25 multiple-choice questions with an item difficulty sufficient to ensure heterogenous performance of the group is sufficient for classroom testing.

Reliability could be measured by giving the same test to the same group and noting the correspondence (test-retest method) or by giving "equivalent" tests to the same group. Both of these methods have major disadvantages for classroom testing and are not generally used by nurse educators. Reliability can be measured with a single test administration by using either the split-half or internal consistency method. The split-half method separately scores responses to odd and even questions and then compares the "odd-question" score to the "even-question" score. The internal consistency of a test can be calculated by using one of the Kuder-Richardson formulas, as described by Popham (1999). Many computer grading programs supply a test reliability coefficient as part of the results (Fig. 26-1).

Reliability is measured on a scale of 0 to 1.00. A reliability coefficient of 1.00 would represent 100% correspondence between two tests or measures. Many standardized tests have reliability coefficients of 0.9 or higher. A reliability coefficient in the range of 0.7 to 0.8 is acceptable for classroom tests. For the test results shown in Figure 26-1, the reliability coefficient is 0.844, indicating good internal consistency of the test. Measures of test reliability are based on the assumption that all students had adequate

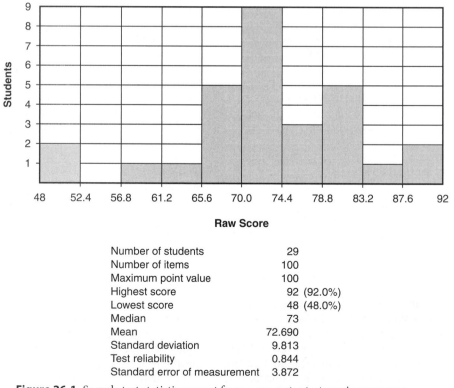

Number of students	29
Number of items	100
Maximum point value	100
Highest score	92 (92.0%)
Lowest score	48 (48.0%)
Median	73
Mean	72.690
Standard deviation	9.813
Test reliability	0.844
Standard error of measurement	3.872

Figure 26-1 Sample test statistics report from a computer test scoring program.

time to answer all questions and that all test items are of about the same difficulty. Because the reliability coefficient functions better when the variability of scores is maximized, tests administered to smaller groups of students (N) may have lower reliability coefficients.

Test Statistics

Various test statistics can be calculated, generated by test-authoring software, or reported from computer scoring services (see Fig. 26-1). These statistics help faculty interpret test results and provide data for item revision. Test grading software typically provides students' raw and percentage scores, individual student reports, and test statistics such as central tendencies and test reliability indices as well as item analysis data.

Raw Score

The raw score is the number of test questions answered correctly. Raw scores are the most accurate test scores but yield limited information. A frequency distribution can be used to arrange raw scores to create class intervals. If tests are scored by computer, a frequency polygon is likely. The percentage score compares the raw score with the maximum possible score.

$$\text{Percent score} = \frac{\text{Raw score (x)}}{\text{Maximum possible score}}$$

Central Tendency

Central tendency is a descriptive statistic for a set of scores. Measures of central tendency include the mean, median, and mode. The mean (or average) has the advantage of ease of calculation. The mean is calculated as the sum of all scores divided by the total number of scores.

$$\text{Mean (m)} = \frac{\text{Sum of all scores (x's)}}{\text{Number of scores (N)}}$$

The median divides the scores in the middle (i.e., 50% of scores fall below the median and 50% of scores are above the median). The median is a better measure of central tendency than the mean if the scores are not normally distributed.

Variability

Variability refers to the dispersion of scores and is thus a measure of group heterogeneity. Variability of scores affects other statistics. For example, low variability (homogeneity of scores) will tend to lower reliability coefficients such as the Kuder-Richardson coefficient (Lyman, 1997). Relative grading scales are most meaningful when they are applied to a wide range of scores. Mastery tests, by design, may show little variability. As groups of students progress in a nursing program, there may be less variability in scores because of attrition of students (failure or withdrawal from the program).

Range

The range is the simplest measure of variability and is calculated by subtracting the lowest score from the highest score. Thus

$$\text{Range} = \text{Highest score} - \text{Lowest score}$$

Standard Deviation

The standard deviation (SD) of scores is the best measure of variability. Most computer scoring programs provide the SD of the scores with the results. There are calculators with statistical functions that can also be used to figure the SD. For more information on formulas and methods for calculating the SD, consult a statistics text. The SD is just the average distance of scores from the mean. In Figure 26-1, the SD is given as 9.8. The SD can be used in making interpretations from the normal curve (Lyman, 1997).

Normal Curve

The normal curve is a theoretical distribution of scores that is bell shaped and symmetrical. The mean, median, and mode are the same score on a normal curve. Also, for a normal curve, 68% of scores will fall within ±1 SD of the mean and 95% of scores will fall within ±2 SDs of the mean. This distribution may be used in assigning grades.

Standard Error of Measurement

The standard error of measurement is an estimate of how much the observed score is likely to differ from the "true" score. That is, the student's "true" score most likely lies between the observed score plus or minus the standard error.

$$\text{True score} = \text{Observed score} \pm \text{Error}$$

The standard error of measurement is calculated by using the SD and the test reliability (Popham, 1999). Many computer scoring programs supply the standard error. Some faculty members give students the benefit of the doubt and add the standard error to each raw score before they assign grades.

Standardized Scores

Standardized scores allow for ease of comparison between individual scores and sets of scores. The z score converts a raw score into units of SD on a normal curve. The z score can be calculated as follows:

$$z = \frac{x - m}{SD}$$

where x = observed score, m = mean, and SD = standard deviation.

For example, for a raw score of 34:

$$z = \frac{34 - 36.8}{6.6} = -0.42$$

Thus a raw score of 34 falls approximately 0.5 SD below the mean.

Because z scores are expressed by using decimals and both positive and negative values, many faculty prefer to use t scores instead. The z score can be used to calculate the t score. Converting raw scores to t scores has the following advantages:
1. The mean of the distribution is set at 50.
2. The SD from the mean is set at 10.
3. t scores can be manipulated mathematically for grading purposes.

$$t = 10z + 50$$

For example, the z score of −.42 would be transformed as follows:

$$t = 10(-.42) + 50 = 45.8$$

Conducting the Item Analysis

Classic test theory is used for this discussion of item analysis and the discrimination index. Classic test theory and related inferences assume a norm-referenced measure. For a critique of classic test theory and an explanation of the newer item response theories, see *Developing and Validating*

Multiple-Choice Test Items (Haladyna, 2004). Item response theories depend on large samples and thus are of limited application to classroom tests.

Item analysis assists faculty in determining whether test items have separated the learners from the nonlearners (discrimination). Many computer scoring programs supply item statistics.

Item Difficulty

The item difficulty index (P value) is simply the percentage correct for the group answering the item. The upper limit of item difficulty is 1.00, meaning that 100% of students answered the question correctly. The lower limit of item difficulty depends on the number of possible responses and is the probability of guessing the correct answer. For example, for a question with four options, $P = 0.25$ is the lower limit or probability of guessing. McDonald (2008) recommends keeping the P values of the items in the range of 0.70 to 0.80 to help ensure that questions separate learners from nonlearners (a good discrimination index). Clifton and Schriner (2010) recommend using 0.50 as a quick reference point, with low limits at 0.30 and high limits at 0.80. Some items may be slightly easier or more difficult, however, and faculty can determine the range of difficulty that is appropriate for their students and tests.

Item Discrimination

Item discrimination refers to the way an item differentiates students who know the content from those who do not. Discrimination can be measured as a point biserial correlation. The point biserial correlation compares each student's item performance with each student's overall test performance. If a question discriminates well, the point biserial correlation will be highly positive for the correct answer and negative for the distractors. This indicates that the "learners," or the students who knew the content, answered the question correctly and the "nonlearners" chose distractors. Popham (1999) rates items with discrimination indices greater than 0.3 as "good" and those with discrimination indices greater than 0.4 as "very good." For example, a point biserial correlation of 0.598 is a very good discriminator because the point biserial correlation is highly positive and the distractors have a negative point biserial correlation. Haladyna (2004) cautions that if the item difficulty index is either too high or too low, the discrimination index is attenuated. The discrimination index is maximized when the item difficulty is moderate ($P = 0.5$). Ultimately, test reliability depends on item discrimination. Inclusion of mastery level material on a norm-referenced test will tend to lower test reliability because that item will tend to be answered correctly by many students and will thus be a poor discriminator.

Distractor Evaluation

In addition to the evaluation of the correct answer to an item for a positive point biserial correlation, each distractor should be individually evaluated. Effective distractors should appeal to the nonlearner, as indicated by negative point biserial correlation values. Distractors with a point biserial correlation of zero indicate that students did not select them and that they may need to be revised or replaced with a more plausible option to appeal to students who do not understand the content. Distractors that were not selected increase the chances that a student could have obtained the correct answer by guessing. One way to develop appealing distractors is to periodically ask open-ended questions to determine the most common errors in thinking. Distractors for questions with numerical answers may need to be "worked out" by following the most typical mistakes that students make.

Revising Test Items

Developing a valid and reliable test is an ongoing process. It is helpful to revise the test immediately after administering it while faculty can recall items and student responses to them. Item revision should be conducted after item analysis. One way to analyze items for revision is to use a test item analysis form (Fig. 26-2). The result of item analysis for each question is entered in the form. Those items falling outside of the "ideal" range should be considered for revision. Items to be revised should include those with the following statistical characteristics:
1. Items with P values that are too high or too low (around 0.5 is ideal)
2. Correct answers with low positive or negative point biserial values (>0.30 is ideal)
3. Distractors with highly positive point biserial values (negative values are ideal)

Assigning Grades

Grades provide both feedback and motivation for students. In the academic setting, assignment of grades may be guided by the institution grading policy or scale. Many computer software programs

Test ___2___
Date ___3/08___

P (Item Difficulty) / D (Item Discrimination)	>.50	.40–.49	.30–.39	.20–.29	.10–.19	.01–.09	Negative	Total
Very difficult P = 50% or less								
Difficult P = 51%–69%	20	10	4	2, 18, 26				6
Average P = 70%–80%	3, 5, 25, 27	9, 14, 19, 24	12, 16, 17, 23, 29					13
Easy P = 81%–100%			6, 8, 11, 15, 21, 28	1, 7, 13, 22, 30				11
Total number of items	5	5	12	8				

X̄ ___75___
KR ___.75___
SD ___3.7___
SEM ___2.8___

Figure 26-2 Sample test item analysis form for a 30-item test.

are available to assist faculty with assigning grades accurately and efficiently (Anema et al., 2002). The two basic methods for assignment are the absolute and the relative ("curved") scales (described in the following sections). Principles of good grading include the following (McDonald, 2008):

1. Informing students of the specific grading criteria at the beginning of the course (stated explicitly in the syllabus)
2. Basing the grades on learning outcomes (not factors such as attendance or effort)
3. Gathering sufficient data (amount and variety) for the assignment of a valid grade
4. Recording data collected for grading purposes quantitatively (e.g., 89%, not B+)
5. Applying the grading system equitably to all students
6. Keeping grades confidential
7. Using statistically sound principles for assigning grades

Absolute Scale

An absolute grading scale rates performance relative to a standard (McDonald, 2008). The student's earned points are compared with the total possible points and are expressed as a percentage earned. The standard should be included in the syllabus at the beginning of the course. Theoretically, all students could receive an A (or an F) with this scale. In reality, the dispersion of the grades depends on the difficulty of the tests. See Table 26-8 for an example of an absolute grading scale.

Relative Scale

A relative grading scale rates students according to their ranking within the group. To assign grades in this system, faculty record scores in order, from high to low. Grades may then be assigned by using a variety of techniques. One method is to assign the grades according to natural "breaks" in the distribution. This method has the disadvantage of being subjective. A better method of assigning grades based on a relative scale is to use the test statistics to create a "curve":

1. Decide whether to use the mean or the median as the best measure of central tendency. If the mean and median are approximately the same, use the mean. If the distribution is skewed, use the median.

TABLE 26-8 Sample Absolute Grading Scale

Percentage Correct	Assigned Grade
90–100	A
80–89	B
70–79	C
60–69	D
<60	F

2. Determine the SD. The C grade will be set as the mean plus or minus one half of the SD (encompassing 40% of the scores). See Table 26-9 for an example of a relative grading scale.

Table 26-10 shows a comparison of the grades assigned to the raw scores with the absolute and relative grading scales described.

Relative grading scales may also be developed by using linear scores such as z scores or t scores (see the section on standardized test scores for directions for calculating these scores). t scores are more commonly used for grading purposes because there are no negative values in this system (Lyman, 1997). The mean score becomes a t score of 50. The z score and t score are figured for each raw score. The faculty member decides what grade to assign to the ranges of t scores. Assuming a normal curve, a t score of 50 would be assigned a grade of C. Computer grading programs that calculate grades according to absolute or relative scales are available. Many experts in assessment and grading do not recommend the use of relative grading scales (Haladyna, 2004; McDonald, 2008).

TABLE 26-9 Sample Relative Grading Scale

Grade	Calculation	Example	Range
A	> Upper B	>45.5	>45.5
B	Upper C + 1 SD	40.5 + 5	40.6 – 45.5
C	Mean ± 0.5 SD	38 ± 2.5	35.5 – 40.5
D	Lower C – 1 SD	35.5 – 5	30.5 – 35.4
F	< Lower D	<30.5	<30.5

Calculated according to Jacobs and Chase (1992).

TABLE 26-10 Comparison of Grades Assigned by Three Methods

Raw Score	Percent Score	Grade (Absolute)	Grade (Relative)
49	98	A	A
45(2)	90	A	B
42(2)	84	B	B
40	80	B	C
39(3)	78	C	C
38(4)	76	C	C
37	74	C	C
35(2)	70	C	D
34(3)	68	D	D
33	66	D	D
30	60	D	F
28	56	F	F

Grading Standards, Grade Inflation, and Grade Indexing

Periodically, faculty, administrators, boards of trustees, or consumers raise questions about the relative meaning of grades and potential or actual grade "inflation." Some possible causes for grade inflation are improved academic readiness of admitted students; student retention programs; competency-based assessments; competitive admission standards; a student population of older, mature, and career-directed students; and pass–fail grading systems.

When there are diverse views about the meaning of grades, faculty may institute *grade indexing*. Grade indexing involves indicating how many students in a given course or section of a course received grades that equaled or exceeded the grade of a given student. This index may appear on the student's transcript.

Nursing faculty as a whole should review grading policies and practices on a regular basis. A consistent philosophy about grading and fair and equitable grading practices communicates concern to the students and competence to nursing's varied publics. Faculty must also continually strive to administer valid and reliable tests that measure students' attainment of course and program competencies.

SUMMARY

Although developing, administering, and analyzing classroom tests may seem like a monumental task, the step-by-step approach presented in this chapter can be used as a guide to simplify this process. By following these guidelines, faculty can create written tests that can be used as effective measures of outcomes in the classroom. Assigning grades is the last step in this process.

REFLECTING ON THE EVIDENCE

1. Compare the six cognitive domains of Bloom (1956) and the six cognitive processes of Anderson and Krathwohl (2001). Notice the relative positioning of evaluation and synthesis and creation in the two taxonomies. What is the evidence for creation as a higher-level cognitive process than evaluation in the newer taxonomy? Hint: Think about the structure of a good literature review.

2. Evaluate an instructor-developed test (your own or another instructor's). What is the evidence for the construct, content, or criterion validity of the test? If such evidence does not exist, how would you go about establishing the evidence for validity?

3. Search the literature for an article about item response theory and an article about classic test theory. Compare the assumptions and usefulness of the two theories. Note: This question is most appropriate for the reader with a strong statistical background or interest.

4. Write a research question about the development or administration of classroom tests. How would you design a study to answer the question?

5. Following the administration of an exam, students tell you that several students were observed cheating. What will you do? How will you respond to the students who reported the incident? What measures can you take to prevent cheating incidents during the next test?

6. The students in your class ask you to "curve" the grades on a classroom test. Write a short explanation of this practice, based on the evidence, in terms understandable to an undergraduate (i.e., what you would tell the students). Take and defend a position on whether you would or would not agree to "curving" the grades.

REFERENCES

American Educational Research Association, American Psychological Association, & National Council on Measurement in Education. (1999). *Standards for educational and psychological testing.* Washington, DC: American Educational Research Association.

Anderson, L. W., & Krathwohl, D. R. (2001). *A taxonomy for learning, teaching, and assessing: A revision of Bloom's taxonomy of educational objectives.* New York, NY: Longman.

Anema, M. G., Anema, C. M., Bass, S. M., Fleming, B. O., Helms, M. A., & Rawls, A., L. (2002). A comparative analysis of computer-based graded programs. *CIN: Computers, Informatics, Nursing, 20*(2), 55–62.

Bloom, B. S., Englehart, M. D., Furst, E. J., Hill, W. H., & Krawthwhol, D. R. (1956). *Taxonomy of educational objectives: The classification of educational goals. Handbook 1: Cognitive domain.* New York, NY: Longman.

Bosher, S. (2003). Barriers to creating a more culturally diverse nursing profession: Linguistic bias in multiple-choice nursing exams. *Nursing Education Perspectives, 24*(1), 25–34.

Clifton, S. L., & Schriner, C. L. (2010). Assessing the quality of multiple-choice test items. *Nurse Educator, 35*(1), 12–16.

DiBartolo, M. C., & Walsh, C. M. (2010). Desperate times call for desperate measures: Where are we in addressing academic dishonesty? *Journal of Nursing Education, 49*(10), 543–544.

Flannelly, L. T. (2001). Using feedback to reduce students' judgment bias on test questions. *Journal of Nursing Education, 40*, 10–16.

Haladyna, T. M. (2004). *Developing and validating multiple-choice test items* (3rd ed.). Mahwah, NJ: Lawrence Erlbaum.

Jacobs, L. C., and Chase, C. I. Developing and Using Tests Effectively: A Guide for Faculty. San Francisco: Jossey-Bass, 1992

Lyman, H. B. (1997). *Test scores and what they mean* (6th ed.). Boston, MA: Allyn & Bacon.

McDonald, M. E. (2008). *The nurse educators' guide to assessing learning outcomes.* Sudbury, MA: Jones & Bartlett.

Miller, M. P., Linn, R. L., & Gronlund, N. E. (2009). *Measurement and assessment in teaching* (9th ed.). Upper Saddle River, NJ: Pearson Education.

Morrison, S., & Free, K. W. (2001). Writing multiple-choice test items that promote and measure critical thinking. *Journal of Nursing Education, 40*, 17–24.

National Council of State Boards of Nursing. (2010). *A test plan for the National Council Licensure Examination for registered nurses.* Retrieved from http://www.ncsbn.org

Oermann, M. H., & Gaberson, K. B. (2009). *Evaluation and testing in nursing education* (3rd ed.). New York, NY: Springer.

Popham, W. J. (1999). *Modern educational measurement: Practical guidelines for educational leaders* (3rd ed.). Boston, MA: Allyn & Bacon.

Su, W. M., Osisek, P. J., Montgomery, C., & Pellar, S. (2009). Designing multiple-choice test items at higher cognitive levels. *Nurse Educator, 34*(5), 223–227.

Wendt, A., & Harmes, J. C. (2009a). Evaluating innovative items for the NCLEX, Part I, Usability and pilot testing. *Nurse Educator, 34*(2), 56–59.

Wendt, A., & Harmes, J. C. (2009b). Developing and evaluating innovative items for the NCLEX, Part 2, Item characteristics and cognitive processing. *Nurse Educator, 34*(3), 109–113.

Wendt, A., & Kenny, L. E. (2009). Alternate item types: Continuing the quest for authentic testing. *Journal of Nursing Education, 48*(3), 150–156.

Wendt, A., Kenny, L., & Riley (2009). NCLEX fairness and sensitivity review. *Nurse Educator, 34*(5), 228–231.

Clinical Performance Evaluation 27

Wanda Bonnel, PhD, RN

In changing health care times, a constant is the importance of clinical evaluation. From patient safety to student confidence as clinicians, getting the clinical evaluation correct is critical. Providing fair and reasonable clinical evaluation is one of the most important and challenging faculty roles. Faculty must discern whether students can think critically within the clinical setting, maintain a professional demeanor, interact appropriately with patients, prioritize problems, have basic knowledge of clinical procedures, and complete care procedures correctly. All the while, faculty need to minimize student anxiety within the complex health care setting so that student clinical performance and not extraneous factors, such as anxiety or fatigue, are being observed.

Assessment of clinical performance provides data from which can be judged the extent to which students have acquired specified learning outcomes. In this chapter, discussion includes general issues in assessment of clinical performance, clinical evaluation methods and tools, and the evaluation process.

General Issues in Assessment of Clinical Performance

When clinical performance is evaluated, students' skills are judged as they relate to an established standard of patient care. Acceptable clinical performance involves behavior, knowledge, and attitudes

that students gradually develop in a variety of settings (Caldwell & Tenofsky, 1996). The ultimate outcome for clinical performance evaluation is safe, quality patient care. Clinical performance evaluation provides information to the student about performance and provides data that may be used for individual student development, assigning grades, and making decisions about the curriculum. Students have the right to a reliable and valid evaluation that assesses achievement of competencies required to take on the role of the novice nurse (Redman, Lenberg, & Walker, 1999). Box 27-1 provides some "quick tips" to be considered at the beginning of the evaluation process.

Good practice includes multidimensional evaluation with diverse evaluation methods completed over time, seeking student growth and progress. All evaluation should respect students' dignity and self-esteem. In addition to the concept of assessment, grading is considered part of a systems approach that includes integrating grading as a component of learning (Walvoord, Anderson, & Angelo, 2010).

Before assessing clinical performance, faculty must consider several issues. These issues include who will be participants in the evaluation, evaluation timing, and evaluation access and privacy.

Participants in Evaluation

Faculty

Faculty have primary responsibility for the student clinical evaluation. Faculty are knowledgeable about the purpose of the evaluation and the objectives that will be used to judge each student's performance. This clarity of purpose provides direction for selection of evaluation tools and processes. Initial faculty

The author acknowledges the work of Dorothy A. Gomez, MSN, RN; Stacy Lobodzinski, MSN, RN; and Cora D. Harwell West, MSN, RN, in the previous edition(s) of the chapter.

BOX 27-1 Quick Tips for Clinical Evaluation

- Define clearly both knowledge and skills that students will need to demonstrate.
- Use multiple sources of data for evaluation.
- Be reasonable and consistent in evaluation of all students.
- Use formative mini evaluations and suggest minor, easy corrections at the time they are needed.
- Present feedback and evaluation in nonjudgmental language, confining comments to a student's behavior.
- Provide evaluation "sandwiches," commenting first on a strength, then on a weakness, then on a strength of the student's behavior.
- Carry an anecdotal record or personal digital assistant (PDA) equivalent for each student, maintaining privacy of data.
- Make specific notes, focusing on specific details of a student's behavior.
- Document student patterns of behavior over time through compilation of records.
- Invite students to complete self-assessments and summarize what they have learned.
- Help students prioritize learning needs and turn feedback into constructive challenges with specific goals for each day.

---

challenges in completing clinical evaluations include factors such as faculty value systems, the number of students supervised, and reasonable clinical opportunities for students. Clinical evaluation is complex, with different students having different learning experiences (Walsh & Seldomridge, 2005). Faculty need to be aware of their own value systems to avoid biasing the evaluation process. When faculty are supervising a group of students in the delivery of safe and appropriate nursing care, faculty can only sample student behaviors. Limited sampling of behaviors or individual biases may result in an inaccurate or unfair clinical evaluation (Orchard, 1994). Because of these limitations, faculty use a variety of evaluation methods to capture the broader picture of student competence. Faculty strive to identify equitable assignments and can consider evaluation input from other sources with potential adjunct evaluators, including students, nursing staff and preceptors, peer evaluators, and patients.

Students

Completion of self-assessments by students provides not only data, as part of the evaluation process, but also a learning experience for the students (Bonnel, 2008; Loving, 1993). Student self-evaluation provides a starting point for reviewing, comparing, and discussing evaluative data with faculty. Initial student involvement in self-assessment tends to facilitate student behavior changes and provides a positive environment for learning and improvement. Participation in their own evaluation also empowers students to make choices and identify their strengths. Self-assessments are further discussed later in this chapter as a component of self-evaluation and self-reflection.

Nursing Staff and Preceptors

Nursing staff may provide input to the evaluation process and tend to provide data from an informed perspective as a result of collaboration with students. Nursing staff should understand their role in student evaluation, with staff expectations in the evaluation process clearly articulated. This includes determining whether staff feedback should be only provided directly to the student or shared with faculty as well. One of the disadvantages of including nursing personnel in the evaluation process is that expectations in the clinical area may differ from course performance objectives. Sharing course objectives, expectations of students, and clinical evaluation forms with staff promotes evaluation partnership. Although evaluation is time consuming for busy nurses, this may be part of a nurse's career development or joint appointment responsibilities.

Preceptors have a specified role in modeling and facilitating clinical education for students, especially for advanced nursing students. Typically preceptors serve a more formal role in evaluation, such as an adjunct faculty role, and provide evaluative data as part of a faculty team. If staff nurses and nurse preceptors provide data for the evaluation process, they should be oriented to the nursing school's evaluation plan. Roles should be clarified, indicating whether staff will be asked to provide occasional comments, to report only incidents or concerns, or to complete a specific evaluation form. Hrobsky and Kersbergen (2002) describe the use of a clinical map to assist preceptors in identifying student strengths and weaknesses. Seldomridge and Walsh (2006) note the importance of adequately preparing adjunct evaluators for their role, teaching these individuals to provide good feedback with tools such as rubrics to promote consistency and specifying clinical activities to evaluate.

Peer Evaluators

There is debate about the appropriateness of having student peers act as evaluators in the clinical setting. Student peers should only evaluate competencies and assignments that they are prepared to judge. There should be clear guidelines for peer review and the student levels of responsibility (McAllister & Osborne, 1997). Peer evaluation can help students develop collaborative skills, build communication abilities, and promote professional responsibility. A potential disadvantage is that peers may be biased in providing only favorable information about student colleagues or may have unrealistic expectations of their student colleagues. Providing students with this peer evaluation opportunity and then appropriately weighting the contribution can be a reasonable practice (Boehm & Bonnel, 2010).

Patients

Patients provide data from the product consumer viewpoint. Patient satisfaction is considered an important marker in quality health care and can be considered as part of student evaluation. Judgments about student performance are made from patients' personal experiences and data should be weighted for their value. Patients often have positive comments to make about their students, which can be positive for the students to hear.

Evaluation Timing

Appropriate timing of evaluation and student feedback should be considered. Formative evaluation focuses on the process of student development during the clinical activity, whereas summative evaluation comes at the conclusion of a specified clinical activity to determine student accomplishment. Formative evaluation can assist in diagnosing student problems and learning needs. Appropriate feedback enables students to learn from their mistakes and allows for growth and improvement in behavior. Summative evaluation attests to competency attainment or meeting of objectives. Each of these concepts has unique contributions to the evaluation process, which is discussed further in Chapter 24.

All parties involved in the clinical performance evaluation should be aware of evaluation time frames at the outset. Timely feedback to students from faculty, both ongoing and formally scheduled, decreases the risk of unexpected evaluation results. Ongoing formative evaluations keep students and faculty aware of the progress toward attainment of learning outcomes and promote opportunities for goal setting. This early intervention by a faculty member may provide needed direction for improvement and prevent a student from receiving an unsatisfactory evaluation in clinical performance.

Evaluation Access and Privacy Considerations

There are both ethical and legal issues relevant to privacy of evaluation data that can affect the student, faculty, and institution. Before conducting clinical evaluations, the educator must determine who will have access to data. In most cases, detailed evaluative data are shared only between the faculty member and the individual student. Program policy should identify who additionally may have access to the evaluation and how evaluative information will be stored and for how long. Evaluative data should be stored in a secure area. As designated by the Family Educational Rights and Privacy Act (FERPA), students 18 years of age or older or in postsecondary schools have the right to inspect records maintained by a school (U.S. Department of Education, 1974). A school's program materials such as catalogues and handbooks can be tools to ensure the creation of reasonable and prudent policies that are in compliance with legal and accrediting guidelines. Privacy of written anecdotal notes and computer documents or personal digital assistant (PDA) notes also need to be maintained. Additionally, anecdotal notes should be objectively written as they have potential to be subpoenaed in legal proceedings. Inadequate security of this information could lead to a breach of student privacy.

Challenges may also exist in evaluating students' use of electronic health records. While protecting health information privacy for patients, the Health Insurance Portability and Accountability Act (HIPAA) may create problems for faculty and students in accessing written clinical data. Since electronic health records are an important component of student learning, faculty need to be familiar with the guidelines and procedures that clinical agencies have developed for students and faculty to access needed patient care documents. Students and faculty may be provided codes, for example, to access electronic data needed for patient care. If clinical access to electronic health records is limited, another way to evaluate the student's ability is to provide simulations using those commercial products designed to teach about the electronic health record. Additional legal considerations are discussed in Chapter 3.

Clinical Evaluation Methods and Tools

Many methods and tools are used to measure learning in the clinical setting. A variety of approaches should be incorporated in clinical evaluation, including cognitive, psychomotor, and affective considerations as well as cultural competence and ethical decision making (Gaberson & Oermann, 2010). Additionally, educators cannot ignore the social connotations of grading, including the impact that evaluation has on the learning process and student motivation (Wiles & Bishop, 2001).

The goal of evaluation is an objective report about the quality of the clinical performance. Faculty need to be aware that potential exists for evaluation of students' clinical performance to be subjective and inconsistent. Even with "objective" instruments based on measurable and observable behavior, subjectivity can still be introduced into a tool that is viewed as objective. Reilly and Oermann (1992) encourage faculty to be sensitive to the forces that contribute to the subjective side of evaluation as they strive for fairness and consistency.

Fair and reasonable evaluation of students in clinical settings requires use of appropriate evaluation tools that are ideally efficient for faculty to use. Any evaluation instrument used to measure clinical learning and performance should have criteria that are consistent with course objectives and the teaching institution's purpose and philosophy. Attention to student clinical progress, not only across semesters but across a program, can be considered with similar, consistent evaluation processes and tools that progress across the program (Bonnel & Smith, 2010).

A faculty group decision about the tools to be used for data collection is typically indicated. Many clinical evaluation tools have been developed and implemented within clinical settings. Faculty must make decisions about using these instruments according to their purpose for clinical evaluation.

Primary strategies for the evaluation of clinical practice include (1) observation, (2) written communication, (3) oral communication, (4) simulation, and (5) self-evaluation. Because clinical practice is complex, a combination of methods used over time is indicated and helps support a fair and reasonable evaluation. See Table 27-1 for a summary of common strategies and clinical evaluation tools by category. These are also discussed in the following paragraphs.

Evaluation Strategies: Observation

Observation is the method used most frequently in clinical performance evaluation. Student performance is compared to clinical competency expectations as designated in course objectives. Faculty observe and analyze the performance, provide feedback on the observation, and determine whether further instruction is needed. A large national survey specific to faculty clinical evaluation and grading practices confirmed the predominance of observation (Oermann, Yarbrough, Saewert, Ard, & Charasika, 2009). Authors noted that continuing issues in clinical evaluation include wide variability

TABLE 27-1 Sample Evaluation Strategies and Tools by Category	
Observation	Anecdotal notes
	Checklists
	Rating scales
	Videotapes
Written	Charting and progress notes
	Concept maps
	Care plans
	Process recordings
	Written tests
	Web-based strategies
Oral	Student interviews and case presentation
	Clinical conferences
Simulations	Interactive multimedia patient simulators
	Role play and clinical scenarios
	Standardized patient examinations
Self-evaluation	Clinical portfolios
	Journals and logs

in clinical environments, increasingly complex patients, and more diverse students.

Real-time observation and delayed video observation are both considered in this discussion. Technology or online cases also provide unique opportunities for enhancing evaluation opportunities and standardization of evaluations. Newer approaches to use of videos in evaluation include online tools such as the National Institutes of Health Stroke Scale training. In this example, video cases were developed based on needed competencies for appropriate use of the Stroke Scale. Students complete testing specific to these competencies as they refer to the online video cases (NIH Stroke Scale, n.d.). This provides a standardized testing approach.

Advantages of observation include the potential for direct visualization and confirmation of student performance, but observation can also be challenging. Sample factors that can interfere with observations include lack of specificity of the particular behaviors to be observed; an inadequate sampling of behaviors from which to draw conclusions about a student's performance; and the evaluator's own influences and perceptions, which can affect judgment of the observed performance (Reilly & Oermann, 1992).

Faculty should seek tools and strategies that support a fair and reasonable evaluation. The more structured observational tools are typically easy to complete and useful in focusing on specified behavior. Although structured observation tools can help increase objectivity, faculty judgment is still required in interpretation of the listed behaviors. Problems with reliability are introduced when item descriptors are given different meanings by different evaluators. Faculty training can help minimize this problem.

Tracking Clinical Observation Evaluation Data

An abundance of information must be tracked in clinical observation. Faculty can benefit from systems to help document and organize this information. Faculty can carry copies of evaluation tools and anecdotal records or can consider the use of a PDA to help facilitate retrieval and use of clinical evaluation records. While a variety of strategies for using PDAs in the clinical setting exist, a particular example is inclusion of anecdotal records and student "check-offs" in the memo function of the PDA

(Lehman, 2003). Privacy in PDA records is also needed.

Common methods for documenting observed behaviors during clinical practice vary in the amount of structure. Examples include anecdotal notes, checklists, rating scales and rubrics, and videotapes.

Anecdotal Notes

Anecdotal or progress notes are objective written descriptions of observed student performance or behaviors. The format for these can vary from loosely structured "plus–minus" observation notes to structured lists of observations in relation to specified clinical objectives. These written notes initially serve as part of formative evaluation. As student performance records are documented over time, a pattern is established. This record or pattern of information pertaining to the student and specific clinical behaviors helps document the student's performance pattern for both summative evaluation and recall during student–faculty conference sessions. Liberto, Roncher, and Shellenbarger (1999) noted the importance of determining which clinical incidents to assess and the need to identify both positive and negative student behaviors.

Checklists

Checklists are lists of items or performance indicators requiring dichotomous responses such as satisfactory–unsatisfactory or pass–fail (Table 27-2). Gronlund (2005) describes a checklist as an inventory of measurable performance dimensions or products with a place to record a simple "yes" or "no" judgment. These short, easy-to-complete tools are frequently used for evaluating clinical performance. Checklists, such as nursing skills check-off lists, are useful for evaluation of specific well-defined behaviors and are commonly used in the clinical simulated laboratory setting. Rating scales, described in the following paragraph, provide more detail than checklists concerning the quality of a student's performance.

Rating Scales and Rubrics

Rating scales incorporate qualitative and quantitative judgments regarding the learner's performance in the clinical setting (Box 27-2). A list of clinical behaviors or competencies is rated on a numerical scale such as a 5-point or 7-point scale

TABLE 27-2 Example of Checklist Items and Format

Professional Domain	Midterm			Final	
	Satisfactory	Unsatisfactory	Not Observed	Satisfactory	Unsatisfactory
Practices within legal boundaries according to standards					
Uses professional nursing standards to provide patient safety					
Follows nursing procedures and institutional policy in delivery of patient care					
Displays professional behaviors with staff, peers, instructors, and patient systems					
Demonstrates ethical principles of respect for person and confidentiality					
Participates appropriately in clinical conferences					
Reports on time; follows procedures for absenteeism					

BOX 27-2 Example of Rating Scale Items and Format

Instructions. On a scale of 1 to 5, rate each of the following student behaviors:
    (Rating Code: 1 = marginal; 2 = fair; 3 = satisfactory; 4 = good; 5 = excellent; NA = not applicable)
____ 1 Serves as patient caregiver (independence when providing patient care, timely completion of all patient care)
____ 2 Functions in the role of team member
____ 3 Uses correct procedure when performing nursing interventions
____ 4 Relates self-evaluation to clinical learning objectives
____ 5 Displays positive behavior when given feedback

with descriptors. These descriptors take the form of abstract labels (such as A, B, C, D, and E or 5, 4, 3, 2, and 1), frequency labels (e.g., *always*, *usually*, *frequently*, *sometimes*, and *never*), or qualitative labels (e.g., *superior*, *above average*, *average*, and *below average*). A rating scale provides the instructor with a convenient form on which to record judgments indicating the degree of student performance. This differs from a checklist in that it allows for more discrimination in judging behaviors as compared with dichotomous "yes" and "no" options. Mahara (1998) noted the benefit of more standardized assessments such as checklists and rating scales but faults these objective scales for failing to capture the complex clinical practice environment and clinical learning. Oermann (1997) emphasized the benefit of asking appropriate patient care questions along with clinical observations to gauge student critical thinking abilities.

Rubrics, a type of rating scale, help convey clinically related assignment expectations to students. They provide clear direction for graders and promote reliability among multiple graders. The detail provided in a rubric grid allows faculty to provide rapid and extensive feedback to students without extensive writing (Walvoord et al., 2010). Typical parts to a rubric include the task or assignment description and some type of scale, breakdown of assignment parts, and descriptor of each performance level (Stevens & Levi, 2005). Rubric examples exist for providing detailed feedback for clinical related assignments such as written clinical plans and conference participation. A web search by topic can provide samples for review.

Rubrics or checklists are beneficial in facilitating both the lab experience and the clinical grading for faculty and students. They promote clear communication as to expectations of best practice in completing skills. Providing skills checklists for students provides direction in their skill learning and practice. Students can use these tools for self-assessments and participate in peer assessments to promote learning. Rubrics can be used within learning management systems as well. These tools can be distributed to students, as well as be completed by faculty, and tracked or monitored over time (Bonnel & Smith, 2010).

Videotapes as Source of Observational Data

Another method of recording observations of a student's clinical performance is through videos. Videos, often completed in a simulated setting, can be used to record and evaluate specific performance behaviors relevant to diverse clinical settings. Advantages associated with videos include their valuable start, stop, and replay capabilities, which allow an observation to be reviewed numerous times. Videos can promote self-evaluation, allowing students to see themselves and evaluate their performance more objectively. Videos also give teachers and students the opportunity to review the performance and provide feedback in determining whether further practice is indicated. Use of videos can contribute to the learning and growth of an entire clinical group when knowledge and feedback are shared (Reilly & Oermann, 1992). Videos are particularly popular for evaluation in distance learning situations. Videos can also be used with rating scales, checklists, or anecdotal records to organize and report behaviors observed on the videos.

Evaluation Strategies: Student Written Communication

Use of written communication, whether paper-based or electronic, enables the faculty to evaluate clinical performance through assessing students' abilities to translate what they have learned to the written word. Review of student nursing care plans or written notes allows faculty to evaluate students' abilities to communicate with other care providers. Through writing assignments, students can clarify and organize their thoughts (Cowles, Strickland, & Rodgers, 2001). Additionally, writing can reinforce new knowledge and expand thinking on a topic. Faculty evaluation focuses on the quality of the content and student ability to communicate information and ideas in written form. The rater can determine the student's perspectives and gain insight into the "why" of the student's behavior. A scoring tool such as a rubric with specified objectives for a designated assignment can promote consistency and efficiency in grading specified assignments (Stevens & Levi, 2005). Written data help support faculty clinical observations.

Documentation and Patient Progress Notes

The value of electronic text-based communication in the changing health care system is evident. Writing cogent nursing and clinical progress notes is an important clinical skill. Reviewing student documentation provides faculty with an opportunity to evaluate students' ability to process and record relevant data. Students' skill in using health care terminology and documentation practices can be examined and critical thinking processes can be demonstrated in these notes (Higuchi & Donald, 2002). With the focus on electronic records as a tool in patient safety, orienting students to these tools and evaluating students' skill in this area is essential (Bonnel & Smith, 2010).

Concept Maps

Concept maps allow students to create a diagram of patient needs and nursing responses, including relationships among concepts. These tools can help students visualize and organize patient-specific data relevant to diagnostic work and nursing and medical diagnoses. Faculty can evaluate students' understanding of concepts and relationships among relevant concepts and assist faculty in clarifying students' misconceptions. These tools also provide faculty with an opportunity to complete a quick review of skills before students perform patient care and to make a quick determination of further learning needs (Castellino & Schuster, 2002; King & Shell, 2002). Concept maps can also serve as worksheets for students and serve as organizing tools for documentation (Schuster, 2000). Kern, Bush, and McCleish (2006) argue that in today's complex health care world, concept maps may better represent care processes than more traditional linear models of documentation.

Nursing Care Plans

Nursing care plans allow faculty to evaluate students' ability to determine and prioritize care needs according to understanding and interpretation of individual patients' health care problems. Historically, nursing care plans have been used by students to document clinical thinking processes, but some would argue that the availability of numerous standardized care plans has minimized the critical thinking component. Some programs report replacing detailed clinical care plans with concept maps or clinical journals and logs. Mueller, Johnston, and Bligh (2001) describe a strategy for modifying care plans and combining them with concept maps to help students clarify the interrelationship of patient problems.

Process Recordings

Process recordings are used to evaluate the interpersonal skills of students within the clinical setting. This form of evaluation requires students to write down their patient–nurse interactions and self-evaluate the communication skills they used. Process recording is a form of self-evaluation that allows students to analyze their own interactive behavior, enabling them to better identify the strengths and weaknesses of their interpersonal communication (Carpenito & Duespohl, 1985). This approach to evaluation has traditionally been used in communication courses and in psychiatric nursing. Additional note has been made of process recording benefits for students working with hospice patients (Hayes, 2005).

Paper-and-Pencil or Electronic Testing Formats

Written testing is frequently used to assess students' basic knowledge for problem solving and decision making in clinical practice. Various test formats (true–false, multiple choice, matching, short answer,

essay) can be incorporated into preclinical or postclinical conferences to gauge students' understanding of specific concepts.

Web-Based Strategies

Newer forms of written evaluation include web-based clinical conferences and electronic case discussions. Faculty may implement postclinical conferences or clinical case discussions within a learning management system. DeBourgh (2001) discusses strategies for incorporating clinical feedback in e-mail correspondence, e-journals, and online threaded discussion boards. Electronic clinical logs can be submitted to monitor ages and diagnoses of patients seen. Written clinical work can be managed via electronic learning management systems. Although not limited to students at a distance, web-based strategies are especially popular for clinical evaluation of students in geographically diverse settings. They may be useful as well for clinical conferences and student evaluation in community health courses with clinical coursework in diverse community settings.

Evaluation Strategies: Verbal Communication Methods

Communication and information sharing are common nursing tasks and important nursing skills. Oral communication strategies such as student interviews, case presentations, and clinical conferences provide evaluative opportunities. These can be used to assess the student's ability to verbalize ideas and thoughts clearly. In addition, these strategies allow faculty to assess a student's critical thinking skills and pose questions to elicit more complex forms of thinking. Evaluation strategies identified as oral communication methods are described in the following paragraphs.

Student Interviews and Case Presentation

In simple interview format, faculty ask questions and students respond. These question-and-answer sessions provide faculty with the opportunity to probe for more detail from students and clarify misconceptions. Faculty can focus on asking "higher-order" questions, moving beyond just factual recall, to better promote student critical thinking (Boswell, 2006; Oermann, 1997). Student case presentations, such as "bullet-point" summaries of patient problems and care strategies, assist students in developing concise presentation skills. Faculty can provide feedback to students and obtain evaluative information about students' thoughts and approaches for patient care.

Clinical Conferences

Clinical conferences provide opportunities for students to integrate theory and practice in terms of their own clinical experiences. Questions, reflections, and discussion within conferences encourage critical thinking and allow for peer feedback. Debriefing of clinical experiences, similar to the debriefing of simulations, provides students with opportunity to reflect and further cement learning. As students debrief, they gain opportunity to assess what happened during their clinical care, compare this to accepted criteria, and consider how well they did. Asking students to engage in further goal setting is an important component of debriefing (Bonnel & Smith, 2010). Oermann (1997) notes that conferences provide an opportunity for faculty to gauge students' abilities to analyze data and critique plans. The multiple student participants in clinical conferences enable faculty to evaluate more than one student at a time.

Multidisciplinary conferences are another form of clinical conference in which the process of problem solving and decision making is a collaborative effort of the group. This group is composed not only of nursing personnel but also of members of other health care disciplines. Evaluation is concerned with the student's active participation within the group and abilities to present ideas clearly in terms of the care plan for the patient. This exercise also promotes working with other disciplines on clinical problem solving. Students may find a degree of risk involved with sharing their knowledge and being evaluated critically by others.

Evaluation Strategies: Clinical Simulations

Simulations can range from simple case role plays to interactions with complex electronic manikins. Through simulations an instructor can identify specific clinical objectives to be demonstrated and focus on student cognitive and psychomotor behaviors defined for the case. Simulations help to create a safe environment for student learning. Benefits of simulations include skill validation and minimal student stress (Miller, Nichols, & Beeken, 2000).

With the changing health care setting, students will likely not have opportunities to care for all types of patients in the various clinical settings for which they will be responsible after graduation. Teaching pattern recognition with cases and scenarios in safe, structured learning environments is becoming an increasingly important strategy. Sample approaches to simulations include technology-based patient simulations, role play and clinical scenarios, and standardized patient examinations.

Technology-Based Patient Simulations

As technology advances, opportunities for clinical evaluation expand. New technologies with digital equipment, such as the Ventriloscope (www.ventriloscope.com), provide opportunities for lab practice and evaluation that include assessing patient abnormal findings as well as the more common normal findings in colleagues acting as pretend patients.

Interactive technology-based cases, with options from low-fidelity to high-fidelity simulation, provide a semirealistic experience for students. Through the use of interactive multimedia, nursing case studies can be presented in a safe setting without clinical environmental distractions or the risk involved in student clinical decision making. Rinne (1994) identifies the following three benefits associated with their use: (1) skills may be demonstrated efficiently; (2) students have unlimited opportunities for practice in a safe environment; and (3) self-evaluation can take place, enabling students to judge their own performance. Novice nursing students report gaining comfort and confidence for clinical care when using simulators as a learning tool (Bremner, Aduddell, Bennett, & VanGeest, 2006). Rhodes and Curran (2005) note the benefits of using patient simulators in teaching clinical judgment as well as decreasing student anxiety in demonstrating clinical skills. A model can be used to guide simulation development for both teaching–learning and testing purposes (Jeffries, 2005). Faculty should clarify for students whether a simulation activity is formative (for teaching purposes) or summative (for outcomes evaluation).

Debriefing and feedback to students, as formative evaluation, are considered to be critical elements in the teaching–learning process with high-fidelity patient simulators (Dearman, 2003; Henneman & Cunningham, 2005; Issenberg, McGaghie, Petrusa, Gordon, & Scalese, 2005). These debriefing sessions can promote critical thinking as students reflect and consider alternate clinical approaches and gain insight into their performance. High-fidelity patient simulators as mechanisms to document student competencies are taking on increasing importance in today's health care settings. Further discussion of simulations as a form of clinical evaluation can be found in Chapter 20.

Role Play and Clinical Scenarios

Role play provides an opportunity for students to try out new behaviors, simulating aspects of nursing care in relation to clinical practice. As students implement the roles called for in specified case guidelines (or scripts for role plays), they gain opportunities to practice competent nurse interactions and behaviors. Students practice interpersonal communication skills and gain opportunity to observe, evaluate, and provide feedback to each other. Making videos of role play can also allow for student self-evaluation.

Additionally, clinical scenarios created with audio or video clips provide students with the opportunity to review an approach to a clinical scenario and actively learn while faculty facilitate the procedure (Dearman, 2003). Students can respond to audiovisual scenarios orally or in writing. The potential for diverse, varied cases promotes relevance to a majority of nursing arenas and can be used in a variety of settings. Additionally, many of these clinical scenarios have potential to be used in online settings.

An advantage that these methods offer is a readily available means of judging specific clinical practices without having to wait for a similar opportunity to arise in the clinical setting. Clinical scenarios can be economically beneficial in the educational setting with large groups of students (Roberts, While, & Fitzpatrick, 1992).

Standardized Patient Examinations

Standardized patient examinations, sometimes referred to as *objective structured clinical examinations* (OSCEs), are another way to evaluate competencies in clinical education. These OSCEs can be described as actors or "pretend patients" in an artificial environment designed to simulate actual clinical conditions (Borbasi & Koop, 1994). A simulation center, modeled as an authentic clinical environment with standardized patients, can provide a safe setting in which to observe and document student competencies.

Standardized patients can provide feedback to students and help ensure competence before students begin practice in the complex "real" world. Potential exists for multiple evaluators to observe and test students in the performance of numerous skills during brief examination periods. The OSCE process, considered an acceptable and powerful approach in clinical performance evaluation, allows rapid feedback to students about identified clinical deficits (Borbasi & Koop, 1994). Specific approaches and satisfaction with the standardized patient experience have been described (Ebbert & Connors, 2004; Gibbons et al., 2002). While many programs use the OSCE as a learning tool with formative feedback, if the OSCE is used as high-stakes testing, then building in a remediation plan should be considered (McWilliam & Botwinski, 2010).

Self-Reflection and Self-Evaluation

Self-reflection and self-evaluation are related concepts. Self-reflection is considered to be an introspective process with self-observation of one's thoughts and feelings. In self-evaluation students complete criteria-based assessments using self-reflection.

Reflecting on one's practice has been described as an integral component of clinical learning (Freshwater, Taylor, & Sherwood, 2010). Self-reflection provides students with an opportunity to think about what they have learned and promotes becoming reflective clinicians. Clinical reasoning depends on both cognitive and metacognitive (thinking about one's thinking) skill development (Kuiper & Pesut, 2004). There are different ways to incorporate reflection into clinical practice, including preactivity, during activity, and postactivity.

Self-evaluation against a standard has been noted as a critical tool for assisting students in gaining lifelong learning skills (Fink, 2003). In self-evaluation, students describe and make qualitative judgments about specified experiences. Self-reflection against a rubric or standard can be a significant tool for student evaluation. Students can examine their progress, identify their strengths and weaknesses, and set goals for improvement in the areas indicated. Good feedback from faculty has been described as a tool for helping students reflect on specified information, gain further self-knowledge, and set further learning goals (Bonnel, 2008).

A potential disadvantage of self-evaluation is that students may not be honest about their level of self-understanding in an effort to protect themselves against potential criticism (Walker & Dewar, 2000). The ability to critically reflect on individual performance may be influenced by the maturity and self-esteem of the student. Students are more likely to share summaries and reflections with faculty if a foundation of trust has been established. If self-evaluation begins at the onset of the students' clinical experience, students can benefit from examining their ongoing progress. Through the teacher–student interaction process, observations and perceptions can be shared, student strengths and weaknesses can be discussed, and self-evaluation strategies can be improved. Student–teacher relationships can become stronger and more constructive as students progress.

Portfolios

Portfolios have been described as collections of evidence, prepared by students and evaluated by faculty, to demonstrate mastery, comprehension, application, and synthesis of a given set of concepts (Slater, 1999). They provide a collage or album of student learning rather than a one-time snapshot. Portfolios allow integration of a number of assessments and can help provide progressive documentation of specified clinical learning outcomes (see Chapter 25). Reflective portfolios are designed to help students consider their progress in clinical learning and also help faculty understand students' clinical learning processes. Faculty can provide portfolio guidelines that help students organize their portfolio components and incorporate reflective summaries (Suskie, 2004). Portfolios can help students learn strategies for documenting clinical competencies as a part of lifelong learning.

Journals and Logs

Journals and logs are, in essence, written dialogues between the self and the designated reader. These written dialogues provide opportunity for students to share values and critical thinking abilities. Journals give students the opportunity to record their clinical experiences and review their progress. This enables students to recall areas of needed improvement and allows them to work on problems and clinical performance weaknesses. The concepts of clinical logs and journals are sometimes used synonymously, but clinical logs can vary in the amount

of detail, ranging from a listing of types of patients and noted student care roles to a more detailed log with a reflection on each patient care experience. Students have described more active learning and thinking about their actions and processes with use of a detailed reflective clinical log (Fonteyn & Cahill, 1998). Sample criteria for written reflections are noted to include description of an event, student's reaction to the event, perceived value of the learning event, learning that occurred, and student's future plans (Blake, 2005).

Faculty should provide specific guidelines as to the amount of detail required in clinical journals or logs and provide clear guidelines as to how (or if) journals or logs will be graded (Kennison & Misselwitz, 2002). If self-reflective materials such as journals are to be graded, concepts such as student depth of thought, making connections between theory and practice, and relating beliefs and behaviors may be developed as an evaluation rubric. Faculty feedback on student self-reflections provides opportunity for further dialogue on learning experiences (Murphy, 2005). Self-reflection and self-evaluation can become part of the process for lifelong, self-directed learning.

Clinical Evaluation Process

Before the evaluation process begins, faculty and students need a clear understanding of the outcomes to be attained at the culmination of the experience. Clinical evaluation is a systematic process that can be considered as having three consecutive phases: (1) preparation, (2) clinical activity phase, and (3) final data interpretation and feedback. A listing of sample tasks within each phase and the roles faculty will assume during each phase are provided in Table 27-3. Additional discussion of selected points in each phase follows.

Preparation Phase

Choosing the Clinical Setting and Patient Assignment as Part of the Evaluation Process

Faculty are responsible for providing each student with ample opportunities to achieve course objectives and must give careful attention to choosing a clinical site that will give students these opportunities. Advance planning is needed because choosing an appropriate clinical site can be challenging. Even in the ideal clinical setting, daily variability exists in

TABLE 27-3 Roles of Faculty Evaluator during the Evaluation Process

PHASE I: PREPARATION

Determine objectives and competencies.
Identify evaluation methods and tools.
Choose clinical site.
Orient students to the evaluation plan.
Focus on objectivity in evaluation.

PHASE II: CLINICAL ACTIVITY

Orient students and staff to the student role.
Provide students clinical opportunities.
Ensure patient safety.
Observe and collect evaluation data from multiple perspectives.
Provide student feedback to enhance learning.
Document findings and maintain privacy of records.
Contract with students regarding any deficiencies.

PHASE III: FINAL DATA INTERPRETATION AND PRESENTATION

Interpret data in fair, reasonable, and consistent manner.
Assign grade.
Provide summative evaluation conference (ensure privacy and respect confidentiality).
Evaluate experience.

terms of patients, providers, and the activity level of the unit, which can complicate evaluation. In addition to unit assignments, specific patient clinical assignments should also be considered as part of a fair evaluation. This includes both the types of patients assigned to students and the duration of clinical assignments.

Teaching and learning in a natural setting provide unique challenges for both students and faculty. Negotiating the balance between student independence and supervision is complex. Faculty must provide adequate supervision to ensure safe delivery of care with the welfare and the safety of patients as the first priority. Before the clinical experience begins, the faculty must develop criteria for what is considered unsafe or inappropriate behavior and what consequences will occur if such behavior is observed. Communication between faculty and students before the clinical experience begins is essential, including orientation to the grading process (Walvoord et al., 2010).

The faculty must be prepared to remove a student from the clinical setting if the student does not meet the minimal level of safety. Students have the right to know the standard used for safe practice and evaluation. Students should also be given an orientation to the clinical facility and to the policies and procedures that will apply to the clinical experience. Unit orientations, as well as orientation to evaluation methods, are important in decreasing the anxiety that can hamper student clinical performance.

Students and faculty are essentially visitors in an established system, and the status of student comfort and support in the clinical environment should be considered in evaluation as well. Chan (2002) noted the importance of a positive clinical learning environment for student learning. A sample form for student evaluation of a clinical setting is provided in Box 27-3.

Determining the Standards and Measurement Tools

Student performance expectations should meet the following criteria: (1) reasonable, (2) consistent and applied equally, and (3) established and communicated before implementation (Orchard, 1994).

Faculty have the responsibility for choosing the appropriate methods and tools for evaluation of the learners' clinical performance. Specific evaluation instruments chosen will be the means of documenting and communicating judgments made about student performance. These tools should document performance expectations relevant to course objectives and be practical and time efficient.

The concepts of interrater reliability (whether results can be replicated by other raters) and content validity (whether a tool measures what is desired) at minimum should be considered in selection of a specific clinical evaluation instrument. More discussion of reliability, interrater reliability, and validity is provided in Chapters 24 and 25.

Inconsistencies in evaluation can result when each course coordinator develops course tools independently. Wiles and Bishop (2001) recommend that faculty work in groups to develop tools that reflect the increasing complexity of competencies required as students progress from program beginners to graduating seniors and to promote consistency from course to course. Often, tools described in the literature or those in use by colleagues can be used or adapted, thus saving time that would be required to develop a new tool. Waltz and Jenkins (2001) have compiled a list of clinical evaluation

---

BOX 27-3 Student Evaluation of Clinical Setting

Name of Agency
Specific Unit

DIRECTIONS

Print the name of the instructor and the name of the agency, the specific unit where you had your clinical experience, and the days of the week you were assigned.

Please respond to the following statements with the rating that best describes your opinion.

A. Strongly Agree
B. Agree
C. Disagree
D. Strongly Disagree

Please qualify any rating of C or D with comments or suggestions. The agency personnel have asked that you make comments because this is the only way they can make improvements or know what is positive. Your ratings and written comments will be used to determine clinical placement for future students and may be shared with individuals in the setting but only in summary form.

APPLICATION OF COURSE MATERIAL

1. The staff facilitated my ability to meet clinical objectives.
2. I was able to meet the objectives of this course in this setting.

POPULATION/PATIENTS

3. Patients presented clinical problems appropriate to the objectives for this course.

4. Culturally diverse patients (e.g., cultural, social, economic) were available in the setting.

HEALTH PROFESSIONALS

5. Nurse managers, staff nurses, and support staff were accepting of students and student learning.
6. Nurse managers, staff nurses, and support staff were available to me to answer questions and provide assistance.
7. The nursing staff were positive role models.
8. Nurses demonstrated professional relationships with other health care professionals.

PHYSICAL ENVIRONMENT

9. The setting was conducive to working with patients and other health care team members.
10. Space was available for conferences with faculty and other students.

OVERALL IMPRESSION OF SETTING

11. I have a positive impression of the quality of care provided in this setting.
12. I would recommend this setting for future students taking this course.
13. Add statements specific to the clinical setting not already covered.

How could your clinical experience have been improved in this clinical setting?

Please use the back of this sheet to make comments and suggestions.

Adapted with permission from a form used by University of Kansas School of Nursing.

---

tools and provide a description and reliability and validity assessments for each.

Clinical Activity Phase

In both obtaining and analyzing clinical evaluation data, faculty need to make professional judgments about the performance of students, being aware of the subjective nature of evaluation. To prevent biased judgments, faculty need to be aware of the factors that can influence decision making and must actively use strategies to prevent biases.

Strategies that can help support trustworthiness of the clinical evaluation data include the following:

- Have specified objectives or competencies on which to base the evaluation.

- Use multiple strategies and combined methods of evaluation for compiling data.
- Include both qualitative and quantitative measures.
- Determine a practical sampling plan and evaluate it over time.
- Provide clear scoring directions for tools to promote consistency between raters in collection and interpretation of data.
- Train faculty in use of specific clinical evaluation tools and approaches for consistency and fairness in grading.
- Be aware of common errors such as the halo effect (assuming that positive behaviors in one evaluated competency will be similar in others).
- Incorporate teacher self-assessment of values, beliefs, or biases that might affect the evaluation process (Oermann & Gaberson, 2009).

Final Data Interpretation and Presentation

Clinical Evaluation Conference

The findings of the clinical evaluation are usually shared with the student individually at the end of the clinical experience or course. No surprises should be presented at this time. The timely feedback of the earlier formative evaluation should provide students with information sufficient to prepare them for this evaluation. A student's self-evaluation is often submitted before the evaluation conference and discussed at this time.

Evaluation results are commonly reported in both written and oral forms. Often, the primary evaluation tool is presented to show student improvement and specifically recall incidents. The faculty should clarify initially that the purpose of the conference is to provide information on the student's clinical performance. The results should be explained, giving specific incidents in which the student had difficulties, excelled, performed adequately, or improved. In addition, the faculty member needs to assist the student in establishing new goals. Finally, the faculty member needs to summarize the conference and end on a positive note.

The environment in which the evaluation conference takes place should be comfortable for the student, and privacy should be maintained. An hour during which the student is responsible for patient care or directly after a tiring clinical experience is not the most conducive time for a conference. An appointment during office hours away from the clinical site provides a more comfortable and private setting for students to listen to constructive criticism or encouraging comments.

Student Response

The student's response to the faculty evaluation typically reflects the fairness with which the results were determined. A student will perceive the results as fair if his or her own appraisal is congruent with that of the faculty. A student self-evaluation submitted before the conference helps faculty gain insight into student perceptions and can give faculty time to prepare a response. However, the best way to ensure congruent results is for faculty to provide the student with a sufficient number of formative evaluations and time to reflect on his or her own performance. Faculty need to be sensitive to the student's needs, emphasizing the student's strengths as well as weaknesses and encouraging goals and aspirations.

Working with Students with Questionable Performance

Supporting At-Risk Students

Developing a positive learning environment is a basic step in promoting positive, supportive student learning relationships. Students have a right to expect respect. Pointing out areas in which students need to improve and specific ways to achieve clinical goals promotes a positive learning environment and minimizes potential legal risks.

Scanlan (2001) discusses the importance of clarifying definitions of safe and unsafe clinical practices and having clear policies and guidelines for working with "problem" students. Minimum patient safety competencies can be observed, checked off, and documented in the learning lab by using the benefits of rehearsal in this setting. School policies can indicate minimum safety competencies that need to be achieved in the learning laboratory before a student moves into the actual clinical setting. Additionally, O'Connor (2006) suggests that faculty can benefit from having a visual image of good, moderate, and poor student behaviors to assist in evaluation.

Zuzelo (2000) summarizes the following key points, which although relevant to all evaluations have particular merit in evaluating a student with questionable clinical performance behaviors.

- Ensure that the criteria for student success (i.e., the written course objectives or competency statements) are clear to all parties.
- If a student is at risk, objectively document a pattern of marginal or failing behavior.
- Report poor performance to students as formative evaluation and provide students with opportunities for remedial work.
- Use strategies such as clinical probation for supporting the at-risk student. Student clinical contracts can be used to document these plans for improvement. The written student contract should clarify student and faculty expectations and what student behaviors need to occur for passing status to be achieved.
- Follow written procedure from school handbooks.

Anecdotal records should be written objectively and used to document a pattern of behaviors. Failing behaviors need to be identified in writing and a contract for corrections should be signed by the faculty member and the student (Osinski, 2003). An annotated record of each counseling session and student evaluation should be signed by both the student and the faculty member and maintained by the faculty member.

Unsatisfactory Performance

Boley and Whitney (2003) note that when a student is given a failing grade, faculty must be aware of the standards to meet, grades must not be "arbitrary or capricious," and faculty must be able to explain how grades are determined related to the program and course objectives. When a fair judgment is made that a student's performance is unsatisfactory or failing, strategies should be used to avert interpersonal or legal problems (Caldwell & Tenofsky, 1996). As soon as the decision is made, communication with the student is essential. Documentation from formative evaluation conferences and student contracts can provide support for this decision. Published school policies and procedures should be followed, including documentation that decisions were made carefully and deliberately. Support from the university or college is essential when performance is determined to be unsatisfactory, and the administration should be notified of impending problems early in the grading process.

Final evaluations that result in unsatisfactory or failing performance require special tact and concern. Faculty need to share specific findings that resulted in a student not meeting the expected clinical objectives. Student contracts not fulfilled need to be identified. Students need time to process the information and should not feel rushed. Faculty need to listen attentively, with a strong show of concern and support, to the student's perceptions. The student may need time to reflect and return for another conference after adjusting to the facts.

Student Reactions

The failing student may react in a variety of ways. Caring faculty will recognize these behaviors and provide empathetic support. Students may respond with denial, providing their own perception of how a specified incident did or did not occur and offering excuses. Faculty need to steer the conversation to the student's not meeting the clinical course objectives and provide support for the student's emotional needs.

A student may attempt to bargain for a passing grade. Faculty need to stand firm and focus on the evaluation results. Faculty can be prepared to provide information about any program options that are available to students who fail a clinical course. As the reality of the loss is recognized, the student may respond with despair, confusion, lack of motivation, indecision, and tears. Faculty should provide support, listen attentively, and generally convey caring behaviors; in some cases faculty may also need to recommend professional counseling. The student may come to terms with the outcome and begin to make plans for the future. Assistance from the faculty in considering further options is often sought by the student. How well the student adapts to the final evaluation typically depends on how well he or she has been prepared for the results.

The student may respond with anger. The student may become demanding or accusing and may have the potential to become violent. In this case, faculty need to take steps to ensure their own safety and that of the student. Faculty should not take the anger personally but provide guidance about feelings and focus on the anger as a part of loss. Thomas (2003) has recommended handling anger with a "professional deep breath."

Additionally, an established grievance policy should be available. Both students and faculty share responsibility for knowing about and appropriately employing such a policy. Students have a right to respond appropriately to grievances. See Chapter 3 for further discussion of legal issues.

Dismissing an Unsafe Student from Clinical Practice

Behaviors unsafe for patient care such as lack of preparation, violence, and substance abuse need to be addressed. Pierce (2001) notes the importance of a broad and thorough policy that allows for safe and appropriate actions to protect both the patient and the student. School policies and procedures need to be followed. Clear policies help prevent arbitrary or capricious responses to an incident. O'Connor (2006) summarizes key points related to the student who is unsafe to care for patients, noting that safety of the patient is the first priority in removing a student but that faculty have an obligation to ensure that all students are returned to an area of safety as well. The student unprepared to care for an assigned clinical patient should be sent to the library or laboratory to prepare. Student orientation to clinical practice should include a review of relevant policies and clarification of professional student behaviors.

Evaluation of the Evaluation

After the final student conference, the student and faculty need to evaluate the entire experience as a whole. The clinical site is evaluated on how well it met the learning and practice needs of the students. Was the philosophy of the staff congruent with that of the faculty and students? Were the students given the opportunity to meet all objectives? As these questions are answered, the preparation phase for evaluation begins again. A continuous quality improvement process for clinical evaluation should be considered, with attention given to structure (appropriate evaluation tools with appropriate clinical environment and patient care opportunities), process (appropriate plans for sampling and evaluating clinical behaviors and for sharing feedback and results of evaluation), and outcome (satisfactory evaluative outcomes indicating safe, competent graduates). Questioning ongoing evaluation practices and including new approaches that further incorporate students' perspectives is recommended (Rankin, Malinsky, Tate, & Elena, 2010).

SUMMARY

Clinical evaluation is important to both patients' safety and students' skill and confidence. Good practice includes multidimensional evaluation with diverse evaluation methods completed over time, seeking student growth and progress (Astin et al., n.d.). All evaluations should respect students' dignity and self-esteem. Nursing students have the unique opportunity to practice skills in natural settings with supervision by experienced nurses. The clinical evaluation provides both subjective and objective data that permit formative and summative analysis of the entire learning experience. Advances in technology are promoting new opportunities for clinical evaluation. Clinical performance evaluation provides students with a means for critical reflection on their future nursing roles. An appropriate evaluation process sets the stage for productive assessment of student learning.

REFLECTING ON THE EVIDENCE

1. How do you currently provide formative feedback to students? What strategies do you use to challenge students to self-reflect and set further learning goals? How do these strategies contribute to active learning and critical thinking?

2. How can selected methods described in this chapter be incorporated into documentation of students' clinical competency? For example, how can students' written assignments best be used to contribute to clinical evaluation? What other approaches that you read about will you incorporate into your evaluation practices?

3. What is your current process for completing a clinical evaluation? In what ways do you incorporate multiple clinical indicators into evaluation (e.g., data from interview, observation, and document review)? How do you then synthesize these diverse pieces of clinical evaluation data? How will you evaluate the success of these approaches?

4. What are the benefits of anecdotal records and rubrics in the clinical evaluation documentation process? How does your faculty team currently use these tools? Are there ways you could expand or improve the use of these tools? How will you determine whether these approaches improve your efficiency and effectiveness in clinical evaluation?

5. What is the state of the science in terms of technologies and clinical evaluation? For example, what are best practices in using high-fidelity patient simulators as part of clinical evaluation? How are clinical learning laboratories and tools such as high-fidelity patient simulators best incorporated into clinical evaluations? What models are there to guide us? What processes are most efficient and effective? What research supports these practices?

REFERENCES

Astin, A. W., Banta, T. W., Cross, K. P., El-Khawas, E., Ewell, P. T., Hutchings, P., . . . Wright, B. D. (n.d.). *AAHE assessment forum: 9 principles of good practice for assessing student learning.* American Association of Higher Education. Retrieved from http://www.assessment.tcu.edu

Blake, T. (2005). Journaling: An active learning technique. *International Journal of Nursing Education Scholarship, 2*(1), Article 7.

Boehm, H., & Bonnel, W. (2010). The use of peer review in nursing education and clinical practice. *Journal for Nurses in Staff Development, 26*(3), 108–115.

Boley, P., & Whitney, K. (2003). Grade disputes: Considerations for nursing faculty. *Journal of Nursing Education, 42*(5), 198–203.

Bonnel, W. (2008). Improving feedback to students in online courses. *Nursing Education Perspectives, 29*(5), 290–294.

Bonnel, W., & Smith, K. (2010). *Teaching technologies in nursing and the health professions.* New York, NY: Springer.

Borbasi, S. A., & Koop, A. (1994). The objective structured clinical examination: Its appreciation in nursing education. *The Australian Journal of Advanced Nursing, 11*(3), 33–40.

Boswell, C. (2006). The art of questioning: Improving critical thinking. In M. Oermann & K. Heinrich (Eds.), *Annual review of nursing education innovations in curriculum, teaching, and student and faculty development, 4,* 291–304. New York, NY: Springer.

Bremner, M., Aduddell, K., Bennett, D., & VanGeest, J. (2006). The use of human patient simulators: Best practices with novice nursing students. *Nurse Educator, 31*(4), 170–174.

Caldwell, L. M., & Tenofsky, L. (1996). Clinical failure or clinical folly? A second opinion on student performance. *Nursing and Health Care Perspectives, 17*(1), 22–25.

Carpenito, L. J., & Duespohl, T. A. (1985). *A guide for effective clinical instruction* (2nd ed.). Rockville, MD: Aspen.

Castellino, A., & Schuster, P. (2002). Evaluation of outcomes in nursing students using clinical concept map care plans. *Nurse Educator, 27*(4), 149–150.

Chan, D. (2002). Development of the clinical learning environment inventory. *Journal of Nursing Education, 41*(2), 69–75.

Cowles, K. V., Strickland, D., & Rodgers, B. L. (2001). Collaboration for teaching innovation: Writing across the curriculum in a school of nursing. *Journal of Nursing Education, 40*(8), 363–367.

Dearman, C. N. (2003). Using clinical scenarios in nursing. In M. Oermann & K. Heinrich (Eds.), *Annual review of nursing education* (pp. 341–356). New York, NY: Springer.

DeBourgh, G. A. (2001). Using web technology in a clinical nursing course. *Nurse Educator, 26*(5), 227–233.

Ebbert, D., & Connors, H. (2004). Standardized patient experiences: Evaluation of clinical performance and nurse practitioner student satisfaction. *Nursing Education Perspectives, 25*(1), 12–15.

Fink, L. D. (2003). *Creating significant learning experiences: An integrated approach to designing college courses.* San Francisco, CA: Jossey-Bass.

Fonteyn, M., & Cahill, M. (1998). The use of clinical logs to improve nursing students' metacognition: A pilot study. *Journal of Advanced Nursing, 28*(1), 149–154.

Freshwater, D., Taylor, B., & Sherwood, G. (2010). *International textbook of reflective practice in nursing.* Indianapolis, IN: Sigma Theta Tau International.

Gaberson, K. B., & Oermann, M. H. (2010). *Clinical teaching strategies in nursing* (3rd ed.). New York, NY: Springer.

Gibbons, S. W., Adamo, G., Padden, D., Ricciardi, R., Graziano, M., & Levine, E. (2002). Clinical evaluation in advanced practice nursing education: Using standardized patients in health assessment. *Journal of Nursing Education, 41*(5), 215–221.

Gronlund, N. (2005). *How to make achievement tests and assessments* (8th ed.). Needham Heights, MA: Allyn & Bacon.

Hayes, A. (2005). A mental health nursing clinical experience with hospice patients. *Nurse Educator, 30*(2), 85–88.

Henneman, E., & Cunningham, H. (2005). Using clinical simulation to teach patient safety in an acute/critical care nursing course. *Nurse Educator, 30*(4), 172–177.

Higuchi, K. A., & Donald, J. G. (2002). Thinking processes used by nurses in clinical decision making. *Journal of Nursing Education, 41*(4), 145–153.

Hrobsky, P. E., & Kersbergen, A. L. (2002). Preceptors' perceptions of clinical performance failure. *Journal of Nursing Education, 41*(12), 550–553.

Issenberg, S., McGaghie, W., Petrusa, E., Gordon, D., & Scalese, R. (2005). Features and uses of high-fidelity medical simulations that lead to effective learning: A best evidence medical education systematic review. *Medical Teacher, 27*(1), 10–28.

Jeffries, P. (2005). A framework for designing, implementing, and evaluating simulations used as teaching strategies in nursing. *Nursing Education Perspective, 26*(2), 96–103.

Kennison, M. M., & Misselwitz, S. (2002). Evaluating reflective writing for appropriateness, fairness, and consistency. *Nursing Education Perspectives, 23*(5), 238–242.

Kern, C. S., Bush, K. L., & McCleish, J. M. (2006). Mind-mapped care plans: Integrating an innovative educational tool as an alternative to traditional care plans. *Journal of Nursing Education, 45*(4), 112–119.

King, M., & Shell, R. (2002). Teaching and evaluating critical thinking with concept maps. *Nurse Educator, 27*(5), 213–216.

Kuiper, R., & Pesut, D. (2004). Promoting cognitive and metacognitive reflective reasoning skills in nursing practice: Self-regulated learning theory. *Journal of Advanced Nursing, 45*(4), 381–391.

Lehman, K. (2003). Clinical nursing instructors' use of handheld computers for student recordkeeping and evaluation. *Journal of Nursing Education, 42*(1), 41–42.

Liberto, T., Roncher, M., & Shellenbarger, T. (1999). Anecdotal notes: Effective clinical evaluation and record keeping. *Nurse Educator, 24*(6), 15–18.

Loving, G. L. (1993). Competence validation and cognitive flexibility: A theoretical model grounded in nursing education. *Journal of Nursing Education, 32*(9), 415–421.

Mahara, M. (1998). A perspective on clinical evaluation in nursing education. *Journal of Advanced Nursing, 28*(6), 1339–1346.

McAllister, M., & Osborne, Y. (1997). Peer review: A strategy to enhance cooperative student learning. *Nurse Educator, 22*(1), 40–44.

McWilliam, P., & Botwinski, C. (2010). Developing a successful nursing objective structured clinical examination. *Journal of Nursing Education, 49*(1), 36–41.

Miller, H. K., Nichols, E., & Beeken, J. E. (2000). Comparing videotaped and faculty-present return demonstrations of clinical skills. *Journal of Nursing Education, 39*(5), 237–239.

Mueller, A., Johnston, M., & Bligh, D. (2001). Mind-mapped care plans: A remarkable alternative to traditional nursing care plans. *Nurse Educator, 26*(2), 75–80.

Murphy, J. I. (2005). How to learn, not what to learn: Three strategies that foster lifelong learning in the clinical setting. In M. Oermann & K. Heinrich (Eds.), *Annual review of nursing education strategies for teaching, assessment, and program planning* (pp. 37–58). New York, NY: Springer.

NIH Stroke Scale (NIHSS) training—Online or mobile. (n.d.). American Heart Association. Retrieved from http://www.strokeassociation.com

O'Connor, A. B. (2006). *Clinical instruction and evaluation* (2nd ed.). Boston, MA: Jones & Bartlett.

Oermann, M. H. (1997). Evaluating critical thinking in clinical practice. *Nurse Educator, 22*(5), 25–28.

Oermann, M. H., & Gaberson, K. (2009). *Evaluation and testing in nursing education* (3rd ed.). New York, NY: Springer.

Oermann, M. H, Yarbrough, S. S., Saewert, K. J., Ard, N., & Charasika, M. E. (2009). Clinical evaluation and grading practices in schools of nursing: National survey findings Part II. *Nursing Education Perspectives, 30*(6), 352–357.

Orchard, C. (1994). The nurse educator and the nursing student: A review of the issue of clinical evaluation procedures. *Journal of Nursing Education, 33*(6), 245–251.

Osinski, K. (2003). Due process rights of nursing students in cases of misconduct. *Journal of Nursing Education, 42*(2), 55–58.

Pierce, C. S. (2001). Implications of chemically impaired students in clinical settings. *Journal of Nursing Education, 40*(9), 422–425.

Rankin, J. M., Malinsky, L., Tate, B., & Elena, L. (2010). Contesting our taken-for-granted understanding of student evaluation: Insights from a team of institutional ethnographers. *Journal of Nursing Education, 49*(6), 333–339.

Redman, R., Lenberg, C., & Walker, P. (1999). Competency assessment: Methods for development and implementation in nursing education. *Online Journal of Issues in Nursing, Topic 10.* Retrieved from http://www.nursingworld.org/MainMenuCategories/ANAMarketplace/ANAPeriodicals/OJIN/TableofContents/Volume41999/No2Sep1999/InitialandContinuingCompetenceinEducationandPracticeCompetencyAssessmentMethodsforDeve.aspx

Reilly, D. J., & Oermann, M. H. (1992). *Clinical teaching in nursing education* (2nd ed.). New York, NY: National League for Nursing.

Rhodes, M., & Curran, C. (2005). Use of the human patient simulator to teach clinical judgment skills in a baccalaureate nursing program. *Computers, Informatics, Nursing, 23*(5), 256–262.

Rinne, C. H.(1994). The SKILLS system: A new interactive video technology [Electronic version]. *T H E Journal, 21*(8), 81–82. Retrieved from http://thejournal.com

Roberts, J. D., While, A. E., & Fitzpatrick, J. M. (1992). Simulation: Current status in nurse education. *Nurse Education Today, 12*(6), 409–415.

Scanlan, J. M. (2001). Learning clinical teaching: Is it magic? *Nursing and Health Care Perspectives, 22*(5), 240–246.

Schuster, P. (2000). Concept mapping: Reducing clinical care plan paperwork and increasing learning. *Nurse Educator, 25*(2), 76–81.

Seldomridge, L., & Walsh, C. (2006). Evaluating student performance in undergraduate preceptorships. *Journal of Nursing Education, 45*(5), 169–177.

Slater, T. F. (1999). Classroom assessment techniques: Portfolios. *Field-tested learning assessment guide* (Screen 1 of 6). Retrieved from http://www.flaguide.org/cat/

Stevens, D., & Levi, A. (2005). *Introduction to rubrics: An assessment tool to save grading time, convey effective feedback and promote student learning.* Sterling, VA: Stylus.

Suskie, L. (2004). *Assessing student learning: A common sense guide.* San Francisco, CA: Anker.

Thomas, S. P. (2003). Handling anger in the teacher–student relationship. *Nursing Education Perspective, 24*(1), 17–24.

U.S. Department of Education. (1974). *The Family Educational Rights and Privacy Act.* Retrieved from http://www.ed.gov/

Walker, E., & Dewar, B. (2000). Moving on from interpretivism: An argument for constructivist evaluation. *Journal of Advanced Nursing, 32*(3), 713–720.

Walsh, C., & Seldomridge, L. (2005). Clinical grades: Upward bound. *Journal of Nursing Education, 44*(4), 162–168.

Waltz, C. F. &. Jenkins, L. S. (2001). *Measurement of nursing outcomes. Volume 1: Measuring nursing performance in practice, education, and research* (2nd ed.). New York, NY: Springer.

Walvoord, B., Anderson, V., & Angelo, T. A. (2010). *Effective grading: A tool for learning and assessment.* San Francisco, CA: Jossey-Bass.

Wiles, L., & Bishop, J. (2001). Clinical performance appraisal: Renewing graded clinical experiences. *Journal of Nursing Education, 40*(1), 37–39.

Zuzelo, P. R. (2000). Clinical issues, clinical probation: Supporting the at-risk student. *Nurse Educator, 25*(5), 216–218.

Educational Program Evaluation 28

Marcia K. Sauter, PhD, RN

Nancy Nightingale Gillespie, PhD, RN

Amy Knepp, NP-C, MSN, RN

The purpose of this chapter is to provide information on how to conduct comprehensive evaluation of nursing education programs. A brief history of program evaluation and examples of models for program evaluation will be followed by a description of a theory-driven approach to program evaluation, which has served as a framework for the evaluation of nursing education programs at a private university since 2000. The evaluation plan was originally adapted from Chen's (1990) theory-driven model for program evaluation, which provides a mechanism for evaluating all program elements, for determining the causal relationships between program elements, for determining program effectiveness, and for identifying strategies to improve program quality. The evaluation plan has demonstrated long-term sustainability and has been easily adapted to changes in accreditation requirements. The evaluation plan has been refined during the past decade while maintaining the overall framework.

Definition of Terms

A *nursing education program* is any academic program in a postsecondary institution leading to initial licensure or advanced preparation in nursing. *Program evaluation* is systematic assessment of all components of a program through the application of evaluation approaches, techniques, and knowledge in order to improve the planning, implementation, and effectiveness of programs (Chen, 2005).

The authors acknowledge the work of Margaret H. Applegate, EdD, RN, FAAN, and David R. Johnson, PhD, APRN, BC, in the previous edition(s) of the chapter.

Program evaluation theory is a framework that guides the practice of program evaluation. A *program evaluation plan* is a document that serves as the blueprint for the evaluation of a specific program. *Program theory* is a set of assumptions that describes the elements of a program and their causal relationships.

Purposes and Benefits of Program Evaluation

The purpose of program evaluation is to improve program effectiveness and demonstrate accountability. Evaluation may be developmental, designed to provide direction for the development and implementation of a program, or outcome-oriented, designed to judge the merit of the total program being evaluated. The focus of program evaluation is dependent on the stage of program implementation, beginning with program planning, through early implementation, and ending in mature program implementation (Chen, 2005). The more advanced a program is in its implementation, the more complex becomes the program evaluation. Specific purposes of program evaluation are as follows:

1. To determine how various elements of the program interact and influence program effectiveness
2. To determine the extent to which the mission, goals, and outcomes of the program are realized
3. To determine whether the program has been implemented as planned
4. To provide a rationale for decision making that leads to improved program effectiveness
5. To identify efficient use of resources that are needed to improve program quality

Relationship of Program Evaluation to Accreditation

Accrediting bodies exert considerable influence over nursing programs. Accrediting bodies include the state board of nursing, the National League for Nursing Accrediting Commission (NLNAC), the Commission on Collegiate Nursing Education (CCNE), and regional accrediting bodies such as the Higher Learning Commission. Nursing education programs must be approved by the state board of nursing to be able to operate and by the regional accrediting body to seek national accreditation. National accreditation by NLNAC or CCNE is voluntary, but the public perception of the school is linked, in part, to this accreditation. Certainly, schools that have a mission to prepare students for graduate education and schools that wish to compete for external funding as a part of their mission will want to meet all levels of accreditation.

Nursing programs have historically been too dependent on accreditation processes to guide program evaluation efforts (Ingersoll & Sauter, 1998). Some nursing programs do not fully engage in program evaluation until preparation of the self-study for an accreditation site visit has begun. To fulfill its purposes, program evaluation must be a continuous activity. Program evaluation built solely around accreditation criteria may lack examination of some important elements or understanding of the relationship between elements that influences program success. Nevertheless, building the assessment indicators identified by these bodies into the evaluation process ensures ongoing attention to state and national standards of excellence.

Historical Perspective

The earliest approaches to educational program evaluation were based on Ralph Tyler's (1949) behavioral objective model, which focused on whether learning experiences produced the desired educational outcomes. Tyler's behavioral objective model was a simple, linear approach that began with defining learning objectives, developing measuring tools, and then measuring student performance to determine whether objectives had been met. Because evaluation occurred at the end of the learning experience, Tyler's approach was primarily summative. Formative evaluation, which includes testing and revising curriculum components during the development and implementation of educational programs, became popular during the 1960s. This trend continued into the 1970s, when the Phi Delta Kappa National Study Committee on Evaluation concluded that meaningful educational evaluation was rare and encouraged educational institutions to continue formative evaluation by focusing on the process of program implementation (Stufflebeam, 1983).

Outcomes assessment became the focus of educational evaluation in the 1980s. In 1984 the National Institute of Education Study Group on the Conditions of Excellence in American Postsecondary Education endorsed outcomes assessment as an essential strategy for improving the quality of education in postsecondary institutions (Ewell, 1985). By the mid-1980s numerous state legislatures began mandating outcomes assessment for public postsecondary institutions (Halpern, 1987) and the regional accrediting agencies began mandating outcomes assessment in their accreditation criteria (Ewell, 1985). Although the focus on outcomes assessment was growing rapidly, initial efforts at implementing outcomes assessment were not successful because educators experienced difficulty in developing appropriate methods for performing outcomes assessment and in obtaining adequate organizational support to implement assessment (Terenzini, 1989). The focus on outcomes assessment led some institutions to confuse outcomes assessment with comprehensive program evaluation. Nursing educators were also influenced by the outcomes assessment movement. Publications from the National League for Nursing (NLN) called for measurement of student outcomes (Waltz, 1988) and described measurement tools for assessing educational outcomes (Waltz & Miller, 1988).

By the early 1990s some of the issues surrounding outcomes assessment had been addressed and successful efforts in outcomes assessment had occurred. As nursing education continued to follow the trend in higher education, the NLN added assessment of learning outcomes to its accreditation criteria in 1991. The CCNE also included outcomes assessment in its initial accreditation standards, first published in 1997.

The Wingspread Group on Higher Education (1993) challenged providers of higher education to use outcomes assessment to improve teaching and learning. Nevertheless, outcomes assessment was not the final solution to improving program quality.

Many postsecondary institutions continued to struggle with outcomes assessment, and those that were able to implement it were often unable to identify any academic improvements as a result of the assessment program (Tucker, 1995). Toward the end of the decade, approaches to organizational effectiveness, especially Deming's continuous quality improvement model, began to influence a more comprehensive approach to program evaluation (Freed, Klugman, & Fife, 1997).

As a result of the growing emphasis on program evaluation in the 1980s and 1990s, university programs were developed to prepare individuals in program evaluation (Shadish, Cook, & Leviton, 1991). As program evaluation became a distinct field of study, theories were developed to guide the practice of evaluation. Some of these theories include Borich and Jemelka's (1982) systems theory; Stufflebeam's context, input, process, and product (CIPP) model (1983); Guba and Lincoln's fourth-generation evaluation framework (1989); Patton's qualitative evaluation model (1990); Chen's theory-driven model (1990); Veney and Kaluzny's cybernetic decision model (1991); and Rossi and Freeman's social research approach (1993). Perhaps because of the nursing profession's emphasis on use of theory to guide practice, the need for program evaluation theory to guide evaluation practices in nursing education was identified in the nursing literature as early as 1978. Friesner (1978) reviewed five evaluation models: (1) Tyler's behavioral objective model, (2) the NLN accreditation model, (3) Stufflebeam's CIPP model, (4) Scriven's goal-free evaluation model, and (5) Provus's discrepancy evaluation. Friesner (1978) concluded that no single model could effectively guide the evaluation of nursing education and recommends that nursing educators blend elements from one or more of the models.

In the early 1990s several articles about program evaluation theory appeared in the nursing literature. Watson and Herbener (1990) reviewed Provus's discrepancy model, Scriven's goal-free evaluation model, Stakes' countenance model, Staropolia and Waltz's decision model, and Stufflebeam's CIPP model. These authors concluded that any of these models could be useful and recommended that nursing educators choose a model that best fits their needs. In contrast, Sarnecky (1990) explicitly recommended Guba and Lincoln's (1989) responsiveness model after comparing it with Tyler's behavioral objective model, Stake's countenance model, Provus's discrepancy model, and Stufflebeam's CIPP model. Sarnecky believed that the other models did not adequately address the plurality of values among stakeholders and the importance of stakeholder involvement. Bevil (1991) proposed a theoretical framework she adapted from several evaluation theories. Ingersoll (1996) reviewed Borich and Jemelka's systems approach, McClintock's conceptual mapping approach, and Chen's theory-driven model. Addressing issues about the reliability and validity of assessment activities, Ingersoll recommended that program evaluation be viewed as evaluation research and that program evaluation theory be used to guide the development and implementation of program evaluation. Ingersoll and Sauter (1998) reviewed Guba and Lincoln's fourth-generation evaluation, Scriven's goal-free approach, Norman and Lutenbacher's theory of systems improvement, Rossi and Freeman's social science approach, and Chen's theory-driven model. The authors suggested that Rossi and Freeman's model and Chen's model had the most potential for guiding the evaluation of nursing education programs. Ingersoll and Sauter also expressed concern that nursing faculty commonly use accreditation criteria to form the framework for evaluation of nursing education programs. They recommended that program evaluation theory serve this purpose. Ingersoll and Sauter (1998) presented an evaluation plan developed from Chen's theory-driven model that incorporated the NLNAC's criteria for baccalaureate programs.

Sauter (2000) surveyed all baccalaureate nursing programs in the United States to determine how they develop, implement, and revise their program evaluation plans. Few nursing programs reported using program evaluation theory to guide program evaluation. However, those educators that did use program evaluation theory were more satisfied with the effectiveness of their evaluation practices.

In the past decade most of the nursing literature related to program evaluation has focused on specific elements of program evaluation, rather than on comprehensive evaluation. Only one article reported a theory-based approach to program evaluation. In 2006 Suhayda and Miller reported on the use of Stufflebeam's CIPP model in providing a framework for comprehensive program evaluation that would serve undergraduate and graduate nursing programs.

Program Evaluation Theories

Program evaluation theories are either method-oriented or theory-driven, depending on their underlying assumptions, preferred methodology, and general focus. Method-oriented theories emphasize methods for performing evaluation, whereas theory-driven approaches emphasize the theoretical framework for developing and implementing evaluation. The more popular approaches have been method-oriented (Chen, 1990; Shadish et al., 1991).

Method-oriented approaches usually focus on the relationship between program inputs and outputs and include an emphasis on a preferred method for conducting program evaluation. Many of the method-oriented approaches emphasize quantitative research methods. A few method-oriented approaches recommend naturalistic or qualitative methods for performing program evaluation.

An example of a quantitative method-oriented program evaluation theory is Rossi and Freeman's (1993) social science model. These authors believe that the use of experimental research methods will produce the most effective program evaluation. The advantage of this approach is that measurement techniques must be reliable and valid, even if experimental design is not used to conduct the evaluation. One of the major limitations of this approach is that the focus on methodology may divert evaluators from other issues, such as recognizing the importance of stakeholder perspective. In addition, experimental designs are often difficult to apply to some aspects of educational evaluation.

An example of a qualitative method-oriented program evaluation theory is Guba and Lincoln's (1989) fourth-generation evaluation. Guba and Lincoln advocate naturalistic methods for program evaluation. A special focus of their approach is the emphasis they place on integrating multiple stakeholders' viewpoints into program evaluation. A major advantage of their approach is that using qualitative methodology allows evaluators to achieve a greater depth of understanding of program strengths and limitations within a specific context. The approach is limited because it tends to overlook outcomes assessment, which usually requires more quantitative methodology.

Theory-driven approaches to program evaluation begin with the development of program theory. Program theory is the framework that describes the elements of the program and explains the relationships between and among elements. When this approach is used, program evaluation is intended to test whether the program theory is correct and whether it has been implemented correctly. If the program is not successful in achieving outcomes, a theory-driven approach allows the evaluator to determine whether the program's failure is due to flaws in the program theory or failure to implement the program correctly. The theory-driven approach often calls for a variety of research methods because evaluators choose the methodology that is best suited to answering the evaluation questions (Chen, 1990).

Chen's (1990) theory-driven model is one of the most comprehensive models for program evaluation. Although the model was intended for evaluation of social service programs, it is adaptable to educational programs. A brief overview of Chen's model is included here. The remainder of the chapter describes a nursing education program evaluation plan that was developed from Chen's theory-driven model. The evaluation plan has been in continuous use since 2000 and has been applied to undergraduate and graduate nursing programs. For a more detailed description of how the evaluation plan was created from Chen's original theory-driven model, see Sauter, Johnson, and Gillespie (2009).

Theory-Driven Program Evaluation

Chen (1990) defines program theory as a framework that identifies the elements of the program, provides the rationale for interventions, and describes the causal linkages between the elements, interventions, and outcomes. According to Chen, program theory is needed to determine desired goals, what ought to be done to achieve desired goals, how actions should be organized, and what outcome criteria should be investigated. Program evaluation is the systematic collection of empirical evidence to assess congruency between the program's design and implementation and to test the program theory. Through this systematic collection of evidence, program planners can develop and refine program structure and operations, understand and strengthen program effectiveness and utility, and facilitate policy decision making (Chen, 1990).

Adapting Chen's Theory-Driven Model to Program Evaluation for Nursing Education

The following section describes a program evaluation plan for nursing education programs adapted from Chen's (1990) theory-driven model. The components of the evaluation plan are organized into six evaluation types, which were modified and adapted from Chen's model. Table 28-1 lists the evaluation types defined by Chen, provides a brief description of the elements of the evaluation type, and demonstrates how Chen's model was adapted to the evaluation of nursing education programs.

The Program Evaluation Plan

The program evaluation plan provides a road map for organizing and tracking evaluation activities. The plan is a written document that contains the

---

TABLE 28-1 Comparison of Chen's Theory-Driven Model for Program Evaluation and a Model for Nursing Education

Chen's Evaluation Types	**Components for Evaluation of Nursing Education Programs**
Normative outcome evaluation • Develop program theory. • Define appropriate activities to achieve the goals. • Explain the linkages between program activities and goals. • Identify and prioritize desired program goals and outcomes.	Mission and goal evaluation • Develop mission, philosophy, and conceptual framework. • Identify program goals and outcomes. • Ensure that program goals and outcomes are congruent with professional standards.
Normative treatment evaluation • Evaluate congruency between the expected and implemented treatment.	Curriculum evaluation Evaluation of teaching effectiveness
IMPLEMENTATION ENVIRONMENT EVALUATION Participant dimension • Evaluates the participants' characteristics, demographics, roles.	*ENVIRONMENT EVALUATION* Student dimension • Assesses recruitment, student qualifications, retention
Implementer dimension • Assesses whether the implementers possess the qualities desired and the kind of relationships they have with participants	Faculty dimension • Assesses faculty qualifications and scholarship
Delivery mode dimension • Determines whether the program can be delivered effectively and in agreement with stakeholder expectations	Delivery mode dimension • Assesses facilities, course delivery, instructional technology, support services
Implementing organization dimension • Determines how organizational culture influences program implementation • Examines authority structures and operating procedures for how they support or inhibit the program's effectiveness	Organization dimension • Assesses leadership, governance, financial resources
Interorganizational relationship dimension • Evaluates the relationship of the organization to other agencies	Interorganizational relationship dimension • Evaluates the relationship of the organization to other agencies, including clinical agencies and accrediting bodies
Micro context dimension • Assesses interpersonal relationships and factors that have immediate impact on the program	Micro context dimension • Assesses admission policies and procedures, student orientation, academic advising
Macro context dimension • Assesses cultural, social, political factors that may influence program success	Macro context dimension • Assesses trends and issues in health care and higher education
Impact evaluation • Determines whether program is successful in achieving its desired outcomes	Outcomes assessment • Assesses learning outcomes

Continued

TABLE 28-1 Comparison of Chen's Theory-Driven Model for Program Evaluation and a Model for Nursing Education—cont'd

Chen's Evaluation Types	Components for Evaluation of Nursing Education Programs
Intervening mechanism evaluation • Determines the causal processes that link the program activities with the program outcomes	Intervening mechanism evaluation • Determines the causal processes that link the program activities with the program outcomes
Generalization evaluation • Determines how evaluation results can be generalized to similar situations, evaluation of the reliability and validity of assessment strategies	Generalization evaluation • Evaluates the reliability and validity of assessment strategies

evaluation framework, activities for gathering and analyzing data, responsible parties, time frames, accreditation criteria and standards, and the means for using information for program decisions. The program evaluation plan provides the mechanism for maintaining continuous evaluation of program effectiveness.

Mission and Goal Evaluation

Program evaluation must begin by determining that appropriate mission, philosophy, program goals, and outcomes have been defined. The expectations of both internal and external stakeholders must be considered. Internal stakeholders include administrators, faculty, and governing boards. External stakeholders include religious organizations for private schools with religious affiliations, regional accrediting bodies, national discipline-specific accrediting bodies, state education commissions and boards of nursing, the legislature, and professional organizations. There should be congruency between the expectations of stakeholders and the program's mission, philosophy, goals, and outcomes. For private institutions with religious affiliations, some perspectives may be prescribed and must be included in mission, philosophy, goals, or outcomes.

The mission of the nursing department should be congruent with the university's mission. Comparison of key phrases in the department's mission with key phrases in the university's mission may be done to assess congruency between mission statements. The identification of gaps between the two mission statements provides information about areas where attention is needed. The assessment should be performed periodically and whenever changes are made to either mission statement.

There should be consensus among the faculty regarding the nursing school's mission and philosophy. A modified Delphi approach to determine the level of agreement among the faculty for each statement in the mission and philosophy is a useful strategy. The Delphi approach is useful for both the development and the evaluation of belief statements (philosophy). This approach seeks consensus without the need for frequent face-to-face dialogue in a manner that protects the anonymity of participants. In this method, questionnaires that list proposition statements about each of the content elements of the belief statement are distributed. A common breakdown of Delphi responses is a five-point range from "strongly agree" to "strongly disagree" so that respondents can indicate their level of support for each proposition. Respondents are provided with feedback about the responses after the first round of questionnaire distribution, and a second round may occur to determine the intensity of agreement or disagreement with the group median responses (Uhl, 1991). After several rounds with interim reports and analyses, it is usually possible to identify areas of consensus, areas of disagreement so strong that further discourse is unlikely to lead to consensus, and areas in which further discussion is warranted. In the evaluation of an established belief statement, the same process will provide data about which propositions continue to be supported, which no longer garner support, and which need to be openly debated (Uhl, 1991). The result provides a consensus list of propositions that either supports the belief statement as it is or suggests areas for revision. Chapter 7 provides further information on development of mission and philosophy.

All accrediting bodies have expectations about mission, philosophy, program goals, and outcomes. The NLNAC (2008) defines Standard I, Mission and Governance, in which it requires that the nursing program provide clear statements of mission, philosophy, and purposes. In addition, the NLNAC has indicated both required and optional outcomes that nursing programs must measure over time to provide trend data about student learning. For example, the required outcomes in the criteria for baccalaureate and higher degree programs are graduation rates, job placement rates, licensure and certification pass rates, and program satisfaction (NLNAC, 2008). The CCNE (2010) also includes in Standard I, Mission and Governance, expectations regarding congruency of the program's mission, goals, and outcomes with those of the parent institution, professional nursing standards, and the needs of the community of interest.

Professional organizations include the American Nurses Association (ANA), American Association of Colleges of Nursing (AACN), and National Organization of Nurse Practitioner Faculties (NONPF). Program goals and outcomes in baccalaureate degree programs should be congruent with the ANA's Standards of Practice (ANA, 2010) and the AACN's Essentials of Baccalaureate Education for Professional Nursing Practice (AACN, 2008a). The same consideration should be given to the AACN's Essentials of Master's Education of Advanced Practice Nursing (AACN, 1996) and the Criteria for Evaluation of Nurse Practitioner Programs (NONPF, 2008) for master's degree programs. The AACN (2006) also provides indicators of quality in doctoral programs in nursing in Essentials of Doctoral Education for Advanced Nursing Practice.

Other important stakeholders include local constituencies, such as health care agencies, that provide clinical learning experiences or employ graduates of the program. A survey of current and potential employers of graduates will help faculty to determine the knowledge and skill requirements of the marketplace. Many institutions establish advisory committees to provide additional information and selected focus groups to add richness to the information. This information is used to ensure that program goals and outcomes are appropriate, to provide input for curriculum planning, and to develop evaluation questions and tools for determining whether market needs are being met.

The mission and program goals should be clearly and publicly stated. Nursing schools that offer several different nursing programs will need to clearly articulate the purpose and program goals of each of these programs. Public announcement of mission and program goals should be available through the Internet and in printed program brochures and catalogues.

Box 28-1 lists the theoretical elements for mission and goal evaluation. Table 28-2 provides a sample evaluation plan for mission and goal evaluation applied to a nursing education program. This sample demonstrates how all elements of the program evaluation plan may be articulated, including the program's theoretical elements, assessment activities, responsible parties, time frames, and related accreditation criteria. For the remaining evaluation components presented in this chapter, only examples of theoretical elements and methods for gathering and analyzing assessment data relevant to the identified theoretical elements are provided. The theoretical elements and assessment strategies that are suggested here are not all-inclusive but may assist nursing faculty in further development of their own program theory and program evaluation plan.

BOX 28-1 Theoretical Elements for Mission and Goal Evaluation

- The mission of the nursing department is congruent with the university's mission.
- There is consensus among the faculty regarding the mission and philosophy.
- There is congruency between the nursing mission, philosophy, conceptual framework, goals, and outcomes for each program.
- Expectations of the state board of nursing, NLNAC, and CCNE are known and considered in the program's mission, goals, philosophy, and outcomes.
- The goals of the program are congruent with professional standards of practice.
- The Nursing Program Advisory Committee has meaningful input into program goals and outcomes.
- Documents and publications accurately reflect mission/goals.

CCNE, Commission on Collegiate Nursing Education; *NLNAC,* National League for Nursing Accrediting Commission.

TABLE 28-2 Mission and Goal Evaluation

Program Theory	Assessment Strategies	Responsible Parties	Time Frame	Recording and Reporting	Accreditation Criteria
The mission of the nursing department is congruent with the university's mission.	Complete a thematic analysis comparing key phrases in the department's mission with the university's mission.	Program evaluation committee	Every 5 years or whenever change occurs in either statement	Update document "Comparison of Departmental and University Mission."	CCNE Standard I, Mission and Governance NLNAC Standard I, Mission and Governance
There is consensus among the faculty regarding the nursing mission and philosophy.	Use Delphi technique to determine level of agreement among the faculty. Number each statement in mission and philosophy. Faculty indicate level of agreement with each statement. Faculty recommend change. If consensus does not occur, make changes and repeat process until consensus is reached. Complete final report summary to include changes that were made, areas for improvement.	Chair	Every 5 years or whenever change occurs in either statement	Update document "History and Revision of Program Mission and Philosophy."	CCNE 1-B: The mission, goals, and expected student outcomes are reviewed periodically and revised, as appropriate, to reflect: professional standards and guidelines and the needs and expectations of the community of interest. Elaboration: There is a defined process for periodic review and revision of program mission, goals, and expected student outcomes. The review process has been implemented and resultant action reflects professional nursing standards and guidelines. The community of interest is defined by the nursing unit. The needs and expectations of the community of interest are reflected in the mission, goals, and expected student outcomes. Input from the community of interest is used to foster program improvement. The program afforded the community of interest the opportunity to submit third-party comments to CCNE, in accordance with accreditation procedures. (See Macro environment.)

Statement	Task	Responsible	Frequency	Data Source	Accreditation Standards
There is congruency between the nursing mission, philosophy, conceptual framework, goals, and outcomes for each program.	Prepare a content map for each element to assess congruency.	Curriculum committee	Every 3 years	Curriculum committee minutes	NLNAC Standard 4 4.1 The curriculum incorporates established professional standards, guidelines, and competencies, and has clearly articulated student learning and program outcomes. 4.6 The curriculum and instructional processes reflect educational theory, interdisciplinary collaboration, research, and best practice standards while allowing for innovation, flexibility, and technological advances.
Expectations of the state board of nursing, NLNAC, and CCNE are known and considered in the program's mission, goals, philosophy, and outcomes.	Review state Nurse Practice Act and educational rules and NLNAC and CCNE accreditation standards and criteria.	Program evaluation committee	Yearly	Program evaluation committee minutes	
The nursing advisory board provides meaningful input into the goals and outcomes of the program.	Review mission, philosophy, conceptual framework, and goals and outcomes for each program with the nursing advisory board and seek feedback (see section titled "Environment Evaluation: Interorganizational Dimension" for additional assessment of advisory board).	Chair	Every 3 years	Nursing advisory board meeting minutes	CCNE I-B from above fits here Or NLNAC Standard 1.3 Communities of interest have input into program processes and decision making.

Continued

TABLE 28-2 Mission and Goal Evaluation—cont'd

Program Theory	Assessment Strategies	Responsible Parties	Time Frame	Recording and Reporting	Accreditation Criteria
The goals of the program are congruent with professional standards.	Compare the BSN program goals with the ANA standards of practice and essentials of baccalaureate education as defined by AACN.	BSN program director			**CCNE I-A** The mission, goals, and expected student outcomes are congruent with those of the parent institution and consistent with relevant professional standards and guidelines for the preparation of nursing professionals. I-A Elaboration: The program identifies the professional standards and guidelines it uses, including those required by CCNE and any additional program-selected guidelines. A program preparing students for specialty certification incorporates professional standards and guidelines appropriate to the specialty area. A program may select additional standards and guidelines (e.g., state regulatory requirements), as appropriate. Compliance with required and program-selected professional nursing standards and guidelines is clearly evident in the program. III-C. The curriculum is logically structured to achieve expected individual and aggregate student outcomes. The baccalaureate curriculum builds upon the foundation of the arts, sciences, and humanities. Master's curricula build on a foundation comparable to baccalaureate level nursing knowledge. DNP curricula build on a baccalaureate and/or master's foundation, depending on the level of entry of the student. Elaboration: Baccalaureate program faculty and students articulate how knowledge from courses in the arts, sciences, and humanities is incorporated into nursing practice. Postbaccalaureate entry programs in nursing incorporate the generalist knowledge common to baccalaureate nursing education as delineated in *Essentials of Baccalaureate Education for Professional Nursing Practice* (AACN, 2008a) as well as advanced course work. III-B. Expected individual student learning outcomes are consistent with the roles for which the program is preparing its graduates. Curricula are developed, implemented, and revised to reflect relevant professional nursing standards and guidelines, which are clearly evident within the curriculum, expected individual student learning outcomes, and expected aggregate student outcomes. Elaboration: Each degree program and specialty incorporates professional nursing standards and guidelines relevant to the program or area. The program clearly demonstrates where and how content, knowledge, and skills required by identified sets of standards are incorporated into the curriculum.

| Documents and publications accurately reflect mission and goals. | Check all publications for accuracy: • Undergraduate and graduate catalogue • School of nursing brochure • Nursing student handbook • Program fact sheet | Recruitment committee | Annually | Recruitment committee meeting minutes | CCNE Standard I Documents and publications are accurate. References to the program's offerings, outcomes, accreditation/approval status, academic calendar, recruitment and admission policies, transfer of credit policies, grading policies, degree completion requirements, tuition, and fees are accurate. NLNAC Standard 3.5 Integrity and consistency exist for all information intended to inform the public, including the program's accreditation status and NLNAC contact information. |

AACN, American Association of Colleges of Nursing; *ANA,* American Nurses Association; *BSN,* bachelor of science in nursing; *CCNE,* Commission on Collegiate Nursing Education; *DNP,* doctorate in nursing practice; *NLNAC,* National League for Nursing Accrediting Commission.

Curriculum Evaluation

One of the most critical elements of program effectiveness is curriculum design. Curriculum design is an organizing framework that arranges the curriculum elements into a program of study. Curriculum design provides direction to both the content of the program and the teaching and learning processes involved in program implementation. Curriculum content involves both discipline-specific knowledge and the liberal arts foundation. Before the curriculum design can be developed, faculty must first determine their definition of the discipline of knowledge so that they may select courses that will best serve the students to prepare to practice. Faculty must determine what ways of knowing, or methods of inquiry, are characteristic of the discipline and what skills the discipline demands. Program goals and outcome statements provide a guide for the development of the program of study. The program goals link the mission and faculty belief statements (philosophy) to the curriculum design, teaching and learning methods, and outcomes. Consequently, the evaluation of the curriculum builds on the evaluation of mission and goals.

Evaluation of Curriculum Organization

Curriculum must be appropriately organized to move learners along a continuum from program entry to program completion. The principle of *vertical organization* guides both the planning and the evaluation of the curriculum. This principle provides the rationale for the sequencing of curricular content elements (Schwab, 1973). For example, nursing faculty often use depth and complexity as sequencing guides; that is, given content areas may occur in subsequent levels of the curriculum at a level of greater depth and complexity. This is supported by the work of Gagné (1977), who developed a hierarchical theory of instruction based on the premise that knowledge is acquired by proceeding from data and concepts to principles and constructs. In evaluation of the curriculum, faculty must assess for increasing depth and complexity to determine whether the sequencing was useful to learning and progressed to the desired outcomes. Determination of whether course and level objectives demonstrate sequential learning across the curriculum can be used as a test of vertical organization. The analysis can be performed with Bloom's (1956) taxonomy as a guide for determining whether objectives follow a path of increasing complexity.

The principle of *internal consistency* is important to the evaluation of the curriculum. The curriculum design is a carefully conceived plan that takes its shape from what its creators believe about people and their education. The intellectual test of a curriculum design is the extent to which the elements fit together. Four elements should be congruent: objectives, subject matter taught, learning activities used, and outcomes (Doll, 1992). Evaluation efforts should include examination of the extent to which the objectives and outcomes are linked to the mission and belief statements. Program objectives should be tracked to level and course objectives. One method of assessing internal consistency is through the use of a curriculum matrix (Heinrich, Karner, Gaglione, & Lambert, 2002). The matrix is a visual representation that lists all nursing courses and shows the placement of major concepts flowing from the program philosophy and conceptual framework. Another approach to assessment of internal consistency is through a curriculum audit (Seager & Anema, 2003). Similar to a curriculum matrix, the curriculum audit provides a visual representation that matches competencies to courses and learning activities.

The principle of *linear congruence*, sometimes called *horizontal organization*, assists faculty in determining which courses should precede and follow others and which should be concurrent (Schwab, 1973). The concept of sequencing follows the principle of moderate novelty in that new information and experiences should not be presented until existing knowledge has been assimilated (Rabinowitz & Schubert, 1991). An appropriate question is: "What entry skills and knowledge does the student need as a condition of subsequent knowledge and experiences?" How faculty answer this question will determine curriculum design and implementation. The evaluation question would address the extent to which students have the entry-level skills needed to progress sequentially in the curriculum. This is a critical question in light of the changing profile of students entering college-level programs. It is often difficult to determine which prerequisite skills should be required for entry and which should be acquired concurrently. Computer skills are a good example. Students enter programs with varying ability in using computers. It is necessary to determine the prerequisite skills needed and the sequence in which advanced skills should be acquired during the program of learning.

Some nursing programs use a specific conceptual framework that identifies essential program "threads" and provides further direction to curriculum development and implementation. Congruency between program threads, program goals, course objectives, and course content will also need to be assessed. Further information on curriculum development and curriculum frameworks can be found in Unit 2.

Course Evaluation

Individual courses are reviewed to determine whether they have met the tests of *internal consistency*, *linear congruence*, and *vertical organization*. A triangulation approach to course evaluation is useful. This approach uses data from three sources—faculty, students, and materials review—to identify strengths and areas for change (DiFlorio, Duncan, Martin, & Meddlemiss, 1989). Each course is evaluated to determine whether content elements, learning activities, evaluation measures, and learner outcomes are consistent with the objectives of the course and the obligations of the course in terms of its placement in the total curriculum.

Faculty should clearly articulate the sequential levels of each expected ability to determine what teaching and learning strategies are needed to move the student to progressive levels of ability and to establish the criteria for determining that each stage of development has been achieved. This need is important in relation not only to abilities specific to the discipline or major but also to the transferable skills acquired in the general education component of the curriculum (Loacker & Mentkowski, 1993). Some faculty achieve this by creating content maps for each major thread or pervasive strand in the curriculum with related knowledge and skill elements. The content maps chart the obligation of each course in facilitating student progression to the expected program outcome. The maps also provide a guide for the evaluation of whether the elements were incorporated as planned.

Angelo and Cross (1993) have developed a teaching goals inventory tool that is useful in individual course evaluation. The purpose is to assist faculty in identifying and clarifying their teaching goals by helping them to rank the relative importance of teaching goals in a given course. The construction of the teaching goals inventory began in 1986 and involved a complex process that included a literature review, several cycles of data collection and analysis, expert analysis, and field testing with hundreds of teachers (Angelo & Cross, 1993). In the process, Angelo and Cross developed a tool that clusters goals into higher-order thinking skills, basic academic success skills, discipline-specific knowledge and skills, liberal arts and academic values, work and career preparation, and personal development. This tool can assist the faculty in determining priorities in the selection of teaching and learning activities designed to advance the student toward the desired goals and in evaluating whether teaching goals and strategies are congruent with course objectives.

Evaluation of Support Courses and the Liberal Education Foundation

Liberal education is fundamental to professional education. Expected outcomes for the liberal arts component of professional programs have received much attention in recent years (Association of American Colleges and Universities, 2002). Expected outcomes for today's college students include effective communication skills; the use of quantitative and qualitative data in solving problems; and the ability to evaluate various types of information, work effectively within complex systems, manage change, and demonstrate judgment in the use of knowledge. In addition, students should demonstrate a commitment to civic engagement, an understanding of various cultures, and the ability to apply ethical reasoning. Nursing faculty should work collaboratively with faculty across disciplines to ensure that the general education curriculum supports the expectations of a twenty first-century liberal education.

Evaluation questions about general education courses should address the extent to which the courses selected enable student learning and contribute to the expected outcomes. They should also be examined for sequencing to ensure that the support courses are appropriately placed to ground and complement the major and enrich the data mix for the organization and use of knowledge in practice. To develop evaluation questions related to the general education courses, faculty must first articulate what the rationale is for each course, what the expected outcomes are from the courses, and how the courses support the major to provide a broad, liberal education. When the expectations are clear, it is easier to select the measures needed to determine whether expectations have been met. Evaluation of the outcomes of the general education courses will be discussed in the section on outcomes.

External accrediting agencies have expectations about liberal education. The NLNAC (2008) states that no more than 60% of courses in associate degree curricula may be in the nursing major. The remainder of coursework should be in general education. The criteria for baccalaureate and higher-degree programs do not indicate a desired ratio. Box 28-2 provides a summary of the theoretical elements associated with curriculum evaluation.

Evaluation of Teaching Effectiveness

Evaluation of teaching effectiveness involves assessment of teaching strategies (including instructional materials), assessment of methods used to evaluate student performance, and assessment of student learning. Teaching strategies are effective when students are actively engaged, when strategies assist students to achieve course objectives, and when strategies provide opportunities for students to use prior knowledge in building new knowledge. Teaching effectiveness improves when teaching strategies are modified on the basis of evaluation

---

BOX 28-2 Theoretical Elements of Curriculum Evaluation

- Course and level objectives demonstrate sequential learning across the curriculum (vertical organization).
- Course objectives are congruent with level objectives, which are congruent with the program goals (internal consistency).
- Course sequencing is defined with appropriate rationale for prerequisites and corequisites (horizontal organization).
- Course content (coursework and clinical experiences) provides graduates with the knowledge and skills needed to fulfill course and level objectives, the program's goals, and defined competencies.
- Support courses enhance learning experiences and provide a foundation in the arts, sciences, and humanities.

---

data. See Chapter 11 for information on designing teaching strategies and student learning activities.

To demonstrate and document teaching effectiveness, faculty need multiple evaluation methods (Johnson & Ryan, 2000). Evaluation methods may include student feedback about teaching effectiveness obtained through course evaluations and focus group discussions, feedback provided through peer review, formal testing of teaching strategies, and assessment of student learning.

Student Evaluation of Teaching Strategies

The institution or nursing department may develop course evaluations to obtain student feedback on teaching effectiveness. The advantage of internally developed evaluations is that they can be customized to the program. The primary disadvantage of internally developed tools is that they may lack reliability and validity. Standardized evaluation tools, such as those found in Individual Development and Educational Assessment (IDEA), offered by the Individual Development and Educational Assessment Center at Kansas State University, and the National Study of Student Engagement (NSSE), offered by the Indiana University Center for Postsecondary Research and Planning, have documented reliability and validity and provide opportunities to compare results among and between academic programs, departments, schools with the institutional score, and a national benchmark.

Although focus groups have been used extensively in marketing and social research, they have the potential to serve as powerful tools for program evaluation (Loriz & Foster, 2001). A focus group discussion with students can provide a qualitative assessment of teaching effectiveness. Focus groups provide an opportunity to obtain insights and to hear student perspectives that may not be discovered through formal course evaluations. The focus group leader should be an impartial individual with the skill to conduct the session. The leader should clearly state the purpose of the session, ensure confidentiality, provide clear guidelines about the type of information being sought, and explain how information will be used (Palomba & Banta, 1999). The reliability and validity of information obtained from a focus group discussion is enhanced when the approach is conducted as research with a purposeful design and careful choice of participants (Kevern & Webb, 2001).

Peer Review of Teaching Strategies

Peer and colleague review may provide information on teaching effectiveness through classroom observation and assessment of course materials. In this context, a peer is defined as another faculty member within the same discipline with expertise in the field, and a colleague is an individual outside of the discipline with expertise in the art and science of teaching. Peer review can serve to promote quality improvement of teaching effectiveness and as documentation for performance review. Before peer review is implemented, there is a need to be clear about what data will be gathered, who will have access to the data, and for what purposes they will be used. Faculty and administrators, as stakeholders in the endeavor, should collaborate to establish the norms and standards. Data from peer review may be used prescriptively to assist faculty in developing and improving teaching skills. At some point, peer review data may be needed for performance review and administrative decision making. Some schools require both classroom visits and opportunities to observe master teachers for all new faculty and periodic classroom visits for all faculty thereafter. In some schools the observation of teaching is voluntary. The age of the classroom as the private domain of the teacher is disappearing rapidly, and both accountability and the opportunity to demonstrate the scholarship of teaching are causing colleges and universities to require increased documentation of teaching as a routine part of the evaluation process.

Although classroom observation has been used as a technique for the peer review of teaching for a number of years, the reliability and validity of this method has been suspect. The validity and reliability of classroom observation as an evaluation tool is increased by (1) including multiple visits and multiple visitors, (2) establishing clear criteria in advance of the observation, (3) ensuring that participants agree about the appropriateness and fairness of the assessment instruments and the process, and (4) preparing faculty to conduct observations (Seldin, 1980; Weimer, Kerns, & Parrett, 1988). Before classroom teaching visits are made, the students should be advised of the visit and should be assured that they are not the focus of the observation. Peer reviewers should meet with the faculty member before the visit and review the goals of the session, what has preceded and what will follow the session, planned teaching methods, assignments made for the session, and an indication of how this class fits into the total program. This provides a clear image for the visitors and establishes a beginning rapport. Some faculty have particular goals for growth that can be shared at this time as areas for careful observation and comment. Finally, a postvisit interview should be conducted to review the observation and to identify strengths and areas for growth. This may include consultation regarding strategies for growth with the scheduling of a return visit at a later date. Many visitors interview the students briefly after the visit to determine their reaction to the class and to ascertain whether this was a typical class rather than a special, staged event. Unless there is a designated visiting team, the faculty member to be visited is usually able to make selections or at least suggestions about the visitors who will make the observation. Peer visits to clinical teaching sessions should follow the same general approach as classroom visits, although specific criteria for observation will be established to meet the unique attributes of clinical teaching and learning. An additional requirement is that the visitor be familiar with clinical practice expectations in the area to be visited.

Evaluation of Teaching and Learning Materials

The review of teaching and learning materials is another element of evaluation of teaching effectiveness that may be conducted through peer review. Materials commonly included for review are the course syllabus, textbooks and reading lists, teaching plans, teaching or learning aids, assignments, and outcome measures. In all cases, the materials are reviewed for congruence with the course objectives, appropriateness to the level of the learner, content scope and depth, clarity, organization, and evidence of usefulness in advancing students toward the goals of the course.

The syllabus is reviewed to determine whether expectations are clear and methods of evaluation are detailed. It is especially important that students understand what is required to "pass" the course. Grading scales and weighting of each of the evaluation methods used in the course should be explained.

In the review of textbooks for their appropriateness for a given course, multiple elements may be considered. The readability of a text relates to the extent to which the reading demands of the textbook match the reading abilities of the students. This assumes that the faculty member has a profile of student reading scores from preadmission testing. Readability of a textbook is usually based on measures of word difficulty and sentence complexity. Other issues of concern include the use of visual aids; cultural and sexual biases; scope and depth of content coverage; and size, cost, and accuracy of the data contained within the text (Armbruster & Anderson, 1991). Another factor of importance is the structure of the textbook. This element relates to the organization and presentation of material in a logical manner that increases the likelihood of the reader's understanding of the content and ability to apply the content to practice. A review should determine the ratio of important and unimportant material and the extent to which important concepts are articulated, clarified, and exemplified. Do the authors relate intervening ideas to the main thesis of a chapter and clarify the relationships between and among central concepts (Armbruster & Anderson, 1991)? The ease with which information can be located in the index is important so that students can use the book as a reference. Because of the high cost of textbooks, it is useful to consider whether the textbook will be a good reference for other classes in the curriculum. A review of a textbook must also include consideration of whether the content has supported student learning. When student papers or other creative products are used for evaluation purposes, it is common to review a sample of these papers or products that the teacher has judged to be weak, average, and above average to provide a clearer view of expectations and how the students have met those expectations. This review provides an opportunity to demonstrate student outcomes. If a faculty member wants to retain copies of student papers and creative works to demonstrate outcomes, he or she should obtain informed consent from the students. Accrediting bodies often wish to see samples of student work, and faculty may use them to demonstrate learning outcomes for purposes of their own evaluation. Each student's identity should be protected and consent should be obtained.

The review of teaching and learning aids depends on the organization and use of these materials. The organization may be highly structured in that all are expected to use certain materials in certain situations or sequences, or materials may be resources available to faculty and students for use at their discretion according to the outcomes they wish to achieve (Rogers, 1983). Students may be expected to search for and locate materials, to create materials to facilitate their learning, or simply to use the materials provided in a prescribed manner. The emphasis will determine whether evaluation questions related to materials are based on variety, creativity, and availability or whether the materials have been used as intended. Regardless of the overall emphasis, teaching and learning materials should be evaluated for efficiency and cost-effectiveness. Efficiency can be evaluated by determining whether the time demands and effort required to use the materials are worth the outcomes achieved. Cost-effectiveness can be determined by considering whether the costs of the materials justify the outcomes.

Formal Measures for Evaluating Teaching Strategies

Formal, objective measures of teaching strategies may include experimental or quasi-experimental designs, with randomization of subjects and control of treatments. For example, a teacher may establish a control group and a treatment group to try different teaching techniques and to evaluate outcomes to prove or disprove predetermined hypotheses. This technique is often used when there are multiple sections of a given course, although it can be accomplished within a section. A common method is to use the traditional strategy with the control group and the new strategy with the experimental group. A common examination or other assessment measure is used with both groups. Analysis may include checking for a significant difference in the scores of the two groups, as well as checking areas in which the most questions were missed for congruence or no congruence between the two groups (Short, 1991). A weakness of some of these efforts is that they are context bound and not generalizable. A strength of these testing strategies is the provision of feedback of value to evaluation questions within a given curriculum.

Another measure for evaluating teaching strategies is to have faculty complete a course report. The course report provides a record of the types of instructional methods used, the rationale for choosing these methods, and results of changes to these methods. Course reports can be reviewed annually through a peer review process or by program administrators. See Figure 28-1 for a sample of a didactic course report for the evaluation of teaching strategies and Figure 28-2 for a sample of a clinical course report for the evaluation of teaching strategies.

Assessment of Student Learning

It is unacceptable to claim that teaching strategies are effective unless there is evidence that links the teaching transaction with student learning. Assessment within the classroom provides evidence for interim outcome evaluation. Interim evaluation refers to outcomes of specific learning episodes, course outcomes, or level outcomes as opposed to outcomes assessed at the conclusion of the program of learning. Glennon (2006) notes that outcomes relate

directly to professional practice and differentiates this from objectives that relate to instruction. Course grades are insufficient and therefore real outcomes are needed not only to assist students in learning better but also to aid faculty in assessing student learning better (Glennon, 2006).

Both formal and informal methods may be used in the classroom to assess student progress and to evaluate the effectiveness of teaching strategies. Chapters 16, 24, and 25 cover these methods in detail. The Angelo and Cross (1993) model of classroom assessment is designed to evaluate teaching strategies with the goal of improving learning. Informal classroom assessment is useful to the teacher for determining how well students are learning, and data from the assessment can be used by the teacher in making changes to improve that learning. This form of classroom assessment is almost never graded and is often anonymous. It is based on the assumptions that student learning is directly related to quality teaching,

---

Example: Course Report—Theory

Program Evaluation Plan: Teaching Strategies Evaluation
The Program Evaluation Plan asks the following questions about teaching strategies and curriculum evaluation: (1) "Are we doing what we meant to do?" (2) "Are we doing the right things right?" This part of the program evaluation plan examines (a) teaching strategies, (b) the ability of chosen teaching strategies to accomplish course objectives, (c) opportunities to expand students' knowledge base, and (d) evaluation of student performance.

TEACHING STRATEGIES
1. Teaching strategies facilitate achieving course objectives.
2. Rationale can be identified for all major teaching strategies.
3. Teaching strategies provide opportunities to use prior knowledge in building new knowledge.
4. Teaching strategies are modified based on evaluation data.

List each course objective.

1. List the teaching strategies for each objective.

2. Identify the rationale for each strategy.

3. Identify how prior knowledge is used in building new knowledge. Examples of strategies include textbooks, assignments, presentations, homework, supplemental assigned readings, lectures, discussions in class or in online discussion forums, audiovisuals, group activities, guest speakers, web-based/web-supported courses, other.

4. Describe the effectiveness of each strategy. Include student comments where appropriate.

What will be changed the next time you teach this course?

Figure 28-1 Example: Course Report—Theory

Example: Course Report—Clinical

Program Evaluation Plan: Teaching Strategies Evaluation
1. Teaching strategies facilitate achieving clinical objectives.
2. Rationale can be identified for all major teaching strategies.
3. Teaching strategies provide opportunities to use prior knowledge in building new knowledge.
4. Teaching strategies are modified based on evaluation data.

List each course objective.

1. List the teaching strategies used for each objective.

2. Indicate the rationale for each strategy.

3. Identify how prior knowledge is used in building new knowledge. Examples of strategies include daily data sheets, journaling, nursing process papers/care plans, instructor skill demonstration (lab or clinical), student return demonstration (lab), direct observation of skill performance and nursing care given, questioning, observational experiences, planned teaching projects, post conferences, role play activities, case studies, computer-based activities/study modules, math competency testing, skills testing in lab, purposeful teaching assignments, and other.

4. Describe the effectiveness of each strategy. Include student comments where appropriate.

What will be changed the next time you teach this course?

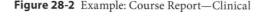

Figure 28-2 Example: Course Report—Clinical

objectives are explicit and monitored, feedback is focused and frequent, assessment is problem focused and context focused, assessment provides the impetus for change, assessment does not require specialized training, and assessment enhances student and faculty learning and satisfaction (Angelo & Cross, 1993). See Chapter 16 for a detailed discussion of classroom assessment methods.

At this juncture, unintended outcomes become apparent and must be analyzed and corrected or incorporated according to the results of analysis. Faculty must determine whether students had the prerequisite skills needed to succeed in the course and whether they left the course with the knowledge and skills necessary to move into the next sequence (DiFlorio et al., 1989).

The use of formalized external testing is another option that assists in the evaluation of student learning. For example, Assessment Technology Incorporated (ATI) provides both content mastery and comprehensive predictor examinations that provide indicators of student learning. These assessments provide questions that students will experience on the licensure examination and provide faculty with feedback that indicates need for improvement in specific content areas. Faculty can then provide focused review of content in which students' scores were low. Other external testing options are available through various companies. Tracking student scores in individual nursing courses can be insightful in revising course content as well as curriculum to better student learning outcomes.

Evaluation of individual student performance must be effectively communicated to students. Documentation should provide evidence that evaluation leads to improvement in performance. This is especially important in clinical evaluation. Clinical evaluation tools should provide documentation that students were clearly informed of expectations and received appropriate feedback regarding their performance and information about how students responded.

Evaluating Student Performance Measures

In addition to documenting that teaching methods are effective, methods of evaluating student performance must be valid and reliable. Multiple-choice examinations are a common, cost-effective, and time-efficient method of testing knowledge acquisition both as students progress in a course and at the conclusion of the course and program. This format provides rapid, quantitative data for individual assessment and aggregate data for centralized evaluation. Although few would argue that multiple-choice examinations should be completely eliminated, critics of this form of testing argue that the multiple-choice format serves to narrow the curriculum to reflect the content of the tests (Bersky & Yocom, 1994). They further argue that this form of testing fails to encourage or measure critical, creative, and reflective thought (Moss, 1992). Although faculty can develop multiple-choice questions that measure higher-order thinking, those requiring recall and basic comprehension are more common (Madaus & Kelleghan, 1992). It is also argued that students can choose the wrong option in multiple-choice questions with good rationale and select correct answers for the wrong reasons (Madaus & Kelleghan, 1992).

In response to this criticism, faculty have sought to measure decision making through the use of essay examinations for case analysis, through direct observation of patient care, and through simulation activities in the campus laboratory. A study by Madaus and McNamara (1970) showed that student grades on essay examinations varied widely according to the individual who read and evaluated the examination and that grades also varied even when evaluations were done by the same individual on different occasions. Although this problem can be reduced by more clearly articulated expectations and improved grading techniques, it remains a criticism of essay testing. A second criticism of essay testing is that it is labor intensive and time consuming. These same criticisms apply to project reports and argument or position papers.

These criticisms, in part, can be addressed in practice disciplines by a form of testing called *clinical simulation testing* (CST). CST is an uncued, interactive testing method that allows students to demonstrate simulated clinical decision-making skills. It is uncued in that the student is not presented with a list of decision options from which to choose. Instead, the student responds to a case scenario by indicating nursing actions through "free text" entry (Bersky & Yocom, 1994). Some view this as a more effective measure of problem-solving and decision-making ability. This testing method is discussed in detail in Chapter 26.

Box 28-3 provides a summary of the theoretical elements associated with evaluation of teaching

> **BOX 28-3 Theoretical Elements of Teaching Effectiveness Evaluation**
>
> - Students are satisfied with teaching strategies.
> - Teaching strategies are modified based on evaluation data.
> - Teaching strategies facilitate achieving course objectives.
> - Teaching materials are effective and efficient.
> - Evaluation of individual student performance is communicated to students and leads to improvement in performance.
> - Methods of evaluating student performance are valid.

effectiveness. Figure 28-3 provides an example of a course report related to student performance.

Environment Evaluation: Student Dimension

The evaluation of the student dimension begins with an examination of whether a sufficient number of qualified students are enrolled. Academic and demographic profiles of prospective students are important to consider. A first consideration is the mission and goals of the institution and school. If diversity is a goal, the selection of students will be different than in schools where high selectivity is a goal. State and private schools may differ in the types of students they wish to attract. Trends in health care provide an important database for defining student enrollment goals. For example, health care reform has opened the market for nurse practitioners to the extent that many schools of nursing have targeted this population. Once a determination of the nature of the student to be recruited has been made, the methods of recruitment require attention. Marketing methods and materials should be reviewed in terms of access to catchment targets, clarity of the message delivered, and results of the effort. An entry inquiry as to the source of the student's information about the school is one way to determine the extent to which marketing materials influenced application decisions.

Admission policies should be clearly defined and support program goals. Student profiles are an important way to track trends in the characteristics

Example: Course Report—Theory

Program Evaluation Plan: Teaching Strategies Evaluation

Evaluation of Student Performance

1. Methods of evaluating student performance are valid and consistently applied.

Course Evaluation of Student Performance			
Exams	Data	Describe the effectiveness of these methods. Include student comments where appropriate.	What will be changed the next time you teach this course?
How do you use item analysis to improve your tests?	List range of KR 20 values on unit exams, excluding the final exam. Range Fall _____ Spring _____ Summer _____ (The KR20 has a normal range between 0.00 and 1.00 with higher numbers indicating higher internal consistency. You should not expect a score higher than 0.80 [commercially available tests will approach 0.95]).	Comment on reliability of your tests, difficulty level of the tests, and the ability of questions to discriminate between high/low achievers.	
What percent of the course grade is the final exam/assignment? (specify which)	Fall _____ % Spring _____ % Summer _____ % _____ exam _____ assignment		
Is the final exam/assignment comprehensive?	Fall _____ yes _____ no Spring _____ yes _____ no Summer _____ yes _____ no		
How many students (number and percent of class) did **not** achieve an average exam score of 80%, but passed the course based on written assignments, homework, and/or student presentations?	Fall _____ _____ % Spring _____ _____ % Summer _____ _____ %		

Figure 28-3 Example: Course Report—Theory

Other Methods of Evaluation			
What other methods of evaluation are used in this course?	___ Written assignments ___ Student presentations ___ Homework ___ Blackboard discussion ___ Quizzes ___ Other (List _____)		
Rubrics are used for all other graded work (yes or no). If no, what is used to determine validity and assure consistent application?	___ yes ___ no (explain)		
Grading policies from the Dept. of Nursing Policy Manual are followed in this course (yes or no). If no, describe what and why.	___ yes ___ no (explain)		
External measures of student performance (ATI):			
Identify ATI Content Mastery test given in this course. What was the total number of students that took the Content Mastery Exam? What number and percent of class achieved the benchmark on the test? (Proficiency Level 2 and above)	 Fall ___ Spring ___ Fall _____ % Spring _____ %	What did you learn from test analysis data provided by ATI?	What (and why) will be changed the next time you teach this course?

Figure 28-3, cont'd

of students admitted to programs of learning. Many colleges and universities require entrance examinations related to basic skills, including standardized examinations such as the Scholastic Aptitude Test (SAT) or discipline-specific tests and institutional examinations in mathematics, English, and reading skills. Grade inflation in both secondary and post-secondary schools has rendered transcript review a difficult measure of student ability and clearly indicates the need for a profile of expectations rather than a single criterion for admission. Schools of nursing are also establishing admission criteria that guide the selection of students with attributes suited to the challenges of current health care delivery systems who more closely match the diversity of the populations they serve and therefore are adding essays, interviews, and references to the usual repertoire of standardized tests and grade point averages (Leners, Beardslee, & Peters, 1996).

Admission policies should be checked for discriminatory elements. One must sort those educational discriminators that ensure a fit between the student and the program of learning and those that are clearly discriminatory from the perspective of social justice. For example, it is appropriate to require that students complete any remediation before admission to the program so they will have the basic skills necessary for success, especially if diversity is a goal. It is not appropriate and it is illegal to exclude students on the basis of gender, religion, race or ethnic origin, or lifestyle.

Many states are increasing high school requirements with a concurrent shift in *college entrance requirements*. Individuals who perform evaluation reviews must keep abreast of these changes to maintain congruence and to determine what remediation programs may be needed for students who graduated from high school before the increased requirements were established. Plans must be in place to ensure communication of the changes in a timely fashion. Some programs find it useful to complete correlation studies to determine the relationship of admission criteria to such outcome measures as program completion or success on licensing or certification examinations after graduation. Although this approach does not measure the potential success of those not admitted, it may provide data about criteria that seem to have little relationship to success indicators.

Progression must be fair and justifiable, support program goals, and be congruent with institutional standards. For example, are there conditions for progression related to grade point average at the end of each semester? If a student must drop out of school for any reason, what are the conditions and standards for return? Are they realistic? Are they known to the students? Do they apply equally to all students with exceptions made only in cases that are clearly exceptional?

Records of student satisfaction and formal complaints should be used as part of the process of the student dimension evaluation. An academic appeals process should be in place for students who wish to challenge rulings, and students should know about the process and how to access it. Some form of due process should be in writing and in operation for the review of disputes regarding course grades or progression decisions. Whether these are discipline specific or campus specific is a function of the size and complexity of the institution. An annual review of appeals and the decisions regarding those appeals provides important information for making revisions to policies and processes that are in place or are needed. All stakeholders should participate in appeals reviews. Most programs have an appeals committee composed of

both students and faculty with channels to administrative review.

An internal method of review is to survey or interview students who leave the program. An obvious data set is information about why students are leaving. Common reasons include academic difficulties or academic dismissal, financial problems, role conflicts, family pressure, military service, and health issues. An examination of the underlying reasons for leaving will often suggest alternatives for intervention that will reduce the attrition rate. These alternatives may relate to student services or specific program issues.

Some programs also gather data about antecedent events that may have influenced the potential to complete the program. The extent of data gathered depends on the goals of the review. Data that can be gathered from the student record are not included on the student survey. With the student's permission, data obtained from the record may include preentrance test scores, grade point average, progression point at the time of withdrawal, specific course grades, and any history of withdrawals and returns. These data are extensive but can be used to develop a profile of the student who does not complete a program in an attempt to identify elements within the control of the school for potential intervention strategies. Including a control group of students who completed the program in the study gives more meaning to the findings by identifying success indicators and allowing for determination of significant differences between the two groups. Box 28-4 provides a summary of the theoretical elements associated with evaluation of the student dimension.

BOX 28-4 Theoretical Elements of Environment Evaluation: Student Dimension

- An adequate number of qualified students are recruited to maintain program viability.
- Admission policies are clearly defined and support program goals.
- Progression policies are fair and justifiable and support program goals.
- Records of student satisfaction and formal complaints are used as part of the process of ongoing improvement.

Environment Evaluation: Faculty Dimension

There must be a sufficient number of qualified faculty to accomplish the mission, philosophy, and expected outcomes of the program. The nature of the program, the expectations of the parent institution, and the requirements of accrediting bodies influence the desired number and qualifications of faculty. Qualifications of faculty may be measured from several perspectives: credentials, diversity, and professional experience.

Qualifications of Faculty

Faculty should possess credentials appropriate to their teaching assignment, to the program levels in which they teach, and to the service and scholarship mission of the school. Faculty members' professional experience and specialty certification should be congruent with their teaching assignments. Evaluation of the level of degree preparation of nursing faculty is related to the program level in which they teach. A master's degree in nursing is the minimum expectation for teaching in associate or baccalaureate degree programs. A doctorate in nursing or a terminal degree in a related field with a master's degree in nursing is the expectation for teaching in graduate programs. Many nursing schools also strive to have faculty with terminal degrees teaching in baccalaureate programs. The nursing profession has been challenged to meet these expectations due to the lack of nurses with terminal degrees. As of 2003, AACN identified that less than 1% of nurses in the United States had obtained a terminal degree (AACN, 2003a). In response to the growing shortage of nursing faculty, AACN published a position statement in 2008 calling for continued commitment to doctoral preparation for faculty teaching in baccalaureate and graduate programs, but also recognizing the importance of clinical expertise in preparing graduates for practice (AACN, 2008b). As of 2010, nearly 93% of unfilled nursing faculty positions are still seeking candidates with doctoral degrees in nursing or a related field (AACN, 2010b). To address the shortage of nurses with terminal degrees, some nursing schools may provide additional incentives and support to faculty with master's degrees to assist them in pursuing their doctorates. In this situation, care must be taken to avoid "inbreeding," which may result in a disproportionate number of faculty with degrees from the parent institution or a common regional institution. Representation of a wide variety of educational institutions in the faculty profile demonstrates a commitment to diversity of ideas and openness to creative differences. "Inbreeding" of faculty may perpetuate the status quo.

Evaluation of faculty qualifications should also include the profile of faculty related to rank, classifications for tenure or nontenure track appointments, and the balance of full-time and part-time positions. Assessment of the number and proportion of faculty for each level of rank provides a measure of faculty experience and expertise in their teaching role. If few faculty members within the school have achieved higher ranks, such as associate or full professor, there may be a lack of senior-level faculty. In some universities, there are multiple categories of faculty, including nontenure-track lecturers and clinical instructors, tenure-track faculty, and scientist tracks (see Chapter 1). In some universities, only tenure-track faculty may participate in the governance of the larger institution. Standing committees within both the school and the university may have criteria for rank and tenure as a condition of membership. A goal of full participation in governance issues at the university level can be compromised or enabled by the number of faculty eligible to participate. On the other hand, a faculty composed largely of tenured members could be a barrier to the recruitment of a more diverse faculty or a goal of increasing the number of faculty members with specific areas of expertise. The balance of full-time and part-time faculty is also of concern in ensuring adequate involvement in governance, meeting needs for academic advising, curriculum development, and program evaluation.

Setting goals for faculty qualifications allows the nursing school to measure progress in achieving those goals. Once the goals for qualified faculty have been identified, the faculty profile can be evaluated or analyzed in terms of those goals. Factors that may be interfering with the achievement of the goals will also need analysis. For example, it is also essential to track the profile of faculty who are within 5 to 10 years of retirement and to examine reasons for faculty turnover. Control of the faculty profile is influenced not only by recruitment goals but also by faculty retention factors.

A factor related to both recruitment and retention of qualified faculty is the salary structure. If a goal of the school of nursing is to support quality programs and to achieve national stature, salaries must be competitive to attract the mix of faculty that promotes excellence. There are multiple sources for comparison of salaries. Internally, it is important to demonstrate that faculty salaries in the school are congruent with those in the larger institution for comparable rank and productivity. External data are available from such sources as the AACN, the American Association of University Professors, and regional groups such as the Big Ten universities. AACN provides salary information for full-time administrative and instructional nursing faculty, including mean and median salaries by rank and degree (AACN, 2010a). The College and University Professional Association for Human Resources conducts an annual survey of faculty salaries for public and private institutions offering baccalaureate and higher degrees. The National Faculty Salary Survey for Four-Year Institutions provides salary data by discipline and rank (College and University Professional Association for Human Resources, 2010). The results of this survey are available online. In addition, customized reports that sort data by variables such as region of the country, size of the institution's operating budget, and religious affiliation for private schools can be requested. Customized reports may provide a more accurate comparison in determining how faculty salaries compare to peer institutions. Some nursing schools may be able to obtain salary information by networking with a select cohort of peer institutions that agree to share data.

Faculty Development

Faculty development begins with orientation. The orientation of new faculty to the university or college, school, and department or division is fundamental to program effectiveness. In this orientation, faculty begin the process of socialization into the academy. They are introduced to the mission and goals of the institution and school at each level represented in the structure. Expectations are reviewed and any documents that will reinforce and guide movement toward those expectations are shared. For example, new faculty are usually given the institutional handbook that contains general policies and teaching, service, and research expectations. Support systems and personnel available to maintain them are introduced and a tour of

the physical plant is conducted. More specific orientation occurs at each level.

Once orientation is completed, faculty should receive support for professional development. Some schools have an office of research to assist faculty in research efforts and others have teaching centers or technology experts to assist faculty in their teaching role. Use of travel monies and planning that encourages faculty to attend conferences, seminars, and research colloquia are important parts of development and should be implemented and tracked as a part of the evaluation effort.

An increasing number of schools are developing mentoring programs that may provide generalist mentoring or specific mentoring in research and teaching. Mentoring is a multidimensional activity that consists of highly individualized dyadic processes and relationships. Stewart and Kruger (1996) list the six essential attributes of mentoring as the teaching–learning process, reciprocal relationship, career development, a knowledge differential between participants, duration of several years, and a relationship impact beyond the mentor relationship. Mentors listen, affirm, counsel, encourage, seek input, and help the novice develop status and career direction. Effective mentoring is the result of personal characteristics of the mentor such as approachability, effective interpersonal skills, adopting a positive teaching role, paying appropriate attention to learning, providing supervisory support, and development of ability (Andrews & Wallis, 1999; Shaffer, Tallarica, & Walsch, 2000). Whatever the view of the mentor, the role needs to be clear to the mentor and mentee and allow for individualization. In large schools, the assignment of a mentor may occur at the department level. In smaller schools, the assignment is often the responsibility of a central administrator or a school committee of faculty. It is common for a senior faculty member to be assigned as a mentor for a period of 1 year, with continuing assignment based on individual need or the development plan. Each member of the mentoring dyad should evaluate the nature and effectiveness of the mentoring relationship at the end of the year or at regular intervals if the relationship extends beyond the year.

The role of the mentor may vary by institution, but common functions include advice and counsel, review of course materials, observation of instruction, assistance in processing evaluation data, modeling master teaching, encouragement, and coaching.

Those who provide mentoring for research often assist the faculty member in accessing support systems on campus, identifying funding sources, and developing a research focus and serve as resources as their assigned faculty members progress in meeting promotion and tenure expectations. The purpose of the relationship is generally consultative and constructive; however, some schools may prefer a more directed, prescriptive approach, especially with new faculty (Brinko, 1993). In an effort to create safety and opportunity for faculty development, the mentor does not become an evaluator.

Another form of mentoring can be accomplished in group sessions. In addition to faculty development offerings at the campus and institutional levels, the school or department may offer a series of open and planned sessions for new and continuing faculty. The focus of the sessions may be related to common concerns, concerns identified through a needs analysis, or issues related to changes in the school. For example, many schools are offering regular sessions on the use of new technology as it is acquired. It may be necessary to offer faculty development related to policy changes, curriculum changes, or any other new development in the school or institution.

Finally, larger schools may have their own department of *continuing education*. In those schools, one expectation of that department may be to participate in faculty development. Through continuing education, a department may offer a series of workshops related to teaching strategies, test construction, evaluation, or other issues of concern to faculty in general. These are usually open to others as well to create a more diverse mix of participants and to provide fiscal support to the department. Some continuing education departments assist faculty in hosting conferences related to their areas of expertise and cosponsor research colloquia or other events that serve faculty in their professional development and provide an opportunity for faculty to share their professional expertise as presenters.

Faculty Scholarship

Faculty achievements in scholarly activity should support program effectiveness. Boyer (1990) suggests that the academic role of the professor has four functions, which are the scholarship of *discovery*, *integration*, *application*, and *teaching*. The scholarship of discovery includes independent research that has been published and subjected to peer review. The scholarship of integration involves such efforts as interdisciplinary activities, reading in other fields, writing interpretive essays, and mentoring junior faculty. The scholarship of application includes professional practice, consultation, and service. The scholarship of teaching involves the teaching role, curriculum development, and program evaluation.

Boyer (1990) suggests that faculty should be able to contract for selected profiles of scholarship across the four functions, in which individual faculty members may focus primarily on one area or a combination of areas. Many institutions have adapted the Boyer model by having faculty declare an area of excellence with baseline expectations for each of the scholarship types. Having selected an area of excellence, the faculty member establishes goals to meet the "contract." Some institutions are experimenting with a "balanced case" approach in which faculty meet specified criteria in each category without designating an area of excellence. In any case, the expectations for faculty in a given school should be consistent with those of the parent institution to avoid conflicts with promotion and tenure expectations.

Judging the merit of scholarly activities within each of the four scholarship functions can be done using a consistent approach based on six attributes of good scholarship (Boyer, 1994). These attributes include (1) clarity of goals, (2) thoroughness of preparation, (3) appropriateness of methods, (4) significance of results, (5) effectiveness in communication of the scholarly work, and (6) reflective critique. The documentation that faculty provide regarding scholarship in any of the four functions can be evaluated against these six attributes. Faculty can address these attributes in a self-evaluation or a committee of peers can use the attributes as a rubric for evaluation.

Knowledge and its advancement (the scholarship of discovery) are essential to the academy, and those who select research as the area of excellence will be measured against criteria established within the school or division. Those criteria will need to withstand the scrutiny of peer review both within and beyond the discipline. The volume of research and publications is less important than the quality of the effort. Some committees ask faculty to select two or three of their best research studies and best publications for review rather than submitting the entire body of work for review. This highlights the focus on quality. An additional expectation is that evidence of both external peer review and review by one's department chairperson be included in the work submitted for review. Selection of one's works for publication or presentation is evidence of its value to the reviewers. Where publications appear may also be of importance. Articles in refereed journals and journals held in high esteem in the discipline are considered evidence of quality review. Before publication, it is important to know the standards of the given institution. For example, some schools give greater weight to articles in refereed journals or to entire books as compared with chapters in a book. Sole authorship versus joint authorship or placement in the listing of authors may be weighted as well. Invited works are often considered evidence of their value. Some institutions also consider invited creative works such as radio or television productions, videotapes, musical scores, and choreography evidence of scholarship or excellence. Receipt of major awards and other forms of recognition as a leader in one's field provides compelling evidence of quality.

Funding for research and special projects is widely accepted as evidence of scholarship. Weighting may be assigned on the basis of the source of the monies. Internal funding may not be weighted as heavily as external funding. External funding may be weighted as well. For example, funding from major foundations or federal programs may receive a more favorable review than several small grants from lesser known sources. Whether one is the principal investigator or a participant may be weighted in the review process. A growing value is attached to applied research that has meaning for a wider audience. Keys to the consideration of any scholarly endeavor are evidence of analysis and synthesis in studies grounded in theory, rather than simple descriptive studies. Variations occur according to the mission of the institution so that each school must determine criteria within the context of that mission. In the final analysis, scholarly works are best judged by one's intellectual peers (Braskamp & Ory, 1994).

The scholarship of application is demonstrated through professional practice and service. Practice as professional service is an area of emphasis in some institutions, whereas in other institutions faculty believe it is not valued as highly as research. Again, evidence exists that more and more institutions are attempting to develop criteria to reflect scholarly service and to grant that service the recognition it merits. A common standard of evidence of scholarly clinical practice and clinical competence is national certification in one's field, especially for those faculty who wish to seek recognition and promotion in the clinical track. With some variation based on institutional mission, the focus on service is its connection to the faculty member's professional expertise. Internally, faculty may demonstrate service through participation and leadership in committees and projects within the department or division and, more broadly, at the campus or institutional level. Committees that affect decision making for innovative enterprises or improvement and policy development demonstrate thoughtful participation. Administrative appointments are generally accepted as evidence of professional service within the institution.

Beyond the institution, faculty may demonstrate service through practice and participation in professional, civic, and governmental organizations relevant to their expertise in a manner that reflects the application of knowledge and the extension and renewal of the discovery element of scholarship. Examples include providing technical assistance to an agency and analysis of public policy for governmental agencies or private organizations (Braskamp & Ory, 1994). Joint appointments or contracts with practice agencies that call on professional expertise are other examples. Certainly, faculty-run clinics are a strong example of such service. Some institutions place applied research in this category of review.

In addition to the listing and description of activities in the area of service, faculty are expected to have documented evidence of the merit or worth of that service. In this area as well, letters from external sources and awards based on service are evidence of merit. Within the institution there is a need for more systematic feedback to those who provide valuable service. Often faculty receive perfunctory notes of thanks for service that do little to define the value of that service. A practice of thanking those who serve with comments about the special expertise provided and outcomes achieved as a result of that service is a valuable form of evidence.

The scholarship of integration is demonstrated through interdisciplinary research, interpreting research findings, and bringing new insight to the field of study. Presentations to the lay public that serve to advance public knowledge of discipline-related issues, development of new and creative teaching materials and modes of delivery, and professional presentations and publications are examples of integrative scholarship. The scholarship of integration may be evaluated by determining whether the activity reveals new knowledge, illuminates integrative themes, or demonstrates creative insight (Boyer, 1990).

It is not possible for a given faculty member to excel in all areas subject to review within the institution. The Boyer (1990) model attempts to respond to a need to look at scholarship differently and to provide multiple ways for faculty to demonstrate worthy productivity. Research and publication are important elements of the academy and are critical to comprehensive and research universities. Limiting the focus of faculty evaluation and reward decisions to a single area, however, discounts the valuable work of a diversified faculty. This very diversity and range of expertise enhances the reputation of an institution and enables the wise use of resources. The obligation of faculty is to provide evidence of scholarly productivity in one or more of the scholarship functions. Institutional leaders are obligated to enable that process and reward positive outcomes.

Evaluation of Faculty Performance

Evaluation of faculty performance promotes quality improvement. The focus of faculty performance evaluation is guided by the philosophy, mission, and goals of the parent institution and the school or division in which the nursing program is housed. Faculty evaluations may be structured against specific job descriptions related to classroom or clinical teaching assignments and include expectations for scholarship and service. Junior and community colleges often focus heavily on the teaching and service mission of the institution within the community it serves, and faculty evaluation reflects this emphasis. Research universities share the teaching and service missions but include an emphasis on research and scholarship as well. Colleges and universities with religious affiliations may include expectations for church-related service in faculty review policies and standards.

The policy and process for faculty performance evaluation should be clearly communicated to faculty. A common approach is to require faculty to submit a yearly development plan to the immediate supervisor that is consistent with the university and department missions and the department goals. Individual faculty goals may also be part of the development plan that includes the faculty member's goals as well as those identified by the supervisor. Goals can be short term and long term and should include strategies or activities planned to fulfill the goals and a timeline for completion. Periodic meetings with the faculty to review progress on development goals should be conducted by the supervisor or administrator.

The faculty member is expected to provide a self-evaluation at the end of the academic year that documents how performance and development goals were obtained, what barriers blocked achievement of goals, and how these barriers will be overcome in the future. A portfolio process may also be used, in which the faculty member includes the development plan, self-evaluation, copies of student course evaluations, examples of scholarly work and service, or other artifacts that demonstrate faculty productivity. During the annual performance review, the supervisor reviews the faculty member's portfolio and provides written feedback on the faculty member's progress in fulfilling the job description. Depending on the processes used throughout the institution, performance evaluation may be done using standard forms with numerical rating scales. The use of standardized forms provides the opportunity to analyze faculty performance across the unit and determine whether the faculty demonstrates development needs in any one particular area. For example, if a number of new faculty are not performing well on a certain measure, additional orientation or training may be needed.

Peer review provides another component for the evaluation of faculty performance. Promotion and tenure review is a well-established form of peer review already in place in most institutions of higher learning. The criteria for the evaluation are developed by faculty and implemented through a faculty committee. Committee reviews usually are composed of both formative and summative evaluation procedures. A common practice is to review faculty at the midpoint of the probationary period, usually in the third year of appointment. A formative review may occur at regular intervals before the summative tenure review is conducted. Formative reviews allow the committee to provide advice to individual faculty members in preparation for the summative review that occurs near the end of the probationary period, usually the sixth year after initial appointment. In larger institutions, a primary committee of peers may do the initial review of a faculty member's final tenure portfolio, along with their recommendation regarding promotion or tenure, before it is forwarded to administration and a campus committee of peers and colleagues for further review. Final recommendations are submitted to institutional administration, the board of trustees, or other institutional governing body for final approval. Variations on this theme relate to the unique features of a given institution.

A common problem in higher education, especially in research universities, is the lack of evaluation plans and criteria for all classifications of faculty. Although the criteria and processes for promotion and tenure of tenure-track faculty are usually in place and subject to ongoing review and refinement, such criteria do not always exist for others beyond the routine annual review. Some schools have nontenure-track faculty serving in lecturer, scientist, or clinical appointments who would benefit from the same careful delineation of criteria for systematic review of their roles consistent with their job descriptions and productivity expectations. Boyer's model of scholarship and the six attributes for evaluation may provide a consistent approach to performance review for nontenure-track faculty (Wood et al., 1998). Another group of faculty that requires evaluation and the opportunity to grow and develop is the part-time faculty cohort. Increasingly, expectations for annual review of part-time faculty with reappointment are contingent on favorable reviews. Adaptation of the tenure-track evaluation format can provide direction to create similar evaluative processes for nontenure-track and part-time faculty.

External factors may influence elements of faculty evaluation. For example, external bodies such as state legislatures and education commissions may establish standards for accountability that must be met by all higher education programs in the state. A common example is in the teaching component of the faculty role. There are often mandates for faculty workload in terms of credit hours or classes taught. There are multiple ways to address this standard. Whatever productivity model is used, certain general standards apply. Faculty workloads should be designed to meet the mission and goals

of the parent institution and the school or division and include those elements of the professional role of faculty emphasized by the institution (teaching, service, research). Although equity of workload expectations is an important standard, so is the flexibility to negotiate assignments to meet the needs of the school. Box 28-5 provides a summary of the theoretical elements associated with evaluation of the faculty dimension.

Environment Evaluation: Delivery Mode Dimension

Classroom and laboratory facilities need to provide an effective teaching and learning environment to support program effectiveness. A review of *instructional space* includes evaluation of support space and a determination of whether classrooms are of sufficient size and comfort to facilitate teaching and learning. *Support space* might include a learning resource center, computer laboratory, and storage for instructional equipment and supplies. Additional support space may include lounges for students, staff, and faculty. In addition, office space and equipment, as well as conference rooms and space to support research, are needed. In some facilities, offices do not have floor-to-ceiling walls so that a goal may be to have sufficient conference space to provide privacy for

---

BOX 28-5 Theoretical Elements of Environment Evaluation: Faculty Dimension

- Faculty members are qualified and sufficient in number to accomplish the mission, philosophy, and expected outcomes of the program.
- Faculty receive orientation that prepares them to be successful.
- Faculty receive adequate support for professional development.
- Faculty achievements in scholarly activity support program effectiveness.
- Evaluation of faculty performance promotes quality improvement.
- Commission on Collegiate Nursing Education now requires: Aggregate faculty outcomes are consistent with and contribute to achievement of the program's mission, goals, and expected student outcomes.

counseling, sensitive advisement, and evaluation conferences. Beyond these basic elements, space requirements are dictated by the mission and goals of the program. The space available should be congruent with the productivity expected of those who use the space, equipment, and supplies. This element is often reviewed through surveys of faculty, students, and staff. Another component of this review is documentation of holdings. It is important not only to have space and equipment but also to know where it is located and how well it is maintained.

Clinical facilities should be evaluated to determine their effectiveness in providing appropriate learning experiences in relation to the mission and goals of the program. This evaluation includes consideration of the patients served by the facility. It is important to assess whether the patient population profile is consistent with the learning objectives of the program and whether the number of patients is sufficient to support the student population. It is equally important for the standard of care provided by the institution to be of high quality so that students will be socialized to high standards. One measure of quality is the accreditation of the facility. Another is the expert judgment of the faculty members who review the facility. The willingness of staff to interact with students in a facilitative manner is important, as is the skill of staff as role models. It is important to know how many other student groups are using the same facility and units within the facility and how easily reservations for these areas can be scheduled. Any special restrictions or requirements may also influence decisions about use of the facility.

Evaluation of the clinical experience may also include review of agency contracts. These contracts should be filed in a central location and should be reviewed on a regular schedule. The conditions of the agreement should be spelled out, and some standards must be met. For example, all contracts should include the process and time frame for canceling or discontinuing the contract with a clause that allows any students scheduled for that facility to complete the current course of study. It is also important that faculty maintain control of student assignments and evaluations within the framework of the agreed-on restrictions and regulations. A review of contracts by legal counsel will ensure that expert judgment has been applied to the legal parameters of the contract.

Some schools have developed and implemented faculty-run clinics that also serve as learning sites for students. Reviews and contracts related to student learning in these clinics should be subject to the same evaluation as any other facility under consideration.

Instructional Technology

Information and instructional technology must be up to date and support the achievement of program goals. Productivity is directly related to the technology available to students and faculty, which enables them to meet their responsibilities and to create a dynamic learning environment. Outcome measures can be specifically stated in this area. For example, one might state that increasing numbers of faculty incorporate virtual simulations into teaching methods until all faculty use virtual experiences to enhance student learning. Another outcome measure might state that virtual technology will be integrated throughout curricula by a stated target date. Assessment of virtual lab usage that includes frequency of use and type of learning experiences from simple to complex simulations can be completed. Faculty and student satisfaction with the virtual lab is another effective outcome measure. Technology needs should be linked broadly to the mission and goals of the school and specifically to the teaching, scholarship, and learning needs of faculty and students.

Also, an assessment of student and faculty skills in the use of information technology at the time of admission or employment should be included. These data provide information for student and faculty development opportunities in the use of both software and hardware in the school itself and in resource facilities such as the library or a computer laboratory. Exciting advances have been made in instructional technology available for the teaching and learning of skills in nursing, but they require planning for availability of the equipment and software and preparation of faculty and students to use these resources. Creating a collaborative relationship with the information system's personnel is necessary to ensure an effective, ongoing dialogue between users of technology (faculty and students) and personnel who maintain the technology equipment.

Distance Education

Distance education is a growing trend in higher education and in nursing education. Distance education is defined as a program of study in which 50% or more of the courses or learning experiences occur through the Internet or other wireless communication devices and that also includes audio conferencing or instruction supported with DVDs or CD-ROMs (Higher Learning Commission, 2010). Internet instruction is the most popular form of distance education. Components of courses, complete courses, or the entire program of study may be offered via the Internet (Cobb & Billings, 2000).

When a program uses distance education for part or all of course delivery, the influence of this delivery mode on program outcomes, teaching–learning practices, and the use of technology must be considered in evaluation (Cobb & Billings, 2000). Methods of data collection may need modification for distance education programs. Because students are not on-site, creative methods such as the use of videotapes, audiotapes, and portfolios may be needed to assess student learning. Recruitment and retention of students require special consideration in distance education because some students may lack the motivation or technological competence to be successful. Other aspects of program implementation that need special consideration for distance education include faculty development and support, student orientation, and learning resources and support services. The appropriate technology, especially Internet delivery modes, and user support must be available to sustain distance education. Costs associated with distance education should be considered in the financial analysis.

Accreditation and Distance Education

As schools of nursing are increasingly offering all or part of their courses by using distance learning strategies such as video conferencing and the Internet, the educational programs must meet quality standards. The Alliance for Nursing Accreditation, a group of organizations charged with the responsibility of monitoring nursing accreditation and certification, has developed a statement on distance education policies (AACN, 2003b). The statement indicates that nursing programs delivered by means of distance learning technologies must meet the same academic standards and accreditation criteria as on-site programs. In addition to meeting existing criteria to ensure quality of educational programs delivered by means of distance learning technologies, generally accepted principles of good practice for distance education have been defined by the eight regional accrediting bodies. The evaluative criteria defined by the regional accrediting bodies address specific elements needed to establish a quality distance education program but are reflective of general accreditation standards. Specifically, the regional accreditors expect distance education programs to demonstrate curricular coherence; sufficient interaction between faculty and students; sufficient opportunities for students to interact and collaborate with each other; instruction provided by qualified and prepared faculty; support for the program through sufficient technological, pedagogical, and student services and resources; and provisions for evaluating student learning and other programmatic aspects and for continuous quality improvement (Higher Learning Commission, 2006).

Library Resources

Library resources must be sufficient to support the programs of learning offered by the institution and the school. Issues of concern in this evaluation include the holdings (books and journals), services, and rates of use. Faculty, students, and librarians are important stakeholders in this review, and each cohort often has a very different perception when the same questions are asked. There is controversy about the relative importance of on-site holdings and access to holdings through interlibrary loan and online databases. Clearly, a core collection of holdings is crucial to students and faculty.

Various standards are used to measure the adequacy of library holdings. Some schools use published source lists as standards for library holdings. The *American Journal of Nursing* list of resources, based on an annual review of books, is a source often used as a standard. Some schools consider it important to include any required textbooks and required readings in the library holdings, at least at the undergraduate level. Graduate programs may require more extensive databases with access to more materials than undergraduate programs because of the scope of reading expectations. Faculty task forces are often assigned to review library holdings in relation to graduate education in specialty majors. Comparisons with the holdings of peer institutions with similar programs are sometimes used in these reviews. Some programs rely on the expertise of the faculty on the task force. Still others survey all faculty in the major for lists of holdings they consider to be critical. The aggregate becomes a point of reference for the review.

Library services are as important as the holdings and are usually assessed by a survey method. Librarians, students, and faculty may indicate their views about services offered and the effectiveness of those services. Surveys may be internally developed and provide very specific information about library services. For example, an internal survey may review the interlibrary loan system to determine both satisfaction and levels of use related to the time frame for borrowing materials. This may be measured against an established goal, such as an average time of 1 week to secure a book. In addition to the quantitative data, an opportunity to comment on the best features and areas of concern related to library holdings and services often provides valuable qualitative data. Some libraries maintain specific use data by school or division. Others do not but can estimate whether a given group of students use the library facilities less, the same, or more than other students. Some libraries have very liberal hours and some do not. This may become an evaluation question, depending on the context.

Most libraries are able to make effective use of technology. The Internet provides access to a wide variety of resources and access to full-text articles and copying services, especially through the World Wide Web. This type of information, ubiquitous because of the Internet, brings new opportunities and challenges to provision of information resources to students over a wide geographic area. Those who make use of this opportunity will establish specific criteria for evaluation geared to access. It is important to identify and review the databases available to faculty and students and methods used to orient them to the use of this service. Box 28-6 provides a summary of the theoretical elements associated with evaluation of the delivery mode dimension.

BOX 28-6 Theoretical Elements of Environment Evaluation: Delivery Mode Dimension

- Classroom and laboratory facilities provide an effective teaching and learning environment.
- Clinical facilities provide effective learning experiences.
- Information and instructional technology is up to date and supports achievement of program goals.
- Library services and holdings are comprehensive and meet needs of students and faculty.

Environment Evaluation: Organization Dimension

The qualifications and leadership skills of program administrators are important to program effectiveness. Formal evaluation of administrators should occur annually or at regularly specified intervals. The specific evaluation of the administrator may include the extent to which the administrator guides the establishment of a clear mission and goals for the unit and the effectiveness with which the administrator represents the department or school, both internally and externally, and contributes to the reputation of the unit within and beyond the institution. Attention should be focused on the administrator's ability to raise funds and to allocate the budget in a fair and effective manner. Evidence of integrity and collegiality is an issue of concern, as are the leadership qualities of conflict resolution, decision making, motivation, and interpersonal skills.

Regardless of the university size and focus, evaluation of administrative effectiveness should be a collaborative process in which faculty members participate. Faculty members should have the opportunity to provide evaluative feedback on the performance of administrative faculty. This collaborative process can be replicated at various levels within the nursing school and the institution. For example, the nursing department chair may be evaluated by the dean of the school and in turn provide evaluative feedback to the dean. This process may be repeated to the level of the vice president for academic affairs who evaluates the dean and in turn receives evaluation feedback from the dean. At all levels, input from supervisors and subordinates is taken into consideration as the faculty or administrator writes his or her own self-evaluation, identifying strengths, plans for improvement, and goals for the upcoming year. In addition to defining the appropriate process for performance review, faculty and administrators should reflect on the effectiveness of the process, including the utility of evaluation forms and the usefulness of evaluation in improving performance.

The use of standard assessment tools, such as those provided by the Individual Development and Educational Assessment Center for the evaluation of department chairs and deans, is another means of obtaining feedback on administrative effectiveness. The advantage of these standardized tools is that they provide the opportunity to compare administrative performance with national benchmarks. The disadvantage of this approach is the cost.

In addition to effective leadership, the structure and governance of the department must provide effective means for communication and problem solving. Bylaws and written policies are two mechanisms for promoting effective department governance. The nursing school's bylaws should be examined for congruence with the constitution and bylaws of the larger institution and the structures included to facilitate faculty governance in relation to academic authority. For example, it is useful to do a comparative analysis of standing committees and the mission and goals of the school. Are the standing committees configured to address major issues related to faculty affairs, student affairs, curriculum, budget, and major thrusts of the mission? In universities with a school of law, consultation is often readily available to review the fit of the bylaws with parliamentary rules and congruence checks. The extent to which stakeholders are included in the committee structures delineated in the bylaws is important as well. For example, are students represented on appropriate committees and how are voting privileges defined? Whether the established mechanisms actually function in the manner described is another issue for evaluation. Minutes of all standing committees should be filed in a central location. These minutes should reflect membership, agenda items, salient discussions, and a precise statement of decisions made and actions taken. It is useful for evaluation follow-up to designate membership annually in the minutes of the first meeting

of each committee. After each name, there should be an indicator of representation (e.g., faculty, student, alumni, consumer). In this way, one can track whether stakeholders indicated in the bylaws are in fact represented on designated committees. Representation is an *intended* means of integration of stakeholders, but attendance and participation are indicators of *actual* participation. Therefore attendance should be recorded for each meeting. Accreditation teams review minutes for these elements and often track membership participation and decisions. Including tracking data is important. For example, the reviewer should state how decisions and documents are channeled for final decision making. If a curriculum committee recommendation was forwarded to the faculty council for deliberation and action, the date it was forwarded should be included. The minutes of the faculty council can then be tracked to ensure that the decision item moved forward in a timely fashion. Accurate record keeping facilitates evaluation tracking.

Policies should be evaluated for their effectiveness in supporting and guiding communication and decision making relevant to program implementation. Policies should be organized in a manual or file and should be available to all to whom they apply. Many schools provide all new faculty with an electronic or written policy manual and send updates to the manual on a regular basis. Students usually receive information related to relevant policies at an appropriate time. For example, some policies are included in the school catalogue. Policies related to specific courses are usually included in course materials. An investigation of how policies are disseminated to those affected by the policies should be a part of the evaluation of policies. Policies should be reviewed annually and updated regularly. The approval documentation that should be present on every policy will demonstrate that all stakeholders had input into their development and approval. Minutes of meetings of appropriate bodies will provide evidence of discussion and action by the stakeholders. Policies need to be clearly stated and widely communicated. Evidence that policies are not followed is cause for analyzing reasons and intervening accordingly.

Program effectiveness is dependent on the availability of adequate fiscal resources. The budget of the nursing unit (school or division) should be reviewed in relation to personnel, equipment and supplies, travel, and infrastructure. As a starting point, *personnel monies* are reviewed in terms of supply and demand. For example, one may have indicated a desired mix of faculty to meet the mission and goals, but that mix depends on the fiscal ability to recruit and attract faculty to meet the mix outcome expectation. If a large percentage of the personnel budget is targeted for part-time faculty, it may be difficult to convert to full-time positions at a desired level to meet broad educational goals in terms of teaching, scholarship, and service. The data gathered in the comparative analysis of salaries noted previously will also have implications for the budget review. If salaries need to be upgraded or compression issues exist, there will be a need for a review of alternatives available to meet competing needs for fiscal support.

As *technology* advances, it becomes increasingly important to identify fiscal support for its use beyond the usual physical environment considerations noted in the physical space section. Although internal and external sources may be found for the acquisition of such technology, funding for maintenance and upgrading is an issue that requires attention. Many programs have received grants for technology hardware only to find that the monies for software, upkeep, and upgrading are not available in the budget. Careful record keeping provides a database for projecting future needs in this area, as well as the cost–benefit evaluation of technology. Decisions must be made regarding the technology that will provide the greatest return for the investment involved. These data also provide supportive evidence when one goes in search of additional funding. Solid data make a stronger case than a wish list. Future acquisitions may depend in part on the data available about the effective use of existing technology. This is a multiple stakeholder issue.

Maintenance and extension of *infrastructure* needs require careful documentation as well. Records of such basic issues as heating, lighting, and telephone service provide trend data for projecting future needs. Building maintenance and expansion for new programs must be documented. When decisions are made—for example, to facilitate faculty communication by installation of voice mail—the cost must be measured against its efficiency. This may also produce evaluation evidence that it is easy to leave a message but difficult to talk to a "live person" or receive follow-up. Data about the potential and actual decrease in support staff realized by advances in infrastructure services may serve to justify their cost or even provide evidence that they save money in the long run. Continuing to request advances without data will ultimately result in the need to make choices that may not be well grounded.

Funding for *faculty development* is important to faculty growth. Input from administration and faculty is needed to target the funds based on the mission and goals of the school and department. For example, if increased scholarship productivity is a goal, a percentage of this budget might be targeted for attending research conferences and giving presentations. A percentage might be targeted for conferences and presentations related to teaching and learning to advance excellence in teaching. Some schools designate some funds to enable students to participate in scholarly conferences or to present papers based on their student research efforts. Evaluation requires a review of the use of the monies for the designated purposes and follow-up in some cases to determine what benefit accrued to the school from the individual's activities funded by the school. Some schools indicate the amount any one person can receive in a specified period and monitor this as an evaluation measure to foster equity.

Fiscal resources may also be dependent on the ability of the nursing school to seek and secure external funding. The size and nature of the parent institution and the school or division will guide outcome expectations in this area. Increasingly, schools are pressed to obtain external funding for programs and scholarship efforts. The sources of stable funding also influence this area. State schools have, in the past, assumed that they would receive their funding in thirds from the state, from tuition, and from external funding. State appropriations are decreasing in most states, and efforts are being made to control increases in tuition and fees to offset this loss. As a result there is a greater need to establish clear goals for *external funding* and to measure progress in this area. Stated goals may be somewhat broad or very specific. For example, some schools may simply indicate that there will be evidence of increased external funding reviewed on an annual basis. In this scenario, any increase is evidence of success. Other schools may set specific goals such as indicating the percentage of increase expected every 1 or 2 years or a 5-year goal of an increase at a stated level with annual targets to achieve the long-term goal. Others indicate specifically where the increases should occur. For example, some schools indicate a desire to increase funding from specific sources such as the National Institutes of Health. These measures provide specific evaluation targets. Trend data over 5- and 10-year periods are useful for analysis of progress over time and as a database for future goals.

Another issue related to fiscal resources is *development monies*. Often resources must be provided to establish a fund-raising program from which returns are expected. For example, many schools support a "friends of (discipline)" advisory group gathered to enable fund-raising campaigns. The goals of the fund-raising should be specified. Some believe that giving is more likely to occur when a specific project that is valued by potential donors is identified. Certainly, a percentage of monies should be designated to be used at the discretion of the school to advance goals, but targeted funding is also critical to success. Evaluation includes measuring the cost of the fund-raising effort against resulting gains. Trend data are critical to this area. It is important to know not only the amount of giving but also the sources of those gifts and the relationship of those sources to marketing efforts.

Many schools have targeted financial incentive projects to encourage donors to engage in the educational mission. Examples include endowed chairs, centers of excellence, technology initiatives, faculty and student recognition programs, library enhancement, and programs for curricular innovations. Evaluation of the success of these initiatives reaches beyond the mere counting of dollars received. It should include the congruence of the initiative to the stated mission and goals, trend data with indicators of performance outcomes for the investment, comparisons with peer institutions, and analysis of the worth of the initiative in meeting the stated goals for that initiative.

The sources of funding are important for review as indicators for future efforts as well. Some schools have relied exclusively on alumni as a source for development monies. Others reach out to corporations and special interest groups. In nursing, for example, hospitals have often provided funding for initiatives of interest to future human resources. They are more likely to continue their interest if evaluation reports are created indicating the efficient and effective use of the monies provided. One of the elements of evaluation often overlooked in this area is the mechanism to inform donors of the outcomes achieved as a result of their generosity. This alone may affect future giving.

Another source of data for analysis and decision making is a review of the goals of *funding groups* and *state initiatives* that may have attached funding. When the goals and initiatives of external agencies are congruent with the mission and goals of the school, this may provide opportunities to apply for funds that will contribute to the desired outcome of increased external funding. These data are usually available through the parent institution, library searches, professional organizations, the office of research and development, or direct contact with the funding group.

Regardless of the sources of funding, nursing programs are facing higher expectations to be cost-effective. As colleges and universities face the need to increase quality and strengthen academic reputation, they also face state and national calls for financial accountability. Because academic programs are the primary driver of costs, it is logical that institutions of higher education examine the cost-effectiveness of academic programs. Dickeson (2010) proposed a process to prioritize academic programs by conducting a simultaneous review of programs using a common set of criteria to determine which programs are most effective, efficient, and central to the mission. The outcome of program prioritization is the strategic allocation of resources and may involve closure of less productive programs to move resources to more productive programs. Nursing schools may find themselves participating in institutional program prioritization projects in the near future. Large nursing schools with multiple nursing programs may need to conduct a school-based prioritization project to determine resource allocation among nursing programs.

An adequate number of qualified staff and professional personnel is necessary to support program effectiveness. For faculty to meet the expectations of teaching, scholarship, and service, the support personnel available to them is critical. The nature of the institution and the mission and goals also influence the standards set in this area. Nursing schools with graduate programs, for example, consider the number of graduate assistants and research assistants to be an issue of importance, and in some cases computer programmers and statisticians may be important to goal achievement.

The level of clerical and professional staff is important to all program levels. Faculty-to-staff ratios and satisfaction surveys to elicit administration, faculty, and staff perceptions about the quality of this support provide baseline data for this review. The analysis of these data may suggest the need for further data to complete a full analysis.

Many institutions of higher education have central evaluation tools and processes for the evaluation of professional and clerical staff. Others rely on school or departmental evaluation. Still others supplement the central evaluation process with unit-specific efforts. The scope of staff under review will vary widely according to the size and complexity of the school. In any event, the evaluation should focus on the job descriptions of the individuals under review and the extent to which the job responsibilities are met in terms of efficiency and effectiveness. As with all other areas of evaluation, the process should include feedback on strengths and areas for growth; the establishment of goals for growth should be appropriate to the evaluation findings. All subsequent evaluations include a review of progress toward the stated goals. A common problem encountered in staff evaluation is the finding that the role of the staff member has drifted, because of changing circumstances, from the job description. This may create tensions that negatively affect evaluation. It is therefore necessary to include a review of the job description for congruence with ongoing expectations. Revisions should occur as needed and as a collaborative effort between the staff member and the appropriate supervisor. Box 28-7 provides a summary of the theoretical

---

BOX 28-7 Theoretical Elements of Environment Evaluation: Organizational Dimension

- Qualifications and skills of program administrators enhance program effectiveness.
- The structure and governance of the department provides effective means for communication and problem solving.
- There are adequate fiscal resources to support ongoing program improvement.
- Nursing faculty participate actively in the university governance system.
- There is an adequate number of qualified staff and professional personnel to support program effectiveness.

---

elements associated with evaluation of the organizational dimension.

Environment Evaluation: Interorganizational Dimension

Program effectiveness is influenced by the relationship of the nursing program with outside agencies. For example, cooperation with health care agencies is essential to providing needed educational experiences. One method of facilitating these relationships is establishing an advisory board that can provide a direct communication link with these important stakeholders. The composition of the advisory board should be evaluated to determine that its membership is appropriate. The purpose and functions of the advisory board should be communicated to members and reviewed periodically for clarity. Effectiveness of the board's function can be determined by surveying board members and nursing faculty regarding their perception of the board's effectiveness in fulfilling its purpose.

Many nursing programs have articulation agreements with other educational institutions that provide mobility pathways for students to complete upper-level degrees. An articulation agreement may define special admissions policies and the type of transfer credits that will be accepted between a community college and a university. For example, an articulation agreement may involve the admission of licensed practical nurses to a 2-year associate nursing degree program. The effectiveness of these articulation agreements can be evaluated by having both institutions review the transfer admission criteria for appropriateness. The nursing program accepting students should conduct a periodic audit of the transcript evaluation process to ensure that transcripts are being accurately evaluated. The final test of the effectiveness of an articulation agreement is an examination of enrollment and various outcomes. Does the articulation agreement support enrollment goals? Are students in the articulation program successful? Comparison of progression, retention, and completion rates of the students in the articulation program with those of students in a more traditional program will provide baseline data from which to determine the effectiveness of the articulation program. Box 28-8 provides a summary of the theoretical elements

> **BOX 28-8** Theoretical Elements of Environment Evaluation: Interorganizational Dimension
>
> - Advisory board provides effective communication link with important stakeholders.
> - Articulation agreements are satisfactory.

associated with evaluation of the interorganizational dimension.

Environment Evaluation: Micro Context Dimension

Micro context evaluation examines the effect of the immediate environment on program implementation, including what happens before students enter the program and after they complete the program. If the program's relationship with prospective students is not satisfactory, students will be discouraged from pursuing admission. A positive relationship with prospective students begins when students receive current and accurate information about the program. Because of the cost of higher education, prospective students need accurate information about financial aid. Transcript evaluation needs to be accurate and performed in a timely manner for all transfer students. New student registration should be run efficiently and provide a welcoming atmosphere. After students are admitted and registered, they will need orientation to the nursing program. Orientation should provide information about nursing program policies, especially requirements for admission into clinical courses and academic progression policies.

Activities at program completion may influence the satisfaction of students and their ongoing relationship as alumni, as well as success in achieving terminal outcomes. The nursing school may offer special workshops in preparing students for licensure examinations. Career services may provide assistance in résumé preparation and job searches.

Academic advising is an important factor in program effectiveness and influences student success from program entry through completion. Some institutions use staff-level student advisers to assist students with registration and ongoing advisement, whereas others assign students to faculty advisers. Programs to educate faculty in effective advising should be evaluated for their utility. Further analysis of advising effectiveness can be determined by surveying students regarding their level of satisfaction with advising. As a component of the advising system, academic advising records are created when a student enters the program. These records should provide a thorough and objective record of student advisement. An audit of student files may be done to determine that files are set up correctly and maintained accurately through program completion.

Other aspects of the immediate environment that influence program success include housing, health services, student academic support services, business office and registrar, and cocurricular activities. One method of evaluating these functions is through student satisfaction surveys, such as the Noel-Levitz Student Satisfaction Inventory (Schreiner & Juillerat, 1993). The survey is designed to measure student satisfaction by comparing students' ratings of what they expected versus what they actually experienced. Results are provided at an institutional level and for each major, and comparisons are made with national norms. Box 28-9 provides a summary of the theoretical elements associated with evaluation of the micro context dimension.

> **BOX 28-9** Theoretical Elements of Environment Evaluation: Micro Context Dimension
>
> - Prospective students receive current and accurate information about program options, admission criteria, and financial aid.
> - Transcript evaluation is accurate and performed in a timely manner for all transfer students.
> - New student registration is run efficiently and provides a welcoming atmosphere.
> - Students receive adequate orientation to the program.
> - Academic advising is effective.
> - Advising records are accurate and maintained from program entry through program completion.
> - Students receive final preparation after program completion for licensure examinations.

Environment Evaluation: Macro Context Dimension

Macro context evaluation seeks to determine effects of the larger environment (social, political, cultural, and economic factors) on program implementation. National trends in health care and changes in local health care delivery should be reviewed and incorporated into program development and revision. Trends in higher education should also be reviewed, and implications for nursing education should be considered in program planning. For example, service learning is a growing trend in higher education. Nursing faculty may need to consider building into the curriculum specific opportunities for service learning. Identification of trends can be done through literature review and through dialogue with advisory board members, community leaders, or elected officials. Box 28-10 provides a summary of the theoretical elements associated with evaluation of the macro context dimension.

Outcome Evaluation

The purpose of outcome evaluation is to determine how well the program has achieved the expected outcomes. At this point, outcomes have already been defined (see Mission and Goal Evaluation). Program outcome measures are those implemented at the conclusion of the program. These may be integrated into the final semester courses or may be applied at exit and during alumni and employer follow-up studies. For each of the outcomes, a simple model provides a framework for assessment and evaluation. The behavior of interest must be

---

BOX 28-10 Theoretical Elements of Environment Evaluation: Macro Context Dimension

- Trends in health care are reviewed and incorporated into program development and revision.
- Changes in local health care delivery are known and incorporated into program development and revision.
- Trends in higher education are known and implications for nursing education are considered in program planning.

---

clearly defined and the attributes of that behavior must be delineated. Faculty must then determine what measures will be used to assess the behavioral attributes with rationale for the selected measures. Finally, faculty must demonstrate how the data from such assessment and evaluation measures have been used to develop, maintain, or revise curricula. To achieve this final objective for outcome evaluation, it must be placed within the context of overall program evaluation. Outcomes assessment in isolation will not provide adequate direction for program revision. Nevertheless, outcome evaluation is critical in that it may be the primary measure by which external stakeholders judge the merit of the program.

Student Outcomes

Student outcomes are measured at multiple levels in the program of learning. *Student learning* outcomes deal with attributes of the learner that demonstrate achievement of program goals. Examples include critical thinking, communication, and therapeutic interventions. Other areas of measurement of learner outcomes occur at the course, clinical practice, and classroom levels. This level of outcome measurement is discussed in detail in Chapters 24 through 27. The level of learner outcome at the broad program level usually involves aggregate data designed to provide general measures of learner success. At this level, one can communicate to the public the extent to which one is preparing well-educated and competent practitioners to meet the human resource needs of the community.

Of particular interest are the *graduation and retention rates* in each program within the school. A clear understanding of the graduation and attrition rates will influence decisions about recruitment and retention methods in the future. The state is interested in the graduation rate from the perspectives of human resource flow and as a measure of return on investment in the educational program. Tracking graduation rates is a measure of the productivity of a program. It is useful to track the absolute attrition of individuals over time, as well as to document the number of graduates compared with the number of program entrants by graduation year. This allows the program to track students who are readmitted and who eventually graduate. In programs with high numbers of adult students, there may be a larger number of students who leave the program because of family problems or job-related issues. They may return and graduate. Thus a given class, when defined by the admission enrollment, may have a lower attrition rate than a class defined by numbers admitted and numbers graduated in the expected time span for program completion. If the school catalogue indicates that a student must complete the program in a given number of years from the time of initial enrollment, the absolute attrition for that group would be calculated based on that time frame.

Many programs use the *pass rate* on national *licensing examinations* or *certification examinations* as a measure of program success. The number of graduates licensed or certified to practice in a given area is seen as a measure of production of qualified human resources. Although a school of nursing has reason to be concerned about pass rates for internal reasons and in response to state mandates in some cases, the use of this measure must be approached with caution. The program is designed to provide students with a general education, as well as to prepare them for competent practice in a profession. The program is not designed to respond to a given examination. Variables other than the program of learning, such as individual preparation or test anxiety, may also influence a graduate's performance on the examination. Certainly, a school should be concerned if the pass rate falls below reasonable norms, and additional assessment measures should be initiated to attempt to determine whether common variables over which the program of learning has control are involved.

Employment rate is an aggregate measure of product demand. The extent to which the graduates are able to find employment may provide both marketing data and a broad measure of employer satisfaction with the product a program produces. Less information may be gleaned in a tight market in which demand exceeds supply. When the demand is high, employment rates may be more an indication of need than selective employment based on the quality of the applicant. When the supply exceeds the demand, the specific applicants the employer selects may provide stronger data. If the graduates of a given program are not in demand or are not marketable, one must question the viability of the program.

Employer: Product Use and Satisfaction

Employer surveys provide a means to determine the extent to which the consumer believes the product (graduate) has the skills necessary for employment expectations. Feedback from employers provides useful data for program review. Brevity is a key to a high response rate on employer surveys, as it is with many others, and is of particular importance during a time of work redesign and increasing demands on the time of employers in health care. Extensive survey tools designed for each program with long lists of questions about skills to which the individual is asked to respond are less likely to be completed. Respondents are more likely to reply to fewer questions that have been well developed to provide useful information.

Several areas are of particular interest. Brief *demographic information* about the nature of the agency is helpful in learning which settings use the program graduates and which expressed concerns or commendations may be specific to a given setting. Whether the employer hires graduates of the program and to what extent are other areas of interest. It is useful to know whether an employer would hire more graduates of the program if they were available. When questions about satisfaction with particular abilities are asked, it is helpful to state them in broad terms rather than providing the traditional laundry list of individual skills. For example, data about satisfaction may be linked to the extent to which an employer believes the graduates of the program are able to problem-solve, think critically, resolve conflicts, communicate effectively, use resources efficiently, and perform essential psychomotor skills safely. These and other broad classifications of behaviors can be selected on the basis of program outcome expectations. Provision of space for comments allows for the addition of qualitative information and the opportunity to identify any specific areas of concern.

Another issue in many employer surveys is the identification of which stakeholders are in the best position to respond to particular questions. Although an administrator may be able to respond more quickly and accurately to demographic questions and inquiries about the number of graduates employed, he or she may not be in the best position to respond to questions about the skills and abilities of graduates. The administrator may respond according to perceptions based on factors other than direct observation. Some employers delegate completion of the survey. Therefore it is helpful to request information about the respondent in the cover letter that accompanies the survey. For example, one might ask the title of the respondent as a guide for determining how likely he or she is to be in a position of interacting directly with graduates. Some schools send employer surveys to graduates and request that they forward the surveys to their immediate supervisors for completion. This practice is problematic in that it usually results in a low return rate and a completed survey often reflects a respondent's reaction to an individual graduate rather than the aggregate of program graduates he or she has observed. Figure 28-4 provides an example of an employer survey and sample questions.

Another method of obtaining ongoing feedback about the graduates of a program is to establish an advisory committee of consumers from agencies that typically employ program alumni. Such committees often provide advice and counsel on multiple matters, but satisfaction with the product and advice about the changing needs of the marketplace are traditional agenda items for such a group.

Alumni: Employment Rates and Profile

There are multiple avenues for obtaining alumni data. One approach is to survey students who are about to become alumni. The exit survey is a method of determining product satisfaction with a program just completed. At this point, students' perceptions are fresh in their minds. Through the exit survey, it is possible to learn which students have found employment at the time of graduation, follow up on entry data collected for comparison purposes, and identify students' perceptions about the strengths and weaknesses of the program they have just completed. The exit survey is usually done within 10 days of graduation and has the advantage of a higher return rate than mailed surveys. A disadvantage is that the exiting students may not have had an opportunity to apply their education in a work setting, which may change their perceptions.

Another method commonly used for exit data is the focus group. A focus group provides an opportunity for a representative group of students in the graduating classes to reflect in more detail about their experiences. Selection of the moderator is important to the collection of rich and valid insights

(Stewart & Shamdasani, 1990). A first concern is that the moderator be skilled in group process and listening. The moderator should have several questions prepared to guide the group discussion yet be able to respond to and facilitate group discussion when other relevant issues emerge. In an end-of-program focus session, more open-ended questions encourage free-flowing responses and invite the participants to provide the amount of information they wish. If specific types of information are desired, the questions may be more structured. The more structured the question, the more reliable the data, but the trade-off may be less richness of data. One may find it useful to begin with open and broad questions and follow with more structured questions as the discussion unfolds.

If the focus group is conducted by someone the students view as a neutral person and if that person is able to facilitate equally the expression of opposing points of view, the participants are more likely to be open in their comments and the content is likely to be more valid. Focus groups have the advantage of providing qualitative data in more detail than is usually obtained in a written survey, but they have the disadvantage of being a representative group that may or may not provide the range of data that a full group survey would provide. Use of both a survey and a focus group may resolve this issue, but students may be reluctant to participate in more than one end-of-program evaluation effort when they are in the process of final examinations and end-of-semester evaluations. Timing is important in this effort.

Alumni surveys may be conducted at regular intervals to obtain long-term data about the products of an educational program. When such surveys are conducted depends on the data desired, the size and complexity of programs in the school, and the cost–benefit ratio of the survey effort. It is common to complete at least 1-year and 5-year surveys. The information sought depends on the level of the program and the outcome measures for which data are sought.

One approach is to provide a *two-part survey* in which one part is devoted to broad outcome measures and the graduates' perceptions of their general education experience on the campus. Questions on this survey may relate to perceptions about the extent to which they acquired skills such as critical thinking and effective written and oral communication; gained an understanding of different

Example: Employer Survey

In order to improve the quality of our academic nursing program, your thoughtful and honest responses to this survey are very important to us. Darken the oval that corresponds to your response.

Section I: Program Goals	Poor	Fair	Good	Excellent
1. Example program goal #1: Value...	0	0	0	0
2. Example program goal #2: Communicate...	0	0	0	0
Section II: Components of Program Goals	**Poor**	**Fair**	**Good**	**Excellent**
3. Example: Manages an environment that promotes clients' self esteem, dignity, safety, and comfort.	0	0	0	0
4. Example: Establishes and maintains effective communication with clients, families, significant others, and health team members.	0	0	0	0
5. Example: Promotes continuity of client care by utilizing appropriate channels of communication external to the organization.	0	0	0	0
Section III: Overall Satisfaction with ASN Nursing Program	**Poor**	**Fair**	**Good**	**Excellent**
6. My overall satisfaction with this employee is:	0	0	0	0

Other Examples of Employer Survey Questions:

7. What is your primary source of information about this graduate?

8. What are your recommendations for strengthening this nursing program?

9. What suggestions do you have to facilitate transition into the professional role?

10. What changes in the health care environment will affect the educational preparation of future graduates?

11. Other comments: Survey completed by: _____
    Position _____

Figure 28-4 Example: Employer Survey

cultures and philosophies; and developed a sense of values and ethical standards, leadership skills, an appreciation of the arts, an ability to view events and phenomena from different perspectives, and an understanding of scientific principles and methods. One can also learn about the alumni's view of services available across the campus and opportunities to interact with students and faculty across disciplines. An advantage to this survey is the opportunity to compare the responses of students across disciplines to determine relative experiences and perceptions.

The second component of an alumni survey is usually *discipline specific*. In addition to general demographic data, the survey seeks information about positions held (title, location, population served, salary), the extent to which alumni believe they were prepared to practice according to the program outcomes, and their general satisfaction with the program. Graduate programs find data related to the scholarship of alumni to be particularly valuable.

Strategies for Improving Alumni Surveys

When surveys are conducted, the questions should be considered carefully in terms of data that will be used in decision making. If surveys are concise and questions are clearly stated, responses are more likely to be received. As a general rule, response rates will be improved if the survey does not exceed four pages. A high response rate increases the credibility of the data in reflecting the perspectives of the population surveyed. The cover letter is an important element of the survey. The letter should be concise yet spell out the importance of the data to the educational program and the value placed on the input received from graduates. The more personalized the letter and the more professional the survey tool, the more likely it is that alumni will respond (Fowler, 1993). The letter should also include a statement about confidentiality and the use of pooled or aggregate data in reports of survey findings to protect the anonymity of the respondents. Although it is useful to have several open-ended questions to obtain qualitative data, the simpler the tool is to complete, the more likely it is that respondents will complete the task. Well-designed questions, for which the respondent can check or circle an item or provide a number as a response, are more likely to be answered. Multiple mailing is

another method of improving the return rate. There are several opinions about the best mailing sequence. One method is to send a second mailing within 2 to 3 weeks of the first, with a second survey tool included in case the first mailing has been misplaced. If cost is an issue, a reminder card may suffice. A third mailing in the form of a postcard should occur between 10 days and 3 weeks after the second mailing, depending on the nature of the survey. If the surveys have been coded, only nonrespondents may be reminded as a cost-saving measure. If the surveys are not coded in an effort to increase the confidence level of the cohort that the survey will be guarded for confidentiality and anonymity, a card can be included with each survey. The card may be coded so that the respondent can send it back separately with a statement that he or she has responded and needs no reminder (Fowler, 1993). Figure 28-5 provides an example of an alumni survey and sample questions. Box 28-11 provides a summary of the theoretical elements associated with outcomes evaluation.

Intervening Mechanism Evaluation

For the purpose of determining how to improve the program's success in achieving outcomes, the intervening variables that influence success must be known and monitored. For example, the intervening variables that influence first-time passage rate on the NCLEX-RN examination may include the following:
1. Qualification of students admitted to the program
2. Definition and implementation of progression policies
3. Quality of the curriculum
4. Quality of instruction
5. Evaluation methods used to determine students' knowledge
6. Preparation of students to take the examination
7. Student anxiety at the time of the examination

The program evaluation plan should be reviewed to determine that each of these intervening variables is identified within the program evaluation plan. A similar process should be followed for all program outcomes. Mapping the relationship between and among intervening variables may help to clarify the role each variable has in influencing outcome achievement.

Potential intervening variables should be reviewed annually and added to the plan as needed. Intervening variables may be identified through

Example: Alumni Survey

As a graduate of our nursing program, you are especially qualified to tell us what works well and what does not. We would like your input and would appreciate any suggestions that you might have. Would you please take a few minutes and complete this survey. The survey is completely anonymous.

Darken the oval that corresponds to your response.

Section I: Perceptions of Attainment of Program Goals. Indicate How Well the Program Prepared You to Fulfill the Following Program Goals.		Poor	Fair	Good	Excellent
1.	Sample program goal #1: Integrate...	0	0	0	0
2.	Sample program goal #2: Utilize...	0	0	0	0
3.	Sample program goal #3: Synthesize...	0	0	0	0
Section II. Satisfaction with Nursing Courses. Indicate How Well Each Course Contributed to Your Attainment of Program Goals.	Course Not Taken— Does Not Apply	Poor	Fair	Good	Excellent
4. Sample Course A	0	0	0	0	0
5. Sample Course B	0	0	0	0	0
6. Sample Course C	0	0	0	0	0
Section III: Overall Satisfaction with BSN Nursing Program		Poor	Fair	Good	Excellent
7. My overall satisfaction with the Nursing Program at University of A.	0	0	0	0	0

Additional Example Survey Questions:

8. What semester and year did you graduate or complete your program at University A?
9. What I liked best about my program was:
10. One thing I believe should be changed is:
11. What suggestions do you have to facilitate transition from the student role to professional practice?
12. Additional Comments

Figure 28-5 Example: Alumni Survey

literature review, program evaluation reports, or internal studies. All intervening variables need to be evaluated at some point in the program evaluation plan. Box 28-12 provides a summary of the theoretical elements associated with intervening mechanism evaluation.

Generalization Evaluation

Generalization evaluation provides the opportunity to examine the program evaluation plan in its entirety and to make revisions to improve its effectiveness. From this perspective, generalization evaluation is a

BOX 28-11 Theoretical Elements of Outcomes Evaluation

- Students achieve all terminal program goals by graduation.
- Students achieve all technical competencies by graduation.
- The program has defined a benchmark for graduation rates.
- The program has defined a benchmark for first-time NCLEX passage rate.
- The program has defined a benchmark for employment rates.
- Students are satisfied with the overall quality of the program.
- Employers are satisfied with the performance of graduates.

BOX 28-12 Theoretical Elements of Intervening Mechanism Evaluation

- Intervening variables are defined for all program outcomes.
- Potential intervening variables are determined each year and added to the plan as needed.
- All intervening variables are evaluated at some point in the program evaluation plan.

type of metaevaluation, or evaluation of evaluation. Generalization evaluation seeks to ensure that program improvement occurs as a result of program evaluation.

The first step is to determine that the program evaluation plan has been implemented correctly. Identifying evaluation activities called for in the plan by responsible parties at the beginning of the academic year will help to ensure that evaluation activities are implemented. Entering the program evaluation plan into an electronic spreadsheet or database may assist faculty in determining responsible parties, activities, and time frames because the plan can be sorted on these categories. Preparation of a year-end report with all completed forms and data sets will help track implementation of evaluation activities.

A record of program changes that are made as a result of evaluation activities should be maintained.

Actions taken to improve program quality can be summarized in a yearly report. This report will serve as a permanent record of the utility of the evaluation plan in bringing about program improvements. Faculty may want to review these summary reports, discuss strengths and limitations of the plan, and propose changes to improve the plan's effectiveness after they have reviewed year-end reports. Questions that will help guide this review include the following: "Does the plan provide information when it is needed for decision making?" "Do the faculty trust the information provided by evaluation strategies?"

Another important factor in the plan's effectiveness is the reliability and validity of evaluation tools. Reliability refers to the accuracy of measurement. Validity means that evaluation tools measure what they intend to measure. Internally developed measurement tools should be evaluated for reliability and validity at the time of their development. If faculty are unable to demonstrate reliability and validity of evaluation tools, they will not be able to trust the results of program evaluation activities. In addition, data need to be appropriately aggregated and trended over time to support decision making. Faculty should be cautious about making decisions based on limited data.

The evaluation of any education program is context specific. Consequently, the results of program evaluation may not be generalized to other programs. Nevertheless, nursing faculty should report successful strategies in program evaluation in the nursing literature. Nursing faculty across the nation may benefit from program evaluation research studies, such as those that report successful assessment strategies or provide insight about intervening variables for common program outcomes. Box 28-13 provides a summary of the theoretical elements associated with generalization evaluation.

BOX 28-13 Theoretical Elements of Generalization Evaluation

- Assessment strategies are reliable and valid.
- Evaluation activities provide meaningful data for program improvement.
- The evaluation plan is reviewed and modified to improve its effectiveness.

Practical Considerations of Theory-Driven Program Evaluation

Creating and implementing theory-driven program evaluation is a rigorous process that includes innumerable benefits and challenges. There are many decision points and a wide diversity of potential ways to create a theory-driven model. The authors, who have implemented and refined a theory-driven model, offer the following practical suggestions for nursing educators who desire to improve their evaluation processes by implementing theory-driven program evaluation.

The first task is to determine faculty satisfaction with the current program evaluation process and assess the readiness of faculty for change. Cultivating a core of interested faculty to spearhead early efforts to change the existing program evaluation paradigm is a valuable strategy to creating openness to this change among the entire faculty. During the initial phase of creating theory-driven evaluation, the enormity of revising the way faculty view program evaluation can be challenging. Faculty who closely follow accreditation standards to create their program evaluation plans may not be able to envision what theory-driven program evaluation has to offer. Faculty may be hesitant to participate in the process because it is new, change is difficult, and they are uncomfortable. Initially, time must be invested in learning about the theory-driven approach to program evaluation.

After faculty become familiar with the theory-driven model, the next step is to define the individual program theory and begin development of the evaluation plan. Using the theory-driven model requires continuous practice, assessment, and refinement to fully integrate the components into a coherent evaluation plan. Introducing individual sections of the model and developing the evaluation plan incrementally helps faculty adjust to the new model. For example, beginning with Mission and Goal Evaluation and developing all elements of the program evaluation plan for that section, including the program theory, criteria for assessment, and assessment tools, will allow faculty to learn this new approach and to experiment through trial and error. This approach may be uncomfortable compared to following a set of prescribed criteria from accreditation standards.

As the plan is being created, data overload can occur because each new section of the plan calls for assessment methods and measurement tools.

Surveys, questionnaires, and other assessment tools need to be found and adapted or created. Created measurement tools may lack reliability and validity, so plans need to include how to address this when tools are constructed, refined, and piloted. Because the process of building a theory-driven evaluation plan is a paradigm shift requiring concentrated attention and continuous refinement, administrative support is essential to the success within the department. Faculty members require time to acclimate to the new theory-based model and relatively new proponents of the theory-driven model need to mentor faculty who were not on the planning committee. As the new theory-driven model is developed, maintain a healthy sense of humor about how the process is "supposed" to work and how long it will take to fully implement. Celebrating small success along the way can renew commitments to continue to use this new paradigm of program evaluation. Keep in perspective that the business of the academy continues unabated by the fact that the department is creating an entirely new evaluation process and format.

Benefits of creating a theory-driven model of evaluation outweigh the challenges and effort. Preparation of accreditation self-study reports is enhanced by having the data in a consistent, available format. Trending data over time is streamlined by the model. The authors experienced the full impact of program improvement after the third year of implementation when it became apparent that the theory-driven model was effective in identifying successful program elements and areas needing improvement.

Flexibility is a by-product of creating a theory-driven model; elements of the program plan may be revised repeatedly. This is not an indication of failure of the process but rather an indication of making the evaluation process unique to each setting. Positive comments and small successes along the way are synergistic to the development process and should be widely shared. Faculty ownership of a theory-driven model increases with the success of the initial processes. An appropriate metaphor for the process of creating a theory-driven model of program evaluation is that it is like a pioneer journey to the New World. The terrain is lush and rich, but it is uneven and unplowed. Pioneers lead the way through new frontiers and smooth the roads along the way so those coming after them can drive cars.

Accountability for Program Evaluation

Responsibility for development and implementation of the program evaluation plan rests with the nursing administration and faculty. The process for development and implementation may vary across nursing schools, depending on such factors as the number of faculty in the nursing school and the institutional resources available to support the evaluation. In some schools, an evaluator position is created to manage program evaluation practices, including the development and implementation of the program evaluation plan. An office of evaluation may be necessary in large schools, providing support staff to coordinate data collection at multiple levels. A common approach in small- and moderate-sized nursing schools is to appoint a standing committee of faculty who provide leadership and coordination of evaluation efforts. Regardless of the plan, the nursing faculty must determine accountability for each element of the evaluation plan. Without clear accountability and firm time frames, it is easy for evaluation efforts to get lost in the press of daily demands on faculty and administration.

Another issue of concern is the reporting and recording of evaluation data. Information is of little value to decision making unless it is channeled to those who are responsible for making decisions. Careful attention to this issue not only increases the likelihood that decisions will be based on actual data but also facilitates analysis of the value of the data. Evaluation data also serve as a rich resource when responses to external reports and accreditation expectations are required. One of the dangers of the theory-based approach is data overload. Because data are used for making decisions, it is best to determine what information is necessary and what is interesting but not important. Over time, a goal of evaluation is to streamline the amount of data collected. Asking questions such as "Why do we need these data or information?" and "How will these data or information assist in making decisions for improvement?" will assist in eliminating data overload.

The location of evaluation information is also important. Access to the information increases the likelihood of its use. An official location for evaluation reports ensures that they can be found when they are needed. Advances in technology have made the development of computer databases an important source of information that can be accessed by multiple stakeholders from a central location or file server.

Finally, the outcome of evaluation efforts in terms of creating change is an element that is sometimes omitted in record keeping. Accrediting bodies are as concerned about the actions that result from analysis of evaluation data as they are that a plan is in place. The best plan loses value if it does not create change when a need for intervention is indicated by the data.

SUMMARY

Program evaluation is a comprehensive and complex process. Use of a theory-driven approach to program evaluation increases the likelihood that all program elements will receive appropriate attention and that evaluation activities will lead to program improvement (Chen, 1990). A theory-driven approach is useful in program planning in addition to evaluation of existing programs. This chapter provided suggestions for developing a theory-driven program evaluation plan appropriate for nursing education programs. The program evaluation plan serves as a road map to ensure that program evaluation activities are appropriately implemented. Development and implementation of a carefully designed theory-driven program evaluation plan will support continuous quality improvement for nursing education programs.

REFLECTING ON THE EVIDENCE

1. How does theory-driven program evaluation differ from method-driven program evaluation?

2. What are the advantages and disadvantages of theory-driven program evaluation?

3. What is the connection between program evaluation and accreditation standards?

4. How can program administrators minimize the challenges of implementing a theory-driven approach to program evaluation?

5. How can theory-driven program evaluation be used in new program development?

6. How does the use of theory-driven program evaluation complement and expand evaluations that emphasize primarily program outcomes?

REFERENCES

American Association of Colleges of Nursing. (1996). *Essentials of master's education for advanced practice nursing*. Retrieved from http://www.aacn.nche.edu

American Association of Colleges of Nursing. (2003a). *Alliance for Nursing Accreditation releases new statement on distance education policies*. Retrieved from http://www.aacn.nche.edu

American Association of Colleges of Nursing. (2003b). *Faculty shortages in baccalaureate and graduate nursing programs: Scope of the problem and strategies for expanding the supply*. Retrieved from http://www.aacn.nche.edu

American Association of Colleges of Nursing. (2006). *Essentials of doctoral education for advanced nursing practice*. Retrieved from http://www.aacn.nche.edu

American Association of Colleges of Nursing. (2008a). *Essentials of baccalaureate education for professional nursing practice*. Retrieved from http://www.aacn.nche.edu

American Association of Colleges of Nursing. (2008b). *The preferred vision of the professoriate in baccalaureate and graduate nursing programs*. Retrieved from http://www.aacn.nche.edu/

American Association of Colleges of Nursing. (2010a). *2009–2010 salaries of instructional and administrative nursing faculty in baccalaureate and graduate programs in nursing*. Retrieved from http://www.aacn.nche.edu

American Association of Colleges of Nursing. (2010b). *Special survey on vacant faculty positions for academic year 2010–2011*. Retrieved from http://www.aacn.nche.edu

American Nurses Association. (2010). *Nursing: Scope and standards of practice*. Retrieved from http://www.nursingworld.org

Andrews, M., & Wallis, J. (1999). Mentorship in nursing: A literature review. *Journal of Advanced Nursing, 29*(1), 201–207.

Angelo, T. A., & Cross, K. P. (1993). *Classroom assessment techniques: A handbook for college teachers*. San Francisco, CA: Jossey-Bass.

Armbruster, B. B., & Anderson, T. H. (1991). Textbook analysis. In A. Lewy (Ed.), *The international encyclopedia of curriculum* (pp. 78–80). Oxford, England: Pergamon Press.

Association of American Colleges and Universities. (2002). *Greater expectations: A new vision for learning as a nation goes to college*. Washington, DC: Author.

Bersky, A. K., & Yocom, C. J. (1994). Computerized clinical simulation testing: Its use for competence assessment in nursing. *Nursing and Health Care, 15*(3), 120–127.

Bevil, C. (1991). Program evaluation in nursing education: Creating a meaningful plan. In M. Garbin (Ed.), *Assessing educational outcomes* (pp. 53–67). New York, NY: National League for Nursing.

Bloom, B. S. (1956). *Taxonomy of educational objectives: The classification of educational goals, Handbook I, Cognitive domain*. New York, NY: McKay.

Borich, G. D., & Jemelka, R. P. (1982). *Programs and systems: An evaluation perspective*. New York, NY: Academic Press.

Boyer, E. L. (1990). *Scholarship rediscovered: Priorities of the professorate*. Princeton, NJ: The Carnegie Foundation for the Advancement of Teaching.

Boyer, E. L. (1994). *Scholarship assessed*. Paper presented at the American Association of Higher Education Conference on Faculty Roles and Rewards, New Orleans, LA.

Braskamp, L. A., & Ory, J. C. (1994). *Assessing faculty work: Enhancing individual and institutional performance*. San Francisco, CA: Jossey-Bass.

Brinko, K. T. (1993). The practice of giving feedback to improve teaching: What is effective? *Journal of Higher Education, 64*(5), 574–593.

Chen, H. (1990). *Theory-driven evaluations*. Newbury Park, CA: Sage.

Chen, H. (2005). *Practical program evaluation: Assessing and improving planning, implementation, and effectiveness*. Thousand Oaks, CA: Sage.

Cobb, K. L., & Billings, D. M. (2000). Assessing distance education programs in nursing. In J. Novotny (Ed.), *Distance education in nursing* (pp. 85–112). New York, NY: Springer.

College and University Professional Association for Human Resources. (2010). *National faculty salary survey for four-year institutions*. Retrieved from http://www.cupahr.org

Commission on Collegiate Nursing Education. (2010). *Standards for accreditation of baccalaureate and graduate nursing education programs*. Retrieved from http://www.aacn.edu/accredition

Dickeson, R. C. (2010). *Prioritizing academic programs and services: Reallocating resources to achieve strategic balance*. San Francisco, CA: Jossey-Bass.

DiFlorio, I., Duncan, P., Martin, B., & Meddlemiss, M. A. (1989). Curriculum evaluation. *Nurse Education Today, 9*, 402–407.

Doll, R. C. (1992). *Curriculum improvement: Decision making and process*. Boston, MA: Allyn & Bacon.

Ewell, P. T. (1985). *Introduction to assessing educational outcomes: New directions for institutional research*. San Francisco, CA: Jossey-Bass.

Fowler, F. J. (1993). *Survey research methods*. Newbury Park, CA: Sage.

Freed, J. E., Klugman, M. R., & Fife, J. D. (1997). *A culture for academic excellence: Implementing the quality principles in higher education* (ASHE-ERIC report vol 25[1], 1088-0042). Washington, DC: Graduate School of Education and Human Development, George Washington University.

Friesner, A. (1978). Five models for program evaluation: An overview. In *Program evaluation* (pp. 1–7). New York, NY: National League for Nursing.

Gagné, R. M. (1977). *The conditions of learning*. New York, NY: Holt-Rinehart.

Glennon, C. D. (2006). Reconceptualizing program outcomes. *Journal of Nursing Education, 45*(2), 55–58.

Guba, E. G., & Lincoln, Y. S. (1989). *Fourth generation evaluation*. Newbury Park, CA: Sage.

Halpern, D. F. (1987). Introduction and overview. In D. F. Halpern (Ed.), *Student outcomes assessment: What institutions stand to gain: New directions for higher education* (pp. 1–30). San Francisco, CA: Jossey-Bass.

Heinrich, C. R., Karner, K. J., Gaglione, B. H., & Lambert, L. J. (2002). Order out of chaos: The use of a matrix to validate curriculum integrity. *Nurse Educator, 27*(3), 136–140.

Higher Learning Commission. (2006). *Best practices for electronically offered degree and certificate programs*. Retrieved from http://www.ncahlc.org

Higher Learning Commission. (2010). *Distance education*. Retrieved from http://www.ncahlc.org

Ingersoll, G. L. (1996). Evaluation research. *Nursing Administration Quarterly, 20*(4), 28–40.

Ingersoll, G. L., & Sauter, M. K. (1998). Integrating accreditation criteria into educational program evaluation. *Nursing and Health Care Perspectives, 19*, 224–229.

Johnson, T. D., & Ryan, K. E. (2000). A comprehensive approach to the evaluation of college teaching. In K. Ryan (Ed.), *Evaluation of teaching in higher education: A vision for the future* (pp. 109–123). San Francisco, CA: Jossey-Bass.

Kevern, J., & Webb, C. (2001). Focus groups as a tool for critical social research in nurse education. *Nurse Education Today, 21*(4), 323–333.

Leners, D., Beardslee, N. Q., & Peters, D. (1996). 21st century nursing and implications for nursing school admissions. *Nursing Outlook, 44*(3), 137–140.

Loacker, G., & Mentkowski, M. (1993). In T. Banta (Ed.), *Making a difference: Outcomes of a decade of assessment in higher education* (pp. 5–24). San Francisco, CA: Jossey-Bass.

Loriz, L. M., & Foster, P. H. (2001). Focus groups: Powerful adjuncts for program evaluation. *Nursing Forum, 36*(3), 31–36.

Madaus, G. F., & Kelleghan, T. (1992). Curriculum evaluation and assessment. In P. W. Jackson (Ed.), *Handbook of research on curriculum* (pp. 119–154). New York, NY: Macmillan.

Madaus, G. F., & McNamara, J. (1970). *Public examinations: A study of the Irish leaving certificate*. Dublin, Ireland: Educational Research Centre, St. Patrick's College.

Moss, P. (1992). Shifting conceptions of validity in educational measurement: Implications for performance assessment. *Review of Educational Research, 62*(3), 229–258.

National League for Nursing Accrediting Commission. (2008). *Accreditation manual with interpretive guidelines*. Retrieved from http://www.nlnac.org

National Organization of Nurse Practitioner Faculties. (2008). *Criteria for evaluation of nurse practitioner programs*. Retrieved from http://www.nonpf.com

Palomba, C. A., & Banta, T. W. (1999). *Assessment essentials: Planning, implementing, and improving assessment in higher education*. San Francisco, CA: Jossey-Bass.

Patton, M. Q. (1990). *Qualitative evaluation and research methods* (2nd ed.). Newbury Park, CA: Sage.

Rabinowitz, M., & Schubert, W. H. (1991). In A. Lewy (Ed.), *The international encyclopedia of curriculum* (pp. 468–471). Oxford, England: Pergamon Press.

Rogers, F. A. (1983). Curriculum research and evaluation. In F. W. English (Ed.), *Fundamental curriculum decisions* (pp. 142–153). Alexandria, VA: Association for Supervision and Curriculum Development.

Rossi, P. H., & Freeman, H. E. (1993). *Evaluation: A systematic approach* (5th ed.). Newbury Park, CA: Sage.

Sarnecky, M. T. (1990). Program evaluation part 1: Four generations of theory. *Nurse Educator 15*(5), 25–28.

Sauter, M. K. (2000). *An exploration of program evaluation in baccalaureate nursing education*. (Unpublished doctoral dissertation). Indiana University, Bloomington, IN.

Sauter, M. K., Johnson, D. R., & Gillespie, N. N. (2009). Educational program evaluation. In D. M. Billings & J. Halstead (Eds.), *Teaching in nursing: A guide for faculty* (3rd ed., pp. 467–515). St. Louis, MO: Elsevier.

Schreiner, L., & Juillerat, S. (1993). *Student satisfaction inventory*. Iowa City, IA: Noel-Levitz.

Schwab, J. (1973). The practical: Translation and curriculum. *School Review, 81*(4), 501–522.

Seager, S. R., & Anema, M. G. (2003). A process for conducting a curriculum audit. *Nurse Educator, 28*(1), 5–6.

Seldin, P. (1980). *Successful faculty evaluation programs: A practical guide to improve faculty performance and promotion/tenure decisions*. New York, NY: Coventry Press.

Shadish, W. R., Cook, T. D., & Leviton, L. C. (1991). *Foundations of program evaluation*. Newbury Park, CA: Sage.

Shaffer, B., Tallarica, B., & Walsch, J. (2000). Win-win mentoring. *Nursing Management, 31*(1), 32–34.

Short, E. C. (1991). *Forms of curriculum inquiry*. New York, NY: State University of New York.

Stewart, B. M., & Kruger, L. E. (1996). An evolutionary concept analysis of mentoring in nursing. *Journal of Professional Nursing, 12*(5), 311–321.

Stewart, D. W., & Shamdasani, P. N. (1990). *Focus groups: Theory and practice*. Newbury Park, CA: Sage.

Stufflebeam, D. L. (1983). The CIPP model for program evaluation. In G. Madaus, M. Scriven, & D. Stufflebeam (Eds.), *Evaluation models: Viewpoints on educational and human services evaluation* (pp. 117–141). Boston, MA: Kluwer-Nijhoff.

Suhayda, R., & Miller, J. M. (2006). Optimizing evaluation of nursing education programs. *Nurse Educator, 31*(5), 200–206.

Terenzini, P. T. (1989). Assessment with open eyes: Pitfalls in studying outcomes. *The Journal of Higher Education, 60*(6), 644–664.

Tucker, R. W. (1995). Outcomes assessment: Bothersome intrusion or efficient path to continuous improvement? *NLN Research & Policy PRISM, 3*(2), 4–5, 8.

Tyler, R. W. (1949). *Basic principles of curriculum and instruction*. Chicago, IL: University of Chicago Press.

Uhl, N. P. (1991). Delphi technique. In A. Lewy (Ed.), *The international encyclopedia of curriculum* (pp. 453–454). Oxford, England: Pergamon Press.

Veney, J. E., & Kaluzny, A. D. (1991). *Evaluation and decision making for health services* (2nd ed.). Ann Arbor, MI: Health Administration Press.

Waltz, C. F. (1988). *Educational outcomes: Assessment of quality—A prototype for student outcome measurement in nursing programs*. New York, NY: National League for Nursing.

Waltz, C. F., & Miller, C. H. (1988). *Educational outcomes: Assessment of quality—A compendium of measurement tools for baccalaureate nursing programs*. New York, NY: National League for Nursing.

Watson, J. E., & Herbener, D. (1990). Programme evaluation in nursing education: The state of the art. *Journal of Advanced Nursing, 15*(3), 316–323.

Weimer, M. G., Kerns, M., & Parrett, J. L. (1988). Instructional observations: Caveats, concerns, and ways to compensate. *Studies in Higher Education, 13*(3), 285–293.

Wingspread Group on Higher Education. (1993). *An American imperative: Higher education for higher education*. Racine, WI: Johnson Foundation.

Wood, S. O., Biordi, D. L., Miller, B. A., Poncar, P., Snelson, C. M., Banks, M. J., & Hemminger, S. A. (1998). Boyer's model of scholarship applied to a career ladder for nontenured nursing faculty. *Nurse Educator, 23*(3), 33–40.

29 Accreditation of Nursing Programs

Marsha Howell Adams DSN, RN, CNE

Accreditation is an ongoing, voluntary process that is pursued by nursing programs to assure quality of those programs. Through the accreditation process, nursing programs are held accountable for establishing appropriate program outcomes and designing effective evaluation systems for measuring those outcomes. This process promotes continuous quality improvement as nursing programs strive to meet those educational outcomes. The National League for Nursing Accrediting Commission (NLNAC) and the Commission on Collegiate Nursing Education (CCNE) serve as the two accrediting organizations for nursing education. Each has been approved by the U.S. Department of Education (USDOE) and is dedicated to maintaining quality nursing programs.

Accreditation and regulation are two distinct, independent entities. Regulation is governed by state boards of nursing. The state boards of nursing develop rules and regulations designated to protect the health, safety, and welfare of the public. In keeping with this mission, nursing programs must comply with the state boards of nursing's administrative code and submit an annual report addressing compliance. While a nursing program can lose its accreditation status and remain operational, state boards of nursing have the legal authority to close nursing programs that do not comply with the criteria as stated in the administrative code (Spector, 2010).

This chapter will provide a general overview of the accreditation process with regional and programmatic accrediting agencies for nursing programs. NLNAC and CCNE will be the two accrediting agencies addressed for the purposes of this discussion. This chapter will provide insight into the nursing program accreditation process, preparing the self-study report, the value of a consultant, and the actual on-site visit. The decision-making

process and follow-up by nursing programs will also be described based on each accrediting agency's processes.

Overview of the Accreditation Process

Accreditation is "a process of external quality review created and used by higher education to scrutinize colleges, universities, and programs for quality assurance and quality improvement" (Eaton, 2009, p. 1). It is a means for assuring quality to stakeholders such as students, families, and the general public by colleges, universities, and programs. Accreditation and quality go hand in hand and can play a significant role in accessibility of funding in both the public and the private sectors, potential employment by college graduates, and transferring program and course credit among colleges and universities. In an effort to hold accrediting organizations accountable, these organizations apply for recognition by the USDOE and the Council for Higher Education Accreditation (CHEA) as a means of external review. Accrediting organizations seek USDOE recognition to become eligible for federal funding. CHEA recognition affords the accrediting organization a standing of quality among the higher education community. According to CHEA, there are four types of accrediting organizations: regional (accredits 2- and 4-year public and private institutions), national faith-related (accredits nonprofit, degree-granting, religious- or doctrine-based institutions), national career-related (accredits single-purpose, for-profit, career-based institutions), and programmatic (accredits specific programs and professions) (Eaton, 2009; USDOE, n.d.).

Institutions that house nursing as a discipline may be regionally accredited. Regional accrediting agencies such as the Southern Association of Colleges and Schools (SACS), the North Central Association of

Colleges and Schools (NCA), and the New England Association of Schools and Colleges (NEASC) accredit 2- and 4-year institutions and are responsible for setting standards and monitoring compliance with those standards by the college or university as a whole. Programmatic accrediting agencies are discipline specific and accredit programs, professions, and schools such as nursing, law, and engineering. The programmatic agencies for nursing programs are NLNAC and CCNE (CHEA, 2010; NLNAC, 2008; Van Ort & Butlin, 2010). In addition to these two entities, there are advanced practice nursing accrediting bodies such as the Council on Accreditation of Nurse Anesthesia Educational Programs and the American College of Nurse-Midwives, Division of Accreditation.

The accreditation model practiced by most accrediting organizations is a combination of a self-study and a site visit by a team of peer evaluators. The self-study is a document addressing the systematic and thorough examination of a program's components in relation to its stated mission created by the program. It is based on the standards and criteria developed by the accrediting organization. The self-study is reviewed by peer evaluators composed of faculty and administrators within the stated profession. A site visit is conducted to verify, clarify, and amplify the self-study content by a team of peer evaluators. The peer evaluators submit a report to the accrediting organization addressing compliance of standards based on information obtained through the self-study and site visit. The accrediting organization's decision-making body composed of elected commissioners makes the final decision whether the program is accredited, reaccredited, or denied accreditation. The accrediting organization publishes a list of all accredited institutions and programs on its website.

The focus of the accreditation process is very similar among accrediting organizations. The basic components addressed include:
- Measurable program outcomes
- Curricula
- Faculty
- Qualified students
- Student support services
- Quality and adequate resources
- Qualified administration
- Policies and procedures
- Formal complaint mechanism
- Systematic program evaluation plan

Programmatic Accrediting Agencies for Nursing Programs

The NLNAC (2008) and the CCNE (2009a) serve as the two accrediting bodies for nursing programs in the United States. Each of these bodies is recognized by the USDOE as a national accrediting agency. This distinct recognition is granted to accrediting agencies who meet specific standards for assuring quality in nursing programs eligible for federal funding and other resources. The NLNAC is recognized as an accrediting body for all types of nursing programs, including practical, diploma, associate, baccalaureate, master's and postmaster's certificate, and clinical doctorate programs. The CCNE is recognized to accredit baccalaureate and higher-degree programs in nursing such as the master's of science in nursing (MSN) and the doctorate in nursing practice (DNP). Doctor of Philosophy (PhD) programs are accredited by regional accreditation agencies. In addition to USDOE recognition, both NLNAC and CCNE are recognized by the CHEA (NLNAC, 2008; CCNE, 2009b).

NLNAC

Accrediting Organization

In 1996 the National League for Nursing (NLN) approved the creation of the NLNAC as an independent entity within the organization; in 1997, with sole authority and accountability, the NLNAC began implementing the accreditation role and responsibilities. The NLNAC's mission is to support nursing education, nursing practice, and the public through accreditation. The commission defines accreditation as "a voluntary, self-regulatory process by which non-governmental associations recognize educational institutions or programs that have been found to meet or exceed standards and criteria for educational quality" (NLNAC, 2008, p. 1).

NLNAC is governed by a 15-member Board of Commissioners composed of individuals representing nursing education (9 commissioners), service (3 commissioners), and the public sector (3 commissioners). The executive director (ED) reports directly to the Board of Commissioners. The remaining organization structure is composed of professional and administrative staff, program evaluators, and support staff. The ED or NLNAC commissioners chair delivers a formal report to NLN, the parent organization, during an NLN Board of Governors meeting annually. While NLN is the parent organization, NLNAC is a wholly owned subsidiary of NLN whose accrediting processes, finances, and administration are separate and independent of NLN to meet compliance requirements of the USDOE. The NLNAC Board of Commissioners is responsible for setting policy and making decisions related to accreditation, policy, finances, and administration (NLNAC, 2008).

Program evaluators (peer reviewers) participate as site visitors, evaluation review panel members, and appeal panel members. These individuals must meet certain criteria related to educational preparation, nursing education expertise, and professional service in addition to attending program evaluator professional development (every 4 years) in order to serve as a program evaluator. Program evaluators are expected to maintain confidentiality regarding nursing programs visited and recommendations made as a result of the self-study and site visit. They also must be from an NLNAC-accredited nursing program. NLNAC provides a detailed accreditation manual that can be downloaded

easily by nursing programs (www.nlnac.org/manuals/Manual2008.htm).

NLNAC Standards and Criteria

There are six designated NLNAC (2008) accreditation standards, including mission and administrative capacity, faculty and staff, students, curriculum, resources, and outcomes. These standards are applicable for all types of nursing programs. The standards and criteria are reviewed every 5 years. Table 29-1 identifies the standards that are defined as "agreed-upon rules for measurement of quantity, extent, value, and quality" (NLNAC, 2008, p. 12). Each standard has specific criteria based on the type of nursing program being evaluated. For example, there are specific criteria (elements that must be addressed in the evaluation of a standard) for the clinical doctorate, master's and postmaster's certificate, baccalaureate, associate, diploma, and practical nursing programs. Distance education is also addressed as a criterion in each of the standards. To aid with preparation of the self-study document, NLNAC provides focus questions for

---

TABLE 29-1 Comparison of NLNAC and CCNE Accreditation Standards

NLNAC Accreditation Standards (NLNAC, 2008)	CCNE Accreditation Standards (CCNE, 2009a)
STANDARD 1	*STANDARD I*
Mission and Administrative Capacity	Program Quality: Mission and Governance
The nursing education unit's mission reflects the governing organization's core values and is congruent with its strategic goals and objectives. The governing organization and program have administrative capacity resulting in effective delivery of the nursing program and achievement of identified outcomes.	The mission, goals, and expected aggregate student and faculty outcomes are congruent with those of the parent institution, reflect professional nursing standards and guidelines, and consider the needs and expectations of the community of interest. Policies of the parent institution and nursing program clearly support the program's mission, goals, and expected outcomes. The faculty and students of the program are involved in the governance of the program and in the ongoing efforts to improve program quality.
STANDARD 2	*STANDARD II*
Faculty and Staff	Program Quality: Institutional Commitment and Resources
Qualified faculty and staff provide leadership and support necessary to attain the goals and outcomes of the nursing education unit.	The parent institution demonstrates ongoing commitment and support for the nursing program. The institution makes available resources to enable the program to achieve its mission, goals, and expected aggregate student and faculty outcomes. The faculty, as a resource of the program, enables the achievement of the mission, goals, and expected aggregate student outcomes.

TABLE 29-1 Comparison of NLNAC and CCNE Accreditation Standards—cont'd

NLNAC Accreditation Standards (NLNAC, 2008)	CCNE Accreditation Standards (CCNE, 2009a)
STANDARD 3	*STANDARD III*
Students	Program Quality: Curriculum and Teaching–Learning Practices
Student policies, development and services support the goals and outcomes of the nursing education unit.	The curriculum is developed in accordance with the mission, goals, and expected aggregate student outcomes and reflects professional nursing standards and guidelines and the needs and expectations of the community of interest. Teaching–learning practices are congruent with expected individual student learning outcomes and expected aggregate student outcomes. The environment for teaching–learning fosters achievement of expected individual student learning outcomes.
STANDARD 4	*STANDARD IV*
Curriculum	Program Effectiveness: Aggregate Student and Faculty Outcomes
The curriculum prepares students to achieve the outcomes of the nursing education unit, including safe practice in contemporary health care environments.	The program is effective in fulfilling its mission, goals, and expected aggregate student and faculty outcomes. Actual aggregate student outcomes are consistent with the mission, goals, and expected student outcomes. Actual alumni satisfaction data and the accomplishments of graduates of the program attest to the effectiveness of the program. Actual aggregate faculty outcomes are consistent with the mission, goals, and expected faculty outcomes. Data on program effectiveness are used to foster ongoing program improvement.
STANDARD 5	
Resources	
Fiscal, physical, and learning resources promote the achievement of the goals and outcomes of the nursing education unit.	
STANDARD 6	
Outcomes	
Evaluation of student learning demonstrates that graduates have achieved identified competencies consistent with the institutional mission and professional standards and that the outcomes of the nursing education unit have been achieved.	

each standard and criteria that facilitate adequately addressing each standard. It is an expectation that all standards will be in compliance for the nursing program to receive initial or continued accreditation. Nursing programs are expected to provide a summary of program strengths, areas in need of development, and an action plan based on the standards and criteria. NLNAC offers self-study forums for nursing programs beginning the accreditation or reaccreditation process. The focus of the forums is an overview of the accreditation process and writing a self-study. Each forum addresses in detail a specific standard that may have been identified as an area needing further nursing program development. For example, Standard 6: Outcomes was identified as an area needing development for fall 2009 and spring 2010, followed by Standard 2: Faculty and Staff (NLNAC, 2010).

NLNAC Accreditation Process

NLNAC follows the accreditation model discussed earlier in the chapter. A four-step process is used that includes a self-study report, an on-site visit, a review by the evaluation panel, and a final decision by the Board of Commissioners. The on-site visit is performed by site visitors composed of professional peers. The team of site visitors looks for congruence between the self-study and the actual functioning of the program. The site visitors make a recommendation to the accreditation status of the nursing program. This report is submitted to NLNAC; a copy is then sent to the nursing program administrator, who has 2 weeks to review the report and clarify any errors noted in it on a response form. The final draft of the report is sent to the site visitors and the nursing program administrator. Next, the report is reviewed by the evaluation review panel, whose role is to validate the site visit team's report and determine that there is strong evidence to support the standards and criteria. This panel is appointed by the NLNAC Board of Commissioners and one of the commissioners serves as a member of the panel. The nursing program administrator may attend the evaluation review panel meeting in person or by conference call. The administrator is in the role of observer only, but may address the panel after deliberations are completed. A recommendation from the panel is made to the Board of Commissioners, which has the sole authority for determining accreditation status of nursing program applicants.

Initial Accreditation and Continuing Accreditation

Nursing programs seeking initial accreditation must comply with certain policies and procedures. The chief executive officer of the college or university initiates the process and authorizes the NLNAC to begin the accreditation process. NLNAC assigns the nursing program a mentor to facilitate the self-assessment process. The nursing program applies for candidacy status by submitting state board of nursing approval documentation, specific fees, and information related to faculty, curriculum, and resources. Once candidacy status is established, the nursing program has 2 years to complete the accreditation process. The nursing program must be in compliance with all standards and criteria to

receive initial accreditation or risk accreditation being denied. Initial accreditation nursing programs are reviewed in 5 years (NLNAC, 2008).

Nursing programs seeking continuing accreditation must be in compliance with all standards and criteria to receive accreditation for 8 years. If a nursing program is found to be noncompliant in one or two standards, the next review is scheduled in 2 years for all types of programs except the practical nurse program, which is reviewed in 18 months. This review can be a follow-up report or a follow-up report with a follow-up site visit. For nursing programs that are noncompliant in three or more standards, the next review, consisting of a site visit with self-study report, is in 2 years for all program types except practical nursing program, which is reviewed in 18 months.

Nursing programs facing possible denial or withdrawal have the opportunity to appeal the decision. Nursing programs have 30 days to begin the appeal process after receiving notification of the adverse accreditation decision. An appeal panel is charged with reviewing all pertinent materials, including any documentation relevant to the adverse accreditation decision and information presented at an appeal hearing where oral presentations are made by two representatives of the nursing program, including the nursing administrator. The final appeal decision is made by the appeal panel. A final decision can be affirmation of the adverse accreditation decision, continuing accreditation with an on-site visit in 8 years, or initial accreditation with an on-site visit in 5 years. All NLNAC accreditation decisions are made available to the USDOE, state boards of nursing, and the public. The NLNAC website (www.nlnac.org) provides extensive information to guide nursing programs in every aspect of the accreditation process.

CCNE

Accrediting Organization

In 1998 the CCNE (initially known as the Nursing Education Accrediting Commission) was created with the sole purpose of accrediting baccalaureate and higher-degree programs, which include MSN and DNP programs. This accrediting organization strives to be mission-driven with a focus on innovation, autonomy, and creativity. Its mission is as follows: CCNE is "an autonomous accrediting agency, contributing to the improvement of the public's health. The Commission ensures the quality and integrity of baccalaureate, graduate, and residency programs in nursing. The Commission serves the public interest by assessing and identifying programs that engage in effective educational practices.

"As a voluntary, self regulatory process, CCNE accreditation supports and encourages continuing self-assessment by nursing programs and supports continuing growth and improvement of collegiate professional education and post-baccalaureate nurse residency programs" (CCNE, 2009a, para 1).

In 2000 the CCNE received initial USDOE recognition, and in 2002 it received CHEA recognition.

The CCNE accreditation process is based on a number of core values (CCNE, 2009c, pp. 3–4). These values are as follows:

- Foster **trust** in the process, in CCNE, and in the professional community.
- Focus on stimulating and supporting **continuous quality improvement** in nursing education programs and their outcomes.
- Be **inclusive** in the implementation of its activities and maintain openness to the **diverse institutional and individual issues and opinions** of the interested community.
- Rely on **review and oversight by peers** from the community of interest.
- Maintain **integrity** through a consistent, fair and honest accreditation process.
- Value and foster **innovation** in both the accreditation process and the programs to be accredited.
- Facilitate and engage in **self-assessment**.
- Foster an educational climate that supports program students, graduates and faculty in their pursuit of **life-long learning**.
- Maintain a high level of **accountability** to the public served by the process, including consumers, students, employers, programs and institutions of higher education.
- Maintain a process that is both **cost-effective and cost-accountable**.
- Encourage programs to develop graduates who are **effective professionals and socially responsible citizens**.
- Assure **autonomy and due process** in its deliberations and decision-making processes.

CCNE is governed by a 13-member Board of Commissioners composed of deans of nursing programs (3 commissioners), faculty (3 commissioners), professional consumers (2 commissioners), public consumers (2 commissioners), and practicing nurses (3 commissioners). CCNE's director reports directly to the Board of Commissioners. In addition to the commissioners, there are standing committees and CCNE staff. The standing committees include the Accreditation Review Committee, Budget Committee, Nominating Committee, Report Review Committee, and Hearing Committee. The staff report to the director and assistant director and are responsible for all board and standing committee activities and for administering the accreditation process and procedures.

The site evaluators are nursing faculty, administrators, and practicing nurses. Each has completed CCNE evaluator training. Site evaluators are expected to maintain confidentiality at all times regarding the accreditation process. Individuals selected as team leaders attend training for leading site visits. The CCNE website provides resources for on-site evaluators (www.aacn.nche.edu/accreditation/EvalResourceBG.htm).

CCNE Standards, Key Elements, and Elaborations

There are 4 CCNE standards with 23 key elements addressing mission and governance, institutional commitment and resources, curriculum and teaching–learning practices, and aggregate student and faculty outcomes. Table 29-1 provides each of the CCNE standards. The standards address expected institutional performance while the key elements provide direction in meeting the overall standard. The rationale for providing key elements is to enable nursing programs to interpret each key element to its broadest sense and allow for creativity and innovation. Elaborations are provided for each key element and are used to help clarify and interpret each key element. At the end of each standard is a list of possible documentation that can be used to support the standard when developing the self-study and preparing for the site evaluation. During the self-assessment process, nursing programs are expected to address strengths, challenges, and an action plan for each standard, noting evidence of the ongoing improvement process in action. The CCNE provides self-study workshops and accreditation updates throughout the year to educate nursing programs regarding the accreditation process.

Nursing programs that are CCNE accredited or in the process of being accredited are required to use the professional standards and guidelines developed by the American Association of Colleges of Nursing (AACN). Each program type has a specific set of "essentials" that guides the nursing program and specifically the curriculum. These essentials outline the expected outcomes needed for graduates of specific programs. For example, *The Essentials of Baccalaureate Education for Professional Nursing Practice* (AACN, 2008) is incorporated in baccalaureate programs and specifies the competencies needed of a baccalaureate graduate. There are also essentials for the MSN and DNP programs.

CCNE Accreditation Process

The accreditation process is very similar to NLNAC and other accreditation organizations. CCNE (2009b) identifies a six-step process as follows:

1. The nursing program develops a self-study report that it uses to perform a self-assessment of how its program meets the CCNE standards and key elements.
2. An on-site visit is conducted, during which a peer evaluation team validates the self-study findings. The peer evaluation team is identified as a fact-finding team. A report is prepared by the team addressing whether the program is in compliance with CCNE standards and key elements.
3. The nursing program is sent the report and the administrator has the opportunity to respond to the report and clarify any areas in question.
4. The Accreditation Review Committee (ARC) reviews the self-study, the evaluation team report, and the nursing program's response. The ARC makes a recommendation to the Board of Commissioners regarding accreditation.
5. The CCNE's Board of Commissioners reviews the ARC recommendation and is solely responsible for deciding whether to grant initial or continuing approval, deny approval, or withdraw accreditation of the program.
6. The Board of Commissioners periodically reviews nursing programs between accreditation terms to monitor continued compliance with the standards.

Initial Accreditation and Continuing Accreditation

The chief executive officer and the chief nursing administrator start the process for nursing programs seeking initial accreditation by requesting applicant status from CCNE. The nursing program must present evidence to support existing institutional accreditation, state board of nursing approval, payment of fees, and potential to meet the accreditation standards. Once applicant status is received, the nursing program has 2 years to complete the accreditation process, including development of a self-study and an on-site visit. Nursing programs receiving initial accreditation are reviewed in 5 years and must submit a continuous progress improvement report at midpoint of the 5 years. Nursing programs that do not comply with the standards are denied accreditation.

Nursing programs seeking reaffirmation of accreditation contact CCNE about 12 to 18 months prior to when the on-site evaluation is due. The chief nursing administrator sends a letter of intent for reevaluation and possible dates for the on-site evaluation. A 10-year continuing accreditation is granted by the CCNE Board of Commissioners for nursing programs that are in compliance with all accreditation standards. CCNE reaffirms these programs based on the self-study and comprehensive on-site visit. Nursing programs that do not comply with the accreditation standards may have their accreditation withdrawn or the programs have the opportunity to "show cause" why a withdrawal should not be made against the program by responding to the Board of Commissioners' concerns related to compliance of standards within a specified time frame. Accreditation decisions are communicated to the USDOE, other applicable institutional accrediting organizations, and the public (if applicable). Nursing programs that face accreditation denials or withdrawals have the opportunity to appeal the decision based on a set procedure. Nursing programs have 10 days to begin the appeal process after receiving notification of the adverse accreditation decision. A hearing committee is appointed by the chair of the CCNE Board of Commissioners. The committee's purpose is to review all written and oral information provided during the appeal process. During the appeal process, the nursing program bears the burden of proof. The hearing committee submits a written decision to the Board of Commissioners to affirm the adverse accreditation decision or to remand the action for reconsideration by the board. Information about all aspects of the CCNE accreditation process is located on the AACN website (www.aacn.nche.edu).

Steps in the Accreditation Process for Nursing Programs

Preparation for the accreditation process should begin 1 to 3 years prior to the planned visit for nursing programs seeking continuing accreditation, in order to have sufficient time to ensure that all aspects of the process are in place. This preparation time may vary based on the number of internal programs to be accredited within the overall nursing program. For example, a nursing program may have baccalaureate, MSN, and DNP programs to be reviewed for accreditation. Other institutions may have single-purpose programs such as only an associate or baccalaureate degree program. For this approach to be successful, some components must be in place as they are developed within the nursing program. A systematic program evaluation needs to be generated that addresses all aspects of the nursing program with specified measurable performance indicators and benchmarks, instruments and tools used for measurement, and the reporting method. Examples of areas to be addressed include aggregate measures such as achievement of program outcomes; quality of instruction and resources for learning; and overall satisfaction with program by students, alumni, faculty, and employers. Nursing programs need to have mechanisms for tracking data to support program outcomes such as graduation rates, NCLEX pass rates, alumni and employer satisfaction, and certification rates. It will serve the institution well to implement databases that can house and retrieve these aggregate data. Three years of data need to be provided in the self-study.

Professional standards and guidelines is another component that needs to be in place. These standards and guidelines serve as building blocks for the nursing curriculum and must be consistent with the program's mission, goals, and expected outcomes. Professional standards and guidelines are developed by professional nursing and specialty organizations, state regulatory agencies, and national recognized accrediting organizations, to name a few. Both NLNAC and CCNE support the use of professional standards and expect that nursing programs can demonstrate how these standards are used within the curriculum and their consistency with overall program outcomes. While CCNE requires certain AACN professional standards based on program type, nursing programs have the opportunity to use other professional standards in addition to those required. Table 29-2 lists some examples of professional standards and guidelines. Table 29-3 describes other components that nursing programs must consider during the accreditation process based on the accrediting organization.

Preparing the Self-Study Report

One of the first steps in preparing the self-study report is to agree on the type of structure and approach to be use when writing it. This can vary according to institution, but it needs to be agreed upon by the faculty and administration so that everyone starts on the same page. Various approaches can be used, such as matching individual standards to specific standing committees to develop first drafts, assignment of one or two faculty to write the self-study, faculty teams assigned to write each

---

TABLE 29-2 Examples of Professional Standards and Guidelines

NLN's Outcomes and Competencies for Graduates of Practical/ Vocational, Diploma, Associate Degree, Baccalaureate, Master's, Practice Doctorate, and Research Doctorate Programs in Nursing (NLN, 2010)

National Association for Practical Nurse Education and Service's (NAPNES) Standards of Practice for Licensed Practical/ Vocational Nurses (NAPNES, 2004)

The Essentials of Baccalaureate Education for Professional Nursing Practice (AACN, 2008)

The Essentials of Master's Education for Advanced Practice Nursing (AACN, 1996)

The Essentials of Doctoral Education for Advanced Nursing Practice (AACN, 2006)

Criteria for Evaluation of Nurse Practitioner Programs (National Task Force on Quality Nurse Practitioner Education, 2008)

ANA's Nursing: Scope and Standards of Practice (ANA, 2010)

Case Management Society of America's (CMSA) Standards of Practice for Case Management (CMSA, 2010)

NLN's Hallmarks of Excellence (NLN, 2004)

TABLE 29-3 Comparison of Accreditation Components

Accreditation Component	NLNAC (2008)	CCNE (2009c)
Annual fees	NLN member: $1875 for one program and $700 for each additional program Non-NLN member: $2875 for one program and $700 for each additional program*	$2195: One program level (e.g., baccalaureate) $2646: Two program levels (e.g., baccalaureate and master's) $3098: Three program levels (e.g., baccalaureate, master's, and DNP)**
Evaluation fees	$1000 application fee for initial and continuing accreditation $835 per evaluator per day*	$1750 per team member**
Composition of site visit team	Three to four visitors representative of program types and one clinician. One of the visitors will be designated as the team chairperson.	Three to four site evaluators including one clinician. One of the site evaluators will be the team leader.
Length of self-study	One program: 200 pages Multiple programs: 300 pages Length is inclusive of all appendices, except for the evaluation plan	One or two programs: 90 pages Three or more programs: 100 pages Length does not include appendices
Length of on-site visit	Minimum of 3 days	Minimum of 3 days
Length of accreditation	Initial accreditation: 5 years Continuing accreditation: 8 years	Initial accreditation: 5 years Continuing accreditation: 10 years
Reporting	Annual report Focused report (if cited for noncompliant standard) Substantive change notification	Annual report Continuous improvement progress report (due at midterm of accreditation period) Special report (if cited for noncompliant standard) Substantive change notification (due 90 days before or after a change)

*Based on 2009–2010 NLNAC fee structure.
**Based on 2010–2011 CCNE fee structure.

standard, hiring an external writer, or developing a steering committee composed of individuals who represent all internal programs and administration. Each representative on the steering committee heads up a writing team of faculty. It is also helpful to identify faculty who have expertise in writing and editing and strategically place them on specific teams. No matter which approach is used, faculty must be knowledgeable and invested in the self-study process and kept abreast of the progress being made. For example, in faculty meetings, accreditation needs to be a routine item on the agenda. Also, a final writer and editor who can take the self-study draft and transform it into a comprehensive, clear, and concise document needs to be identified. This individual is responsible for performing a comprehensive review of the document (removing erroneous materials, deleting duplication of content, and ensuring that each standard has been adequately and accurately addressed).

The development of an accreditation timeline is crucial. Time must be provided to perform a self-review and self-assessment of all components of the nursing program, complete the self-study process, and write the actual document. The more time allowed to develop the self-study, the less pressure on the faculty and staff and the more comprehensive and well-written the document will be. During this self-study process it would not be in a nursing program's best interest to make any major program changes. This has the potential of moving the faculty focus from self-review, self-assessment, and self-study development to implementation of the major change. The need for major changes may be revealed during the self-study process and can be identified as such.

The timeline is created working backward and beginning with the possible dates for the on-site visit. Necessary events to include on the timeline are due dates for multiple drafts of each standard; faculty meetings to discuss standards both during self-study development and in preparation for the on-site visit; program improvement and program outcomes; finalizing self-study; mock visit date with an external consultant; due dates for printing and binding self-study copies for faculty, administration, and visitors; preparation of the resource room; and finalizing the agenda for the site visit.

Interpreting the standards correctly is another component that is important for success. Both NLNAC and CCNE provide self-study workshops and forums for faculty to attend that convey important information related to each standard and offer a format for clarifying any areas of confusion. Faculty writing the self-study need to understand the importance of speaking to the standards, key elements, and elaborations for CCNE or to the standards, criteria, and focus questions for NLNAC. Also, the identification of program strengths, challenges and areas needing development, and an action plan provides the evidence for the program evaluators that an overall quality improvement approach is taking place. It is helpful to have faculty that serve as on-site evaluators who can be used as internal consultants while writing the self-study. These individuals can provide valuable insight into the development and organization of the self-study document.

Accurate documentation is an important component of the self-study. It helps the faculty stay focused while performing a thorough self-assessment and self-review and it provides the evaluation team with a clearer, more concise picture of the program. It is imperative that a "feedback loop" is evident in the documentation demonstrating the decision-making process of the nursing program. Correctly referencing sources such as committee, course and faculty organization minutes, including the committee and course name and meeting dates, throughout the self-study facilitates self-assessment and the evidence of a "feedback loop." Referencing other information such as the catalogue (including page numbers) and data sources also supports a more concise review of the program. The use of tables, charts, and graphs is highly recommended wherever possible. Essential tables and figures should be placed in the body of the self-study. Key documents such as the strategic plan, curriculum evaluation system, and organizational chart should be placed in the appendices, where page limitations are not as much of an issue.

Another component that has been found to be helpful in facilitating the accreditation process as well as self-study development is the use of an external consultant and the scheduling of a mock visit. An external consultant who is knowledgeable about the accreditation process, specifically the processes of the accrediting agency that will be making the site visit, can be instrumental in completion of the self-study document and preparation for the on-site visit. The external consultant can review the self-study document in detail and offer objective recommendations for improvement. In the mock visit, the external consultant can provide opportunities for faculty and administration to engage in a simulated accreditation visit. This allows faculty and administration to practice their responses to questions that may be asked during the actual on-site visit. The mock visit can help faculty identify their knowledge strengths and the areas needing further development related to the self-study content. It can alert faculty to who is better suited to respond to a certain question and show faculty the importance of all faculty engaging with the on-site evaluators during the actual visit. During the mock visit, faculty should be reminded to respond with short answers and use examples to further clarify their points.

Finally, the self-study should be neat, attractive, and easily accessible. It should be professionally printed to ensure an overall attractive appearance. The ability to move from standard to standard and from standard to specific supporting tables and appendices without difficulty is important to on-site evaluators. The use of printed tab dividers between each standard and for each appendix is a good method of promoting accessibility of materials. Also, providing a detail table of contents and a list of all tables and appendices aids in the ease of reading and decreases the time needed to search for specific documents.

The On-Site Visit

The purpose of the on-site visit is to allow the evaluation team time to validate the information provided in the self-study, to assess compliance with the accreditation standards, and to gain insight into the quality improvement plan of the nursing program. The evaluation team accomplishes its purpose by conducting interviews with the communities of interest, both internal and external, such as the faculty, students, central administration, clinical agency representatives, alumni, and any other stakeholders deemed by the nursing program administrators and the team leader of the evaluation team to have a significant impact on the nursing program. The evaluation team will have a designated area called the resource room where documentation to support the self-study is housed. This area will serve as the "home base" for the evaluation team during the site visit.

Preparing for the On-Site Visit

The goal of preparing for the on-site visit is to determine what items the evaluation team will need or want to review, collect this information for them, and make this visit as positive and pleasant as possible for the evaluation team members and the nursing program. The nursing program administrators will develop a draft agenda that will be sent to the team leader or chair of the evaluation team for final approval. It is not unusual for this approval process to go through a number of drafts prior to finalization. In developing this agenda, meeting times need to be designated for the evaluation team to interview significant individuals and groups such as the president, provost, clinical agencies, and alumni. It is important to inform your communities of interest in a timely manner so that scheduling can be manageable. Usually letters are sent out by the chief nursing administrator to the communities of interest detailing the on-site visit and inviting these individuals or groups to submit comments about the nursing program. Notices are placed in college publications, in-class announcements, and electronically through courses and e-mail lists.

The on-site visit agenda should reflect meeting times for the following individuals, groups, and sites to be visited: central administration, such as the president and provost; key individuals on campus, such as the deans of the graduate school, libraries, and distance education, if applicable, as well as the registrar and chief financial officer; students, faculty, alumni, and clinical agency representatives; and clinical and classroom sites. Transportation to and from meetings and clinical sites needs to be finalized based on the agenda.

Faculty need to be notified if the evaluation team will be visiting their clinical sites. Finally, there need to be ample blocks of time designated for the evaluation team to spend in the resource room. While scheduling of the agenda may occur several months in advance, it is a good practice to confirm the agenda with all stakeholders about a week or two before the actual visit.

Preparing the Resource Room

Since the resource room will be considered the "home base" for the evaluation team, it should be equipped in a manner that will meet the needs of the evaluation team. There should be tables and chairs; computers and a printer; office supplies such as pens, pencils, and Post-it Notes; and a listing of all exhibits available for review. It is also good to have water, soft drinks, and snacks available for the team. Everything should be easily accessible to the evaluation team. One approach to successfully prepare the resource room is to assign specific faculty to this area. They would be responsible for ensuring that all documents are labeled and correctly placed in the resource file. The resource file should be categorized according to standard and criteria or key element. One recommendation is to make multiple copies of short documents such as minutes, highlight the information cited in the self-study, and place a copy in each criteria or key element file where the minutes show support within the self-study. This allows more than one team member to access file information at a time.

The resource file should contain documents such as examples of student work, course syllabi, course schedules for the last 3 years, faculty teaching assignments, faculty vitae and accomplishments, evaluation responses from all sources, minutes cited in the self-study demonstrating support of the feedback loop, student formal complaints and grievances list, and letters from communities of interest. Aggregate data tracking NCLEX pass rates, graduation rates, certifications, and employment rates should be available in the resource room for the evaluation team to view. Both NLNAC and CCNE provide information related to documents that should be available in the resource room on their websites at www.nlnac.org/manuals/NLNAC-Manual2008.pdf (NLNAC) and www.aacn.nche.edu/Accreditation/pdf/advice.pdf (CCNE).

Decision-Making Process by the Accrediting Organization

Earlier in this chapter the specific decision-making process was discussed according to each accrediting organization. The process is as follows:

- Peer evaluation team submits a report to the accrediting organization based on compliance with the standards as addressed in the self-study and on-site visit.
- The chief nursing administrator of the nursing program has an opportunity to respond to the evaluation team's report.
- The evaluation team's report, nursing program's response to the report and the actual self-study are sent to the accrediting organization's review panel that makes a recommendation.
- The review panel's recommendation and all relevant materials are sent to the Board of Commissioners, which makes the final decision of whether to grant, reaffirm, deny, or withdraw accreditation.
- The final decision is communicated to the USDOE, the parent institution, and appropriate accrediting and state agencies.

Each accrediting organization has an appeals process that the nursing program may choose to pursue based on an adverse accrediting decision. The nursing program has a certain number of days after receiving notification of the board's decision to begin the appeal process.

SUMMARY

Successful completion of the accreditation process is a worthy achievement for all nursing programs. The components of self-review and self-assessment should be viewed as ongoing rather than sporadic. Being accredited means that the nursing program demonstrates evidence of quality and that a systematic program evaluation with measurable performance indicators is in place. Since both NLNAC and CCNE accredit baccalaureate and higher-degree programs, these types of nursing programs have a choice regarding their accreditation organization. Associate degree and practical nursing programs seeking accreditation use NLNAC since this organization accredits all types of nursing programs. While faculty may view the accreditation process as tedious and time consuming, NLNAC and CCNE provide detailed guidelines for nursing programs to use in their pursuit of initial and continuing accreditation.

REFLECTING ON THE EVIDENCE

1. How can technology be used to advance the accreditation process?

2. Are there other accreditation models that may streamline the accreditation process?

3. Based on your experience with the accreditation process, what are some recommendations for better engagement of faculty in the accreditation process, particularly new or junior faculty?

REFERENCES

American Association of Colleges of Nursing. (1996). *The essentials of master's education for advanced practice nursing.* Retrieved from http://www.aacn.nche.edu/

American Association of Colleges of Nursing. (2006, October). *The essentials of doctoral education for advanced nursing practice.* Retrieved from http://www.aacn.nche.edu/

American Association of Colleges of Nursing. (2008, October 20). *The essentials of baccalaureate education for professional nursing practice.* Retrieved from http://www.aacn.nche.edu/

American Nurses Association. (2010). *Nursing: Scope and standards of practice* (2nd ed.). Silver Spring, MD: Author.

Case Management Society of America. (2010). *Standards of practice for case management.* Retrieved from http://www.cmsa.org/

Commission on Collegiate Nursing Education. (2009a). *CCNE mission statement and goals.* Retrieved from http://www.aacn.nche.edu/

Commission on Collegiate Nursing Education. (2009b). *Procedures for accreditation of baccalaureate and graduate degree nursing programs.* Washington, DC: Author.

Commission on Collegiate Nursing Education. (2009c). *Standards for accreditation of baccalaureate and graduate degree nursing programs.* Retrieved from http://www.aacn.nche.edu/

Council for Higher Education Accreditation. (2010). *Directories.* Retrieved from http://www.chea.org/

Eaton, J. (2009). *An overview of U.S. accreditation.* Washington, DC: Council for Higher Education Accreditation.

National Association for Practical Nurse Education and Service. (2004). *NAPNES standards of practice for licensed practical/vocational nurses.* Retrieved from http://www.napnes.org/

National League for Nursing. (2004). *Hallmarks, indicators, glossary & references.* Retrieved from http://www.nln.org/

National League for Nursing. (2010). *Outcomes and competencies for graduates of practical/vocational, diploma, associate degree, baccalaureate, master's practice doctorate, and research doctorate programs in nursing.* New York, NY: Author.

National League for Nursing Accrediting Commission. (2008). *National League for Nursing Accrediting Commission manual.* Atlanta, GA: Author.

National League for Nursing Accrediting Commission. (2010). *2010 report to constituents.* Atlanta, GA: Author.

National Task Force on Quality Nurse Practitioner Education. (2008). *Criteria for evaluation of nurse practitioner programs: A report of the National Task Force on Quality Nurse Practitioner Education.* Retrieved from http://www.aacn.nche.edu/

Spector, N. (2010). Approval: National Council of State Boards of Nursing. In L. Caputi (Ed.), *Teaching nursing: The art and science* (Vol. 3, pp. 448–477). Glen Ellyn, IL: College of DuPage Press.

U.S. Department of Education. (n.d.). Accreditation in the United States: Criteria and procedures for recognition of state agencies for nursing education. Retrieved from http://www2.ed.gov/admins/finaid/accred/accreditation_pg19.html#CriteriaforNurseEducation

Van Ort, S., & Butlin, J. (Eds.). (2010). *Achieving excellence in accreditation: The first 10 years of CCNE.* Washington, DC: CCNE.

Index

Page numbers followed by "b" indicate boxes; "f" figures; "t" tables.

1-minute papers, 287-288

A

AACN. *See* American Association of Colleges in Nursing.
AAUP. *See* American Association of University Professors.
Absolute grading scales, 482, 482-483t
Abstract conceptualization, 23
Academia-service partnerships, 329
Academic advising, 538
Access, curriculum development and, 97
Accountability, 97, 120-121, 135, 547
Accreditation
  defined, 423
  distance learning and, 532
  on-site visits and, 559-561
  process overview, 550-551, 557
  programmatic agencies for, 551
  regulation vs., 550
  self-study report preparation and, 557-559
  steps in process of, 557
Accreditation model, 429
Accrediting bodies. *See also* CCNE; NLNAC.
  curriculum designs and, 121-122
  curriculum development and, 132-133, 142-143
  decision-making process of, 561
  online learning and, 405, 407
  program evaluation and, 504, 509
Accumulating precedents, 57
Accuracy of evaluation instruments, 433-434
Action verbs, 151, 152t, 465t
Active experimentations, 23
Active learning. *See also* Critical thinking.
  online learning and, 412
  overview of, 172
  student responses to, 261-262
Activist learning style, 23
Acute and transitional care environments, 312-313
ADA. *See* Americans with Disabilities Act.
ADHD. *See* Attention deficit hyperactivity disorder.
Adjunct faculty, 329-330
Administrative violations, 246-247, 246b, 256
Admission policies, 521-523
Adobe Presenter, 395
Adult education theory, 220-223
Advanced organizers, 211-212
Advisory committees, 541
Aesthetics, 230-231
Affective domain of knowledge, 151, 151f, 177-180, 319b
Affordability, curriculum development and, 96-98
Affordable Health Care Act, 99

Aging of population, 94
Alabama Board of Education, Dixon v., 41
Alcoholism, 63-66
Algorithms, 267
ALINE model, 213
Alliance for Nursing Accreditation, 532
Alumni surveys, 541-543, 544f
Ambulatory practice, 102
American Association of Colleges in Nursing (AACN), 143
American Association of University Professors (AAUP), 4
American Commitments: Diversity, Democracy, and Liberal Learning, 294
American Journal of Nursing list of resources, 532-533
American Organization of Nurse Executives (AONE) guiding principles, 122-125
Americans with Disabilities Act (ADA), 55-56
Amplification, media and, 378
Analytic approach to grading, 444-446
Andragogy, 220-223
Anecdotal notes, 433, 489
Animation, overview of, 371-372
Annoying acts, 245-246, 245f, 246b, 256
Antecedents, 427, 524
Anticipatory sets, 263
Anxiety, 66-70, 321
AONE guiding principles, 122-125
Appeal process, 40-44, 42-43b
Application, scholarship of, 7-8, 527-528
Appointment, promotion, and tenure (APT) committees, 6
Appointment process, overview of, 5
Appointments, overview of, 4-5
APT (Appointment, promotion, and tenure) committees, 6
Argument mapping, 272
Argumentation, 267
ARS. *See* Audience response systems.
Art, teaching as, 203
Articulation agreements, 537-538
ASKED model, 20
ASN to BSN programs, 127
Assessment. *See also* Classroom assessment techniques.
  communicating grading expectations and, 444-446, 445-447b
  defined, 422
  evaluation vs., 441
  matching strategy to domain of learning, 444
  of online learning, 408
  overview of strategies for, 448-450t, 448-461
  selecting strategies for, 441-444
  in teaching-learning process, 204-205
  use of simulations for, 356-357

Assessment models, 428
Assessment Technology Incorporated (ATI), 520
Assimilation theory, 211-213
Assisted learning, 217
Associate degree programs, 126
Associate instructors, 5
Astin, Alexander, 112
Asynchronous interactions, 403-404
Asynchronous technologies, 387, 393-396
ATI. *See* Assessment Technology Incorporated.
At-risk students, 498-500
Attention deficit hyperactivity disorder (ADHD), 59-60
Attitude scales, 432
Attitudes, cultural competence and, 304
Attitudinal perspective, 298-299
Audacity, 395
Audience response systems (ARS), 381
Audio conferencing, 387-389, 388t
Audio media, 373
Audio recording, 449, 457-458
Audio test items, 472-473
Authentic learning, 235-237
Avatars, 355

B

Baby Busters (Generation X), 16-17, 17t
Baccalaureate degree programs, 126-127, 152
Back-channel communications, 381-382
Background checks, 70
Ball State University, 343
Banks, James A., 291-292
Behavioral objective model, 504-505
Behaviorism, 110t, 203-204, 206b, 207-209
Behaviorist psychology, 207
Benchmarking, 155-156, 404-405, 429
Bergen Community College, 113-114b
Biased response to scarce resources, 19
Biases, 299, 475-476
Blended courses, 398, 402, 403t
Blocking, 128-129
Bloom's competency taxonomy, 150, 465, 465t
Boards of nursing, curriculum designs and, 121
Bodily-kinesthetic intelligence, 219
Body position, media and, 378
Books, cultural knowledge and, 305-306
Brain-based learning, 236
Breach of contract, 36, 41
Bridging programs, 127
Bring Theory to Practice demonstration program, 123-124
Buckley Amendment, 38, 251-252, 487
Burnout, 67
Buzz groups, 392
Bylaws, 534